Graft-vs.-Host Disease

HEMATOLOGY

Series Editors

Kenneth M. Brinkhous, M.D.

Department of Pathology
University of North Carolina
School of Medicine
Chapel Hill, North Carolina

Sanford A. Stass, M.D.

Hematopathology Program
The University of Texas System Cancer Center
M. D. Anderson Hospital and Tumor Institute
Houston, Texas

Additional Volumes in Preparation

Graft-vs.-Host Disease

Immunology, Pathophysiology, and Treatment

edited by

Steven J. Burakoff
Dana-Farber Cancer Institute
Harvard Medical School
Boston, Massachusetts

H. Joachim Deeg
University of British Columbia
Vancouver General Hospital
Vancouver, British Columbia, Canada

James Ferrara
Dana-Farber Cancer Institute
Harvard Medical School
Boston, Massachusetts

Kerry Atkinson
St. Vincent's Hospital
Sydney, New South Wales
Australia

Marcel Dekker, Inc.   •   New York and Basel

Library of Congress Cataloging-in-Publication Data

Graft-vs.-host disease: immunology, pathophysiology, and treatment /
   edited by Steven J. Burakoff ... [et al.].
      p.   cm. -- (Hematology; v. 12)
     Includes bibliographical references.
     ISBN 0-8247-8188-0 (alk. paper)
     1. Graft versus host disease. I. Burakoff, Steven J. II. Series:
Hematology (New York, N. Y.); v. 12.
     [DNLM: 1. Graft Vs Host Disease--immunology. 2. Graft Vs Host
Disease--physiopathology. 3. Graft Vs Host Disease--therapy. W1
HE873 v. 12 / WO 680 G737]
    RD123.5.G73 1990
    617.4'4--dc20
    DNLM/DLC
    for Library of Congress   90-3188
                                                       CIP

This book is printed on acid-free paper.

MARCEL DEKKER, INC.
270 Madison Avenue, New York, New York 10016

Current printing (last digit):
10 9 8 7 6 5 4 3 2 1

PRINTED IN THE UNITED STATES OF AMERICA

Series Introduction

For most of this century, hematology has followed a pattern of major scientific discoveries, improved understanding of disease, and rapid application of new knowledge in the clinic. The rate of advance continues at an accelerating pace, so that all but the most zealous have difficulty in keeping up with the literature in even a limited area of specialized interest. As the explosive development of knowledge continues apace, it is a continuing challenge to keep abreast of significant new developments as they impact on clinical and laboratory hematology. The Hematology series is designed to help in this respect, by providing up-to-date and expert presentations on important subject areas in our field. It is hoped that these works, both individually and collectively, will become important volumes for updating information and for reference for the clinician, investigator, teacher, and student, and in this manner contribute to the advancement of hematology.

This volume provides a comprehensive coverage of the nature of graft-vs.-host disease (GVHD), its varied clinical manifestations, and its management. With the widespread use of blood marrow transplantation for the treatment of leukemias and other malignancies, radiation sickness, and certain inborn errors of metabolism, combined with the increasing use of allogeneic donors, the high prevalence and increasing significance of GVHD has become widely apparent.

The editors have divided the book into two parts. Part I provides a state-of-the-art presentation of the basic pathophysiology, immunopathology, and other fundamental aspects of acute and chronic GVHD. The study of animal models of the disease has broadened the understanding of GVHD immeasurably, basic to which is the recognition of the several subsets of T lymphocytes and the role they play in elaborating cytokines, with humoral and cell-mediated cellular injury in the target organs, mainly the immune system, intestine, skin, and liver. The importance of the data in this part of the book extends far beyond GVHD, opening up as it does the whole field of lymphocyte patho-physiology. This area is one of rapid advance and great excitement, revealing multiple points for intervention in efforts to prevent or control the GVH diseases. Part II covers the many aspects of clinical GVHD, including pathology, pathophysiology, histocompatibility antigens, opportunistic infections, treatment, and preventive measures. The introduction of Part II includes a brief history of bone marrow transplantation and GVHD.

The book has 39 chapters written by experts in the field. The book is designed in a "user friendly" manner, with a listing of abbreviations and elegant perspectives as introductions to the field as a whole and to each part of the book. This aspect should be especially valuable to the nonexpert in the field. This volume should appeal to a wide audience, including hematologists, immunologists, pathologists, and clinicians in a wide range of specialties dealing with GVHD and related problems, including transfusion medicine. It should be valuable to both teacher and student for reading and reference. The editors, a team of four, with the authors have succeeded admirably in producing a major contribution to the field, for which they should be justifiably proud.

Kenneth M. Brinkhous
Series Coeditor

Foreword

Some four decades ago a wasting symdrome known as "runt disease" was observed in neonatal mice injected with lymphoid cells of foreign origin. Shortly thereafter it was found that adult mice given lethal irradiation and foreign marrow or spleen cells developed a confusing syndrome of radiation damage and burnt-out lymph nodes and spleens called "secondary disease." An immunological basis for these syndromes was indicated by the fact that mice given syngeneic marrow or lymphoid cells do not develop these symptoms which were apparently related to a reaction of the foreign cells (graft) against the recipient (host). The frequency and intensity of these syndromes in inbred mice were found to be dependent on genetic differences between the strains studied.

Marrow transplantation studies in an outbred canine model yielded similar findings, demonstrating that these syndromes were not unique to inbred rodents. The potential application of marrow transplantation to treatment of radiation injuries or fatal hematological dyscrasias in man stimulated intensive research into the immunology and the genetics of these phenomena. Clinical marrow transplantation attempts began in 1957, and a number of reports over the following five years showed how difficult marrow transplantation would be in our species. It was soon recognized that the graft-vs.-host reaction and its consquence, graft-vs.-host disease (GVHD), constituted a major obstacle to the practical application of marrow transplantation in man. In fact, in the early days of clinical marrow transplantation the only successful cases involved patients with an identical twin (syngeneic) marrow donor, and it appeared that allogeneic marrow grafting would never be possible in man because of the severity of GVHD.

During the 1960's increasing knowledge of human histocompatibility typing and experience with supportive care including platelet transfusions, isolation techniques, and antibiotics expanded substantially. These advances made it possible to identify human siblings who had inherited the same two human leukocyte antigen (HLA) haplotypes and to support patients long enough for a marrow graft to begin to function. The use of an

HLA-identical sibling marrow donor for patients with genetic or malignant disease of the marrow or lymphoid system began to result in some long-term healthy survivors of marrow transplantation. However, even with an HLA genetically identical donor, severe GVHD occurred in some patients despite the use of prophylactic immunosuppressive agents after grafting. Further, it was found that severe GVHD was often refractory to treatment with immunosuppressive agents and that these recipients were immunoincompetent because of GVHD, its treatment, or both. Long before AIDS appeared on the scene, the care of marrow transplant recipients provided extensive clinical experience with opportunistic infections—candida, aspergillus, pneumocystis, herpes, and cytomegalovirus. Studies of humoral and cellular immunity in patients with GVHD began to shed light on the pathogenesis of the disorder. These studies along with the recognition of clinical similarities contributed to our understanding of naturally occurring autoimmune diseases such as systemic lupus erythematosus (SLE) and scleroderma.

Fortunately, many recipients of HLA-identical marrow grafts did not develop GVHD or developed it in a mild and controllable form. Those patients with hematological malignancies who became long-term disease-free survivors—some now 20 years postgrafting—demonstrated "cure" of an otherwise fatal disease by high-dose chemoradiation therapy and marrow grafting. Marrow grafting using an HLA-identical sibling is now preferred treatment for a wide variety of malignant and nonmalignant acquired diseases and for genetically determined dyscrasias. Increasing knowledge of human histocompatibility systems has made it possible to use family member donors other than HLA-identical siblings and, more recently, to identify unrelated donors for some patients who lack a family member donor.

Yet, problems remain and these problems are the focus of current research: recurrence of malignancy after grafting; opportunistic infections, especially viral; complications consequent to intensive chemoradiation therapy; late secondary malignancies; and, of course, GVHD. Fortunately, progress has been made not only in our understanding of GVHD but also in its prevention and treatment. Chemical immunosuppression, especially with the combination of methotrexate and cyclosporine, has significantly reduced the incidence and severity of GVHD. Trials with cyclosporine, antithymocyte globulin, and selected monoclonal antibodies show progress in treatment of GVHD. Removal of T cells from donor marrow has had a striking effect in reducing the incidence and severity of GVHD. However, T cell removal has also resulted in an increased incidence of graft failure and, with some diseases, recurrent malignancy. An understanding of the mechanism behind these complications may make it possible to take advantage of a therapeutic benefit of GVHD—the graft-vs.-leukemia phenomenon.

We are now confronted with a rapidly expanding knowledge of interleukins, cytokines and regulators of proliferation and differentiation, low molecular-weight substances that permit cells to communicate with each other and with themselves. These substances and their role in immunology and the rapidly increasing knowledge of the genetic information at the molecular level underlying all these phenomena suggest that we are entering upon a new era of research and understanding. It is reasonable to suppose that this research will increase our knowledge not only of the immunology of the graft-vs.-host reaction but also of the pathogenesis of diseases that involve the marrow and lymphoid systems. This volume provides an overview of what has been achieved and points the way to the next decade of research.

E. Donnall Thomas, M.D.
Fred Hutchinson Cancer Research Center
Seattle, Washington

Preface

There are two major reasons for producing a broad overview of graft-vs.-host disease (GVHD). From a clinical standpoint, GVHD can be a devastating complication of bone marrow transplantation. Significant progress has been made; however, several obstacles remain in overcoming this problem, particularly in patients given histoincompatible grafts. Multiple approaches, discussed in the clinical sections of this book, have been taken, each with advantages and disadvantages. Frequently, those approaches were based on experimental models. Thus, it is only logical that the clinical sections are preceded by a description of preclinical studies. It is these animal models that have been critical in advancing our understanding of the physiology of GVHD. Control of genetic variables as well as the ability to produce GVHD in a variety of models have permitted insights not possible in a strictly clinical context. In addition, these systems have also provided models for understanding lymphocyte development and function in vivo irrespective of GVHD. The increasing sophistication and precision of cellular and molecular probes have initiated an analysis of cellular mechanisms in physiological environments rather than in a petri dish or test tube. The abnormalities of GVHD thus provide a perspective from which to understand the complexities of normal lymphocyte differentiation and activation. The insights from these studies should lead to improved understanding of fundamental lymphocyte biology and thus to new therapeutic strategies, not only in bone marrow transplantation, but in other areas, such as autoimmune diseases. It is our hope that future editions of this book will reflect this increased understanding and will witness further movement from experimental models to clinical realms.

The production of a book this size is a long and complex undertaking, and we are grateful to the many people who have given generously of their time and effort. We would like to thank particularly Joshua Hauser and Michele Fox for their labors in the preparation of the index. We also wish to acknowledge the continued support of our colleagues and teachers who have encouraged us over many years, especially David. G. Nathan, Fred S. Rosen, Baruj Benacerraf, Rainer Storb, and E. Donnall Thomas.

Steven J. Burakoff
H. Joachim Deeg
James Ferrara
Kerry Atkinson

Contributors

Kerry Atkinson, M.D., M.R.C.P., F.R.A.C.P. Senior Staff Specialist, Department of Hematology, Bone Marrow Transplant Program, St. Vincent's Hospital, Sydney, New South Wales, Australia

Patrick G. Beatty, M.D., Ph.D. Associate Professor of Medicine, Department of Medical Oncology, Fred Hutchinson Cancer Research Center, University of Washington School of Medicine, Seattle, Washington

Richard Benjamin, M.D. Division of Immunology, Department of Pathology, University of Cambridge, Cambridge, England

Bruce R. Blazar, M.D. Associate Professor, Division of Bone Marrow Transplantation, Department of Pedriatics, University of Minnesota Hospitals and Clinics, Minneapolis, Minnesota

Raleigh A. Bowden, M.D. Assistant Professor of Pediatrics, and Assistant Member, Division of Hematology-Oncology and Infectious Diseases, Fred Hutchinson Cancer Research Center, Seattle, Washington

Steven J. Burakoff, M.D. Chief, Division of Pediatric Oncology, Dana-Farber Cancer Institute, Harvard Medical School, Boston, Massachusetts

Jean-Yves Cahn, M.D. Assistant, Bone Marrow Transplant Unit, Department of Hematology, Jean Minjoz Hôpital, Besançon, France

Henry N. Claman, M.D. Professor, Departments of Medicine and Microbiology/Immunology, University of Colorado School of Medicine, Denver, Colorado

Mike Clark, M.D. Division of Immunology, Department of Pathology, University of Cambridge, Cambridge, England

Stephen R. Cobbold, M.D. Division of Immunology, Department of Pathology, University of Cambridge, Cambridge, England

Michele Cottler-Fox, M.D. Senior Staff Fellow, Department of Transfusion Medicine, National Institutes of Health, Bethesda, Maryland

H. Joachim Deeg, M.D. Professor, Departments of Pathology and Medicine, University of British Columbia, and Director, Histocompatibility Laboratory, Vancouver General Hospital, Vancouver, British Columbia, Canada

Martin J. S. Dyer, M.D. Department of Haematology, University of Cambridge, Cambridge, England

Michelle V. Felstein, B.Sc., Ph.D.* Research Assistant, Department of Bacteriology and Immunology, Western Infirmary, University of Glasgow, Glasgow, Scotland

James Ferrara, M.D. Assistant Professor of Pedriatrics, Division of Pedriatic Oncology, Dana-Farber Cancer Institute, Harvard Medical School, Boston, Massachusetts

Tariq Ghayur, Ph.D. Research Fellow, Department of Pedriatic Oncology, Dana-Farber Cancer Institute, Harvard Medical School, Boston, Massachusetts

Eliane Gluckman, M.D. Professor, Bone Marrow Transplant Unit, Hôpital Saint Louis, Paris, France

Frances T. Hakim, M.D. Experimental Immunology Branch, National Cancer Institute, National Institutes of Health, Bethesda, Maryland

Geoffrey Hale, M.D. Division of Immunology, Department of Pathology, University of Cambridge, Cambridge, England

Peter J. Heidt, Ph.D., B.M. Head, Department of Microbiology and Gnotobiology, Radiobiological Institute TNO, Rijswijk, The Netherlands

P. Jean Henslee-Downey, M.D. Assistant Professor of Medicine and Pediatrics, and Director, Bone Marrow Transplantation Program, Albert B. Chandler Medical Center, University of Kentucky Medical Center, Lexington, Kentucky

Patrick Hervé, M.D. Professor, Department of Hematology, Bone Marrow Transplant Unit, Hôpital Jean Minjoz, Besançon, France

Allan D. Hess, Ph.D. Associate Professor of Oncology, Oncology Center, The Johns Hopkins University School of Medicine, Baltimore, Maryland

Mary M. Horowitz, M.D. Assistant Scientific Director, International Bone Marrow Transplant Registry, Medical College of Wisconsin, Milwaukee, Wisconsin

Peter Jacobs, M.D., Ph.D. University of Cape Town Leukaemia Centre and Department of Haematology, Groote Schuur Hospital, Cape Town, Republic of South Africa

Jan M. Jeske, B.S. Medical College of Wisconsin, Milwaukee, Wisconsin

Nancy A. Kernan, M.D. Assistant Attending Pediatrician, Bone Marrow Transplantation Service, Memorial Sloan-Kettering Cancer Center, New York, New York

---

Present affiliation: Research Fellow, Department of Transplant Biology, Clinical Research Centre, Harrow, Middlesex, England

Robert Korngold, Ph.D. Associate Professor, Department of Microbiology and Immunology, Jefferson Medical College, Philadelphia, Pennsylvania

Wayne S. Lapp, Ph.D. Professor, Department of Physiology, McGill University, Montreal, Quebec, Canada

Ann V. LeFever, Ph.D. Assistant Professor, Department of Pediatrics, Medical College of Wisconsin, Milwaukee, Wisconsin

Thomas P. Loughran, Jr., M.D. Assistant Member, Division of Clinical Research, Fred Hutchinsin Cancer Research Center, University of Washington School of Medicine, Seattle, Washington

Lawrence G. Lum, M.D.* Bone Marrow Transplantation Program, Medical College of Wisconsin, Milwaukee, Wisconsin

Tom Maier, Ph.D. Assistant Professor, Departments of Medicine and Microbiology/Immunology; University of Colorado School of Medicine, Denver, Colorado

Paul J. Martin, M.D. Associate Professor of Medicine, Human Immunogenetics Program, Fred Hutchinson Cancer Research Center, University of Washington School of Medicine, Seattle, Washington

Tammy M. Martin, B.S. Senior Research Technologist, Department of Pediatrics, Medical College of Wisconsin, Milwaukee, Wisconsin

Fritz Melchers, Ph.D. (Dr.rer.nat) Director, Basel Institute for Immunology, Basel, Switzerland

Allan McI. Mowat, M.D., Ph.D., M.R.C.Path. Lecturer, Department of Bacteriology and Immunology, Western Infirmary, University of Glasgow, Glasgow, Scotland

Robertson Parkman, M.D. Division Head, Division of Research Immunology and Bone Marrow Transplantation, Department of Pediatrics, University of Southern California School of Medicine and Childrens Hospital of Los Angeles, Los Angeles, California

Pierre-Francois Piguet, M. D. Maître d'Enseignement et de Recherche, Department de Pathologie, Centre Medical Universitaire, Geneva, Switzerland

Shixin Qin, M.D. Division of Immunology, Department of Pathology, University of Cambridge, Cambridge, England

Joel M. Rappeport, M.D. Professor of Medicine and Pediatrics, Departments of Medicine and Pediatrics, Yale University School of Medicine, New Haven, Connecticut

Olle Ringdén, M.D., Ph.D. Professor of Transplantation Immunology and Director of Bone Marrow Transplantation, Departments of Clinical Immunology and Transplantation Surgery, Huddinge Hospital, Huddinge, Sweden

Antonius G. Rolink, Ph.D. Member, Basel Institute for Immunology, Basel, Switzerland

Jean E. Sanders, M.D. Associate Member, Fred Hutchinson Cancer Research Center, and Associate Professor, Department of Pedriatrics, University of Washington, Seattle, Washington

---

*Present affiliation: Department of Hematology-Oncology, Wayne State University, Detroit, Michigan

Thomas A. Seemayer, M.D. Professor of Pathology and Pediatrics, Department of Pathology, The Montreal Children's Hospital, McGill University Faculty of Medicine, Montreal, Quebec, Canada

Gene M. Shearer, M.D. Experimental Immunology Branch, National Cancer Institute, National Institutes of Health, Bethesda, Maryland

Charles C.-Y. Shih, Ph.D. Assistant Professor, Department of Pediatrics, Medical College of Wisconsin, Milwaukee, Wisconsin

Howard M. Shulman, M.D. Associate Member of the Clinical Division, Fred Hutchinson Cancer Research Center, and Associate Professor, Department of Pathology, University of Washington School of Medicine, Seattle, Washington

Dale C. Snover, M.D. Department of Laboratory Medicine and Pathology, University of Minnesota Hospital, Minneapolis, Minnesota

Thomas R. Spitzer, M.D. Acting Director, Bone Marrow Transplant Program, Vincent T. Lombardi Cancer Research Center, Georgetown University Hospital, Washington, D.C.

Jonathan Sprent, M.D., Ph.D. Member, Department of Immunology, Research Institute of Scripps Clinic, La Jolla, California

Georg Stingl, M.D. Professor of Dermatology and Head, Division of Cutaneous Immunology, Department of Dermatology, University of Vienna Medical School, Vienna, Austria

Andreas Strasser, Ph.D.* Member, Basel Institute for Immunology, Basel, Switzerland

Keith M. Sullivan, M.D. Associate Professor of Medicine, Department of Medicine, University of Washington School of Medicine, and Associate Member, Division of Clinical Research, Fred Hutchinson Cancer Research Center, Seattle, Washington

Robert L. Truitt, Ph.D. Research Professor, Department of Pediatrics, Medical College of Wisconsin, Milwaukee, Wisconsin

Daniel A. Vallera, Ph.D. Professor and Director, Section on Experimental Cancer Immunology, Department of Therapeutic Radiology, University of Minnesota Hospitals and Clinics, Minneapolis, Minnesota

Georgia B. Vogelsang, M.D. Assistant Professor of Oncology, Department of Oncology, Oncology Center, The Johns Hopkins University School of Medicine, Baltimore, Maryland

Beatrix Volc-Platzer, M.D. Assistant Professor, Division of Cutaneous Immunology, Department of Dermatology, University of Vienna Medical School, Vienna, Austria

Jaak M. Vossen, M.D., Ph.D. Professor of Pediatric Immunology, Department of Pediatrics, University Hospital, Leiden, The Netherlands

Herman Waldmann, M.D. Division of Immunology, Department of Pathobiology, University of Cambridge, Cambridge, England

Paul L. Weiden, M.D.[†] Attending Physician, Section on Hematology-Oncology, The Virginia Mason Clinic, Seattle, Washington

---

Present affiliations:
*Member, The Walter and Eliza Hall Institute of Medical Research, Melbourne, Victoria, Australia
†Affiliate Investigator, Clinical Research Division, Fred Hutchinson Cancer Research Center, Seattle, Washington

Michael B. Widmer, Ph.D.   Senior Staff Scientist, Department of Immunology, Immunex Corporation, Seattle, Washington

Gary C. Yee, Pharm. D.   Associate Professor, Pharmacy Practice, College of Pharmacy, University of Florida, Gainesville, Florida

Contents

Glossary

ANLL	acute nonlymphocytic leukemia
ALL	acute lymphocytic leukemia
ASGM$_1$	asialo GM$_1$
ATG	anti-thymocyte globulin
BFU-E	burst forming unit, erythroid
BMT	bone marrow transplant
CD1, 2 etc.	cluster of differentiation 1, 2 etc.
CFU	colony-forming unit
C-GVHD	chronic graft-vs. host disease
cGy	centi-Gray (1cGy = 1 rad)
Con A	concanavalin A
CML	chronic myelogenous leukemia
CMV	cytomegalovirus
CTL	cytotoxic T lymphocyte
CSF	colony-stimulating factor
CSP, CsA	cyclosporin A; cyclosporin(e)
DLA	dog leukocyte antigen
DTH	delayed-type hypersensitivity
EBV	Epstein-Barr virus
F(ab)	antigen-binding fragment of Ig
FACS	fluorescein-activated cell sorter
FcR	receptor for the common fragment of Ig
FITC	fluorescein isothiocyanate
GI	gastrointestinal
GVHD	graft-vs.-host disease
HLA	human leukocyte antigen
HSV	herpes simplex virus

HVG	host-vs.-graft
IBMTR	International Bone Marrow Transplant Registry
IFNα, β etc.	interferon α, β, etc.
Ig	immunoglobulin
IL 1, 2, etc.	interleukin 1, 2, etc.
i.p.	intraperitoneal
i.v.	intravenous
LDA	limiting dilution analysis
LPS	lipopolysaccharide
mAb	monoclonal antibody
MHC	major histocompatibility complex
MLC	mixed lymphocyte culture
MLR	mixed lymphocyte reaction
mRNA	messenger ribonucleic acid
MTX	methotrexate
NK	natural killer
PBMC	peripheral blood mononuclear cells
PFC	plaque-forming cells
PG	prostaglandin
RIA	radioimmunoassay
r	recombinant
SBA	soybean agglutinine
SCID	severe combined immunodeficiency
SLE	systemic lupus erythematosus
SRBC	sheep red blood cell
TBI	total body irradiation
Th	T helper cell
TNF	tumor necrosis factor
VZV	varicella zoster virus

Graft-vs.-Host Disease

PART I
Experimental
Graft-vs.-Host Disease

Introduction

James Ferrara and Steven J. Burakoff
Dana-Farber Cancer Institute
Harvard Medical School
Boston, Massachusetts

The chapters gathered in the experimental section of this volume represent a broad variety of approaches to the study of Graft-vs.-Host Disease (GVHD). They are eloquent testimony to our increased understanding of the basic pathogenetic mechanisms that underlie the disorder. The use of animal models has been critical to this development. Although large-animal models have made substantial contributions to our understanding of GVHD, most experimental systems have used rodents. The mouse remains the most frequently studied species. Sufficient numbers of animals can be used in each experimental arm, a wide variety of cellular and molecular murine probes are readily available, and the existence of inbred mouse strains has permitted exceptional control over genetic variables that are essential to define the histocompatibility differences that stimulate GVHD.

As one compares the results of these investigations, certain themes emerge in the areas of GVHD pathophysiology, target destruction, and therapeutic interventions. To begin at the beginning, there is now widespread consensus that the fact that T cells initiate GVHD. The role of T-cell subsets in histocompatibility differences between donor and host is reviewed by Korngold and Sprent in Chapter 2. Using highly purified T-cell subsets, the authors have correlated the subset of T cells that causes lethal GVHD with the differences in major and minor histocompatibility antigens between donor and recipient. $CD8^+$ ($Lyt-2^+$) cells are responsible for GVHD directed against MHC class I differences, and $CD4^+$ ($L3T4^+$) cells are responsible for GVHD to MHC class II differences. When entire MHC differences (class I and class II) exist, either $CD4^+$ or $CD8^+$ cells can produce GVHD. GVHD to minor histocompatibility differences are always produced by $CD8^+$ cells, but $CD4^+$ cells may also recognize these antigens in some strain combinations. Mature T cells from the host are sufficient to cause GVHD, and the absence of a host thymus has no effect on GVHD induction.

A second approach to the analysis of the T cells responsible for GVHD is the use of T-cell clones to cause disease as described by Vallera and Blazar (Chapter 4). They

use the Simonsen splenomegaly assay as an index of GVHD, and their results suggest that
GVHD to MHC antigens are consistently induced only by helper independent cytotoxic
T cells ("HIT" CTL), which are able to both manufacture their own IL-2 and lyse their
targets. The necessity of IL-2 for the induction of GVHD was also observed by Parkman
(Chapter 3) when the elimination of IL-2-secreting cells prior to bone marrow transplant
(BMT) prevented the appearance of clonable cytotoxic cells in the spleen of GVHD mice
2 weeks later. Data from our laboratory demonstrate that an antibody to the IL-2 receptor is able to prevent GVHD when given immediately after BMT (Chapter 1). Thus, from
several different experimental models, IL-2 appears to be an essential component in the
pathophysiology of GVHD.

   IL-2 is not the only cytokine that appears to be central to the production of
GVHD. Indeed, the recent availability of purified recombinant cytokines and highly
specific antibodies have initiated an exciting phase of research into the role of soluble
mediators in the pathophysiology of GVHD. The case for tumor necrosis factor (TNF)
as a central mediator of GVHD is detailed by Piguet in Chapter 13. There are three critical observations: first, there is increased mRNA for TNF in mice with GVHD; second,
infusion of TNF causes necrosis and histopathologic changes consistent with GVHD; and
third, passive immunization after BMT with a polyclonal antiserum to TNF prevents
GVHD. Taken together, these findings argue convincingly for a central role of TNF in
GVHD. The author points out that this cytokine is directly cytotoxic to the tissues, and
considers TNF to be the ultimate effector of the apoptotic necrosis observed in GVHD.

   A third lymphokine implicated in GVHD is interferon-γ (IFN-γ). Several different
GVHD systems, particularly those involving immunosuppression, have identified IFN-γ as
a critical GVHD component (see Chapters 1, 5, and 11). The prominent roles of IL-2,
TNF, and IFN-γ in these models suggest that Th1 cells may be a critical cellular subset to
its induction; however, the secretion of other lymphokines in the dysregulated setting
of GVHD is likely and requires further investigation.

   A soluble mediator such as TNF is attractive as an ultimate effector of GVHD because of the paucity of lymphoid cells infiltrating affected organs. The increased appreciation of the role of cytokines in GVHD has led many scholars to consider the possibility of multicellular networks. Whether T cells alone release the relevant cytokines
or whether other cells are recruited in the process is currently an area of controversy.
Piguet suggests that macrophages are the most likely sources of TNF, and notes that a
T-cell-derived cytokine can drive macrophages to produce TNF. The implication of a
second cell such as macrophages as the source of TNF suggests a two-phase model of
GVHD, which is evident in several experimental systems. Other groups have suggested
that a second cellular effector may be an NK-like cell. Our own studies demonstrate
that an activated natural killer (NK) cell is intimately involved at the site of GVHD organ
damage in the skin, liver, and intestine. By electron microscopy, this cell is observed in
what appears to be an effector-target interaction in situ. We have therefore favored a
two phase model in which T cells induce GVHD by interaction with alloantigens and release lymphokines (afferent phase); these lymphokines in turn activate an NK cell, which
mediates tissue damage (efferent phase).

   The importance of NK cells in the effector phase of GVHD is observed in other
systems as well. In Chapter 7, Ghayur and colleagues examine the induction of $ASGM_1^+$
cells with natural killer activity in producing GVHD in a $P \rightarrow F_1$ model. These data demonstrate that the peak of NK activity correlates with the severity of GVHD. Using donor
mice with the beige mutation, which are deficient in natural killer activity, donor NK

cells are shown to be necessary for the tissue destruction (the effector phase) of GVHD. Splenomegaly (an index of the afferent phase) does not require these NK cells. These authors also favor a two-phase pathogenetic mechanism in which lymphokines are released and recruit a number of different cells (including host and donor) during the afferent phase; the efferent phase consists of an induced cell population directly altering tissue destruction, either through cellular contact or through the release of further lymphokines.

Specific target organ destruction of GVHD is examined by several investigators (Chapters 1, 5, 7, 8, and 9). The most closely scrutinized target organ of GVHD in this book is the immune system itself. Because both the anatomic and the functional aspects of the immune system can be analyzed in experimental settings, a dynamic picture of the working immune system can be detailed. Such studies show that GVHD produces both immunosuppression and immunodeficiency. In clinical transplantation, these effects of GVHD on the immune system are more difficult to discern because of the confusion introduced by the use of immunosuppressive drugs necessary to prevent and treat GVHD. In experimental models, these drugs can be avoided and both the immunosuppression and the immunodeficiency induced by GVHD can be observed and distinguished under the proper conditions. It is worth noting that the immune system is the most sensitive GVHD target organ, and immunodeficiencies are often manifest when no other signs or symptoms of GVHD are evident. A deficiency in IL-2-secreting cells in GVHD has been noted by several investigators; of great interest is the decrease in other lymphokines such as colony stimulating factors (CSFs) that may be essential to the proliferation of hematopoietic progenitors as described by Hakim and Shearer (Chapter 8). During GVHD, the number of phenotypically mature T cells may be normal, but there is a decrease in their functional repertoire including precursors of proliferating and cytolytic cells (Chapter 1). This functional incompetence of T cells may persist for extended periods and is possibly related to differentiation factors that cannot be produced by a dysplastic, thymus of mice with GVHD. Thymosin, for example, is able to restore the proliferative abilities of $CD4^+$ cells in animals with GVHD, and in double transplant protocols, the addition of an intact thymus or $CD4^+$ cells was able to restore responses to alloantigens or to modified self antigens (Chapter 8). The damage inflicted by acute GVHD on thymic microenvironment may be important in the development of chronic GVHD (see below).

In Chapter 11, Mowat reviews the effects of GVHD on the intestine. The intestine has a complex compartmental organization (e.g., it is the largest lymphoid organ of the body), and this complexity contributes to GVHD pathophysiology. Histopathologic analysis of intestinal GVHD again suggests a two-phase process. The first phase (proliferative) involves primarily crypt cells and damages epithelial architecture. The second phase (atrophic) affects the villis and results in destruction of the mucosa, although the relationship of this degeneration to the damaged epithelial architecture is uncertain. It is important to note that histocompatibility antigens are probably not primary targets in the intestine; transplanted (fetal) intestines (syngenic with the donor) are injured as innocent bystanders in mice undergoing GVH reactions. Natural killer cells may again play a role, because $ASGM_1^+$ cells are implicated as effector cells, particularly of crypt hyperplasia.

The effects of GVHD on the skin are discussed in two chapters. In Chapter 5, Maier and Claman describe $CD4^+$ infiltrating cells found in skin of mice with chronic GVHD. There is also increased collagen and fibrosis and the presence of activated mast cells. The response of mast cell precursors to IL-3 in their system suggests a multiple phase process in which the effector cells respond to soluble T-cell-mediated products including heparin-binding growth factors. Changes in human skin have been studied by Volc-Platzer and Stingl (Chapter 12). Of special interest is a finding similar to that in the intestine, which is a hyperproliferative appearance of the epidermis. In these studies, the increased expression of DR (MHC class II) antigens correlates with the development of acute GVHD and precedes histopathologic changes in 50% of the cases. Such changes would imply the presence of IFN-γ in the skin as well. The phenotype of the few infiltrating cells seems to be both CD3$^+$CD8$^-$ and CD3$^+$CD8$^+$. The authors suggest that the different maturation characteristics of certain donor lymphocyte populations may lead to dysregulation of cytokines and eventual cytotoxic damage.

A final target population considered is host leukemia. Malignant host cells are obviously a desired target population when transplantation is performed for various forms of cancer. It is essential to understand graft-vs.-host leukemia (GVL) mechanisms in order to distinguish them from GVHD processes and hopefully use these distinctions to therapeutic advantage. In Chapter 10, Truitt uses alloimmunization protocols to obtain T cells that are specific for certain classes of antigens and exert a GVL effect without creating GVHD. Using limiting dilution analysis, a direct correlation between the number of clonal cells injected and their ability to eliminate leukemia in vivo could be demonstrated. GVL effector cells with multiple phenotypes (both CD8$^+$ and CD8$^-$) were isolated; the CD8$^-$ cells seem similar or identical to lymphokine-activated killer cells. Lymphocyte clones that cause GVHD were also isolated, but no single characteristic distinguished clones that caused GVHD from those that did not. In the case of at least two clones, GVL effects were separable from GVH effects. It would thus appear that distinct but overlapping populations mediate GVL and GVHD, but clear identification as a CTL or NK/LAK cell is not yet possible.

Important differences between acute and chronic GVHD are observed clinically, and in Chapter 3, Parkman addresses this distinction when he isolates T-cell clones from mice with GVHD at different times after BMT. In a model of GVHD to minor histocompatibility antigens, during the acute phase of GVHD (14 days after BMT) the majority of isolated clones are cytotoxic and specific for minor histocompatibility antigens of the recipient; these antigens are recognized in association with MHC class I molecules. These findings are in concordance with the conclusions of Korngold and Sprent that CD8$^+$ cells can always induce GVHD to minor histocompatibility antigens. However, when clones from these same mice are isolated during the chronic phase of GVHD (50 days after BMT), none are cytotoxic and they are no longer specific for minor histocompatibility antigens of the host; they recognize a common determinant of MHC class II (Ia) that is present on both donor and host cells because these strains are genetically identical at the entire MHC. Chronic GVHD clones stimulate Ia expression on other cells, and secrete both IL-2 and IL-4. The different antigenic specificities and functional profiles of clones isolated during the acute and chronic forms of the same disease thus suggest that different T cells are involved in their pathogenesis. Autoreactive CD4$^+$ cells may mediate chronic GVHD in the same animal whose acute GVHD was initiated by CD8$^+$ cells directed against minor histocompatibility host antigens. Presumably, new CD4$^+$ cells have arisen in chronic GVHD whose target antigen is a public epitope of the MHC class II molecule, making them autoreactive. Parkman's analysis also suggests that cytokine secretion by these clones may be responsible for the increased collagen deposition and fibrosis observed in chronic GVHD.

A similar autoreactivity has been observed by Rolink and colleagues in their study of chronic GVHD and B-cell function. Fifteen percent of hybridomas cloned from the spleens of mice with chronic GVHD produced autoantibodies. They consider the role of lymphokine-producing T cells in the polyclonal activation of B cells, and how such activation might result in autoimmune phenomena to endogenous antigens. The possibilities are numerous, but they conclude that no single event can reasonably account for all the details of the autoimmune phenomena.

Another view of GVHD pathogenesis has emerged from studies of syngenic GVHD. The chapter by Hess elegantly summarizes what we have learned about this important phenomenon over the last decade. There are histologic similarities between syngeneic and chronic GVHD, and thus the mechanisms elucidated may be separate from the pathophysiology of acute GVHD outlined earlier, which seems to be directed at mostly epithelial targets. Syngeneic GVHD appears to be a consequence of defective autoregulation. Administration of cyclosporine A and radiation of the thymus are both necessary for this phenomenon. Cyclosporine A treatment alters the type of cells in the thymus, producing fewer single positive mature cells, decreased $\alpha\beta$ T-cell receptor (TCR) bearing cells, and greatly increases the number of $\gamma\delta$ TCR cells. These cells are potentially autoreactive. Evidence is presented that supports the following model: first, cyclosporine impairs the clonal deletion of autoreactive cells; second, thymic radiation eliminates an autoregulatory cell from the thymus, which normally would eliminate self-reactive clones. The combination of these events allows increased production of autoreactive cells, which proliferate and migrate to the peripheral blood. If severe thymic damage causes a relatively permanent loss of autoregulatory mechanisms, then autoaggression may continue unchecked and a full-blown (chronic) GVHD may develop. The effector cells of chronic GVHD seem to be CD8[+], directed against a public determinant of Ia. The development of GVHD requires a CD4[+] (? lymphokine producing) cell because although CD8[+] cells are directed during cyclosporine treatment, GVHD develops only when cyclosporine has been stopped and CD4[+] cells can proliferate.

The final chapters review new strategies for preventing and treating GVHD. Herman Waldmann reports on the use of anti-MHC class I and anti-MHC class II antibodies to produce tolerance to minor histocompatibility antigens without host irradiation. Other antibodies have also been able to help create tolerance, such as anti-CD4/CD8 and anti-CD11a (LFA-1). The use of such antibodies with little or no radiation is promising for future clinical attempts to induce tolerance without chronic panimmunosuppression such as occurs with total body irradiation. The use of anti-IL-2 receptor antibodies (Chapter 1) was also able to prevent GVHD and promote tolerance. Two points are particularly noteworthy from Waldmann's clinical data. The incidence of chronic GVHD correlates with cyclosporine use; such an observation is consistent with the data from Hess in the induction of syngeneic GVHD with cyclosporine and its resemblance to chronic GVHD. The use of CAMPATH (a pan-lymphocyte antibody that binds human complement) has also correlated with increased marrow graft failure and increased leukemia relapse. These complications represent substantial obstacles to more widespread use of T-cell depletion, as has been noted in this and other chapters.

Another innovative therapeutic approach has been the use of thalidomide as presented by Vogelsang. Thalidomide has been used in conjunction with cyclosporine A in treating acute GVHD, and there seems to be an additive but not synergistic effect between the two compounds. In chronic GVHD, some synergistic effects between the two drugs were noted, but dosage problems have prevented definitive conclusions. Similarities

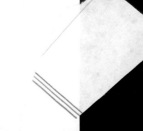

between thalidomide and cyclosporine effects include a decrease in CD4$^+$ cells, the induction of suppressor cells, binding to cyclophilin, and the potential to induce syngeneic GVHD.

Our increased understanding of which T cells initiate GVHD and the role of lymphokines in altering the usual patterns of lymphocyte function have laid the groundwork for the development of more specific therapies for both the prevention and the treatment of GVHD. Increased information about the receptors that control growth, development, and function of T-cell subsets as well as their ligands, will offer new reagents and approaches to the selective abrogation of antihost responses. Such information will also provide insight into the critical cellular and molecular processes of host defense and self tolerance. Studies of GVHD may thus eventually lead to new therapeutic strategies for multiple diseases, including immunodeficiencies and autoimmune diseases.

1

The Pathophysiology of Acute Graft-vs.-Host Disease in a Murine Bone Marrow Transplant Model

James Ferrara and Steven J. Burakoff
Dana-Farber Cancer Institute
Harvard Medical School
Boston, Massachusetts

I. INTRODUCTION

Graft-vs.-Host Disease (GVHD) is a common and often lethal complication of allogeneic bone marrow transplantation (BMT). Although GVHD affects multiple organ systems, its pathophysiologic mechanisms have proven difficult to elucidate in the clinical setting. Many of these difficulties arise from the acuity of the disease, its protean manifestations, and the impracticality of invasive diagnostic procedures, particularly when therapeutic options are limited. We have therefore chosen to study GVHD in a well-defined and carefully controlled murine BMT model initially described by Korngold and Sprent (1). In this model, bone marrow transplants are performed between donor (B10.BR) and recipient (CBA/J) mouse strains that are genetically identical at the major histocompatibility complex (MHC, designated H-2 in the mouse). Although both donor and recipient strains in this model are of the H-2^k haplotype, they differ in their background genes and thus are incompatible for many minor histocompatibility antigens (HA). These minor HA differences are significant enough to induce a severe and often lethal GVHD.

This murine system mirrors the genetics of HLA-identical, allogeneic BMT, currently the most common type of allogeneic marrow transplant performed. The wide disparity in background genes between donor and recipient strains makes this mouse model particularly relevant to transplants from HLA-matched, unrelated donors. Such transplants are now performed with greater frequency because of the increased numbers of HLA-identical individuals who are identified in national and international bone marrow donor registries. Thus, the GVHD produced in this model will hopefully provide insights into the pathophysiology and natural history of an important and complex disease process, as well as lead to novel approaches to its prevention and ultimate cure.

II. INDUCTION OF GVHD

A. BMT Protocol

The BMT protocol of this model is similar to that used in clinical transplantation. CBA/J mice receive a total of 1100 rads whole body irradiation in two doses separated by a 3-hour interval in order to minimize gastrointestinal toxicity. Donor bone marrow is harvested from tibias and femurs of B10.BR mice. T cells are eliminated from the bone marrow by treatment with anti-Thy1.2, a pan T-cell monoclonal antibody, and complement. After two cycles of antibody and complement, 10×10^6 bone marrow cells are injected via tail vein. Animals are housed in clean (but not sterile) conditions and given chlorine (eight parts part million) in their drinking water for the first 2 weeks after BMT. All marrow transplant recipients engraft completely as judged by the presence of only donor forms of erythrocyte enzymes (carbonic anhydrase) and T-cell surface markers (Lyt-1, Lyt-2). The number and self-renewal capacity of hematopoietic stems cells is not affected by treatment with anti-Thy1.2 and complement as judged by CFU-s and R_s of treated BM (2).

A limiting dilution analysis (LDA) reveals that fewer than one in ten thousand functinal T cells remain in the bone marrow after treatment with anti-Thy1.2 and complement. Thus, each mouse that receives T-cell-depleted BM receives less than 10^3 T cells, or less than 4×10^4 T cells per kilogram. This method of T-cell depletion reduces the number of T cells to below the threshold levels at which GVHD to minor histocompatibility antigens has been observed in both experimental and clinical transplantation (3,4). No mice receiving T-cell-depleted bone marrow show clinical evidence of GVHD, and they have nearly 100% long-term survival.

B. Addition of T Cells and T-Cell Subsets to BM

GVHD is induced in this model by the addition of T-cell-enriched splenocytes from donor B10.BR mice to the bone marrow (Fig. 1). After donor splenocytes are passed over a nylon wool column, the nonadherent fraction is approximately 90% Thy 1^+; these Thy 1^+ cells are then added to the bone marrow inoculum (previously depleted of T cells) in order to induce GVHD. This method avoids any variation due to differing numbers of Thy 1^+ cells in the donor bone marrow and allows precise quantitation of the number of T cells injected into each mouse. Recipients of as few as 10^4 Thy 1^+ splenocytes in the donor bone marrow begin to show clinical signs of GVHD after several weeks: inability to gain weight, diarrhea, perianal dermatitis, ruffled fur, and hunched posture. The addition of greater numbers of Thy 1^+ cells to the bone marrow increases the severity of GVHD. When 10^6 T cells or greater are present in the bone marrow, mortality increases to 100% (1,4,5).

The type of mature T cell required to produce GVHD in this system was determined by addition of T-cell subsets to the donor bone marrow (Fig. 1). L3T4 is the murine homolog of T4 (CD4); Lyt-2 is the murine homolog of T8 (CD8). Anti-L3T4 and complement treatment (two cycles) of Thy 1^+ spleen cells produces an L3T4$^-$, Lyt 2^+ population (>90% by FACS). Similarly, Lyt 2^-, L3T4$^+$ cells were prepared by treating Thy 1^+ cells with two cycles of anti-Lyt-2 and complement. Mice were then transplanted with 10^7 T-cell-depleted bone marrow cells alone or with addition of 10^6 Thy 1^+ (unseparated) cells, Lyt-2$^-$ (L3T4$^+$) cells, or L3T4$^-$ (Lyt-2$^+$) cells. Survival and weight after BMT were both monitored, and the results are shown in Figure 1. The Lyt-2$^-$ subset did not produce GVHD either by weight loss or lethality. The L3T4$^-$ subset,

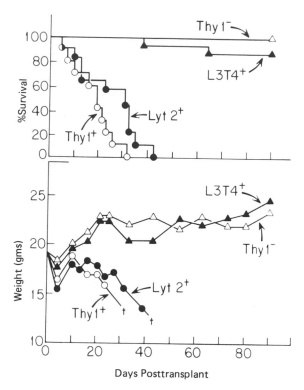

Figure 1   Induction of GVHD to minor HA after BMT (B10.BR → CBA/J) by Thy 1$^+$ Lyt 2$^+$ donor cells. Four groups of 10-12 CBA/J mice were given TBI and transplanted with 10^7 T-cell-depleted B10.BR bone marrow as described in the text. Donor B10.BR splenocytes were enriched for Thy 1$^+$ cells and aliquots were then treated with anti-Lyt 2 or anti-L3T4 and complement or complement alone. Survival and weight are plotted against time after BMT. △, BM only (Thy1$^-$); ○, BM and 10^6 Thy 1$^+$ splenocytes (Thy 1$^+$); ▲, BM + 10^6 L3T4$^+$ splenocytes (L3T4$^+$); ●, BM + 10^6 Lyt 2$^+$ splenocytes (Lyt 2$^+$). From Ref. 43.

on the other hand, produced GVHD as severe as unseparated Thy 1$^+$ cells. Thus, mature Lyt-2$^+$, L3T4$^-$ T cells are responsible for inducing GVHD in this system, an observation that confirms earlier observations of Korngold and Sprent (4). Further experiments using different strain combinations suggest that Lyt-2$^+$ cells can always produce GVHD to minor histocompatibility antigens, but L3T4$^+$ cells are also able to elicit it at times (6). A detailed analysis of the role of T-cell subsets producing GVHD to both minor and major histocompatibility antigens is presented by Korngold and Sprent in Chapter 2.

III. GVHD PATHOPHYSIOLOGY

A. GVHD Target Organs

1. Skin, Intestine, Liver

In clinical transplantation, the three main target organs of GVHD are skin, intestine, and liver. These three organs are also affected in murine GVHD as determined by histopathological analysis. We have carefully examined the organs of affected mice for evidence of GVHD changes, particularly the skin, which is the most commonly biopsied tissue in clinical transplantation. The cutaneous GVHD pathology in this model is extensive and its severity correlates with the number of T cells added to the bone marrow (5). The cutaneous manifestations of GVHD in this model were initially overlooked because CBA/J mice do not lose their fur; alopecia is a prominent aspect of GVHD in other mouse strains, but not in CBA/J (7,8). On closer examination, however, macroscopic manifestations of cutaneous disease such as erythroderma and skin thickening are present. Histologic examination of the skin reveals several abnormalities almost identical to GVHD in humans (Fig. 2). These abnormalities include basal cell hyperplasia, vacuolization, exocytosis of mononuclear cells that have infiltrated the epidermis and satellosis (dying keratinocytes surrounded by infiltrating monunuclear cells). Epidermal and follicular dyskeratosis (cellular degeneration and death defined by nuclear pyknosis or fragmentation and cytoplasmic hypereosinophilia) are also histologically similar to that found in human cutaneous GVHD. Dyskeratosis is a constant feature of the epidermal destruction observed in GVHD, and the dyskeratotic index (the number of dyskeratotic cells per linear millimeter) serves as a semiquantitative measurement of GVHD severity (Fig. 2).

Standard histopathologic changes of GVHD are also seen in this model in two other principal target organs, i.e., the intestine and the liver (Fig. 3). In the intestine, a mononuclear infiltrate into the epithelium of the crypts is noted by 2 weeks after transplantation. Destruction of the crypt epithelium appears simultaneously with this mononuclear infiltrate, increasing in intensity until week 5 when several necrotic cells are visible in each crypt, particularly at the base. Crypts become hyperplastic with increased numbers of mitotic cells, and villi become shortened and edematous. A detailed analysis of the pathophysiology of intestinal GVHD is presented in Chapter 11.

The liver is also affected by GVHD, primarily in the portal tracts. Mononuclear cells infiltrate initially around bile ducts, and by week 5 neutrophils have also invaded the portal space and continued on into the hepatic parenchyma. At this time, necrotic hepatocytes and necrotic bile duct epithelium are evident. The inflammatory infiltrate subsides after 6 weeks but does not totally disappear and leaves substantial portal fibrosis in its wake.

The pathologic changes in the target organs of skin, gut, and liver in this mouse model correspond closely to the changes observed in human GVHD. We have noted that the most intense epithelial destruction appears to be in areas of increased proliferation or of great potential for self-renewal. In the skin, this region is the rete ridge; in the intestine, the base of the crypts; and in the liver, the periductular epithelium. In all these tissues, dying epithelial cells are often observed adjacent to infiltrating mononuclear cells. Epithelia in these regions may possess a common antigenic determinant that serves as a target for the mononuclear effector cells. All three of these areas are considered as regions of self-renewal where stem cells are most likely to reside. Therefore a common element of GVHD pathophysiology in the skin, liver, and intestine may be an actively proliferating, immature cell which serves as the target of the GVH response.

2. Lymphopoiesis

The systemic effects of GVHD are not restricted to the skin, liver, and intestine. Experimental GVHD models have demonstrated defects in many organ systems, including lymphopoiesis and hematopoiesis (10-14). The immune system seems more sensitive to dam-

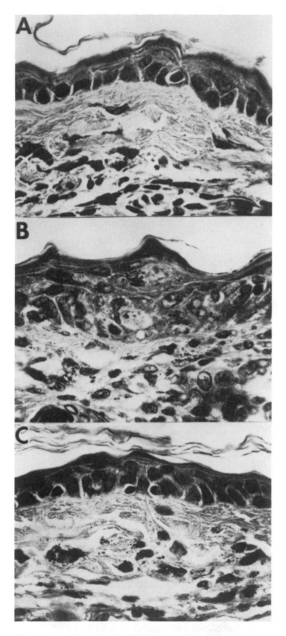

Figure 2 Cutaneous GVHD and its prevention with an anti-IL-2 receptor MAb. Ear skin was obtained 16 days after BMT from CBA/J mice that had been transplanted with 10^7 T-cell-depleted B10.BR bone marrow cells (A) or 10^7 T-cell-depleted bone marrow cells plus 10^6 Thy 1$^+$ splenocytes (B,C). Immediately after BMT, mice were given five daily intraperitoneal injections of 0.4 mg of a control IgM MAb (B) or of anti-IL-2 receptor antibody (C). Histologic changes characteristic of GVHD include basal cell hyperplasia and vacuolization, mononuclear infiltrates, epidermal maturation disarray, and epidermal dyskeratosis. Dyskeratotic index (number of dyskeratotic cells per 10 linear mm epidermis): A, 1.3 ± 0.47; B, 16.3 ± 4.45; C, 6.1 ± 1.61. From Ref. 43.

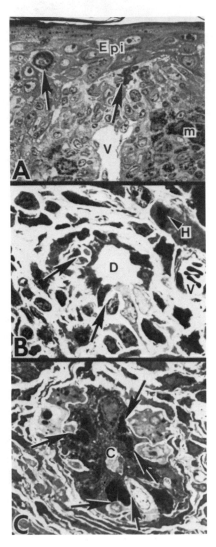

Figure 3 Acute GVHD in skin, liver, and intestine day 16-20 after BMT. A, skin. The dermis and lower portion of the epidermis (EPI) are infiltrated by numerous mononuclear cells, many of which are in apposition to degenerating epidermal cells (arrows). Degenerative changes consisted of focal basal cell layer vacuolization, often initially involving the infundibula of hair follicles and epidermal dyskeratosis as previously reported (5). Dermal vessels (V) are dilated, and numerous melanin-containing macrophages (m), the residual of previous epidermal injury, are seen. B, liver. Bile duct (D) of hepatic portal tract is surrounded and focally infiltrated by numerous mononuclear cells, many of which have elaborate microvilli. Sites of apposition (arrows) between mononuclear cells and ductular epithelial cells are characterized by condensed, darkly stained cytoplasm and nuclear pyknosis of the latter cell type. Neighboring hepatocytes (H) show evidence of cellular degeneration (intracellular edema and distortion) as well as occasional mitotic figures. C, intestine (colon). The base of intestinal crypt (C) is infiltrated by numerous lightly stained mononuclear cells, some of which contain cytoplasmic granules. Points of direct contact (arrows) with densely stained, degenerating crypt epithelial cells are observed. From Ref. 23.

age induced by GVHD than visceral organs such as the gastrointestinal tract (see Chapter 11), but such studies have usually been carried out in unirradiated recipients whose lymphohematopoietic systems were initially normal. The relevance of GVHD-induced changes in these models to the effects of GVHD on lymphohematopoietic reconstitution after BMT is unclear. For example, the rapid proliferation and differentiation of engrafting marrow makes the demonstration of GVHD-specific effects after BMT quite difficult. In human transplantation, these variations are further complicated by the heterogeneity of pretransplant disease states and chemotherapy regimens, both of which may alter critical aspects of the lymphohemopoietic microenvironment. We have therefore used this murine radiation BMT model to examine the effects of GVHD on immunologic and hematologic reconstitution. As described below, GVHD produces a complex set of changes in these reconstituted organs, changes that are often more apparent in the function rather than the phenotype of mature lymphoid, erythroid, and myeloid cells.

The reconstitution of the immune system after BMT is a complex and dynamic process. There are conflicting reports on the effects of GVHD on the appearance of mature lymphocytes in the peripheral blood after human BMT (15,16). To examine effects of GVHD on immunologic reconstitution in this model, splenocytes from mice with and without GVHD were phenotypically analyzed for a panel of cell surface antigens found both on normal, mature T cells (Thy1, Lyt-1 (CD5), Lyt-2 (CD8), and L3T4 (CD4)) and on mature B cells (surface Ig, mu heavy chain, kappa light chain, and Ia (which is not expressed on T cells in the mouse)). When examined over time, there is only a slight delay (1-2 weeks) in the recovery of mature lymphocytes compared to mice without GVHD (Fig. 4). After 3-4 weeks, phenotypically mature lymphocytes are present in spleens of all transplanted mice; normal numbers of lymphocytes are achieved by approximately 2 months after transplant (17).

The function of these newly developed lymphocytes, however, does not correlate well with their mature phenotype, particularly from mice with GVHD (Fig. 5). The functional repertoire of T cells during immune reconstitution was assessed by determining the number of reactive precursors in a given population using limiting dilution analysis (LDA), a sensitive and highly quantitative technique. The frequency estimate generated from these analyses defines cellular function as the number of functional cells, not the amount of function per cell. In these experiments, lymphocytes were stimulated with the T-cell mitogen, Con A, and the number of T-cell precursors was measured for two principal T-cell functions: lymphokine (IL-2) production and cell mediated cytotoxicity (Fig. 5). T-cell functions return to normal levels only after several months, and this delay was exacerbated in animals with GVHD where function deficits persist at 12-16 weeks after BMT. These deficits were not obvious in standard high density cultures where normal functional indices can be generated despite low numbers of precursors (19). Such "normal" function by a few precursors in high density cultures might be due to a simultaneous loss in regulatory (suppressor) cells in those same cultures. Besides defects in lymphokine production and cytotoxicity (Fig. 5), there is a defect in proliferative T-cell precursors as well (19). These data thus suggest that the functional capacity of T cells after BMT lags behind their acquisition of a mature T-cell phenotype.

Previous studies have ascribed the impaired lymphocyte function observed in acute GVHD primarily to defective helper T-cell activity (10,11). Recent data suggest that a GVHD-induced helper cell deficit is engendered by thymic dysfunction (11,12) (these findings are discussed in detail in Chapter 8). However, the functional analysis by limiting dilution in this model demonstrates deficits not only in lymphokine secretion

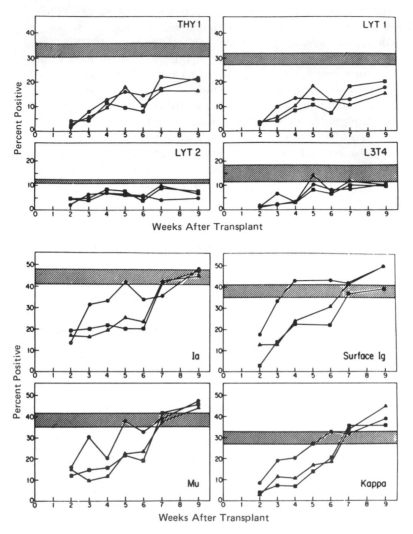

Figure 4 Recovery of T- and B-cell surface phenotype after BMT. CBA/J mice were transplanted as described in the text and graded numbers of Thy1[+] donor splenocytes were added to the donor BM (●, 0 T cells; ▲, 10^4 T cells; ■, 10^5 T cells). Mice (2-4 from each group from four separate transplants) were sacrificed every one to two weeks after BMT and splenocytes were stained with MAb directed at the various cell surface antigens. Staining of normal donor splenocytes is shown in the horizonal bar (mean ± S.D.). From Ref. 7.

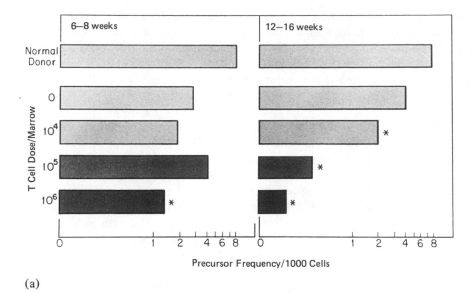

(a)

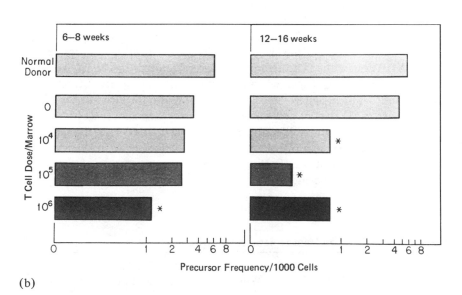

(b)

Figure 5 Diminished lymphocyte precursors in GVHD. CBA/J mice were transplanted as described in the text, and graded numbers of Thy 1$^+$ donor splenocytes (10^4, 10^5, 10^6) were added to the BM cells at the time of transplant. BMT recipients were sacrificed and analyzed for splenic T-lymphocyte function at 6-8 weeks or 12-16 weeks after BMT by limiting dilution analysis (LDA). Frequencies for helper T-lymphocyte (pHTL) and cytolytic T-lymphocyte (pCTL) precursors were determined as described in the text. *, significant difference (p ⩽ 0.05) from BMT plus 0 T cells control. From Ref. 18.

but also in lymphocyte proliferation and cytotoxicity, the assays for which are conducted under conditions of (exogenous) lymphokine excess. Thus, during reconstitution after BMT, deficits in all T-cell functions occur despite their mature phenotype, and these deficits are more profound and of longer duration in the presence of GVHD. These functional abnormalities are subtle and not observable in standard high density cell cultures and are most clearly discerned in highly quantitative LDA assays.

3. Hematopoiesis

Studies in unirradiated, P-into-F_1 rodent models of GVHD have demonstrated that GVHD can have a deleterious effect on bone marrow function and hematopoiesis (13,14). The studies of immunologic reconstitution after BMT outlined above demonstrate that GVHD delays functional T-cell reconstitution, particularly when analyzed by sensitive assays such as LDA. In order to investigate whether the donor hematologic reconstitution might be affected by GVHD, hematopoiesis was evaluated in mice with or without GVHD at several time points following BMT. Peripheral blood counts, bone marrow cellularity, progenitor cell numbers and stem cell (CFU-s) content were measured simultaneously (20). Results are summarized in Table 1. GVHD had no effect on peripheral blood indices at any time after transplant. Bone marrow cellularity and numbers of hematopoietic progenitor cells were also not significantly different in GVHD and non-GVHD mice, although they were clearly lower than normal donor controls. GVHD did induce significant differences in the number of stem cells (CFU-s) present in both the bone marrow and spleen. GVHD reduced the stem cell number as early as 2 weeks after BMT, and this deficit continued to be noted 5 months later. The number of hematopoietic stem cells was lower than normal in all transplanted mice, but it was suppressed even further by GVHD despite the fact that multilineage progenitors and peripheral blood counts seemed unaffected. These results suggest that GVHD damages hematopoietic stem cells, but that such damage may not be discernible in the levels of mature, circulating cells or even at the level of progenitor cells. Cell cycling data suggest that both stem cells and progenitors are proliferating faster in mice with GVHD. This more rapid cell cycling may be a compensatory effect for the lower number of stem cells in hematopoietic organs of mice with GVHD, thereby allowing for production of normal numbers of circulating peripheral cells.

Table 1 The Effect of GVHD on Hemopoietic Reconstitution

		Hct	WBG	BM ($\times 10^{-6}$) per 2 hind limbs	CFU-s per 10^6 BM
No GVHD	1 mo.	40.5 ± 3.4	1.84 ± 0.38	21.0 ± 17.8	153 ± 16
	5 mo.	32.5 ± 3.1	2.60 ± 1.45	40.6 ± 4.8	240 ± 40
GVHD	1 mo.	34.8 ± 12.4	1.58 ± 0.64	23.4 ± 13.2	48 ± 19
	5 mo.	38.0 ± 4.6	2.73 ± 0.38	48.8 ± 4.0	134 ± 32
N1 donor		41.3 ± 5.0	4.40 ± 0.33	51.1 ± 7.9	450 ± 40

CBA/J mice were irradiated (1100 rad) and transplanted with 5×10^5 T-cell-depleted B10.BR BM alone (no GVHD) or BM plus 1×10^5 B10.BR splenocytes (GVHD). Four to six animals in each group were sacrificed at both 1 and 5 months after BMT and assayed for peripheral blood values (Hct and WBC), BM cellularity ($\times 10^6$) and CFU-s (day 8). Age-matched B10.BR donor mice served as normal controls.

GVHD delays or impairs reconstitution of hematopoiesis as measured by CFU-s in this model. Detailed analysis of hematopoietic progentors was required to reveal such defects, a situation similar to the impairment observed in T-cell reconstitution. In the clinic, severe clinical GVHD is often accompanied by a return to dependence on blood product transfusions. However, this phenomenon is often attributed to increased consumption and destruction of mature blood elements in patients with multisystem disease, not decreased hematopoiesis. The murine data suggest that deficits in hematologic reconstitution production may also be induced by GVHD, although these deficits are not discernable by standard laboratory techniques. Recent data from Seattle on patients with thrombocytopenia after severe GVHD also suggest that GVHD may adversely affect hematopoiesis (21). Such observations agree with the abnormal stem cell values seen in this model and suggest that GVHD has a chronically deleterious effect on the hematopoietic graft.

Both hematopoietic and lymphopoietic organs appear to be targets of GVHD in this BMT model. These findings challenge our usual notions of GVHD because all transplant recipients are completely engrafted with donor lymphohematopoiesis. The *donor* graft is affected, despite the fact that the donor CFU-s in the graft are genetically identical to the T cells that induce GVHD. It is possible that the newly engrafting marrow is an innocent bystander of nonspecific cytotoxicity induced by the GVH reaction, a phenomenon which has been observed in other GVHD target organs such as the intestine (see Chapter 11). Further studies of effector cells in this model also support this hypothesis.

B. GVHD Effector Cells

Mononuclear cell infiltrates in GVHD target organs are often found in close proximity to dead or necrotic epithelial cells, which seem to be the target cells in the damaged tissue. The simultaneous appearance of necrotic epithelial cells and infiltrating mononuclear cells occurs in all three target organs: skin, intestine, and liver. In the skin, the earliest histologic alterations are seen in the epidermis at approximately day 12, followed by progressive epidermal cell necrosis, which peaks 4-5 days later when satellosis (the apposition of dying keratinocytes to infiltrating mononuclear cells) is often observed (5). The membranes of these mononuclear cells extend in multiple pseudopodia and interdigitate extensively with the dying keratinocytes. The visual relationship of these two cell types therefore has the classic appearance of a target-effector interaction and is also seen in the intestine and in the liver (Figs. 3 and 6).

Attempts to identify more precisely these presumed mononuclear effector cells led to surprising results (Fig. 6). Because Lyt-2$^+$ cells in the bone marrow inoculum correlated with clinical and histologic GVHD, the initial expectation was to find the Lyt-2$^+$ mononuclear cells in the skin. However, immunohistochemical analysis revealed instead that these cells have the following surface phenotype: Thy 1$^+$, Mac 1$^+$, ASGM$_1$$^+$, Lyt-2$^-$, Ia$^-$ (22). This surface phenotype is more consistent with natural killer (NK) cells than mature T cells. Transmission electron microscopy confirmed that the infiltrating mononuclear cells were large granular lymphocytes (LGLs), a morphologic characteristic of NK cells. These LGLs exhibit many features of activated cells including: (1) elaborate cell surfaces with numerous elongated projections, (2) coarsely clumped chromatin with indented nuclei, (3) dense, membrane-bound cytoplasmic vacuoles, and (4) parallel arrays of tubules. None of the cells showed cytoplasmic characteristics of macrophages such as phagolysosomes. Despite their appearance as activated cells, they remain Ia$^-$, which also strongly suggests that these cells are not scavenger macrophages attracted to

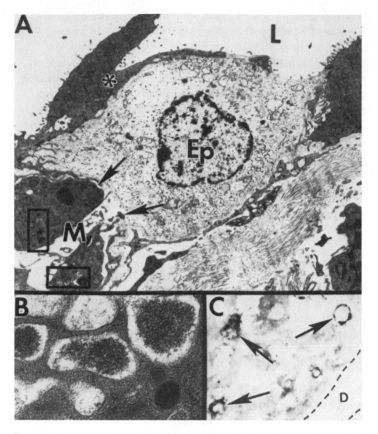

Figure 6 LGL phenotype of acute GVHD infiltrate (day 16). A, hepatic bile duct epithelium (day 16). Mononuclear cells (M) are in apposition to a degenerating ductular epithelial cell (Ep), which is partially covered by attenuated normal epithelial cells (*), which maintain an almost continuous viable lining of the duct (L = ductular lumen) (X 10,000). B, large granular morphology of mononuclear infiltrate. The granules of mononuclear cells exhibited variable diameters, ranging from 200-800 nm. Morphological features of monocytes or macrophages, including cytoplasmic phagolysosomes, were never observed in these cells (X56,000). C, immunohistochemistry analysis. Liver sections were stained with anti-asialo GM_1 antibody. Positively labeled cells (arrows) are present in the vicinity of a longitudinally sectioned bile-duct (D). (Immunoperoxidase technique, X400). From Ref. 23.

the site of epithelial necrosis. Evidence further supporting the identification of these LGLs as NK cells was derived from functional analysis of splenocytes from animals in the first month after transplant (23). NK activity (lysis of the YAC tumor target) was increased in all BMT recipients, but especially in animals with GVHD . At the same time, fewer cytolytic T-cell precursors (pCTL) were seen in the GVHD group, as noted in other models (24). Thus, both by in situ phenotype and by functional analysis, mature cytolytic T lymphocytes were scarce in GVHD mice, whereas LGLs with an NK phenotype and activity predominated.

Further studies regarding the origin of these mononuclear cells were performed by inducing GVHD in CBA/J recipients with spleen and bone marrow cells from a second MHC-identical strain, AKR (23). The AKR strain expresses a different Thy1 allele (Thy1.1) from the CBA/J strain (Thy1.2) and thus offered an opportunity to identify the mononuclear infiltrating cells as of donor or host origin. Immunoperoxidase staining of the skin showed that no cells reacted with the host-specific allele (Thy1.2), even though they were Thy1$^+$ (using a pan-Thy 1 antibody). Thus, the infiltrating cells appeared to be of donor origin.

C. Two-Phase Model of GVHD

As data accumulated in this GVHD system, it was increasingly difficult to reconcile them all with a model of a Lyt-2$^+$ effector cell. Such a model postulated that B10.BR Lyt-2$^+$ cytotoxic T lymphocytes recognize minor HA of the CBA/J host and destroy host tissues with those antigens. Data regarding impaired lymphohemopoietic reconstituting could be explained in this model by donor CTL destruction of host stromal and/or epithelial elements critical to the reconstituting graft. But direct histologic examination of visceral target tissues suggested that Lyt-2$^+$ cells were not primarily responsible for GVHD target destruction. First, Lyt-2$^+$ were rarely found among the infiltrating mononuclear cells in skin, intestine, and liver. Second, these mononuclear cells had the morphology of LGLs on electron microscopy and possessed the surface markers of NK cells by immunohistochemistry. Third, increased NK activity was observed in the spleen of GVHD mice, whereas CTL were diminished. As discussed above, proliferation and lymphokine-producing T cells were also decreased, as were donor hematopoietic stem cells. Once activated, NK cells are less specific than T cells in their cytotoxicity, and this lack of specificity may explain the damage to donor CFU-s. The cumulative weight of these observations suggested that GVHD activates a nonspecific LGL effector mechanism that can damage the donor graft itself as well as the host.

NK cells have been observed as GVHD effector cells in other experimental systems, particularly the P $\rightarrow$ F$_1$ model studied by Ghayur and colleagues (25,26). In that system, splenic NK cells of donor origin mediate the tissue damage of GVHD and splenocytes from NK-defective beige mice are unable to elicit the full spectrum of GVHD pathology. Although initially unexpected, the importance of NK cells in two widely different experimental models of GVHD suggests that their relevance is not limited by the idiosyncratic constraints of a particular experimental system. However, the importance of T cells in producing GVHD has also been clearly demonstrated, and LGLs must be activated or induced before they are capable of eliciting GVHD tissue damage (26). We have therefore proposed an interactive model of GVHD pathogenesis with both an afferent and an efferent phase (27). According to this interpretation, the afferent phase of acute GVHD commences when donor T cells react with alloantigens of the host. These Lyt-2$^+$ T cells release a variety of lymphokines, such as interleukin-2, tumor necrosis factor, and interferon-γ, all of which have been shown to activate LGLs (28-30). The Lyt-2$^+$ phenotype of these cells is most probably due to the fact that these cells recognize minor histocompatibility antigens in association with MHC class I antigens rather than MHC class II antigens. In the efferent phase of acute GVHD, ASGM$_1$$^+$ LGLs are activated by the released lymphokines and engage in tissue destruction. The exact identity of these LGLs is still unclear. Lymphokine activated killer (LAK) cells are a heterogeneous population of cells with LGL morphology and which exhibit MHC-unrestricted cytotoxicity. The recently described $CD3^+\gamma\delta$ cells express both $ASGM_1$ and the $\gamma\delta$ receptor on their cell surfaces and have been found in murine skin as an endogenous lymphocyte population (31-33). They can exhibit NK. Recently, lymphocytic infiltrates in GVHD skin have been determined to possess a novel T-cell phenotype: $CD3^-CD4^+$ (H. Sakamoto, manuscript in preparation). activity and would therefore seem to be attractive candidates for GVHD effector cells. Further studies are in progress to determine what role, if any, these cells play in the pathogenesis of GVHD.

This two-phase model accounts for the ability of both anti-T-cell and anti-NK-cell antibodies in vivo to prevent GVHD (34,35). The phenomenon of syngeneic GVHD may also be accounted for by this model. A clinical syndrome, consistent with GVHD and supported by classic hsitological features on skin biopsy, has been reported in syngeneic transplants (autologous or identical twins) (36,37). Whether this represents authentic GVHD has been questioned because of the lack of any allogeneic stimulus. However syngeneic, IL-2-activated peripheral blood cells have produced a GVHD-like reaction when they are administered as a form of antitumor therapy (38), and these LAK cells can recognize both syngeneic and allogeneic lymphoblast targets (39). Such IL-2-activated cells may also reduce the number of stem cells when cocultivated with syngeneic bone marrow (40). The mechanism of cytotoxicity of syngeneic tissue remains unclear, but it is consistent with damage being caused by NK-like cells. A convincing argument is also made by Hess (Chapter 6) that syngeneic GVHD results from the failure to delete autoreactive T cells during immune reconstitution. Such autoreactive T cells may represent another possible but not necessarily mutually exclusive mechanism of syngeneic GVHD.

IV. GVHD IMMUNOSUPPRESSION AND LYMPHOKINE DYSREGULATION

Consistent with the two-phase model proposed above, lymphokine dysregulation is an essential component of GVHD pathogenesis. We have begun to investigate this dysregulation by analyzing the role(s) of lymphokines in creating the functional deficits in immunologic reconstitution observed in GVHD (18). Suppression of lymphocyte responses in GVHD have been noted in both clinical and experimental BMT. At 4-6 weeks after BMT, splenic lymphocytes from transplanted mice are capable of responding to polyclonal activators such as Concanavalin A (Con A) or lipopolysaccharide (LPS). However, lymphocytes from transplanted mice with GVHD (GVHD lymphocytes) are unable to proliferate to these mitogens. This inhibition of proliferation occurs in spite of the presence of phenotypically mature T cells and B cells. Although GVHD lymphocytes cannot proliferate to Con A, they can produce lymphokines such as IL-2. To investigate the mechanism of this unresponsiveness, GVHD lymphocytes are cocultured with normal donor B10.BR lymphocytes. Normal lymphocyte proliferation of Con A was suppressed (Table 2). Suppression could be eliminated by creating the GVHD lymphocytes with anti-Thy 1 MAb and complement, but not by treatment with a combination of anti-Lyt-2 and anti-L3T4 and complement. Pretreatment of GVHD lymphocytes with leucine methyl ester (LME), a compound that destroys cells containing cytoplasmic granules, also reversed the suppression.

Several lines of evidence suggest that this suppression of cocultures normal lymphocytes also contributes to the inability of GVHD lymphocytes to proliferate. First, as Table 2 demonstrates, suppressor cells can be removed from GVHD splenocytes, allowing normal donor lymphpcytes in coculture to proliferate normally to both Con A and LPS. Second, although unseparated GVHD lymphocytes are unresponsive to LPS,

Table 2　Characteristics of GVHD Suppressor Cells

	Donor lymphocyte proliferation	
Pretreatment of GVHD Cell	T cell (Con A)	B cell (LPS)
No treatment	−	−
Anti-Thy1 and complement	++	++
Anti-Lyt 2 + anti-L3T4 and complement	−	−
LME	++++	++++

GVHD was induced in CBA/J mice by transplantation of 10^7 B10.BR T-cell-depleted BM cells plus 10^5 Thy1[+] spleen cells. Four to six weeks after transplantation splenocytes from GVHD were irradiated (1500 rad) and cultured with donor B10.BR splenocytes in the presence of 2.5 μg/ml Con A or 10 μg/ml LPS. Prior to coculture, GVHD splenocytes were pretreated with anti-Thy1.2 and complement, anti-Lyt 2[+] anti-L3T4 and complement, or leucine methyl ester (LME) for 40 minutes. From Ref. 7.

if B cells are isolated, they are capable of proliferating and secreting immunoglobulin. Third, when suppressor cells are removed from GVHD spleen with LME treatment (removing 5-10% of the cells), the remaining lymphocytes can proliferate to both Con A and LPS (18). These suppressor cells have many of the characteristics of "natural" suppressor cells: they are Lyt-2⁻, L3T4⁻, surface Ig⁻, nonadherent to plastic, relatively radioresistant, and their suppression is not MHC-restricted. One notable difference is that the suppressor cells observed here are Thy 1[+], whereas other natural suppressors are Thy 1⁻ (41). Some natural suppressor cell lines have been found to express the mRNA for the γ-chain of the T cell receptor (42). Although it is not yet clear whether the suppressor lymphocytes in GVHD spleen are related to such natural suppressors, it is possible that CD3-$\gamma\delta$ cells may be involved in both the immunologic deficiencies and the solid organ destruction in this model and may therefore represent a final common effector mechanism of GVHD.

Table 3　Anti-γ-IFN Reverses GVHD Immunosuppression

	^{3}H-Thymidine incorporation (cpm)	
BMT group	No antibody	Anti-γ-IFN
A. Simple culture		
No GVHD	123,076 ± 15,030	226,937 ± 578
GVHD	9,651 ± 5,042	169,710 ± 12,701
B. Coculture		
No GVHD	96,235 ± 1,055	128,963 ± 18,180
GVHD	2,309 ± 1,090	50,048 ± 2,473

Splenocytes from mice with and without GVHD were obtained four weeks after BMT and were stimulated for 3 days in culture by Con A (3 μg/ml) either alone (A) or irradiated (1500 rad) and then added to normal B10.BR splenocytes in coculture (B). Monoclonal anti-γ-IFN (1 μg/ml) was added to half the cultures on day 0. From Ref. 17.

Interferon-γ (IFN-γ) also appears to play an important role in the suppressive effects of GVHD lymphocytes. The addition of anti-γ-IFN antibody to cultures of GVHD splenocytes stimulated with Con A substantially improved their proliferation (Table 3). Anti-γ-IFN also reversed the suppression of normal donor lymphocytes by GVHD splenocytes. This reversal of suppression was also observed for LPS stimulation (B-cell proliferation) in identical culture conditions (18). Thus γ-IFN secretion seems to be dysregulated by GVHD lymphocytes when stimulated in culture, and this lymphokine appears to suppress the proliferative response of other normal cells. A role for IFN-γ in GVHD immunosuppression has also been reported in other experimental models (41). Further studies are in progress to examine other lymphokines which may be dysregulated in GVHD and which may also contribute to abnormalities in immunologic reconstitution.

V. MONOCLONAL ANTIBODY THERAPY FOR GVHD

According to the model proposed here, the elimination of T cells from the bone marrow abolishes GVHD by eliminating the afferent (T cell) arm of the GVHD response. Another approach to the prevention of GVHD is to eliminate the active cell population by administerion of antibodies in vivo. Monoclonal antibodies (MAbs) have been generated against multipe T-cell surface proteins, many of which are functional receptors, and these MAbs can block T-cell function in vitro. MAbs are potentially attractive therapeutic agents for GVHD prophylaxis because they can prevent cellular activity independently of the elimination of targeted cells via complement lysis or removal in the reticuloendothelial system. In this murine model, we have tested in vivo MAb directed against the interleukin-2 receptor (IL-2R) as prophylaxis for GVHD (43). The proliferation of T cells is dependent on IL-2, and the number of IL-2R increases up to ten thousand-fold when a T cell is activated (44,45). The anti-IL-2R antibody used in these experiments was chosen for its ability to block the binding of IL-2 and therefore the proliferation of T cells in vitro. In vivo injections of this antibody might therefore prevent the clonal expansion of T cells as well as marking them for elimination through lysis by serum complement or removal from the circulation by the reticulo-endothelial system. Results of these experiments are shown in Figure 7. GVHD was induced in CBA/J mice by the transplantation of 10^7 T-cell-depleted B10.BR bone marrow cells plus 10^6 B10.BR splenic T cells. Daily injections of the antibody (0.1 mg) were given intraperitoneally for the first 5 days following BMT. Control groups received an irrelevant monoclonal antibody or saline. Survival in the anti-IL-2R group at 100 days was 60% compared to 0% in control groups. Other clinical parameters of GVHD such as weight loss and diarrhea were also significantly improved. The histologic severity of GVHD was measured by the number of dyskeratotic cells present in skin biopsies, and the severity of cutaneous GVHD was significantly diminished in the anti-IL-2R group (see Fig. 2). Thus, an antibody administered in vivo can prevent GVHD even with large numbers of T cells in the bone marrow. This long-term clinical effect was achieved despite the fact that the antibody was administered only for a short time after transplant, consistent with a "window of tolerance" in the early posttransplant period, which is critical to the balance between host and graft tissues.

Although the administration of large doses of anti-IL-2R MAb therapy was able to prevent GVHD in the majority of animals tested, it was not able to completely prevent GVHD. There are several possible explanations for this partial effect. First, incomplete

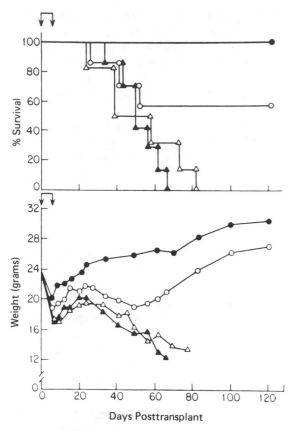

Figure 7 The effect of anti-IL-2 receptor MAb on clinical GVHD. Survival (top) and weight (bottom) curves of CBA/J recipients of B10.BR BM and 0 donor T cells (●) or 10^6 donor T cells (○,▲,△). Five daily intraperitoneal injections (↓↓) of 0.75 ml normal saline contained 0.4 mg of anti-IL-2 receptor (○), control Ig (△), or no antibody (▲).

recognition of the targeted cell population could result from only partial penetration of antibody into tissues or compartments where the cells have already infiltrated, such as the spleen or lymphatic system. Second, the affinity of the antibody for the IL-2 receptor might be lower than that of the natural ligand, IL-2, and thus incomplete inhibition of proliferation would result. Third, antibodies might be capped and endocytosed after binding to the cell surface but before the targeted cells are eliminated through either complement-mediated lysis or general clearance via the reticulo-endothelial system. If the efficacy of the antibody arises largely through the blockade of function rather than through the elimination of cells, this last possibility is least probable. The use of MAbs conjugated to immunotoxins such as ricin to prevent GVHD presents another approach to this problem, as discussed by Vallera et al. in Chapter 3.

The reasons noted above for a partial antibody effect assume that the targeted cell surface protein identifies the principal GVHD effector cell and that the elimination or functional impairment of these cells will prevent GVHD. A second possibility for the partial effect of antibodies in vivo is that the cell population identified is only partially responsible for GVHD. Thus, cells bearing the IL-2R may not be the only cells involved in GVHD pathogenesis. In fact, when the skin from mice with GVHD was examined by immunohistochemical analysis, no consistently IL-2R positive population was identified. The anti-IL-2R MAb may only be directed at cells in the afferent arm of GVHD, and this antibody may not inhibit or eliminiate previously activated effector cells. Antibodies directed against functional cell surface receptors on both T cells and NK cells, such as anti-LFA-1, are currently being evaluated. These studies will help to clarify the cell populations involved and their mechanism(s) of action.

Future monoclonal antibody therapy in vivo is likely to concentrate not only on cell surface antigens by on lymphokines themselves which are released during GVHD. As discussed earlier, the point of continuity between the afferent and efferent arms of the acute GVHD response is the dysregulated release of lymphokines, which may play an important, central role in the pathogenesis of GVHD. A neutralizing antibody to IFN-γ has been successful in reversing the immunosuppression of proliferating lymphocytes in vitro, and its efficacy in vivo is currently being evaluated. The in vivo administration of polyclonal antibodies to tumor necrosis factor (TNF) has recently been demonstrated to reduce GVHD in vivo and further underscores the importance of lymphokines to this reaction. With availability of these antibodies, we may begin to understand which specific lymphokines are important in GVHD and in what sequence they work. The importance of secondary cellular effectors such as NK cells or CD3-$\gamma\delta$ cells can also be more critically analyzed. Further experiments using these and other newly developed monoclonal antibodies will not only further our understanding of the basic physiologic processes that occur during GVHD but may offer potentially useful therapies in the clinic.

VI. CONCLUSIONS

The pathophysiology of GVHD is a complex process with several interactive components. In this chapter, we have reviewed our studies of GVHD in a murine BMT model across minor HA. Lyt-2$^+$ T cells in the bone marrow induce GVHD; infiltrating effector cells in target organs do not share this phenotype, however, and instead they have the appearance of LGLs by electron microscopy and immunohistocytochemistry. NK activity is increased in BMT recipients with GVHD, and CTL precursors are diminished. We suggest that these data are most consistent with a two-phase model of acute GVHD in which mature T cells react to foreign host antigens and release lymphokines, which then activate NK cells. These NK cells are less specific in their cytotoxicity and they damage recipient skin, intestine, and liver; they may also damage the donor graft in an innocent bystander.

Lymphokine dysregulation is a pivotal event in the induction of GVHD. IFN-γ is one lymphokine that is at least partially responsible for immunosuppression observed in the GVHD induced in this model. IL-2 is also an essential mediator in the early phases because anti-IL-2R monoclonal antibody therapy has been able to prevent GVHD despite the presence of large numbers of T cells in the donor inoculum. Further experiments are in progress to dissect which lymphokines are important in the induction of NK (CD3-$\gamma\delta$) effector cells and what, if any, lymphokines are in turn released by these effectors to cause tissue destruction. The pathological spectrum of GVHD may eventually be explained by a variety of cellular mediators, activated by a cascade of cytokines and interleukins. Specificities for various targets may then be due to the tissue tropism of these cellular mediators (e.g., CD3-$\gamma\delta$ cells home to skin and intestine). These findings may not only help us understand the dysregulated cellular interactions which can occur after bone marrow transplantation, but help to clarify various autoimmune and immunodeficient states as well.

ACKNOWLEDGMENTS

This work was supported by NIH grants K11 AI 00653-03 and 2P01-CA39542-04 and a grant from the Dyson Foundation. We thank Pim van Dijken, Abul Abbas, Donna Wall, and George Murphy for their helpful discussions and Carolyn Gregory for preparation of the manuscript.

REFERENCES

1. Korngold R, Sprent J: Lethal graft-versus-host disease after bone marrow transplantation across minor histocompatibility barriers in mice: Prevention by removing mature T cells. J Exp Med 1978;148:1687.
2. Ferrara J, Lipton J, Hellman S, et al.: Engraftment following T cell depleted marrow transplantation. I. The role of major and minor histocompatibility antigens. Transplant 1987;43:461.
3. Kernan NA, Collins NH, Juliano L, et al.: Clonable T lymphocytes in T cell depleted bone marrow transplants correlate with development of graft-versus-host disease. Blood 1986;68:770.
4. Korngold R, Sprent J: Lethal graft-versus-host disease across minor histocompatibility barriers in mice. Clin Haematol 1983;12:681.
5. Ferrara J, Guillen FJ, Sleckman B, et al.: Cutaneous acute graft-versus-host disease to minor histocompatibility antigens in a murine model: Histologic analysis and correlation to clinical disease. J Invest Dermatol 1986;86:371.
6. Korngold R, Sprent J: Variable capacity of L3T4$^+$ T cells to cause lethal graft-versus-host disease across minor histocompatibility barriers in mice. J Exp Med 1987;165:1552.
7. Charley MR, Bougert JL, Hamilton BL, et al.: Murine graft-versus-host disease: A chronologic and quantitative analysis of two histologic patterns. J Invest Dermatol 1983;81:412.
8. Hamilton BL, Parkman R: Acute and chronic graft-versus-host disease induced by minor histocompatibility antigens in mice. Transplant 1983;36:150.
9. Rappaport H, Khalil A, Halle-Pannenko O, et al.: Histopathologic sequence of events in adult mice undergoing lethal graft-versus-host reaction developed across H-2 and/or non-H-2 histompatibility barriers. Am J Pathol 1979;96:121.
10. Mori T, Tsoi S, Gillis E, et al.: Cellular interactions in marrow grafted patients. 1. Impairment of cell-mediated lympholysis associated with graft-versus-host disease and the effect of interleukin 2. J Immunol 1983;131:1771.
11. Moser M, Miznochi JT, Sharrow SO, et al.: Graft-versus-host reaction limited to a class II MHC difference results in a selective deficiency in L3T4$^+$ but not in Lyt2$^+$ T helper cell function. J Immunol 1987;138:1355.
12. Fukuzawa M, Via CS, Shearer GM. Defective thymic education of L3T4$^+$ T helper cell function in graft-versus-host mice. J Immunol 1988;141:430.
13. Rolink AG, Radaszkiewicz T, Pals ST, et al.: Allosuppressor and allohelper T cells in acute and chronic graft-versus-host disease. I. Alloreactive suppressor cells rather than killer T cells appear to be decisive effector cells in lethal graft-versus-host disease. J Exp Med 1982;155:1501.
14. Iwasaki T, Fujiwara H, Shearer GM: Loss of proliferative capacity and T cell immune development potential by bone marrow in mice undergoing a graft-versus-host reaction. J Immunol 1986;137:3100.

15. Ault K, Antin JH, Ginsberg D, et al.: Phenotype of recovering lymphoid cell populations after marrow transplantation. J Exp Med 1985;161:1483.

16. Friedrick W, O'Reilly RJ, Koziner B, et al.: T lymphocyte reconstitution in recipients of bone marrow transplants with and without GVHD: Imbalances of T cell subpopulations having unique regulatory and cognitive functions. Blood 1982;59: 696.

17. Wall DA, Hamberg SD, Reynolds DS, et al.: Immunodeficiency in graft-versus-host disease. I. Mechanism of immune suppression. J Immunol 1988;140:2970.

18. Ferrara JLM, Daley JP, Burakoff SJ, et al.: Functional T cell deficits after bone marrow transplantation across minor histocompatibility barriers: Effects of graft-versus-host disease on precursor frequency of reactive cells. J Immunol 1987;138: 3598.

19. Ferrara JLM, Wall DA, van Dijken PJ, et al.: Graft versus host disease: Mechanisms of immunodeficiency and monoclonal antibody therapy. In: *Bone Marrow Transplantation. Current Controversies.* Edited by Gale, RP and Champlin RE. Alan R Liss, Inc., New York, 1989.

20. Van Dijken, PJ, Wimperis J, Ferrara JLM: The effect of graft-versus-host disease on hematopoiesis in mice. Manuscript submitted.

21. Sullivan KM, Witherspoon RP, Storb R, et al.: Prednisone and azathioprine compared with prednisone and placebo for treatment of chronic vs host disease: Prognostic influence of prolonged thrombocytopenia after allogeneic marrow transplantation. Blood 1988;72:546.

22. Guillen FJ, Ferrara J, Hancock WW, et al.: Acute cutaneous graft-versus-host disease to minor histocompatibility antigens in a murine model. Evidence that large granular lymphocytes are effector cells in the immune response. Lab Invest 1986;55:35.

23. Ferrara JLM, Guillen FJ, Van Dijken PJ, et al.: Evidence that large granular lymphocytes of donor origin mediate acute graft-versus-host disease. Transplant 1989;47:50.

24. Jadus MR, Peck AB: Lethal murine graft versus host disease in the absence of detectable clonable T lymphocytes. Transplant 1983;36:281.

25. Ghayur T, Seemeyer TA, Konghsavn, PAL, et al.: Graft-versus-host reactions in the beige mouse. An investigation of the role of host and donor natural killer cells in the pathogenesis of graft-versus-host disease. Transplant 1987;44:261.

26. Ghayur T, Seemeyer TA, Lapp WS: Prevention of murine graft-versus-host disease by inducing and eliminating $ASGM_1{}^+$ cells of donor origin. Transplant 1988;45:586.

27. Ferrara J, Marion A, Murphy G, et al.: Acute graft-versus-host disease: Pathogenesis and prevention with a monoclonal antibody in vivo. Transplant Proceed 1987;19: 2662.

28. Peters PM, Ortaldo JR, Shalaby MR, et al.: Natural killer-sensitive targets stimulate production of TFN-α but not TNF-β (lymphotoxin) by highly purified human peripheral blood large granular lymphocytes. J Immunol 1986;137:2592.

29. Svedersky LP, Sherphard HM, Spencer SA, et al.: Augmentation of human natural cell-mediated cytotoxicity by recombinant interleukin-2. J Immunol 1984;133:714.

30. Svedersky LP, Nedwin GE, Goeddel DV, et al.: Interferon-γ enhances induction of lymphotoxin in recombinant interleukin-2 stimulated peripheral blood mononuclear cells. J Immunol 1985;134:1604.

31. Brenner MB, McLean J, Schaft H, et al.: Two forms of the T cell receptor gamma protein on peripheral blood cytotoxic T lymphocytes. Nature 1987;325:689.

32. Romani N, Stingl G, Tschachler E, et al.: The Thy-1 bearing cell of murine epidermis. A distinctive leukocyte perhaps related to natural killer cells. J Exp Med 1985; 161:1368.

33. Stingl G, Gunter KC, Tschachler E, et al.: Thy 1^+ dendritic epidermal cells belong to the T cell lineage. Proc Natl Acad Sci USA 1987;84:2430.
34. Charley HR, Mikhael A, Bennett M, et al.: Prevention of lethal minor determinant graft-versus-host disease in mice by the in vivo administration of anti-asialo GM_1. J Immunol 1983;131:2101.
35. Cobbold S, Martin G, Waldmann H: Monoclonal antibodies for the prevention of graft-versus-host disease and marrow graft rejection. The depeletion of T cell subsets in vitro and in vivo. Transplant 1986;42:239.
36. Rappeport J, Mihm M, Neiherz E, et al.: Acute graft-versus-host disease in recipients of bone marrow transplants from identical twin donors. Lancet 1979;2:717.
37. Hood AF, Vogelsang GB, Black LP: Acute graft-versus-host disease. Development following autologous and syngeneic bone marrow transplantation. Arch Dermatol 1987;123:745.
38. Rosenberg SA, Lotze MT, Muul LM, et al.: Observations on the systemic administration of autologous lymphokine activated killer cells and recombinant interleukin-2 to patients with metastatic cancer. New Engl J Med 1985;313:1485.
39. Sondel PM, Hank SA, et al.: Destruction of autologous human lymphocytes by interleukin 2-activated cytotoxic cells. J Immunol 1986;137:502.
40. Long GS, Hiserodt JC, Harnaha JB, et al.: Lymphokine activated killer (LAK) cell purging of leukemia cells from bone marrow prior to syngeneic transplantation. Transplant 1900;45:in press.
41. Holda JH, Maier T, Claman HN: Evidence that IFN-γ is responsible for natural suppressor activity in GVHD spleen and normal bone marrow. Transplant 1988; 45:772.
42. Hertel-Wulff B, Lindsten T, Schwadron B, et al.: Rearrangement and expression of T cell receptor genes in cloned murine natural suppressor cell lines. J Exp Med 1987;166:1168.
43. Ferrara JLM, Marion A, McIntyre JF, et al.: Amelioration of acute graft-versus-host disease due to minor histocompatibility antigens by in vivo administration of anti-interleukin 2 receptor antibody. J Immunol 1986;137:1874.
44. Cotner T, Williams JM, Christenson L, et al.: Simultaneous flow cytometric analysis of human T cell activation, antigen expression and DNA content. J Exp Med 1983; 157:461.
45. Smith KA, Cantrell DA: Interleukin-2 regulates its own receptors. Proc Natl Acad Sci USA 1985;82:864.

2

T-Cell Subsets in Graft-vs.-Host Disease

Robert Korngold
Jefferson Medical College
Philadelphia, Pennsylvania

Jonathan Sprent
Research Institute of Scripps Clinic
La Jolla, California

I. INTRODUCTION

Allogeneic bone marrow transplantation (BMT) has advanced in recent years to the point of becoming a primary therapeutic procedure for several fatal diseases, including aplastic anemia, severe combined immunodeficiency, and leukemia (1). However, this procedure also has the potential for application in numerous other hematologic, metabolic, and oncologic disorders, provided that the risk factors associated with transplantation can be substantially reduced. The most life-threatening complication in BMT patients is Graft-vs.-Host Disease (GVHD), which can occur in as many as 30-70% of HLA-identical sibling transplants, with approximately 50% fatality. A high percentage of those patients that do survive the acute form of GVHD may also later develop the chronic form of the disease, which can persist for several years and result in serious debilitation. Recipients of marrow from unrelated HLA-matched or partially matched donors exhibit even higher susceptibility to the development of GVHD, despite the use of such potent immuno-suppressive drugs as methotrexate and cyclosporine.

Several laboratories working with rodent models have shown that mature T cells contaminating the bone marrow inoculum are responsible for the development of GVHD, both for major histocompatibility complex (MHC) (2-7) and non-MHC genetic differences (8-10). Based on these studies, clinical transplantation trials have been initiated to evaluate the advantages of T-cell depletion of donor marrow for allogeneic BMT. The results have shown a markedly reduced incidence of GVHD in the marrow recipients (1,11-14). Unfortunately, several transplant centers have also reported an associated increased incidence of marrow graft failures (11,15) following T-cell depletion, and, in the case of leukemic patients, there appears also to be an increase in the rate of tumor relapse (11,12,16,17). Graft failure is probably mediated by residual host components that are usually kept under control by donor GVH-reactive T cells (16). Donor T cells in the marrow inoculum may also enhance stem cell engraftment and hematopoiesis by production of such lymphokines as IL-3 and GM-CSF (18). With regard to the increased incidence of leukemia relapse, it is argued that GVH-reactive T cells attack residual tumor cells through recognition of alloantigens and/or tumor-specific antigens (16,19). T-cell depletion of marrow grafts thus promotes outgrowth of the tumor cells. Another serious disadvantage of T-cell depletion protocols is that, because of the lack of either mature donor or host T cells, patients face a prolonged period of immunoincompetency and for this reason are often more susceptible to such opportunistic infections as cytomegalovirus pneumonitis (20).

One possible means of addressing the problem of avoiding GVHD while maintaining some of the advantages associated with the presence of T cells in the donor inoculum (enhancing engraftment, mediating an antileukemia effect and providing adoptive immunocompetency) may be to selectively deplete only one subpopulation of T cells. The ideal approach would be to remove T cells bearing specific antihost receptors. Since this approach is currently technically unfeasible, a simpler option is to deplete one of the two major subdivisions of T cells, either the helper-type or cytotoxic-type T cells, expressing the $CD4^+$ or $CD8^+$ phenotypes, respectively. In this respect, much of our recent work has concentrated upon analysis of the ability of these two major subsets to cause GVHD in relation to different genetic barriers. This article is primarily devoted to a discussion of our own data (published and unpublished) concerning this topic; for a broader review of this area refer to Ref. 21.

II. FEATURES OF T-CELL SUBSETS AND THEIR PURIFICATION

In mice, mature T cells can be separated on the basis of their expression of the cell surface molecules Lyt-2 (CD8) and L3T4 (CD4) (22). Whereas a high proportion of immature thymocytes express both molecules, peripheral T cells express either Lyt-2 or L3T4 molecules, but rarely both. Although the physiological function of CD4 and CD8 molecules is still unclear, it is well established that the expression of these molecules correlates with T-cell responses to class I vs. class II MHC gene products (H-2 products in the mouse) (22,23). It is well accepted that T cells generally recognize antigen in association with self-MHC molecules (22). Lyt-2^+ T cells recognize antigen in the context of H-2 class I (K/D) molecules, whereas L3T4$^+$ T cells respond to antigen plus class II (Ia) H-2 molecules. The same rules apply to T-cell recognition of allogeneic H-2 molecules, i.e., Lyt-2^+ cells respond to stimulator cells expressing allogeneic class I determinants, and L3T4$^+$ cells respond to stimulator cells expressing allogeneic class II determinants. It should also be noted that it has recently become apparent that the L3T4$^+$ T-cell subset can be further subdivided by analysis of lymphokine production into the Th1 and Th2 subclasses, defined by release of either interferon and IL-2, or IL-4, respectively (24). As these helper subsets are extremely difficult to differentiate on the basis of any phenotypic markers, they have yet to be examined for their possible roles in GVHD.

Early attempts to assess the role of T-cell subsets in GVHD were based on negative selection procedures with antibody plus complement and often yielded contradictory results due to the inefficiency of the reagents utilized (25,26). This was particularly evident with the lethal GVHD assay, where contamination with low numbers of residual T cells can lead to significant mortality. We have now turned to a rigorous approach for purifying T-cell subsets combining both negative and positive selection procedures. For preparation of purified Lyt-2$^+$ donor T cells, we initially treat lymph node cells with a mixture of monoclonal antibodies (MAb) specific for B cells (J11d) and L3T4 molecules plus complement. Surviving cells are then panned over anti-Lyt-2 MAb-coated plates, the nonadherent cells removed, and the bound cells retrieved and analyzed for purity by FACS analysis (27). A similar approach is used for preparation of purified L3T4$^+$ cells, i.e., treatment of LN cells with anti-Lyt-2 MAb plus complement followed by panning over anti-L3T4 MAb-coated plates. The purified T-cell subsets are then added to donor T-cell-depleted (anti-Thy 1 MAb plus complement-treated) bone marrow (ATBM) inoculum and injected intravenously into appropriate lethally irradiated recipients for study of GVHD across either H-2 or non-H-2 genetic barriers.

III. GVHD DIRECTED TO H-2 DIFFERENCES

A. Full H-2 Differences

It has been recognized for many years that the transfer of T cells across a full MHC barrier can result in a very severe GVHD response (2-7). Yet, it was relatively recently realized that isolated Lyt-2$^+$ and L3T4$^+$ T-cell subsets are each capable of causing GVHD (27).

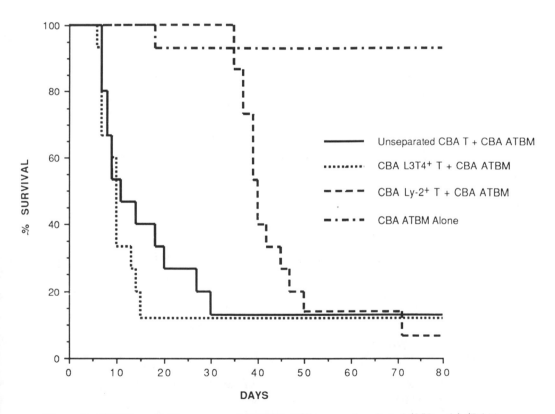

Figure 1 GVHD mortality across a full MHC difference. Irradiated (850 rads) (B6 × CBA)F$_1$ mice were injected with semi-allogeneic CBA ATBM (4 × 10^6) along with either CBA unseparated, L3T4$^+$, or Lyt-2$^+$ T cells (10^6).

As exemplified in Figure 1, the injection of unseparated CBA (H-2^k) T cells (along with donor ATBM) into lethally irradiated semi-allogeneic (CBA × B6(H-2^b))F$_1$ mice results in an acute form of GVHD with high recipient mortality and a short median survival time (MST) of 20 days. Equally severe GVHD is induced by transfer of purified CBA L3T4$^+$ T cells. On the other hand, purified Lyt-2$^+$ T cells, although clearly capable of inducing GVHD leading to 100% mortality, exhibit significantly slower response kinetics, with an MST of 48 days in the experiment illustrated. The relative potency of L3T4$^+$ and Lyt-2$^+$ T cells, however, seems to be dependent on the particular strain combination tested. Thus, with the C3H → (C3HxDBA/2 (H-2^{kxd})F$_1$ combination, Lyt-2$^+$ cells were found to be more potent than L3T4$^+$ cells. In the B6 → (CBA × B6)F$_1$ strain combination, both T-cell subsets responded equivalently (28). A more precise appreciation of the capacity of individual T-cell subsets to cause GVHD across H-2 barriers can be gained by using donor-host combinations differing at isolated class I and class II H-2 loci.

B. Class I H-2 Differences

The capacity of purified T cells and T-cell subsets plus ATBM to cause GVHD in hosts expressing allelic class I differences is illustrated in Table 1. In each of the three strain combinations tested, high mortality was seen with both unseparated T cells and with purified Lyt-2$^+$ cells. On the other hand, purified L3T4$^+$ T cells were completely ineffective at mediating disease. This finding is in agreement with the dogma concerning the restriction patterns of the T-cell subsets, i.e., that class I differences are recognized solely by Lyt-2$^+$ T cells. Similar findings apply to GVHD directed to mutant class I differences, e.g., with transfer of B6 (bbbb) T cells to mutant class I (H-2K) different bm1 (bm1bbb) mice (Fig. 2). As for allelic class I differences, lethal GVHD to mutant class I differences is caused solely by Lyt-2$^+$ T cells and not by L3T4$^+$ T cells (27). Using the B6 → bm1 strain combination, we explored several features of Lyt-2$^+$ T-cell-mediated GVHD (29).

   First, it was found that transfer of B6 donor Lyt-2$^+$ T cells in a dosage between 3×10^5 to 2×10^7 cells resulted in equivalent GVHD with close to 100% mortality and an MST of about 35 days. Thus, regardless of the number of Lyt-2$^+$ T cells injected,

Table 1   Anti-Class I GVHD

Strain combination	Class I difference	Donor cells	Mortality	
			% Dead	MST (days)
B10.A → B10.TL (700 rad)	K	Whole T	100	32
		L3T4$^+$	0	>80
		Lyt-2$^+$	88	37
		ATBM alone	0	>80
B10.A → (B10.A × B10.TL)F1	K	Whole T	75	63
(800 rad)		L3T4$^+$	0	>80
		Lyt-2$^+$	100	34
		ATBM alone	0	>80
B10.A → B10.BR (800 rad)	D	Whole T	100	36
		L3T4$^+$	13	>80
		Lyt-2$^+$	88	44
		ATBM alone	38	>80

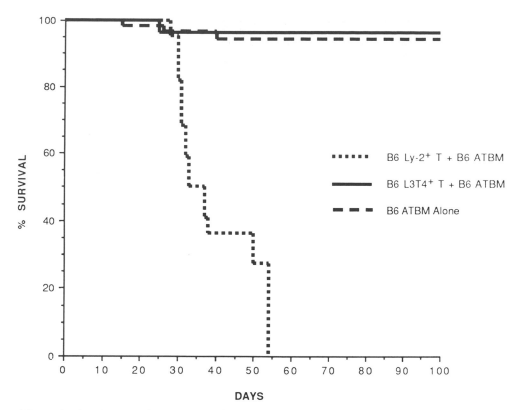

Figure 2 GVHD mortality across a class I H-2K difference. Irradiated (1000 rad) (B6 × bm1)F_1 mice were injected with B6 ATBM (2 × 10^6) along with either B6 L3T4$^+$ or Lyt-2$^+$ T cells (10^6).

most of the recipients died from a late-onset chronic form of GVHD. Especially with higher cell dosages, the mice exhibited physical symptoms of illness early after the first week of transplant with typical signs of GVHD such as weight loss. However, over the next 2 weeks, most of the mice appeared to recover from this early phase of disease, but then relapsed into progressive deterioration and eventual fatality within the next 2 weeks. We considered the possibility that this biphasic pattern of disease might be due to some dependence of the donor B6 Lyt-2$^+$ T cells upon the presence of exogenous sources of IL-2. Perhaps the initial responses were supported by the presence of residual radio-resistant host L3T4$^+$ T cells and, as IL-2 was depleted, the activity of the GVH-reactive donor Lyt-2$^+$ T cells waned? As newly derived donor-type L3T4$^+$ T cells began to emerge from the thymus after 4 weeks, there might be enough "bystander" production of IL-2 (e.g., in response to third-party antigens) to allow for the continuation of the Lyt-2$^+$ T-cell-mediated GVHD response.

The possible dependence of donor Lyt-2$^+$ cells upon residual host L3T4$^+$ cells was tested by conducting the transplant in conjunction with in vivo treatment of the recipient mice with anti-L3T4 MAb given in multiple injections. Control experiments indicated that this treatment effectively eliminated not only residual host cells, but also the capa-

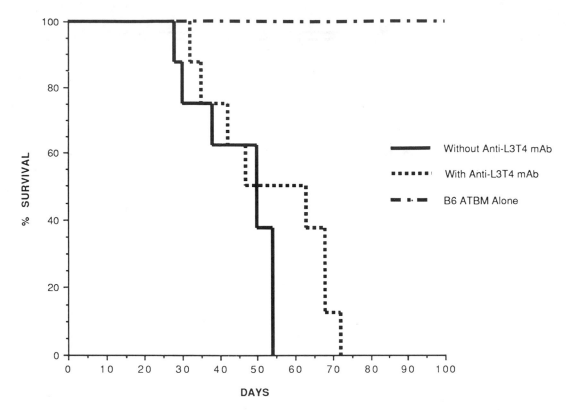

Figure 3 Effect of in vivo anti-L3T4 MAb treatments upon GVHD mortality across a class I H-2K difference. Irradiated (1000 rad) (B6 X bm1)F_1 mice were transplanted with B6 ATBM (2 X 10^6) along with 10^6 B6 Lyt-2$^+$ T cells. Recipient mice were then injected intraperitoneally with 0.2 ml undiluted anti-L3T4 MAb (GK1.5 ascites fluid) on days 1, 3, and 7 and then 0. 1 ml at weekly intervals thereafter.

city of donor L3T4$^+$ T cells to mediate an anti-class II GVHD. As shown in Figure 3, the course of anti-L3T4 MAb injections had little effect upon the GVHD potential of B6 Lyt-2$^+$ T cells in irradiated (B6xbm1)F_1 mice, suggesting that the early phase of GVHD reactivity was not dependent upon exogenous IL-2 from residual host L3T4$^+$ T cells. Since anti-L3T4 MAb injections were administered for up to 6 weeks after transplant, a mandatory role for newly derived donor-type L3T4$^+$ T cells from the thymus would also appear unlikely. To further substantiate this argument, anti-class I GVHD was assessed in thymectomized (Tx) irradiated (B6xbm1)F_1 recipients. As shown in Figure 4, the relative GVHD potential of donor B6 Lyt-2$^+$ T cells was not significantly different in recipients which were thymectomized versus those that were sham thymectomized (STx).

It thus appears that donor B6 Lyt-2$^+$ T cells, or at least a subpopulation of these cells, do indeed function in vivo without exogenous sources of IL-2, either from residual host cells or from de novo generated donor-derived L3T4$^+$ T cells. Is the reverse situation true, i.e., does an exogenous source of IL-2 enhance GVHD development? Two ap-

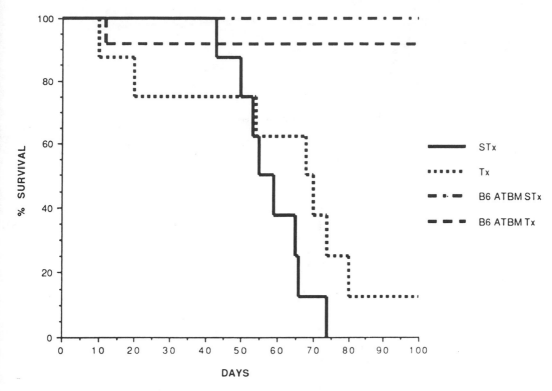

Figure 4 Effect of thymectomy upon GVHD mortality across a class I H-2K difference. Irradiated (1000 rad) (B6 × bm1)F_1 mice were transplanted after B6 ATBM (2 × 10^6) along with 5 × 10^6 B6 Lyt-2$^+$ T cells. Recipient mice were used at 4-8 weeks after thymectomy (Tx) or sham thymectomy (STx).

Table 2 Effect of Exogenous Sources of IL-2 on Anti-Class I GVHD

Dose of B6 Lyt-2$^+$ T cells	In vivo injection	Dose of B6 L3T4$^+$ T cells	Mortality	
			% Dead	MST (days)
2 × 10^6	mock IL-2	—	100	49
	rIL-2	—	100	29
ATBM alone	rIL-2	—	10	>100
5 × 10^6	—	—	100	50
	—	1 × 10^6	100	17
	—	2 × 10^5	100	16
2 × 10^6	—	—	100	37
	—	1 × 10^6	100	33

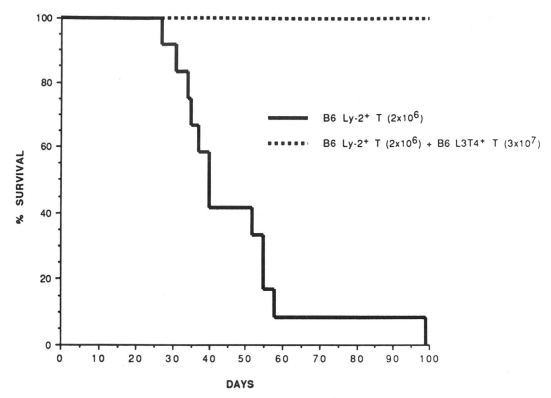

Figure 5 Protective effect of high dose donor L3T4$^+$ cells in GVHD across a class I H-2K difference. Irradiated (1000 rad) (B6 × bm1)F$_1$ mice were transplanted with B6 ATBM (2 × 10^6) along with either 2 × 10^6 B6 Lyt-2$^+$ T cells, alone, or with 3 × 10^7 B6 L3T4$^+$ T cells.

proaches were used to address this question. First we injected irradiated (B6xbm1)F$_1$ mice with a dose of 2 × 10^6 B6 Lyt-2$^+$ T cells followed by multiple i.p. injections of large doses of rIL-2 (6 × 1000 U/injection, 2 days apart, beginning on day 8 postirradiation). As shown in Table 2, this treatement significantly lowered the MST compared to control mice given mock rIL-2. The second approach was to inject irradiated (B6xbm1)F$_1$ mice with B6 Lyt-2$^+$ T cells together with a small dose (<10^6) of B6 L3T4$^+$ T cells. With high doses (5 × 10^6) of Lyt-2$^+$ cells, the addition of small doses of L3T4$^+$ cells considerably accelerated the onset of GVHD. Collectively, these findings suggest that although Lyt-2$^+$ cells can function in the absence of L3T4$^+$ cells, the presence of these cells or their products (IL-2) can potentiate the function of Lyt-2$^+$ cells.

An interesting, and rather unexpected, result occurs when high dosages of donor B6 L3T4$^+$ T cells (3 × 10^7) are added to the Lyt-2$^+$ T cell plus donor ATBM inoculum. As shown in Figure 5, heavily irradiated (B6xbm1)F$_1$ recipients of this cell combination exhibited no mortality and except for weight loss in the first 2 weeks had no other visible symptoms of an ongoing GVHD. A similar finding occurred following transfer of high doses of unseparated donor B6 spleen cells (0.8-1.0 × 10^8) into either irradiated (B6xbm1)F$_1$ or homozygous bm1 mice. In these situations, the recipients often become

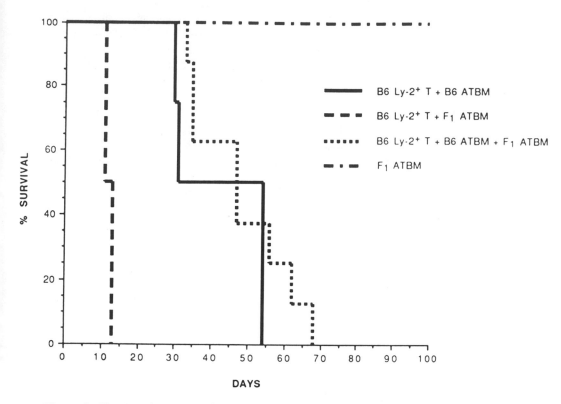

Figure 6 Varying the source of bone marrow in anti-class I GVHD. Irradiated (1000 rad) (B6 × bm1)F_1 mice were transplanted with 10^6 B6 Lyt-2$^+$ T cells along with 2 × 10^6 of either B6, F_1 host, or a mixture of both types of ATBM.

quite ill and express symptoms of GVHD, but then recover without fatality. One explanation for this phenomenon is that the "protective" effect afforded by L3T4$^+$ T cells reflects T helper function, which counters the often fatal bacteremia that accompanies GVHD. This idea is consistent with the evidence that germ-free mice are comparatively resistant to lethal GVHD (30). The possibility that L3T4$^+$ T cells act by suppressing anti-class I responses of the donor Lyt-2$^+$ T cells is unlikely because sublethal symptoms of GVHD are apparent, at least transiently, and preliminary histological analysis suggests the presence of typical GVHD lesions in the recipients.

The pattern of chronic lethal GVHD caused by Lyt-2$^+$ cells is seen with both high (1000 rad) and low (600 rad) irradiation of the host and with a wide dose range of Lyt-2$^+$ cells (2.5×10^5 to 5×10^6) (29). These findings apply with donor ATBM. With host-type ATBM, very rapid mortality occurs. This is illustrated by the experiments shown in Figure 6. It can be seen that transfer of 10^6 B6 Lyt-2$^+$ T cells with B6 ATBM to irradiated (B6xbm1)F_1 mice led to 100% fatality with an MST of 43 days. Substituting the recipient F_1 ATBM for donor type marrow resulted in an acute form of GVHD with an MST of 12 days. At the time of death, the mice exhibited extensive tissue pallor and the spleens were markedly atrophied, indicative of hematopoietic failure. Combining both donor and recipient ATBM in the transplant inoculum gave a survival pattern similar to the group given just donor ATBM. This finding suggests that B6 Lyt-2$^+$ T cells attack the F_1 marrow cells directly rather than by means of a bystander effect, e.g., the release of inhibitory or cytotoxic lymphokines. Further support for the ability of donor Lyt-2$^+$ T cells to destroy host-type hematopoietic cells came from experiments in which B6 Lyt-2$^+$ T cells were transplanted to lightly irradiated (500 rad) (B6xbm1)F_1 mice. When 2 X 10^6 B6 Lyt-2$^+$ cells were cotransferred with donor ATBM, the recipients all died with an MST of 32 days. In contrast, when the B6 Lyt-2$^+$ T cells were injected without added bone marrow cells, the recipients succumbed to rapid fatality (MST of 15 days) from apparent hematopoietic failure. Thus, at least in the B6 → bm1 combination, the form of GVHD observed depends largely upon whether the hosts receive donor marrow cells. These cells counteract the early loss of residual host hematopoietic cells destroyed by the donor Lyt-2$^+$ T cells. The recipients are thus able to survive for several weeks before succumbing to typical GVHD-associated complications.

C. Class II H-2 Differences

The transfer of purified donor B6 L3T4$^+$ T cells to irradiated class II (I-A)-different (B6xbm12)F_1 mice leads to fatal GVHD directed to the class II antigens of the host (27).

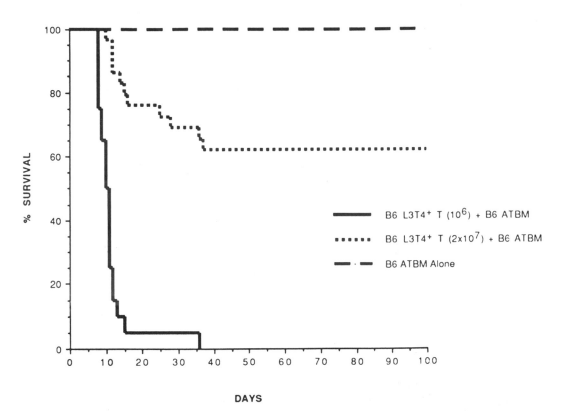

DAYS

Figure 7 GVHD mortality across a class II difference. Irradiated (1000 rad) (B6 X bm12)F_1 mice were transplanted with B6 ATBM (2 X 10^6) along with either a low dose (10^6) or high dose (2 X 10^7) of B6 L3T4$^+$ T cells.

The anti-class II GVHD mediated by L3T4$^+$ T cells supplemented with donor ATBM has the following features. First, with recipient mice exposed to heavy irradiation (1000 rad), low dosages of donor B6 L3T4$^+$ T cells, e.g., 10^5 cells, induce a severe acute form of lethal GVHD with an MST of < 21 days (Fig. 7). Lower dosages of L3T4$^+$ cells commonly lead to the development of a more chronic type of GVHD with a lower mortality rate. On the other hand, as the dosage of L3T4$^+$ T cells is increased, e.g., to 2 × 10^7 cells, an appreciable number of recipient mice survive with no obvious symptoms of on-going GVHD. This effect may be similar to the protection seen when high dosages of L3T4$^+$ T cells are transferred with Lyt-2$^+$ cells to class I-different hosts. With class II-different hosts, however, L3T4$^+$ T cells are potent mediators of GVHD. Even so it seems possible that L3T4$^+$ cells in large doses provide sufficient T helper function to tip the balance towards "protection" against opportunistic bacteriemia and allow survival. The protective effect of L3T4$^+$ cells can also be observed with transfer of high dosages (10^8 cells) of unseparated B6 spleen cells, whereas lethal GVHD is observed at lower dosages. It should be noted that the protective effects of high doses of L3T4$^+$ T cells may depend upon environmental factors and/or the extent of target antigen expression.

A second distinguishing feature of anti-class II GVHD is that, in contrast to anti-class I GVHD, hosts given intermediate doses of irradiation (e.g., 700-800 rad) plus donor marrow, show quite limited mortality, irrespective of the donor L3T4$^+$ T cell dosage utilized. This finding only applies to the transfer of L3T4$^+$ T cells with donor-type marrow cells. With transfer of host-type marrow, severe acute lethal GVHD can be induced in recipients given even quite low doses of irradiation (600 rad). This form of GVHD presumably reflects hematopoietic failure as the result of donor L3T4$^+$ cells attacking the host stem cells. This acute lethal GVHD fails to occur when the donor L3T4$^+$ cells are transferred with a mixture of donor and host marrow.

IV. GVHD DIRECTED TO NON-H-2 DIFFERENCES

Early studies with depletion of T cells from donor marrow inoculum by anti-Thy 1 plus complement pretreatment supported the role of T cells in development of GVHD directed to multiple minor histocompatibility antigens (minor HA) (8,31). In some strain combinations, such as in B10.BR ↔ CBA mice, the transfer of low dosages of T cells (e.g., 10^4 cells) can lead to high mortality associated with a chronic form of GVHD. Increasing the dosage of T cells added to donor ATBM results in a shortened MST and a more acute severe form of disease (8). Initial observations with a single strain combination (B10.BR → CBA) and with donor T-cell subsets prepared by negative selection (MAb plus C treatment) indicated that Lyt-2$^+$ T cells were responsible for GVHD directed to minor HA; L3T4$^+$ T cells did not seem to play a detectable role, either as effector cells or helper cells (31). We have recently reinvestigated this question using six different minor HA combinations and employing highly purified T-cell subsets (32). As summarized in Table 3, the combined results indicated that: (1) in every strain combination expressing multiple minor HA differences, donor Lyt-2$^+$ T cells were capable of mediating lethal GVHD, though with variable potency; (2) in four of the strain combinations (C3H.SW → B6, B10.BR → CBA, DBA/2 → B10.D2, and B10.S → SJL) Lyt-2$^+$ T cells appeared to be the only mediators of GVHD, transfer of L3T4$^+$ T cells caused no mortality or any of the typical clinical symptoms of GVHD; and (3) in two strain combinations (B10.D2 → BALB/c and B10.D2 → DBA/2), it is of interest that donor L3T4$^+$ T cells were able to

Table 3 Summary of GVHD in H-2-Compatible, Minor HA-Different Strain Combinations

Donor → Recipient (Irradiation [rads]) (H-2 haplotype)	80-d mortality [% dead (MST)] with donor cells			
	Whole T	L3T4$^+$ T	Lyt-2$^+$ T	ATBM alone
C3H.SW → B6 (750) H-2^b	48% (58d)	5% (>80d)	77% (45d)	0% (>80d)
B10.BR → CBA (750) H-2^k	96% (38d)	35% (73d)	96% (39d)	8% (>80d)
DBA/2 → B10.D2 (820) H-2^d	26% (>80d)	11% (>80d)	73% (53d)	8% (>80d)
B10.S → SJL (800) H-2^s	88% (34d)	13% (>80d)	88% (35d)	0% (>80d)
B10.D2 → BALB/c (750) H-2^d	93% (20d)	78% (24d)	75% (39d)	0% (>80d)
B10.D2 → DBA/2 (800) H-2^d	92% (38d)	85% (45d)	42% (58d)	8% (>80d)

cause a high incidence of GVHD, the potency of these cells being greater than that of Lyt-2$^+$ T cells. These observations raise several interesting questions.

First, does the inability of donor L3T4$^+$ T cells to mediate GVHD in the majority of minor HA-different strain combinations simply reflect a low frequency of minor HA-specific L3T4$^+$ T cells in the (unprimed) donor inoculum? To address this possibility, donor C3H.SW mice were presensitized to recipient B6 antigens by intraperitoneal injection of 2 × 10^7 B6 splenocytes 3 weeks before their use in the GVHD assay. Cell subsets purified from these donor mice exhibited increased GVHD potential for both the unseparated T and Lyt-2$^+$ T-cell groups, but there was no increased activity in the L3T4$^+$ T cell group in comparison to that found with unprimed cells (32).

Second, although L3T4$^+$ T cells did not lead to fatal GVHD in most strain combinations, subclinical signs of disease might be evident at the histopathological level. Sequential histological analysis following transplantaton was performed on the C3H.SW → B6 combination and revealed typical patterns of developing GVHD lesions in the spleen, gut, liver, and lymph nodes of mice receiving either donor whole T or Lyt-2$^+$ T cells. However those mice given purified donor L3T4$^+$ T cells did not exhibit any histological expression of GVHD in any target organ and appeared identical to the ATBM control group. This lack of response by L3T4$^+$ T cells was true for all timepoints from day 3 up to one year after initial injection.

Third, can in vitro assays predict whether L3T4$^+$ T cells induce GVHD across minor HA barriers? Thus far, our results on this question have been negative. For example, the ability of either unprimed or presensitized donor L3T4$^+$ T cells to proliferate in response to stimulation by antigen-presenting cells of the recipient strain in culture does not predict their behavior in vivo. Thus unprimed B10.D2 L3T4$^+$ T cells do not respond at all to stimulation by BALB/c irradiated spleenocytes in vitro, but are very potent in mediating GVHD; conversely, B10.BR L3T4$^+$ T cells respond very strongly to CBA stimulators (largely because of the MIs difference) in culture, but fail to induce GVHD (32). Likewise, we have found no correlation between GVHD induction and the ability of L3T4$^+$ plus IL-2 to generate cytotoxic T cells specific for minor HA in vitro

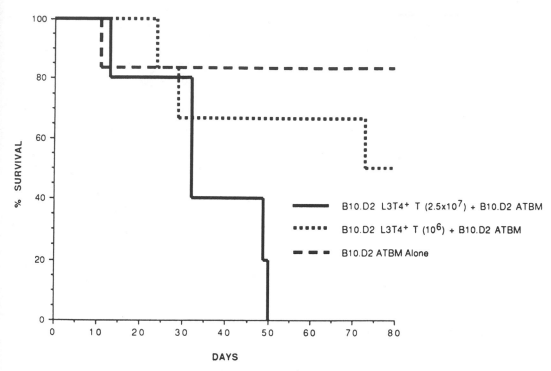

Figure 8 Effect of high dosages of donor L3T4$^+$ T cells upon GVHD mortality across a B10.D2 → DBA/2 multiple minor histocompatibility antigen difference. Irradiated (800 rad) DBA/2 mice were transplanted with 4 × 10^6 B10.D2 ATBM along with B10.D2 L3T4$^+$ T cells.

(33). The role of the Th1 and Th2 L3T4$^+$ T-cell subsets in relation to anti-minor HA GVHD has yet to be investigated, but is hampered by the lack of reliable markers for these cells (24). At present, the explanation for the marked strain variability seen in the capacity of L3T4$^+$ cells to mediate GVHD to minor HA is obscure.

It is worth mentioning that, in apparent contrast with GVHD directed to H-2 differences, we have thus far seen no evidence that large doses of L3T4$^+$ T cells protect mice against GVHD to minor HA. In fact in the B10.D2 → DBA/2 combination large doses of L3T4$^+$ T cells cause greater mortality than small doses (Fig. 8). The significance of this finding is unclear.

As for anti-class I GVHD, the capacity of purified Lyt-2$^+$ T cells to mediate GVHD to minor HA does not seem to depend on helper function from radio-resistant host L3T4$^+$ T cells. As shown in Figure 9, the MST observed when B10.BR Lyt-2$^+$ T cells are transferred to irradiated (750 rad) CBA recipients, plus donor ATBM is not significantly altered when anti-L3T4 MAb is administered at the time of transplant. It thus appears that purified Lyt-2$^+$ T cells can mediate anti-minor HA GVHD independent of exogenous help. This finding is consistent with previous reports of in vitro responses to minor HA where some cytolytic clones were able to provide their own IL-2 (34). It also fits with observations on the phenotype of the cells required for the generation of CTLs in vitro

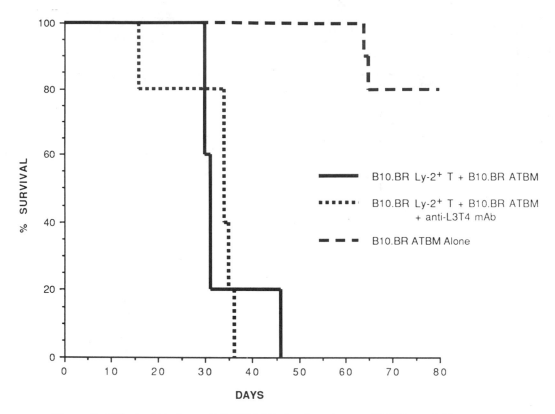

Figure 9   Effect of in vivo anti-L3T4 MAb treatment upon GVHD mortality across a B10.BR → CBA multiple minor histocompatibility antigen difference. Irradiated (750 rad) (CBA) mice were transplanted with 4×10^6 B10.BR ATBM along with 2×10^6 B6 Lyt-2^+ T cells. Recipient mice were injected intraperitoneally with 25 μl undiluted anti-L3T4 MAb (GK1.5 ascites fluid) 6 hr before transplant.

directed against single minor HA specificities (35). We have recently reexamined the question of the requirement for "helper" T cells for in vitro CTL development using either single or multiple minor HA differences (R. Korngold and P. Wettstein, unpublished data). The data indicates that Lyt-2^+ T cells from B6 mice presensitized in vivo to either H-3, H-4, or H-Y antigens are fully capable of generating CTL activity after secondary stimulation in vitro, in the absence of presensitized B6 L3T4$^+$ T cells. In marked contrast, B6 Lyt-2^+ CTL responses to multiple minor HA-different BALB.B cells are highly dependent upon the presence of presensitized B6 L3T4$^+$ T cells in the restimulated culture. A possible explanation of this data is that, during the phase of presensitization to minor HA in vivo, Lyt-2^+ CTL precursors at the population level may be selected for dependence upon the exogenous "help" of L3T4$^+$ T cells. This dependence is more likely to be generated in the multiple minor HA situation since there is a higher probability that L3T4$^+$ T cells would also be stimulated, thereby providing suffi-cent quantities of IL-2. In the case of a single minor H antigen, immunodominance ef-fects (36) may limit stimulation to only Lyt-2^+ CTL precursors, and thus favor selection of helper-independent cells, i.e., those Lyt-2^+ cells which can produce their own IL-2.

A similar phenomenon may account for the ability of unprimed purified donor Lyt-2$^+$ T cells to mediate anti-multiple minor HA GVHD, in the presumed absence of exogenous sources of IL-2. The environmental conditions in the host may selectively direct these cells towards "helper" independence. Further analyses of these responses are currently in progress as well as investigation into whether the phenomenon of immunodominance has any physiological relevance for GVHD responses to minor H antigens.

V. DISCUSSION

The combined data on the role of T-cell subsets in lethal murine GVHD are summarized in Table 4. For H-2-compatible strain combinations disparate for multiple minor HA, Lyt-2$^+$ T cells regularly cause lethal GVHD, whereas L3T4$^+$ T cells are only active in a minority of situations. Lyt-2$^+$ T cells are the sole mdiators of anti-class I GVHD, whereas L3T4$^+$ T cells control anti-class II GVHD. In combinations exhibiting a full mismatch at the H-2 complex, isolated populations of Lyt-2$^+$ and L3T4$^+$ T cells are each capable of causing lethal GVHD, the relative potency of each subset depending upon the particular H-2 differences involved.

Since Lyt-2$^+$ and L3T4$^+$ T cell subsets tend to express different functions, i.e., cell-mediated lympholysis and lymphokine production, respectively, one might expect the pattern of GVHD mediated by each subset to be different. However, it should be emphasized that, at the population level, both T-cell subsets show functional overlap. Thus, some L3T4$^+$ cells exhibit cytolytic activity (33), while Lyt-2$^+$ T cell clones are capable of releasing various lymphokines, including IL-2 and IFN-γ (34,37) and can also mediate DTH responses (38). It should also be borne in mind that the primary target organs for GVHD, such as the spleen, lymph nodes, liver, and gut, express both class I and class II antigens and hence provide targets for the T-cell subsets. Although the tissue distribution of class II molecules is normally limited to only a few cell types, e.g., macrophages, B cells, and dendritic cells, local production of IFN-γ could cause induction or upregulation of class II expression on many other cell types (39). Preliminary histopathology analysis of H-2 mutant mice with anti-class I and anti-class II GVHD suggests that Lyt-2$^+$ and L3T4$^+$ cells do cause the development of quite similar, though not identical, lesions in the gut tissue (A. Mowat, R. Cheney, R. Korngold, and J. Sprent, unpublished data). Whether the same applies for GVHD across multiple minor HA barriers is currently under investigation.

Under certain conditions, especially in H-2 mutant mice, L3T4$^+$ and Lyt-2$^+$ cells elicit quite different patterns of GVHD. Lyt-2$^+$ T cells are very potent mediators of

Table 4 Summary of the Role of T-Cell Subsets in GVHD

Genetic difference between donor and recipient	T-cell subset involved
Non-H-2 (Minor HA)	Lyt-2$^+$ T cells in *all* cases L3T4$^+$ T cells in *some* cases
Class I	Lyt-2$^+$ T cells
Class II	L3T4$^+$ T cells
Full H-2	L3T4$^+$ and/or Lyt-2$^+$ T cells

lethal GVHD in class I-different mice (B6 → bm1), and severe mortality applies even with light irradiation of the host (500 rad) and with transfer of quite small doses of Lyt-2$^+$ T cells (10^5/mouse). Although mortality rates approach 100%, recipients of Lyt-2$^+$ cells tend to die only after a period of several weeks. With L3T4$^+$ T cells, by contrast, GVHD leads to rapid death, many of the recipients dying within 2 weeks. Interestingly, this pattern of acute lethal GVHD seen in class II-different recipients of L3T4$^+$ cells (B6 → bm12) is seen only with relatively high doses of irradiation, i.e., >800 rad. With lower doses of irradiation, only mild GVHD results and mortality rates are low. These findings apply to the transfer of donor L3T4$^+$ of Lyt-2$^+$ cells plus either *donor* ATBM or a mixture of donor plus host marrow, Lyt-2$^+$ cells (B6 → bm1) and L3T4$^+$ cells (B6 → bm12); both cause death from hematopoietic failure within 2–3 weeks, even in lightly irradiated mice. These findings suggest that Lyt-2$^+$ T cells and L3T4$^+$ T cells are each capable of direct cytolytic attack against host lymphohematopoietic cells. CTL attack appears to be antigen-specific because hematopoietic failure is not observed in recipients given a mixture of donor plus host marrow.

The relevance of these findings in mice to the present clinical situation for BM transplantation is still unclear. As mentioned earlier, patients transplanted with HLA-compatible bone marrow depleted of T cells have a dramatic reduction in the incidence of GVHD, but exhibit a significant increase in failure of engraftment and relapse of leukemia (11,15-17). The simplest explanation for these findings is that the donor T cells mediating GVHD are able to attack the host cells, which contribute to graft rejection and also attack residual host leukemia cells. Since in the majority of multiple minor HA-different murine strain combinations assayed, L3T4$^+$ (CD4$^+$) cells do not mediate GVHD, one could make a case for selective depletion of CD8$^+$ cells from human marrow so that CD4$^+$ cells can facilitate engraftment and, in the case of leukemic patients, possibly mediate antileukemic activity. Another potential advantage of this approach is that leaving CD4$^+$ cells in the marrow suspension could provide an immediate source of immunocompetency, thereby enabling the recipient to counteract the threat of opportunistic infectious agents. As suggested from results for anti-class I GVHD in mice (see Fig. 5), the presence of donor CD4$^+$ cells in substantial numbers can protect the hosts against lethal GVHD mediated by CD8$^+$ cells (although such protection has yet to be shown for MHC-compatible strain combinations). The major problem, however, is that very little is known about minor H antigens in man and hence it is difficult to assess whether, in a given clinical situation, CD4$^+$ cells will act as effector cells for GVHD. Nevertheless, preliminary data from a small nonrandomized clinical trial for the selective depletion of CD8$^+$ cells from marrow inoculum has indicated only minimal problems with GVHD in the transplanted patients (R. Champlin, personal communication; 40). Unfortunately, the complications of graft failure and leukemic relapse in this study were still quite evident. Larger randomized trials are needed to clarify these issues. Eventually, it might be feasible to supplement the marrow inoculum with additional donor CD4$^+$ T cells (derived from donor PBL, for example), which might also be manipulated in vitro to improve their responsiveness (e.g., presensitizing the cells to the leukemia cells of the host). We stress, however, that the protective effect of CD4$^+$ cells in mice is by no means an invariable finding. Hence, until the precise conditions for the protective effects of CD4$^+$ cells can be established, the clinical potential of this approach is difficult to assess.

Since the availablity of an HLA-matched sibling donor is often very limited, the option of performing marrow transplantation across partial HLA barriers will presumably receive increasing attention (12,17,41). Based on studies in mice, transplantation across a full HLA barrier would probably necessitate depletion of both $CD4^+$ and $CD8^+$ T-cell subsets from the marrow inoculum. However, this approach is likely to be complicated by the above mentioned problems of engraftment, leukemic relapse, and associated immunoincompetency. For donor/recipient patient combinations involving only a class I or class II difference, however, appropriate selective depletion of $CD8^+$ or $CD4^+$ cells, respectively, might avoid GVHD while reducing the other major risk factors of transplantation. Further experimental work on understanding the nature and involvement of T-cell subsets in GVHD and these other complications is obviously necessary.

ACKNOWLEDGMENT

This work was supported by U. S. Public Health Service Research Grants CA-38951 and CA-38355 from the National Cancer Institute.

REFERENCES

1. Gale RP, Champlin R, eds.: Bone Marrow Transplantation: Current Controversies. Alan R Liss Inc, New York, 1988.
2. Tyan ML: Modification of severe graft-versus-host disease with antisera to the theta antigen or to whole serum. Transplantation 1973;15:601.
3. Trentin JJ, Judd KP: Prevention of acute graft-versus-host (GVH) mortality with spleen-absorbed antithymocyte globulin (ATG). Transplant Proc 1973;5:865.
4. Rodt H, Thierfelder S, Eulitz E: Anti-lymphocytic antibodies and marrow transplantation: III. Effect of heterologous anti-brain antibodies on acute secondary disease of mice. Eur J Immunol 1974;4:25.
5. Muller-Ruchholtz W, Wottge H-U, Muller-Hermelink HK: Bone marrow transplantation in rats across strong histocompatibility barriers by selective elimination of lymphoid cells in donor marrow. Transplant Proc 1976;8:357.
6. Onoe K, Fernandes G, Good RA: Humor and cell-mediated immune responses in fully allogenic bone marrow chimera in mice. J Exp Med 1980;151:115.
7. Vallera DA, Soderling CCB, Carlson GJ, Kersey JH: Bone marrow transplantation across major histocompatibility barriers in mice. Transplantation 1981;31:218.
8. Korngold R, Sprent J: Lethal graft versus-host-disease following bone marrow transplantation across minor histocompatibility barriers in mice: Prevention by removing mature T cells from marrow. J Exp Med 1978;148:1687.
9. Hamilton BL, Bevan MJ, Parkman R: Antirecipient cytotoxic T lymphocyte precursors are present in the spleens of mice with acute graft-versus-host disease due to minor histocompatibility antigens. J Immunol 1981;126:621.
10. OKunewick JP, Meredith RF, Raikow RB, Buffo MJ, Jones DL: Possibility of three distinct and separable components to fatal graft-versus-host reaction. Exp Hematol 1982;10:277.
11. Franceschini F, Butturini A, Gale RP: In: Progress in Bone Marrow Transplantation. Gale RP, Champlin R, eds. Alan R Liss Inc, New York, 1987, p. 323.
12. Henslee PJ, Thompson JS, Romond EH, et al. T cell depletion of HLA and haploidentical marrow reduces graft-versus-host disease but it may impair a graft-versus-leukemia effect. Transplant Proc 1987;19:2701.
13. Filipovitch AH, Vallera DA, Youle RJ, et al.: Ex vivo T cell depletion with immunotoxins in allogenic bone marrow transplantation: The pilot clinical study for prevention of graft-versus-host disease. Transplant Proc 1985;17:442.
14. O'Reilly RJ, Collins NH, Kernan N, et al.: Transplantation of marrow-depleted T cells by soybean lectin agglutination and E-rosette depletion: Major histocompati-

bility complex-related graft resistance in leukemic transplant recipients. Transplant Proc 1985;17:455.

15. Gale RP, Reisner Y: Graft rejection and graft-versus-host disease: mirror images. Lancet 1986;2:1468.

16. Gale RP, Champlin RE: How does bone-marrow transplantation cure leukemia? Lancet 1984;2:28.

17. Storb R: Critical issues in bone marrow transplantation. Transplant Proc 1987; 19:2774.

18. Blazar BR, Widmer MB, Soderling CCB, et al.: Augmentation of donor bone marrow engraftment in histoincompatible murine recipients by granulocyte/macrophage colony-stimulating factor. Blood 1988;71:320.

19. Truitt RL, Shih C-Y, Kaehler DA, et al.: Graft-versus-leukemia and graft-versus-host reactivity following alloimmunization of MHC-compatible donor mice. In: Recent Advances in Bone Marrow Transplantation. Gale RP, ed. Alan R Liss Inc, New York, 1983; p. 243.

20. Weiner RS, Dicke KA: Risk factors for interstitial pneumonitis following allogenic bone marrow transplantation for severe aplastic anemia: a preliminary report. Transplant Proc 1987;19:2639.

21. Korngold R, Sprent J: T cell subsets and graft-versus-host disease. Transplant 1987;44:335.

22. Sprent J, Webb S: Function and specificity of T cell subsets in the mouse. Adv Immunol 1987;41:39.

23. Dialynas DP, Wilde DB, Marrack P, et al.: Characterization of the murine antigenic determinant designated L3T4a, recognized by monoclonal antibody GK1.5: expression of L3T4a by functional T cell clones appears to correlate primarily with class II MHC antigen-reactivity. Immunol Rev 1983;74:29.

24. Kurt-Jones EA, Hamberg S, Ohara J, Paul WE, Abbas AK: Heterogeneity of helper/inducer T lymphocytes. I. Lymphokine production and lymphokine responsiveness. J Exp Med 1987;166:1774.

25. Vallera DA, Soderling CCB, Kersey JH: Bone marrow transplantation across major histocompatibility barriers in mice: III. Treatment of donor grafts with monoclonal antibodies directed against Lyt determinants. J Immunol 1982;128:871.

26. Korngold R, Sprent J: Surface markers of T cells causing lethal graft-versus-host disease to class I versus class II H-2 differences. J Immunol 1985;135:3004.

27. Sprent J, Schaeffer M, Lo D, Korngold R: Properties of purified T cell subsets. II. In vivo responses to class I vs. class II H-2 differences. J Exp Med 1986;163: 998.

28. Korngold R, Sprent J: Purified T cell subsets and lethal graft-versus-host disease in mice. In: Progress in Bone Marrow Transplantation, edited by Gale RP, Champlin R. Alan R Liss Inc, New York, 1987; p. 215.

29. Sprent J, Schaeffer M, Gao E-K, Korngold R: Role of T cell subsets in lethal graft-versus-host disease (GVHD) directed to class I versus class II H-2 differences. I. L3T4[+] cells can either augment or retard GVHD elicited by Lyt-2[+] cells in class I-different hosts. J Exp Med 1988;167:556.

30. Pollard M, Chang LF, Srivastava KK: The role of microflora in development of graft-versus-host disease. Transplant Proc 1976;8:533.

31. Korngold R, Sprent J: Features of T cells causing H-2 restricted lethal graft-vs-host disease across minor histocompatibility barriers. J Exp Med 1982;155:872.

32. Korngold R, Sprent J: Variable capacity of L3T4[+] T cells to cause lethal graft-versus-host disease across minor histocompatibility barriers in mice. J Exp Med 1987;165:1552.

33. Golding H, Munitz TI, Singer A: Characterization of antigen-specific, Ia-restricted

L3T4$^+$ cytolytic T lymphocytes and assessment of thymic influence on their self specificity. J Exp Med 1985;162:943.

34. Roopenian DC, Widmer MC, Orosz GG, Bach FH: Helper cell-independent cytolytic T lymphocytes specific for a minor histocompatibility antigen. J Immunol 1983;130:542.

35. Wettstein P, Frelinger J: T lymphocyte responses to non-H-2 histocompatibility antigens. I. Role of Ly-1$^+$2$^+$ T cells as cytotoxic effectors and requirement for Ly-1$^+$2$^+$ T cells for optimal generation of cytotoxic effectors. J Immunol 1981; 127:43.

36. Wettstein PJ, Bailey DW: Immunodominance in the immune response to "multiple" histocompatibility antigens. Immunogenetics 1982;16:47.

37. Von Boehmer H, Turton K: Autonomous proliferating K/D restricted cytolytic T cell clones. Eur J Immunol 1983;13:176.

38. Von Boehmer H, Kisielow P, Weiserson W, Haas W: Lyt-2$^-$ T cell-independent functions of Lyt-2$^+$ cells stimulated with antigen or concavalin A. J Immunol 1984;133:59.

39. Skoskiewicz MJ, Colvin RB, Scheeberger EE, et al.: Widespread and selective induction of major histocompatibility complex-determined antigens in vivo by gamma interferon. J Exp Med 1985;162:1645.

40. Champlin R, Gajewski J, Feig S, et al.: Selective depletion of CD8 positive T-lymphocytes for prevention of graft-versus-host disease following allogeneic bone marrow transplantation. Transplant Proc 1989;21:2947.

41. Beatty PG, Clift RA, Mickelson EM, et al.: Marrow transplantation from related donors other than HLA-identical siblings. N Engl J Med 1985;313:765.

3

Clonal Analysis of Graft-vs.-Host Disease

Robertson Parkman
University of Southern California School of Medicine and
Childrens Hospital of Los Angeles
Los Angeles, California

I. INTRODUCTION

The two principal reasons for research into Graft-vs.-Host Disease (GVHD) is that, first, GVHD remains a major problem in human bone marrow transplantation and, second, GVHD is a unique model in which to study the regulation of the immune system. Depending upon the scientific questions to be asked, various models of GVHD have been studied. The parent-F_1 model may be most appropriate when studying cellular interactions, the effect of GVHD on thymic maturation, the production of auto-antibodies and other questions in which the investigator does not wish to cytoreduce or alter the recipient by the use of irradiation or chemotherapy. If, on the other hand, questions related to human GVHD and its clinical complications are addressed, then models in which the donor-recipient pairs are histocompatible, the recipients are cytoreduced prior to transplantation, and both clinically detectable acute and chronic GVHD occur, are most appropriate.

Many of the disagreements that occur in discussions concerning GVHD are due to the fact that the different models may involve different effector mechanisms. The present discussion will center on a murine model of histocompatible GVHD that is as analogous as possible to human histocompatible bone marrow transplantation. The donor and recipient combination is identical at both class I and class II histocompatibility antigens, differs at minor histocompatibility antigens, is irradiated prior to transplantation, and develops both clinically detectable acute and chronic GVHD (1).

We have evaluated the cellular and cytokine mechanisms involved in this model of histocompatible murine GVHD by the development of T-lymphocyte clones from the recipients. The T-lymphocyte clones have allowed a more complete determination of the mechanisms involved in GVHD. The results demonstrate that the pathogenesis of acute and chronic GVHD differ significantly and that both cellular and cytokine mechanisms are involved in both acute and chronic GVHD. In addition, the clonal analysis of GVHD has revealed that both recipient-restricted and auto-antigens (histocompatibility antigens shared by the donor-recipient) play a role in GVHD.

II. THE MURINE MODEL

The basic model used for these studies is the transplantation of C57Bl/6 (B6) recipient mice with histocompatible LP bone marrow and spleen cells. The mice are $H-2^b$, $I-A^b$, and M1s identical and are mutually nonstimulatory in mixed lymphocyte culture. Lethally irradiated (950-1050 R) recipient animals can be hematopoietically reconstituted with as few as 5×10^6 anti-Thy 1.2-treated LP spleen cells. The development of GVHD is dependent upon the transplantation of donor (LP) T lymphocytes in addition to hematopoietic stem cells (2). The incidence and characteristics of GVHD are dependent upon the number of T lymphocytes transplanted. The transplantation of less than 5×10^6 LP spleen cells results in no significant GVHD. The transplantation of 20×10^6 LP spleen cells results in the development of both acute and chronic GVHD. Clinically acute GVHD is characterized by a hunched back appearance and anasarca; most affected animals die. Animals that do not die by day 30 from acute GVHD are at risk of developing chronic GVHD, which is characterized by alopecia, dermal fibrosis, and wasting (Table 1). If 50×10^6 LP spleen cells are transplanted, then 80-90% of animals developed fatal acute GVHD. Thus, the LP-B6 model, like human histocompatible GVHD, can present as two discrete clinical syndromes, acute and chronic GVHD. The LP-B6 model, therefore, differs from other models like the C3H-CBA model, in which the animals do not develop the clinical and pathological findings of chronic GVHD (3).

III. ESTABLISHMENT OF T-LYMPHOCYTE CLONES

T-lymphocyte clones were established from animals with acute GVHD (14-19 days following transplantation) and clinically detectable chronic GVHD (50 days) following transplantation. Routinely, the recipient's spleen cells were stimulated with irradiated (5000R) recipient B6 spleen cells in mixed lymphocyte culture without exogenous IL-2. After one week, the viable lymphoblasts were isolated and cloned by limiting dilution with irradiated B6 stimulators and exogenous IL-2. The resultant clones were individually expanded and characterized for (1) their antigenic specificity, (2) their phenotype, (3) their cytokine dependency, (4) their cytotoxic capacity, (5) their ability to stimulate collagen synthesis, and (6) their cytokine production. The characterization of the clones has permitted us to characterize the subpopulations of clonagenic T lymphocytes present in animals with GVHD and has allowed us to determine some of the cellular interactions involved in GVHD. In some experiments to determine potential cellular interactions in GVHD, LP spleen cells were treated in vitro with monoclonal antibodies to CD4 (anti-L3T4) or CD8 (anti-Lyt 2) and complement prior to transplan-

Table 1   Comparison of GVHD in Human BMT Recipients and Murine Model (LP → B6)

	Class I	Class II	MLC	Acute GVHD	Chronic GVHD
Human	Identical	Identical	Nonreactive	+	+
Murine	Identical	Identical	Nonreactive	+	+

tation. The terminology used in the studies is the following: Clones derived from animals with acute GVHD are termed G clones; clones derived from animals receiving Lyt-2-depleted spleen cells are L2 clones, clones derived from animals receiving L3T4-depleted spleen cells are L3 clones, and clones derived from animals with clinically detectable chronic GVHD are CG clones.

A. Antigenic Specificity

The antigenic specificity of G, CG, L2, and L3 clones was determined using both donor (LP) and recipient (B6) spleen cells as stimulator cells in the presence of exogenous IL-2 (Table 2). Of 31 G clones analyzed, 20 clones were specifically stimulated by recipient (B6) but not donor (LP) spleen cells (4). The remaining 11 clones were stimulated equally by LP and B6 spleen cells. Thus, the majority of the G clones were specific for recipient restricted minor histocompatibility antigens while the minority of G clones had specificity for histocompatability antigens shared by donor-recipient cells. When the CG clones from chronic GVHD mice were analyzed, they were all stimulated equally by donor and recipient spleen cells. No recipient-specific clones were identified.

To determine the minor histocompatibility antigens that stimulated the recipient-specific clones, clones were stimulated in vitro with B6 congenic mice. The recipient-specific clones were stimulated only by $H-2^v$ mice, and the stimulating minor antigens were D^b restricted (Table 3). Multiple patterns of stimulation were seen, suggesting that multiple D^b restricted minor histocompatibility antigens were involved.

When the G and CG clones, which were stimulated equally by donor-recipient spleen cells, were analyzed with the same recombinant mice, a different pattern was seen. The autoreactive clones were stimulated by all strains expressing $I-A^b$ (Table 4). Thus, T-lymphocyte clones derived from animals with acute GVHD consisted of T lymphocytes

Table 2 Histocompatibility Antigen Specificity of T-Lymphocyte Clones from Recipients with Acute and Chronic GVHD

| Clone | Medium | Stimulating Spleen Cells (CPM) | |
		Donor (LP)	Recipient (B6)
		ACUTE GVHD	
G-1	3,225	4,340	13,463
G-2	818	1,999	4,503
G-3	2,818	4,631	24,896
G-93	364	834	12,051
G-7	3,441	14,332	9,439
G-10	1,025	5,135	9,070
G-17	1,163	13,625	19,825
G-100	597	6,261	9,784
		CHRONIC GVHD	
CG-46	1,364	18,677	19,338
CG-47	1,757	11,870	10,265
CG-52	59	6,181	10,313

Clones stimulated for 3 days with irradiated spleen cells in the presence of exogenous IL-2.

Table 3 D^b Restriction of Recipient-Specific Acute GVHD Clones

		Stimulating Spleen Cells (CPM)				
Clone	Medium	LP *bbbb*	B6 *bbbb*	B10.A(2R) kkk*b*	B10.A(5R) *bb*kd	219 *bbbb*
G-6	508	1450	*21,252*	*11,951*	801	1711
G-9	675	2016	*39,645*	*9,596*	1289	2303
G-81	741	4557	*102,585*	*58,030*	6340	5335
G-93	604	1044	*5,097*	*3,213*	549	1218

Clones stimulated for 3 days with irradiated spleen cells in the presence of exogenous IL-2.

with specificity for multiple B6 restricted minor histocompatibility antigens and auto-reactive T lymphocytes with specificity for the shared class II histocompatibility antigen, I-A^b. The only clonagenic T lymphocytes (CG clones) identified in animals with clinically detectable chronic GVHD had specificity for the shared I-A^b. Thus, the only clonagenic T lymphocytes in mice with chronic GVHD were autoreactive T lymphocytes.

B. Cell-Mediated Lysis

It has been assumed that the major effector mechanism in GVHD is cytotoxic T lymphocytes (5). To determine whether the T lymphocyte clones derived from animals with acute and chronic GVHD were cytotoxic, the clones were assayed in a CML assay using Con A-stimulated donor and recipient lymphoblasts as target cells. Of six G clones with blastogenic specificity for B6 restricted minor histocompatibility antigens, five clones were specifically cytotoxic for B6 targets while one was noncytotoxic (Table 5). Of the autoreactive clones derived from animals with acute GVHD, all were noncytotoxic except one clone, which specifically lysed B6 target cells even though its blastogenic specificity was I-A^b. All of the autoreactive clones derived from animals with chronic GVHD were

Table 4 Ia Specificity of Autoreactive T-Lymphocyte Clones from Recipients with Acute and Chronic GVHD

		Stimulating spleen cells (CPM)					
Clone	Medium	LP *bbbb*	B6 *bbbb*	B10.A(2R) kkk*b*	B10.A(5R) *bb*kd	129 *bbbb*	B10.MBR *b*kkq
			Acute GVHD				
G-96	823	*8,687*	*5,622*	1,211	*5,123*	4,956	–
G-100	963	*13,047*	*13,148*	5,166	*15,387*	–	4658
G-102	10,535	*40,571*	*58,673*	18,987	*50,032*	–	–
			Chronic GVHD				
CG-46.2	463	*38,714*	*51,529*	2,021	*42,730*	–	1739
CG-52	321	*14,221*	*8,529*	337	*3,778*	*15,801*	–

Clones stimulated for 3 days with irradiated spleen cells in the presence of exogenous IL-2.

Table 5 Cell Mediated Lysis by GVHD T-Lymphocyte Clones

Clone	Blastogenic specificity	Target (% specific lysis)	
		Recipient (B6)	Donor (LP)
Acute GVHD			
G-1	B6 restricted minor	13.2	1.6
G-2	B6 restricted minor	−3.0	−17.0
G-3	B6 restricted minor	56.8	0.1
G-6	B6 restricted minor	29.0	−13.6
G-81	B6 restricted minor	57.1	−7.7
G-17	I-A	51.2	0.1
Chronic GVHD			
CG-46	I-A^b	0.0	3.5
CG-47	I-A^b	−6.1	−0.3
CG-51	I-A^b	−6.5	7.7

Specific lysis determined using ^{51}Cr-labeled Con A–stimulated spleen cells as target cells in a 4-hour assay.

noncytotoxic for both donor and recipient targets. Thus, cytotoxic cells with specificity for minor histocompatibility antigens uniquely expressed on recipient cells were found in animals with acute GVHD, while cytotoxic T lymphocytes were not identified in animals with chronic GVHD. The absence of cytotoxic T lymphocytes in mice with chronic GVHD is consistent with previous experiments using whole spleen cells (6).

C. Phenotypic Analysis

The phenotypic characteristics of acute and chronic GVHD T-lymphocyte clones were determined (Table 6). The cells, whose blastogenic specificity was for recipient-restricted

Table 6 Phenotype of Acute and Chronic GVHD T-Lymphocyte Clones

Blastogenic specificity	Frequency	Phenotype
ACUTE GVHD		
B6 restricted minor histocompatibility antigen	20/31	Thy 1.2$^+$, Lyt 2$^+$, L3T4$^-$
I-A^b	11/31	Thy 1.2$^+$, Lyt 2$^-$, L3T4$^+$
CHRONIC GVHD		
I-A^b	8/8	Thy 1.2$^+$, Lyt 2$^-$, L3T4$^+$

minor histocompatibility antigens, all displayed a Thy 1.2^+, Lyt 2^+, and L3T4$^-$ phenotype with variable expression of Lyt-1. The autoreactive T-lymphocyte clones, regardless of whether they were derived from animals with acute or chronic GVHD, expressed a Thy 1.2^+, Lyt-2$^-$, L3T4$^+$ phenotype. Thus, the majority of cells with specificity for recipient restricted minor histocompatibility antigens were classic cytotoxic T lymphocytes (CD8$^+$), while most of the helper (CD4$^+$) T lymphocytes were autoreactive with specificity for the shared I-A^b.

D. IL-2 Dependency

When the T-lymphocyte clones were characterized for their dependency upon exogenous IL-2 for in vitro growth, it was found that all of cytotoxic T lymphocytes required exogenous IL-2 for their in vitro growth (Table 7). Of 23 autoreactive clones tested from animals with acute GVHD, (i.e., G and L2 clones), 14 were capable of in vitro proliferation without exogenous IL-2, suggesting that they were capable of in vivo growth without exogenous IL-2.

Since the autoreactive clones did not require exogenous IL-2, it suggested that they secreted cytokines capable of supporting their autocrine growth, i.e., IL-2 and/or IL-4. To determine which cytokines were produced by the clones, the supernatants of the stimulated clones were assayed for the presence of IL-2 and IL-4 using HT2 cells as an indicator system with and without the presence of antibodies to IL-2, IL-2R, and IL-4 (Table 8). Autoreactive T-lymphocyte clones capable of IL-2-independent growth were shown to produce IL-4 alone (Table 8) and in some cases, IL-2 alone or IL-2 and IL-4 (data not shown).

Table 7 In Vitro IL-2 Dependency of GVHD T-Lymphocyte Clones

Clone	Addition of IL-2	Stimulating spleen cells (CPM)			Specificity
		Media	LP	B6	
G-1	−	126	390	566	B6 restricted
	+	3,225	4,340	*13,463*	minor
G-3	−	222	831	526	B6 restricted
	+	2,818	4,631	*24,896*	minor
G-10	−	364	*4,146*	*4,666*	I-A^b
	+	1,025	*5,135*	*9,070*	
G-17	−	67	368	41	I-A^b
	+	1,163	*13,625*	*19,825*	
G-19	−	45	105	147	I-A^b
	+	793	*4,373*	*9,806*	
L2.21	−	217	*22,769*	*14,888*	I-A^b
	+	158	*16,043*	*11,406*	
CG-46	−	820	*16,933*	*13,094*	I-A^b
	+	787	*25,790*	*17,997*	

GVHD T-lymphocyte clones stimulated for 3 days with irradiated spleen cells with and without exogenous IL-2.

Table 8 IL-2/IL-4-Supported In Vitro Autocrine Growth by Autoreactive T-Lymphocyte Clones

Clone	Antibody added	Stimulating spleen cells (CPM)		
		Medium	LP	B6
L2.30	—	311	11,622	30,035
	αIL-2	1,765	13,964	44,576
	αIL-4	1,713	1,625	6,029
L2.31	—	264	22,173	44,891
	αIL-2	403	15,211	58,042
	αIL-4	411	714	3,577
L2.37	—	81	8,080	28,357
	αIL-2	116	9,683	29,887
	αIL-4	927	1,498	3,790

Autoreactive GVHD clones stimulated for 3 days with irradiated spleen cells without exogenous IL-2 with and without the addition of antibodies to IL-2 and IL-4.

Murine helper T-lymphocyte clones can be divided into those that are type I helper T lymphocytes (T_H1), producing IL-2 and γ-interferon, and type 2 helper cells (T_H2), producing IL-4 (6). The presence of T lymphocytes capable of producing both IL-2 and IL-4 was, therefore, surprising, although human T lymphocyte clones capable of producing both IL-2 and IL-4 have been identified (7). The results indicate that some murine autoreactive T-lymphocyte clones are capable of producing both IL-2 and IL-4 in vitro and potentially in vivo. The autoreactive helper T lymphocytes might, therefore, be the source of the IL-2 required for the proliferation and differentiation of the IL-2-dependent cytotoxic T lymphocytes.

To determine if the autoreactive helper T-lymphocyte clones were necessary for the in vivo growth of recipient-specific cytotoxic T lymphocytes and other effector cells, the donor LP spleen cells were depleted of L3T4$^+$ T lymphocytes. When the spleen cells from the transplant recipients were cloned on day 14, no clonagenic Lyt-2$^+$ T-lymphocyte clones were isolated. The few clones that were isolated had Thy 1.2$^+$, L3T4$^+$, Lyt 2$^-$ and required exogenous IL-2 for their in vitro growth, suggesting their relative immaturity. Thus, the elimination of mature L3T4$^+$ autoreactive helper T lymphocytes prior to transplantation results in the lack of detectable Lyt-2$^+$ B6-specific cytotoxic T lymphocytes following transplantation and suggests that the autoreactive helper T lymphocytes are required for the in vivo growth of cytotoxic T lymphocytes presumably due to their production of IL-2/IL-4 which are required for the in vivo growth and differentiation of cytotoxic T lymphocytes.

E. Collagen Deposition

Chronic GVHD is characterized histopathologically by increased collagen deposition. The mechanism of the increased collagen deposition is unclear. The increased collagen deposition may be due to increased collagen production secondary to an increased number of fibroblasts or an increase in the amount of collagen synthesized per fibroblast. To determine if the GVHD clones were capable of stimulating collagen production, clone supernatants were assayed for their capacity to stimulate fibroblast proliferation and col-

Table 9 Stimulation of Fibroblast Collagen Production by GVHD T-Lymphocyte Clones

Clone	Total collagen production	Fibroblast number	Collagen production/ Fibroblast
Acute GVHD			
G-1	2.18	2.39	0.91
G-3	1.63	1.95	0.83
G-7	2.04	1.17	1.75
G-19	1.45	0.95	1.53
G-81	1.04	1.07	0.83
Chronic GVHD			
CG-43	1.05	1.01	1.02
CG-46	2.13	0.91	2.03
CG-52	2.09	1.10	1.90

Results presented as the ratio of fibroblasts stimulated with clone supernatants/fibroblasts stimulated with control supernatants.

lagen production (Table 9). Acute GVHD clones, primarily the cytotoxic T-lymphocyte clones, were able to stimulate total collagen production primarily by stimulating fibroblast proliferation although some autoreactive clones were able to stimulate total collagen production through increasing the amount of collagen produced per fibroblast (8). When the autoreactive clones from animals with chronic GVHD were analyzed, none of the clones stimulated fibroblast proliferation although some autoreactive clones did stimulate total collagen production by increasing the amount of collagen synthesized per fibroblast. Thus, it appears that autoreactive clones stimulated fibroblast collagen production on a per cell basis while the cytotoxic T-lymphocyte clones stimulate collagen production secondary to increased fibroblast proliferation.

A characterization of the cytokines produced by the GVHD clones revealed that the B6-specific cytotoxic T-lymphocyte clones produce both γ-interferon and TNF-β, both of which were able to stimulate fibroblast proliferation. So far, none of the cytokines studied (IL-1, IL-2, IL-3, IL-4, TNF-α, and γ-interferon) were able to stimulate fibroblast collagen production on a per cell basis. Thus, the cytokine produced by the autoreactive T lymphocytes from mice with clinically detectable chronic GVHD that stimulates collagen production on a per cell basis has not been identified.

F. Ia Expression

Increased expression of class II histocompatibility antigens (Ia) is seen in kerotinocytes, the gastrointestinal tract, the liver, and the kidneys of both human and murine bone marrow transplant recipients (9-10). Because γ-interferon has been shown both in vitro and in vivo to stimulate Ia expression, it has been assumed that γ-interferon is responsible for the increased Ia expression. The supernatants of both acute and chronic GVHD clones were analyzed for their capacity to stimulate macrophage Ia expression. Eight of 17 acute GVHD clones were able to stimulate Ia expression (Table 10). Six of the Ia-inducing supernatants contained significant amounts (53-1200 IU/ml) of γ-interferon. Of the γ-interferon-producing clones, five were B6-specific cytotoxic T lymphocytes and one was an autoreactive clone. Of 10 chronic GVHD clones analyzed, only two clones were capable of stimulating Ia expression; both clones produced significant

Table 10 Cytokine Production by GVHD T-Lymphocyte Clones

Clone	Ia expression[a]	γ-INF[b]	TNF[c]	CML[d]
Acute GVHD				
G-1	+	+	+	+
G-2	+	−	−	−
G-6	−	−	−	−
G-81	+	+	+	+
G-93	+	+	−	+
L2.18	−	−	+	−
L2.18	−	−	+	−
Chronic GVHD				
CG-46	−	−	+	−
CG-47	+	+	−´	−
CG-52	+	+	−	−

[a]Increased Ia expression by P388D1 macrophages following incubation with clone supernatants.

[b]Presence of γ-INF detected by inhibition of VSV replication.

[c]Presence of TNF determined by 50% lysis point of L929 fibroblasts.

[d]CML with % specific release >10% considered positive.

amounts of γ-interferon. Thus, the cells responsible for γ-interferon production during acute and chronic GVHD differ significantly: During acute GVHD, γ-interferon is produced primarily by CD8$^+$ cytotoxic T lymphocytes, while during chronic GVHD, γ-interferon is produced by CD4$^+$ autoreactive helper T lymphocytes.

G. Tumor Necrosis Factor

Tumor Necrosis Factor (TNF) has been implicated as a cytokine potentially involved in the pathogenesis of acute GVHD (11). The administration of exogenous antibodies to TNF reduce mortality and eliminate the histopathological features of acute GVHD. When the supernatants of the GVHD clones were analyzed for the presence of TNF, both CTL and autoreactive T lymphocytes were demonstrated to produce TNF-β, suggesting that TNF-β in addition to cytotoxic T lymphocytes may be an important effector mechanism in the pathogenesis of acute GVHD.

IV. CONCLUSIONS

Clonal analysis of the recipients of histocompatible bone marrow transplants has revealed a heterogenous population of clonagenic T lymphocytes, including recipient-specific, IL-2-dependent cytotoxic T lymphocytes; recipient-specific, IL-2-dependent helper T lymphocytes, autoreactive, IL-2-dependent T lymphocytes; and autoreactive, IL-2/IL-4-producing T lymphocytes. In addition to the production of IL-2, the production of γ-interferon and TNF-β by both autoreactive and recipient-specific clones has been demonstrated. These cytokines, besides being involved in the direct destruction of recipient tissues, may be involved in the increased expression of class II histocompatibility antigens, which can stimulate the autoreactive T lymphocytes. Of interest is the fact that clinical GVHD is restricted primarily to those organs in which increased class II histocompatibility antigen expression is found.

Although cytotoxic cells (cytotoxic T lymphocytes and NK) may be involved in the pathogenesis of acute GVHD, cytokines, especially TNF-β, may also play an important role. The clonal analysis of GVHD has demonstrated a lack of clonagenic cytotoxic T lymphocytes in mice with chronic GVHD and suggests that chronic GVHD is due primarily to cytokines produced by autoreactive helper T lymphocytes; in the present model there is no established role for either cytotoxic T lymphocytes or T lymphocytes with specificity for recipient-restricted minor histocompatibility antigens in the pathogenesis of chronic GVHD. The model states that chronic GVHD is essentially an autoimmune disease, i.e., the effector mechanisms are directed against histocompatibility antigens expressed on donor cells (12). Chronic GVHD in the murine model, like its human analogue, has many features in common with autoimmune diseases. The establishment of T-lymphocyte clones has given increased insight into the complex events involved in the pathogenesis of histocompatible GVHD.

ACKNOWLEDGMENT

This work was supported by NIH Grants CA35971 and AR37394.

REFERENCES

1. Hamilton BL, Parkman R: Acute and chronic graft-versus-host disease induced by minor histocompatibility antigens in mice. Transplantation 1983;36:150-155.
2. Hamilton BL, Bevan MJ, Parkman R: Anti-recipient cytotoxic T lymphocyte precursors are present in the spleens of mice with acute graft-vs-host disease due to minor histocompatibility antigens. J Immunol 1981;126:621-625.
3. Korngold R, Sprent J: Lethal graft-versus-host disease after bone marrow transplantation across minor histocompatibility barriers in mice: Prevention by removing mature T cells from marrow. J Exp Med 1978;148:1687-1698.
4. Parkman R: Clonal analysis of murine graft-vs-host disease. I. Phenotypic and functional analysis of T lymphocyte clones. J Immunol 1986;136(10):3543-3548.
5. Bevan MJ: The major histocompatibility complex determines susceptibility to cytotoxic T cells directed against minor histocompatibility antigens. J Exp Med 1975; 142:1349-1364.
6. Mosmann TRH, Cherwinski MW, Bond MA, et al.: Two types of murine helper T cell clone. I. Definition according to profiles of lymphokine activities and secreted proteins. J Immunol 1986;136:2348-2357.
7. Paliard X, Malefijt RDW, Yssel H, et al.: Simultaneous production of IL-2, IL-4, and IFN-γ by activated human CD4[+] and CD8[+] T cell clones. J Immunol 1988;141:849-855.
8. Sullivan KM, Parkman R: The pathophysiology and treatment of graft-versus-host disease. Clin Haematol 1983,12:775-789.
9. Mason DW, Dallman M, Barclay AN: Graft-versus-host disease induces expression of Ia antigen in rat epidermal cells and gut epithelium. Nature 1981;293:150-151.
10. Breathnach SM, Katz SI: Keratinocytes synthesize Ia antigen in acute cutaneous graft-vs-host disease. J Immunol 1983,131:2741-2750.
11. Piguet PF, Grau GE, Allet B, et al.: Tumor necrosis factor/cachectin is an effector of skin and gut lesions of the acute phase of graft-vs-host disease. J Exp Med 1987; 166:1280-1289.
12. Graze PR, Gale RP: Chronic graft versus host disease: a syndrome of disordered immunity. Am J Med 1979;66:611-620.

4

T-Cell Clones in Graft-vs.-Host Disease

Daniel A. Vallera and Bruce R. Blazar
University of Minnesota Hospitals and Clinics
Minneapolis, Minnesota

Michael B. Widmer
Immunex Corporation
Seattle, Washington

I. INTRODUCTION

Graft-vs.-Host Disease (GVHD) is a disease that occurs when T cells in transplanted donor bone marrow respond against major and/or minor histocompatibility antigens on the surface of the recipient's cells. This definition does not reflect the complexity of the disease, since the exact nature of cells that mediate GVHD and the antigens that these cells recognize are still not completely understood. Moreover, our traditional understanding of GVHD as a graft-vs.-host event has been complicated by the description of syngeneic GVHD (1). A large volume of published evidence demonstrates that histocompatibility antigens on murine host tissues (H-2 and non-H-2) induce donor T lymphocytes in the donor bone marrow inoculum to proliferate and differentiate (2). Perhaps the first indication that T cells could cause GVHD was that the disease occurred in mice given high doses of H-2 disparate thymus cells (3,4). Studies in an H-2 identical, minor antigen mismatched model of GVHD showed that even as few as 0.3% (3×10^4) T cells returned to a T-cell-depleted suspension of murine bone marrow induced GVHD-related mortality (5). Moreover, in human HLA-matched transplant patients, a correlation was observed between the number of T cells determined by limiting dilution analysis and the development of GVHD (6). Although these findings are somewhat controversial, a threshold dose of 10^5 T cells was identified beyond which a majority of patients developed GVHD.

Recent technology shows immense potential for clarifying the mechanisms of GVHD including the cells and factors that induce the disease, the antigens that trigger it, and the effector cells that carry out pathological destruction. One useful development is the ability to isolate and propagate T-cell clones. A second is the availability of monoclonal antibodies for more discriminative analyses of cell populations. This review will address clonal analysis primarily for the study of GVHD mechanisms. We will present some of our data that represent the first analysis of various clonotypic T cells and their ability to induce GVHD-related splenomegaly. The role of monoclonal antibodies in determining GVHD mechanisms through cell population studies will then be described. Finally, we will discuss the potential of monoclonal antibodies, primarily linked to toxins (i.e., immunotoxins), for elimination of GVHD-causing T cells.

II. CLONAL T-CELL STUDIES

A. T-Cell Clones from Mice with GVHD

Limiting dilution and micromanipualtion technologies have allowed investigators to propagate and isolate T-cell clones (7-11), which has permitted a more precise evaluation of GVHD. T-cell clones were isolated from C57BL/6 murine recipients of LP spleen cells in an attempt to determine whether or not acute and chronic GVHD represent two distinct processes (12). Studies showed that T cells cloned 10-14 days posttransplant (time of acute GVHD) differed from cells cloned 50 days posttransplant (time of chronic GVHD). These cells differed in their antigenic specificity, cytotoxic capacity, and surface phenotype. The studies further suggested that acute GVHD was primarily due to recipient specific cytotoxic T cells, whereas chronic GVHD was due to autoreactive helper T lymphocytes. Furthermore, some evidence indicates that certain autoreactive T-cell clones are capable of interleukin-4 (IL-4) production, and IL-4 may have a central role in the pathogenesis of acute and chronic GVHD (13). These investigators point out that certain properties of IL-4, including the ability to induce IgE synthesis, synergistic reactivity with INF-gamma to induce Ia, support of autoreactive T-cell growth, and stimulation of fibroblast collagen production as well as B-cell proliferation, correlate with as yet unexplained clinical observations associated with chronic GVHD. Such findings illustrate the utility of clonal analysis for determining the nature of cell populations that contribute to GVHD and the biological characteristics (such as IL-4 production) that influence the activity of these cells.

B. Clonal Addback Experiments

Although the analysis of clones isolated from animals with GVHD has been informative, the cells studied may or may not have a causal relation to GVHD. Another strategy involves the propagation of T-cell clones in vivo to directly assess their ability to mediate GVHD. Investigators have studied (14) the ability of injected clones to mediate a cutaneous GVH response in an immune lymphocyte transfer test (2,15). In this assay, alloreactive lymphocytes are injected intradermally and recipient mice are examined for a cutaneous GVHD lesion resembling a delayed type hypersensitivity (DTH) reaction. Several T-cell clones were evaluated with intradermal injection of control day 6 C57BL/6 anti-DBA/2 clones into semiallogeneic (C57BL/6 $\times$ DBA/2)F1 mice. One of seven helper clones demonstrated activity. The active clone was directed against H-2^d (presumably Ia of the recipient) while the inactive clones were directed against background (mls), H-2^d, or H-1.3. Four of eight cytotoxic T-cell clones were active and recognized H-2K^d and H-2D^d.

Using a similar assay, Shiohara et al. (16) reported comparable findings using allo-Ia reactive T-cell clones but went a step further. Clones were established from mixed lymphocyte cultures of I-congenic strain combinations. Similar to Biel et al. (14), local intradermal injections of helper or cytotoxic T-cell clones caused cutaneous DTH-like responses against appropriate Ia antigens in all cases. However, histopathologic studies showed that only two of six clones examined induced local changes consistent with grades 2-3 cutaneous GVHD 48-72 hours after inoculation. Interestingly, both clones were capable of functioning as helpers for antibody production, were cytolytic against appropriate I-A targets, and could mediate lysis via the release of the cytotoxic lymphokines, lymphotoxin, and interferon-gamma. In one case, not only the clones, but host Lyt-1$^+$ cells were involved in local GVHD induction, suggesting that lymphokines secreted from the clones may be responsible for T-cell recruitment. The cytolytic ability of the cloned T cells was not sufficient to induce GVHD. Examination of the epidermis with monoclonal antibodies an immunoperoxidase revealed Lyt-1$^+$ cloned cells preferentially located in the area of severe epidermal cell damage. Thus, the identification of an Lyt-1$^+$ effector cell agrees with findings in murine skin graft rejection models at both the population (17) and clonal (18) level, which also suggests a role for Lyt-1$^+$ helper T cells. These studies have certain limitations in that the cells used to generate cutaneous GVH responses were injected locally into footpads and read after 48 hours. This may or may not correlate to the events of a systemic GVH response. Also, the time interval from injection of clones to measurement of activity was rather short.

Addback experiments have also been used by Truitt et al. to analyze the potential of T-cell clones to mediate a graft-vs.-leukemia effect in vivo (19). A T-cell clone was made from primed B10.BR responders. The clone recognized a minor histocompatibility antigen encoded outside the H-2 complex but present on both normal and leukemic AKR cells. The clone prevented the transfer of a lethal leukemia cell response when injected into AKR recipients along with AKR leukemia cells. When analyzed independently for GVH responses, this T-cell clone also mediated the GVH response of body weight loss, indicating that the same T cells that mediate antileukemia effects can cause GVH responses. A different clone, also isolated from B10.BR responders and reactive with Qa-1-encoded class II-like molecules, also mediated an antileukemia effect. But unlike the previous clone, it did not express GVH activity, suggesting that different subpopulations of T cells may be responsible for antileukemia and GVH reactivity. This may relate to the fact that the Qa-1 target molecule is expressed on leukemia cells but has limited expression on normal host tissues. These findings underscore the importance of clonal analysis for determining GVHD mechanisms and perhaps for developing GVHD therapy.

C. Bifunctional T-Cell Clones

The above clonal studies suggest that different subtypes of T cells, helper and/or cytotoxic, are involved in GVHD. Although some researchers believe that the induction of GVHD depends on cooperative interaction between these subpopulations, alternate explanations exist. It is possible that cells regarded as limited to the helper or cytotoxic subsets are not truly restricted. In a functional sense, helper cells are defined as noncytolytic and IL-2 independent. In contrast, cytotoxic cells are defined as cytotoxic, as well as IL-2 dependent since they are unable to proliferate in the absence of exogenous IL-2. Clonal analyses in functional assays suggests that we can no longer restrict ourselves to these terms. The existence of a lymphocyte that exhibits the IL-2-independent proliferation of helper T cells and cytolytic activity of conventional cytotoxic T lymphocytes (CTL) has been documented (20). Our data support the hypothesis that these cells operate in the induction of splenomegaly across a whole H-2 histocompatibility difference and may represent a pathway for GVHD pathogenesis.

We have used the Simonsen splenomegaly assay to measure GVH activity for in vivo clonal analysis of GVHD (21). We chose the Simonsen assay because it takes advantage of the reproducible splenic hypertrophy that occurs as part of the GVH reaction (22). In general, splenomegaly of neonatal F_1-type recipients reaches a peak 8-10 days after inoculation of parental-type donor lymphocytes. Thus, the assay can be considered a longer-term analysis of GVHD activity than the lymphocyte transfer test. After 10 days, spleens may be either atrophic or enlarged and the measure of splenomegaly unreliable. In the assay, there is a logarithmically linear relationship between the dosage of immunocompetent lymphocytes injected and splenomegaly (23,24).

1. T-Cell Clones

T-cell clones were derived by limiting dilution from day 5 C56BL/6 anti-DBA/2 mixed lymphocyte cultures (MLC) as previously described (25). The cells were seeded at 0.25 cells/well in the presence of 10^6 irradiated DBA/2 spleen cells and 25-50% secondary MLC supernatant (2°MLC SN). Subcloning was accomplished by seeding cloned cells at 0.1 cells/well under identical conditions. Cells from positive wells were expanded and subcultured in the presence of irradiated DBA/2 splenocytes and 20% 2°MLC SN.

Three functional types of clones resulted: (1) cytotoxic T-cell clones that were capable of mediating alloantigen-specific cytolytic activity against ^{51}Cr-labeled target cells but were unable to proliferate autonomously in vitro in the absence of an added source of IL-2 (2°MLC SN); (2) helper T-cell clones that were noncytotoxic but able to proliferate upon coculture with allogeneic cells in the absence of exogenous growth factors; and (3) helper independent bifunctional T-cell clones capable of both specific cytotoxicity and proliferation in the absence of exogenous growth factors.

Cytolytic activity against DBA/2 alloantigen was measured by a standard technique (26). Cloned cells were mixed with 2×10^3 ^{51}Cr-labeled targets at several effector:target cell ratios. DBA/2 targets were either P815 mastocytoma cells maintained in vitro or concanavalin A-stimulated spleen cells. The percentage of ^{51}Cr release was determined for duplicate reaction mixtures. The proliferative response of cloned cells to allogeneic stimulating cells was determined by incubating 10^6 cloned cells obtained 7 days after previous subculture with 10^4 irradiated (2 Gray) allogeneic spleen cells (7,25). Cultures were pulsed for 6 to 8 hours on day 2 with 2 μCi tritiated thymidine. Cultures were harvested onto glass fiber filters, and thymidine incorporation was determined by standard liquid scintillation counting techniques.

2. Clonal Analysis of GVHD-Induced Splenomegaly

Simonsen activity was measured by injecting C56BL/6 anti-DBA/2 clones intraperitoneally into nonirradiated (C57BL/2 $\times$ DBA/2)F_1 neonates, 6 to 8 days old. Spleen and body weight was determined 8 days later. The spleen to body weight ratio (S:B wt. ratio) was calculated as:

$$\frac{\text{Spleen weight in grams}}{\text{Body weight in grams}} \times 1000$$

Positive and negative controls were performed in all experiments. For a positive control, normal C56BL/6 splenocytes were injected. For a negative control, (C57BL/6 $\times$ DBA/2) F_1 splenocytes were injected into the (C57BL/6 $\times$ DBA/2)F_1 neonates. Percent control Simonsen activity was determined as follows:

Table 1 Simonsen Activity of Various Types of T-Cell Clones[a]

T-cell clones	Type	Cytotoxic	Proliferative	% Simonsen activity
C2-11	Bifunctional	+	+	45
BD6-13	Bifunctional	+	+	11
C2-16	Helper	−	+	2
C1-2	Helper	−	+	15
5-9	Helper	−	+	18
C2-15	Helper	−	+	14
C2-10	Cytotoxic	+	−	10
5-11	Cytotoxic	+	−	7
5-26	Inactive	−	−	14
5-33	Inactive	−	−	0
−	MLC[b]	+	+,	100
−	MLC	+	+	59

[a]C57BL/6 neonates were injected with 6-8 $\times$ 10^6 T-cell clones. Eight days later the spleen:body ratio was determined. Percent Simonsen activity was calculted based on positive and negative control values as described.

[b]Cells obtained from a mixed lymphocyte culture of C57BL/6 splenocyte responder cells and irradiated DBA/2 stimulator cells.

$$\frac{\text{test S:B wt. ratio} - \text{negative control S:B wt. ratio}}{\text{positive control S:B wt ratio} - \text{negative control S:B wt. ratio}} \times 100$$

Several T-cell clones of helper, cytotoxic, and bifunctional origin were injected at a dose of 6-8 $\times$ 10^6 cells into F_1s (Table 1). The bifunctional clone, C2-11, showed the highest percent Simonsen activity of any clone tested in independent experiments. The S:B wt. ratio was statistically higher for C2-11-injected mice as compared to that obtained following the injection of F_1-negative control cells (determined by Student t-test analysis). In contrast, BD6-13, another bifunctional clone, did not show remarkable Simonsen activity. We considered this background activity since inactive clones showed 0-5% activity.

Four helper T-cell clones were tested with activities ranging from 2 to 18% when 6-8 $\times$ 10^6 cells were injected. Three cytotoxic clones were tested with activities ranging from 7 to 14% when 6-8 $\times$ 10^6 cells were injected. None of the helper or cytotoxic clones tested were active in the Simonsen test. As an additional positive control, cells obtained from 5-day C57BL/6 anti-DBA-2 MLCs were injected. Greater than 59% control response was obtained in two experiments when 6 $\times$ 10^6 cells were injected.

3. Phenotypic Analysis of T-Cell Clones

Cells from the bifunctional clones C2-11, BD6-13, and BD6-28 were studied for the expression of various T-cell markers by indirect immunofluorescence on a Becton-Dickinson FACS IV (Table 2). Lyt-2 is the murine homologue of CD8 in man (27) and recognized by anti-Lyt-1. Although it is considered a pan-T marker (29), a higher antigen density on helper cells may explain its usefulness as a helper cell-specific marker. All bifunctional clones expressed the Lyt-2 antigen, but did not express the L3T4 antigen,

Table 2 Expression of Different Antigens on the Surface of Various T-Cell Clones[a]

Clone	Percent positive cells				
	L3T4	Lyt-2.2	Lyt-1.2	Thy 1.2	Mac-1
Bifunctional					
C2-11	3	42	2	92	1
BD6-13	2	58	1	91	0.5
BD6-28	5	60	2	82	NA
Helper					
C2-16	87	2	48	82	NA
Cytotoxic					
C2-10	1	42	4	87	NA

[a]Cloned T cells were incubated with saturating concentrations of the monoclonal antibodies GK1.5, anti-Lyt-2, anti-Lyt-1, and anti-Thy 1.2, or M1/70 for 30 min at 4°C to study the surface expression of L3T4, Lyt-2.2, Lyt-1.2, Thy 1.2, or Mac-1, respectively. After 30 min, FITC-labeled goat anti-mouse gammaglobulin (FITC-GAMG) was added for 30 min. The cells were washed and evaluated for surface expression on a Becton-Dickinson FACS IV. Background expression was determined following incubation with control ascites fluid and FITC-GAMG. Histograms were generated by an Apple II computer program. Control histograms were subtracted from test histograms for the final result.

[b]NA = data not available.

nor the Lyt-1.2 antigen. As a positive control, the clones were reacted with Thy 1.2 (anti-pan-T) and all were positive. As a negative control, neither C2-11 nor BD6-13 were positive for the myeloid marker, Mac-1. As anticipated, the helper clone C2-16 was positive for L3T4, Lyt-1.2, and Thy 1.2, but not Lyt-2.2, while the cytotoxic clone C2-10 was positive for Lyt-2.2 and Thy 1.2, but negative for L3T4 and Lyt-1.2. Since all bifunctional clones were Lyt-2$^+$, L3T4$^-$, Lyt-1$^-$, and since CTL precursors are Lyt-2$^+$, Lyt-1$^+$ (29), we believe that bifunctional cells are more closely related to cells of CTL lineage.

Detailed phenotypic and functional analyses of clonal cells capable of mediating GVHD have been possible in this study and studies by others (12). Parkman identified 23 clones obtained from the splenocytes of mice undergoing a GVHD reaction due to the minor histocompatibility differences of the donor inocula. Seven of the 23 clones were remarkably similar to our bifunctional clones in that they exhibited both antihost cytolytic antihost proliferative responses, and had the identical phenotype of Lyt-2$^+$, L3T4$^-$. Therefore, it is possible that some or all of the clones isolated by Parkman were bifunctional cells, and that bifunctional cells may be important mediators of GVHD not only in nonirradiated neonatal recipients of major H-2 disparate T cells, but also in irradiated adult recipients of minor H-2 disparate T cells.

III. MONOCLONAL ANTIBODIES IN GVHD STUDIES AND THERAPY

A. The Use of Monoclonal Antibodies for Establishing GVHD Mechanisms

More complete and specific donor cell depletion studies are possible since the development of monoclonal antibodies (30). Monoclonal antibodies have advantages over polyclonal antisera in their specificity, homogeneity, and availability. Earlier depletion studies with polyclonal antisera supported the notion that T cells were involved in GVHD induction (31-34). However, the reagents were often cross-reactive with other cell populations. Other studies suggested that murine T-cell subpopulations could be distinguished with antisera (27,35). Anti-Lyt-1 was reactive against helper cells, while anti-Lyt-2 was reactive against cytotoxic T cells. Lyt-1 expression was not entirely restricted to helper cells in another investigation (9). More restrictive monoclonal antibodies (anti-L3T4) were produced that react against Lyt-2$^-$ helper T cells (28). Using monoclonal antibodies against Lyt-2 and L3T4, it is possible to separate T cells into nonoverlapping cytotoxic and helper subpopulations. These reagents have been paramount in determining the role of T-cell subpopulations in GVHD induction.

Although various models have shown that different subtypes of T cells can mediate GVHD, monoclonal antibodies have been useful for comprehension of the relationship between target histocompatibility antigens and GVHD induction in mice. In depletion studies using monoclonal anti-Thy 1, mature T cells induced GVHD to multiple minor (5,36-38) and major (39,40) histocompatibility antigens. Using monoclonal antibodies raised against cytotoxic and helper T-cell subpopulations, investigators have shown that GVHD across minor histocompatibility differences is induced mostly by cytotoxic cells (41), although helper cells do play a role in certain strain combinations (42). Regarding whole H-2 differences, early depletion studies with monoclonal antibodies indicated that GVHD was largely controlled by Lyt-1$^+$ helper T cells (43). In these studies using two different models of GVHD, BALB/c into C57BL/6 and C3H/HeN into C57BL/6, Lyt-2$^+$ cytotoxic cells played a slight role in GVHD induction. In a semiallogeneic transplant model of CBA into (CBA × B6)F$_1$ (44) and a fully allogeneic transplant model of BALB/c into C57BL/6 (45), GVHD was caused mostly, but not entirely, by L3T4$^+$, Lyt-2$^-$ helper T cells. Depletion studies (44) showed that GVHD generated across class II histocompatibility differences involved only L3T4$^+$ cells, while GVHD generated across class I histocompatibility differences appears to be mediated by Lyt-2$^+$ cells which may be aided by L3T4$^+$ cells. The involvement of both helper and cytotoxic cells in GVHD induction across whole H-2 or class I differences may be a function of the independent subpopulations or perhaps due to the presence of bifunctional T cells.

1. Role of NK Cells in GVHD Induction

Depletion studies have also been used to clarify the role of NK cells in GVHD induction. The lack of reagents that selectively eliminate mature NK cells and their immediate precursors while preserving T and accessory populations previously hindered a definitive analysis of donor NK cells in GVHD. Depletion of NK donor cells using an NK lineage restricted monoclonal antibody, NK1.1 (46), showed that NK cells do not contribute to the generation of GVHD across whole H-2 differences (47).

B. Monoclonal Antibodies Linked to Toxins for In Vivo Therapy of GVHD

Investigators have shown that GVHD can be ameloriated in mice following the injection of anti-T-cell monoclonal antibodies (48,49), and an anti-IL-2 receptor monoclonal antibody has demonstrated potential against GVHD (50). Our group believes that monoclonal antibodies can be even more effective when used to deliver cytotoxic molecules. Our desire to test this hypothesis is based on the fact that (1) in vivo monoclonal antibody therapy has not been completely effective (51,52); (2) current therapies for GVHD employ nonspecific and often deleterious agents, and (3) GVHD prophylaxis using T-cell depletion has side effects that have not been overcome (53).

As a cytotoxic agent, we have employed a potent catalytic toxin extracted from the seeds of the castor bean plant *Ricinus communis*. Ricin is a glycoprotein consisting of a 30 kDa A chain and a 30 kDa B chain. The A chain is an enzyme and the portion of the molecule involved in cell kill. A single molecule of ricin A chain in the cytosol can kill a cell (54) by inhibiting protein synthesis at the level of the 28S component of the 60S ribosome (55). The A chain of ricin, once inside the cell cytosol, can inactivate up to 1500 ribosomes per minute (56). The B chain is the portion of the molecule that binds to terminal nonreducing galactose residues on the cell. When ricin is linked to antibody, lactose must be present to block the native galactose binding site of B chain and render the conjugate antibody specific. Our laboratory has evaluated intact ricin immunotoxins for GVHD prophylaxis in mice (57,58) and used them clinically in humans (59,60). The presence of B chain is advantageous in vitro because it somehow facilitates the translocation of A chain into the cytosol (61). Also, intact ricin immunotoxins have different trafficking properties compared to immunotoxins devoid of B chain (62). However, lactose does not entirely block B chain binding in vivo (63). Thus, intact ricin immunotoxins have limited value for systemic in vivo therapy. For in vivo therapy of GVHD, we have studied immunotoxins devoid of B chain in a murine model of bone marrow transplantation across the major histocompatibility barrier (64). We found that immunotoxins made with anti-Lyt-1 monoclonal antibody linked to ricin A chain when injected intravenously 8 days after GVHD induction increased median survival time, but some animals still died of GVHD. Toxicities associated with immunotoxins in irradiated mice included weight gain, pleural effusions, peritoneal effusions, and hypoproteinuria. The model should prove useful to optimize treatment and minimize immunotoxin-related toxicities.

Ricin A chain immunotoxins have been used clinically (65-69). Anti-CD5, recognizing the human equivalent to murine Lyt-1 (27), was linked to ricin A chain and used to treat a patient with severe grade 3-4 steroid-resistant acute GVHD after an allogeneic, human leukocyte antigen-identical, bone marrow transplant (69). Immunotoxin therapy produced a complete clinical response in the skin and gastrointestinal tract. The patient tolerated a 14-day course without signs of toxicity. However, months later, the patient developed chronic GVHD. Although these findings are preliminary, they have led to a multi-institutional phase 2 trial and underscore the potential of immunotoxin therapy.

IV. CONCLUDING REMARKS

The studies presented in this review highlight the utility of T-cell clones, monoclonal antibodies, and immunotoxins for research directed toward overcoming GVHD. The complexity of GVHD is reflected in our failure to establish a single mechanisms of pathogenesis. Negative depletion studies using monoclonal antibodies have established that (1) the nature of responding T cells is related to the type of histocompatibility antigens expressed on the surface of host cells, and (2) more than one type of cell is involved in GVHD. When crossing the whole H-2 barrier, helper as well as cytotoxic cells are involved, and investigators have been able to clone different T cells from mice undergoing acute and chronic GVHD.

Our data suggest that previous attempts to establish GVHD mechanisms may have been complicated by the existence of an autonomously proliferating (helper-independent) cytolytic T cell with properties of both helper and cytolytic T cells. This bifunctional cell has been defined by clonal analysis. In addback experiments, these cells can mediate GVHD activity. Our examination of 12 T-cell clones of which two were bifunctional showed only one capable of causing convincing, reproducible Simonsen activity. This was indeed a bifunctional clone, and in our opinion, a role for these cells in GVHD is indicated. However, we do not believe that the bifunctional cells alone account for all instances of GVHD pathogenesis since not all bifunctional cell clones injected were capable of inducing splenomegaly. In our past studies of GVHD prevention across the whole H-2 barrier, anti-Lyt-2 as compared to anti-Lyt-1 monoclonal antibodies have been only slightly, albeit reproducibly, effective in preventing GVHD. Thus, these bifunctional cells may represent a small portion of the total T-cell fraction and only a minor pathway for GVHD induction across the whole H-2. Since anti-Lyt-2 is more effective in preventing GVHD across non-H-2 histocompatibility differences, bifunctional cells may play a more important role in minor antigen GVHD.

Pathological GVHD can exist in syngeneic bone marrow transplants (1), investigators have cloned host cells reactive against host antigens in models of chronic GVHD (12), and recipient-derived T cells are responsible for the destruction observed in cutaneous GVHD (16). Together, these findings suggest that an autoimmune component of GVHD could mediate tissue damage, while simultaneously sustaining the proliferation of other unifunctional and bifunctional T cells through IL-2, or perhaps, as demonstrated in clonal studies, through other lymphokines such as IL-4 (13). Factors independent of cytolysis and proliferation, such as the capacity to home and the production of appropriate interleukins, may also affect the ability of a T-cell clone to induce activity in vivo.

T-cell clones are important tools for assessing all of these factors. Addback experiments, in particular, will yield important information as to whether different or similar populations of T cell are responsible for GVH reactivity, engraftment promotion, and antileukemia effects. Monoclonal antibodies linked to toxins could prove useful as cell-specific probes for delineating the cells involved in the GVHD network. Immunotoxins might also be developed into powerful and specific reagents for elimination of GVHD-causing cells. T-cell clones, monoclonal antibodies, and immunotoxins are currently contributing to the design and evaluation of new strategies for GVHD prevention and therapy.

ACKNOWLEDGMENTS

Supported in part by U.S. Public Health Service Grants Nos. R01-CA-31618, R01-CA-36725, P01-CA-21737, T32-CA-09445, and R23-AI-19254 awarded by the National Cancer Institute, DHHS, by American Cancer Society Research Grant No. IM-502, by the Minnesota Medical Foundation, and by the Children's Cancer Research Fund. Drs. Vallera and Widmer are Scholars of the Leukemia Society of America. Dr. Blazar is a

Fellow of the Leukemia Society of America and recipient of Clinical Investigator Award
No. K08-AM1509 from the National Institutes of Health. We thank Dr. L. Biel for providing clones 5-9, 5-11, 5-26, and 5-33. This is Center for Experimental Transplantation
and Cancer Research No. 48.

REFERENCES

1. Glazier A, Tutschka PJ, Farmer ER, Santos GW: Graft-versus-host disease in cyclosporin A-treated rats after syngeneic and autologous bone marrow reconstitution. J Exp Med 1983;158:1-8.
2. Grebe SC, Streilein WJ: Graft-versus-host reactions: a review, in *Advances in Immunology*, vol. 22, edited by Dixon FJ and Kunkel HG. Academic Press, New York, 1976; pp. 119-221.
3. Vos O, De Vries MJ, Collenteur J-C, van Bekkum DW: Transplantation of homologous and heterologous lymphoid cells in x-irradiated and non-irradiated mice. J Natl Cancer Inst 1959;23: 53-73.
4. Billingham RE, Silvers WK: Quantitative studies on the ability of cells of different origin to induce tolerance of skin homografts and cause runt disease in neonatal mice. J Exp Zool 1961;146:113-129.
5. Korngold R, Sprent J: Lethal graft-versus-host disease after bone marrow transplantation across minor histocompatibility barriers in mice: prevention by removing mature T cells from marrow. J Exp Med 1978;148:1687-1698.
6. Kernan NA, Collins NH, Juliano L, Cartagena T, Dupont B, O'Reilly RJ: Clonable T lymphocytes in T cell-depleted bone marrow transplants correlate with development of graft-vs-host disease. Blood 1986;68:770-773.
7. Glasebrook AL, Fitch FW. Alloreactive cloned T cell lines: I. Interactions between cloned amplifier and cytolytic T cell lines. J Exp Med 1980;151:876-895.
8. Fathman CG, Hengartner H: Crossreactive mixed lymphocyte reaction determinants recognized by cloned alloreactive T cells. Proc Natl Acad Sci. USA 1979;76:5863-5866.
9. MacDonald HR, Cerottini J-C, Ryser JE, Maryanski JL, Taswell C, Widmer MB, Brunner KT: Quantitation and cloning of cytolytic T lymphocytes and their precursors. Immunol Rev 1980;51:93-123.
10. Nabholz M, Engers HD, Collavo D, North M: Cloned T cell lines with specific cytolytic activity. Curr Top Microbiol Immunol 1978;81:176-187.
11. von Boehmer H, Hengartner H, Nabholz M, Lernhardt W, Schreier M, Haas W: Fine specificity of a continuously growing killer cell clone specific for H-Y antigen. Eur J Immunol 1979;9:592-597.
12. Parkman R: Clonal analysis of murine graft-vs-host disease. I. Phenotypic and functional analysis of T lymphocyte clones. J Immunol 1986;136:3543-3548.
13. Parkman R, Champagne J, DeClerck Y, Cooper M, Draper V, Walker S: Cellular interactions in graft-vs-host disease. Transplant Proc 1987;19:52-54.
14. Biel LW, Roopenian DL, Widmer MB, Bach FH: Induction of immune skin lesions by T lymphocyte clones of particular subclasses. Transplant Proc 1985;17:610-611.
15. Tyler JD, Steinmuller D, Galli SJ, Waddick KT: Allospecific graft-versus-host lesions mediated in MHC-restricted fashion by cloned cytolytic T lymphocytes. Transplant Proc 1983;15:1441-1445.
16. Shiohara T, Narimatsu H, Nagashima M: Induction of cutaneous graft-versus-host disease by allo- or self-Ia-reactive helper T cells in mice. Transplantation 1987;43: 692-698.
17. Loveland BE, Hogarth PM, Ceredig R, McKenzie IFC: Cells mediating graft rejection in the mouse. I. Lyt-1 cells mediate skin graft rejection. J Exp Med 1981;153:1044-1057.

18. Kim B, Rosenstein M, Weiland D, Eberlein TJ, Rosenberg SA: Clonal analysis of the lymphoid cells mediating skin allograft rejection. Mediation of graft rejection in vivo by cloned Ly-1$^+$2$^-$ proliferative, noncytotoxic long-term cell lines. Transplantation 1983;36:525-532.
19. Truitt RL, LeFeber AV, Shih CC-Y: Analysis of effector cells in the graft-versus-leukemia reaction and their relation to graft-versus-host disease, in *T-Cell Depletion in Allogeneic Bone Marrow Transplantation*, edited by Martelli MF, Grignani F, Reisner Y. Serono Symposia Review No. 13, Ares-Serono Symposia, Rome, Italy, 1988, pp. 73-85.
20. Widmer MB, Bach FH: Antigen-driven helper cell-independent cloned cytolytic T lymphocytes. Nature 1981;294:750-752.
21. Vallera DA, Blazar BR, Soderling CCB, Clinchy C, Widmer MB: Induction of graft-versus-host reactivity in mice using cloned T cells, submitted.
22. Simonsen M, Jensen E: in *Biological Problems of Grafting*, edited by Albert F, Medawar PB. Blackwell, Oxford, 1959; pp. 214-266.
23. Simonsen M. Graft versus host reactions. Their natural history, and applicability as tools of research. Progr Allergy 1962;6:349-467.
24. Billingham RE: The biology of graft-versus-host reactions. Harvey Lect 1968;62:21-78.
25. Cerottini JC, Engers HD, MacDonald HR, Brunner KT: Generation of cytotoxic T lymphocytes in vitro: I. Response of normal and immune mouse spleen cells in mixed leukocyte cultures. J Exp Med 1974;140:703-717.
26. Cerottini JC, MacDonald HR: Limiting diultion analysis of alloantigen-reaction T lymphocytes. V. Lyt phenotype of cytolytic T lymphocyte precursors reactive against normal and mutant H-2 antigens. J Immunol 1981;126:490-496.
27. Ledbetter JA, Rouse RV, Micklem HS, Herzenberg LA: T cell subsets defined by expression of Lyt-1,2,3 and Thy-1 antigens: Two-parameter immunofluorescence and cytotoxicity analysis with monoclonal antibodies modifies current views. J Exp Med 1980;152:280-295.
28. Dialynas DP, Wilde DB, Marrack P, Pierres A, Wall KA, Havran W, Otten G, Loken MR, Pierres M, Kappler J: Characterization of the murine antigenic determinant, designated L3T4a, recognized by monoclonal antibody GK1.5: Expression of L3T4a by functional T cell clones appears to correlate primarily with class II MHC antigen-reactivity. Immunol Rev 1983,74:29-56.
29. Kohler G, Milstein C: Continuous cultures of fused cells secreting antibody of a pre-defined specificity. Nature 1975,256:495-497.
30. Tyan ML: Modification of severe graft-versus-host disease with antisera to the theta antigen or to whole serum. Transplantation 1973;15:601-604.
31. Rodt HV, Thierfelder S, Eulitz M: Suppression of acute secondary disease by heterologous anti-brain serum. Blut 1972;25:385-389.
32. von Boehmer H, Sprent J, Nabholz M: Tolerance to histocompatibility determinants in tetraparental bone marrow chimeras. J Exp Med 1975;141:322-334.
33. Cantor H: The effects of anti-theta antiserum upon graft-versus-host activity of spleen and lymph node cells. Cellular Immunol 1972;3:461-469.
34. Cantor H, Boyse EA: Functional subclasses of T-lymphocytes bearing different Ly antigens: I. The generation of functionally distinct T-cell subclasses is a differentiative process independent of antigen. J Exp Med 1975;141:1376-1389.
35. Cantor H, Boyse EA: Functional subclasses of T lymphocytes bearing different Ly antigens: II. Cooperation between subclasses of Ly$^+$ cells in the generation of killer activity. J Exp Med 1975;141:1390-1399.
36. Halle-Pannenko O, Pritchard LL, Motta R, Mathe G: Non-H-2 antigens can induce high GVH mortality in adult recipients of normal cells. Biomedicine 1978;29:253-255.

37. Hamilton BL, Bevan MJ, Parkman R: Anti-recipient cytotoxic T lymphocyte precursors are present in the spleens of mice with acute graft versus host disease due to minor histocompatibility antigens. J Immunol 1981;126:621-625.
38. OKunewick JP, Meredith RF, Raikow RB, Buffo MJ, Jones DL: Possibility of three distinct and separable components to fatal graft-versus-host reaction. Exp Hematol 1982;10:277-291.
39. Vallera DA, Soderling CCB, Carlson GJ, Kersey JH: Bone marrow transplantation across major histocompatibility barriers in mice. Effect of elimination of T cells from donor grafts by treatment with monoclonal Thy-1.2 plus complement or antibody alone. Transplantation 1981;31:218-222.
40. Norin AJ, Emeson EE, Veith FJ: Long-term survival of murine allogeneic bone marrow chimeras: effect of anti-lymphocyte serum and bone marrow dose. J Immunol 1981;126:428-432.
41. Korngold R, Sprent J: Features of T cells causing H-2 restricted lethal graft-vs-host disease across minor histocompatibility barriers. J Exp Med 1982;155:872-883.
42. OKunewick JP, Buffo MJ, Kociban DL: Evidence for two distinct mechanisms in acute fatal graft-versus-host reaction across minor histocompatibility barriers. Exp Hematol 1987,15:365-372.
43. Vallera DA, Soderling CCB, Kersey JH: Bone marrow transplantation across major histocompatibility barriers in mice: III. Treatment of donor grafts with monoclonal antibodies, directed against Lyt determinants. J Immunol 1982;128:871-875.
44. Korngold R, Sprent J: Surface markers of T cells causing lethal graft-vs-host disease to class I vs class II H-2 differences. J Immunol 1985;135:3004-3010.
45. Pietryga DW, Blazar BR, Soderling CCB, Vallera DA: The effect of T-subset depletion on the incidence of lethal graft-vs-host disease in a murine MHC-mismatched transplantation system. Transplantation 1987;43:442-444.
46. Koo GC, Peppard JR: Establishment of monoclonal anti-NK-1.1 antibody. Hybridoma 1984;3:301-303.
47. Blazar BR, Soderling CCB, Koo GC, Vallera DA: Absence of a facilitory role for NK 1.1-positive donor cells in engraftment across a major histocompatibility barrier in mice. Transplantation 1988;45:876-883.
48. Thierfelder S, Cobbold S, Kummer U, Waldmann H, Schuh R: Antilymphocytic antibodies and marrow transplantation. VII. Two of nine monoclonal anti-Thy-1 antibodies used for pretreatment of donor marrow suppressed graft-versus-host reactions without added complement. Exp Hematol 1985;13:948-955.
49. Cobbold S, Martin G, Waldmann H: Monoclonoal antibodies for the prevention of graft-versus-host disease and marrow graft rejection. The depletion of T cell subsets in vitro and in vivo. Transplantation 1986;42:239-247.
50. Ferrara JLM, Marion A, McIntyre JF, Murphy GF, Burakoff SJ: Amelioration of acute graft vs host disease due to minor histocompatibility antigens by in vivo administration of anti-interleukin 2 receptor antibody. J Immunol 1986;137:1874-1877.
51. Ritz J, Schlossman SF: Utilization of monoclonal antibodies in the treatment of leukemia and lymphoma. Blood 1982;59:1-11.
52. Scheinberg DA, Houghton AN: Current status of antitumor therapy with monoclonal antibodies. Oncology 1987;44:31-37.
53. Maraninchi D, Gluckman E, Blaise D, Guyotat D, Rio B, Pico JL, Leblond V, Michallet M, Dreyfus F, Ifrah N, Bordigoni A: Impact of T-cell depletion on outcome of allogeneic bone-marrow transplantation for standard-risk leukaemias. Lancet 1987; 2:175-178.
54. Eiklid K, Olsnes S, Pihl A: Entry of lethal doses of abrin, ricin, and modeccin into the cytosol of HeLa cells. Exp Cell Res 1980;126:321-326.

55. Endo Y, Kazuhiro M, Motizuki M, Tsurugi K: The mechanisms of action of ricin and related toxic lectins on eukaryotic ribosomes. The site and characteristics of the modification in 28S ribosomal RNA caused by toxins. J Biol Chem 1987;262: 5908-5912.

56. Olsnes S, Fernandez-Puentes C, Carrasco L, Vasquez D. Ribosome inactivation by the toxic lectins abrin and ricin. Kinetics of the enzymic activity of the toxin A-chains. Eur J Biochem 1975;60:281-288.

57. Vallera DA, Youle RJ, Neville Jr. DM, Kersey JH: Bone marrow transplantation across major histocompatibility barriers. V. Protection of mice from lethal graft-versus-host disease by pretreatment of donor cells with monoclonal anti-Thy-1.2 coupled to the toxin ricin. J Exp Med 1982;155:949-954.

58. Vallera DA, Youle RJ, Neville Jr. DM, Soderling CCB, Kersey JH: Monoclonal antibody-toxin conjugates for experimental graft-versus-host disease prophylaxis: Reagents selectively reactive with T cells and not murine stem cells. Transplantation 1983,36:73-80.

59. Filipovich AH, Vallera DA, Youle RJ, Haake R, Blazar BR, Neville Jr. DM, Ramsay NKC, McGlave P, Kersey JH: Graft-versus-host disease prevention in allogeneic bone marrow transplantation: A pilot study using immunotoxins for T cell depletion of donor bone marrow. Transplantation 1987;44:62-69.

60. Vallera DA: Immunotoxins for ex vivo bone marrow purging in human bone marrow transplantation, in *Immunotoxins*, edited by Frankel AE. Kluwer Academic Publishers, Boston, 1988; pp. 513-583.

61. Youle RJ, Neville Jr. DM: Kinetics of protein synthesis inactivation by ricin anti-Thy 1.1 monoclonal antibody hybrids. J Biol Chem 1982;257:1598-1601.

62. Manske JM, Buchsbaum DJ, Vallera DA: The role of ricin B chain in the intracellular trafficking of anti-CD5 immunotoxins. J Immunol 1989;142:1755-1766.

63. Weil-Hillman G, Uckun FM, Manske JM, Vallera DA: Combined immunochemotherapy of human solid tumors in nude mice. Cancer Res 1987;47:579-585.

64. Vallera D, Byers V, Smith J, Chang C, Blazar B: In vivo use of monoclonal antibody immunotoxins (ITs) for therapy of acute graft-versus-host disease (GVHD) across a major histocompatibility barrier in mice. J Cellular Biochem 1988;suppl 12C:115.

65. Hertler AA, Schlossman DM, Borowitz MJ, Laurent G, Jansen FK, Schmidt C, Frankel AE: A phase I study of T101-ricin A chain immunotoxin in refractory chronic lymphocytic leukemia. J Biol Response Mod 1988;7:97-113.

66. Laurent G, Pris J, Farcet J-P, Carayon P, Blythman H, Casellas P, Poncelet P, Jansen FK: Effects of therapy with T101 ricin A-chain immunotoxin in two leukemia patients. Blood 1986;67:1680-1687.

67. Spitler LE, del Rio M, Khentigan A, Wedel NI, Brophy NA, Miller LL, Harkonen WS, Rosendorf LL, Lee HM, Mischak RP, Kawahata RT, Stoudemire JB, Fradkin LB, Bautista EE, Scannon PJ: Therapy of patients with malignant melanoma using a monoclonal antimelanoma antibody-ricin A chain immunotoxin. Cancer Res 1987; 47:1717-1723.

68. Spitler LE: Clinical studies: solid tumors, in *Immunotoxins*, edited by Frankel AE. Kluwer Academic Publishers, Boston 1988; pp. 493-514.

69. Kernan NA, Byers V, Scannon PJ, Mischak RP, Brochstein J, Flomenberg N, Dupont B, O'Reilly RJ: Treatment of steroid-resistant acute graft-vs-host disease by in vivo administration of an anti-T-cell ricin A chain immunotoxin. JAMA 1988;259:3154-3157.

5

Experimental GVHD Across Minor Histocompatibility Barriers

Tom Maier and Henry N. Claman
University of Colorado School of Medicine
Denver, Colorado

I. INTRODUCTION

Graft-vs.-Host Disease (GVHD) was once believed to be a curiosity from the immunologist's laboratory. Since the development of "immunologic engineering," in particular the use of bone marrow (BM) transplantation in the treatment of leukemias and aplastic anemia, GVHD has risen to be a major clinical problem.

The focus of this chapter is the analysis of GVHD produced in experimental animals which differ in their minor histocompatibility antigens (MiHA). We might combine the abbreviations to call this phenomenon, MiHA-GVHD. In virtually all situations, the identities of the various minor antigen mismatches are not known. This is primarily because typing antisera for MiHA are not generally available.

There are two major reasons for the interest in MiHA-GVHD, aside from the general biological inquisitiveness about immunological reactions to non-major MHC.

- It is a model for human BM transplantation. In most clinical situations, the BM donor and the BM recipient are matched at the HLA-A,B,C and DR regions (i.e, they are "HLA identical"). Furthermore, the donor and recipient peripheral blood (T) cells neither stimulate nor respond to each other in the one-way or two-way mixed leukocyte reaction (MLR). Thus, donor and recipient are "MLR nonreactive." In many mouse systems, these same conditions often apply, i.e., the donors and recipients are "MHC-identical, MLR nonreactive," provided they are identical at the mls (minor lymphocyte stimulating) locus. Thus, animal systems of MiHA-GVHD are good models for GVHD across minor histocompatibility barriers in man.
- Some animal systems of MiHA-GVHD resemble human idiopathic autimmune syndromes. This is particularly true in one mouse model we have studied in detail. This model system resembles scleroderma and primary biliary cirrhosis (PBC) and will be discussed later.

II. MURINE MODELS OF MiHA-GVHD

Most models of MiHA-GVHD have been worked out in mice because we know the most about the transplantation antigens of this species. However, there are many variables involved in any given model, and one model system may differ from another in more ways than just the two strains used. Thus, one needs to consider whether the mls is involved, whether parental cells are given to F_1 recipients or to another parental strain, the age of the recipient, and whether it is irradiated or chemically immunosuppressed. Finally, various assays are used to assess the type and degree of MiHA-GVHD. These range from lethality (a crude but very definite endpoint) to subtleties of cellular immune function.

Table 1 (1-28) summarizes a variety of models in mice with attention being paid to the variables just mentioned. One can see that the most popular models involve the infusion of cells from parent-1 donors into irradiated adult parent-2 recipients. In such a system, it is obvious that recipient irradiation (or a suitable cytoreductive substitute) is necessary to diminish or eliminate the P_2 anti-P_1 (host-vs.-graft) component. It is worthwhile to note, however, that most $P \to F_1$ models of MiHA-GVHD also use recipient irradiation. While the "orthodox" (Medawarian) laws of transplantation suggest that there should be no host-vs.-graft activity in $P_1 \to (P_1 \times P_2)F_1$ combinations, the fact is that host irradiation greatly enhances the GVHD. This may be partly or wholly because there are F_1 antiparent reactions, which are radiosensitive (29). The most frequently studied

Table 1 Murine Models of GVHD Across Minor Histocompatibility Barriers

Barrier		Genetic direction	X-ray	Age of recipient newborn	Assays[a]	References
MiHA	mls					
+ (single)	?	$P_1 \to P_2$	+	Newborn	D, Spl, Skn	1
+	+	$P_1 \to F_1$	+	Adult	D, Hist	2
+	+	$P_1 \to F_1$	+	Adult	D, Hist, Supp, Spl	3-6
+	±	$P_1 \to P_2$	+	Adult	D, CTL	7-10
+	−	$P_1 \to P_2$	+	Adult	D, CTL, Hist	11-15
+	±	$P_1 \to P_2$	+	Adult	CTL	16
+	+	$P_1 \to P_2$	+	Adult	CTL, DTH	17
+	+	$P_1 \to P_2$	+	Adult	D, Hist	18
+	+	$P_1 \to P_2$	+	Adult	CTL, Supp	19
+	−	$P_1 \to P_2$	+	Adult	Hist, Wt	20
+	−	$P_1 \to P_2$	+	Adult	Supp, MLR	21,22
+	−	$P_1 \to F_1$	+	Adult	Cytokines	23,24
+	?	$P_1 \to P_2$	+	Adult	D, Hist	25
+	+	$P_1 \to P_2$	±	Adult	PLN	26
+	−	$P_1 \to P_2 \to F_1$	±	Adult	PLN	27
+	+	$P_1 \to P_2$	−	Adult	PLN, Spl	28

[a]Assays: D = death, DTH = delayed type hypersensitivity, Hist = histology, MLR = mixed leukocyte reaction, PLN = popliteal lymph node, Skn = skin graft rejection, Spl = splenomegaly, Supp = suppressor phenomena, Wt = body weight.

features of MiHA-GVHD have been lethality and lymphoid depeletion. In addition, anti-recipient cytotoxic T lymphocytes (CTL) and noncytotoxic T cells have been found as well as suppressor T and non-T cells and excesses and deficiencies in various cytokines. Histological results have been interesting in that they resemble not only the human pictures of acute and chronic GVHD but also the idiopathic autoimmune syndromes, scleroderma and PBC.

A.   Acute vs. Chronic MiHA-GVHD

The distinction between acute and chronic GVHD is somewhat arbitrary. Although the changes, particularly the histopathological appearances, differ between the acute and the chronic syndromes, it is wise to consider these two aspects of GVHD as a continuum. Furthermore, it is almost certain that any chronic MiHA-GVHD can be converted into an acute GVHD by changing any number of variables which would aggravate the donor-anti-host reactivity and alleviate the host-antidonor reactivity. These maneuvers include raising the number of grafted cells, increasing the proportion of mature T cells in the graft, increasing the immunosuppression of the recipient and possibly preimmunizing the donor against the recipient.

B.   The Nature of T Cells Initiating MiHA-GVHD

It is useful to know which donor T cells are critical for the induction of GVHD. (This subject is discussed at length in Chapter 00.) In MHC-GVHD, it is clear that donor $CD4^+$ cells are most important in GVHD across class II MHC barriers and donor $CD8^+$ cells are most important in GVHD across class I MHC barriers (8-10,30). The situation in MiHA-GVHD is not as clear. The importance of various subsets of donor T cells depends upon the strains of mice and the protocol. In the C57BL/6 → LP model, $CD8^+$ cells were critical. In the reverse model, both $CD8^+$ and $CD4^+$ cells were needed. In the B10.D2 → BALB/c combination, $CD4^+$ cells are far more important than $CD8^+$ cells (13). Another approach, again using lethality as a readout, showed that MiHA-GVHD induced by lymph node cell suspensions was more dependent on Lyt 2^+ cells, while that induced by spleen cell suspensions was more dependent on Lyt-1^+ cells (31).

   The reasons for these results escape us as yet because most of the current work is descriptive. Another unsolved problem is the degree of chimerism in these models. Because antibodies and markers which identify MiHA differences are not readily available or known, these studies cannot yet be done completely.

C.   Mechanisms of Tissue Damage in MiHA-GVHD

It is likely that different subsets of donor T cells will mediate different types of tissue damage in the various MiHA-GVHD systems. This has not been explored systematically. Often a group of investigators describes a GVHD model using one or several of a variety of assays to determine the degree of reaction. Rarely is there a comprehensive attempt to discover which mechanisms may be important for tissue damage and which may be irrelevant. Among the parameters measured are delayed-type hypersensitivity (17), Thy^+ suppressor cells (32), and natural suppressor (NS) cells (21-24). Cytotoxic T cells have been extensively investigated. Some appear to be donor antihost cells (12), while Parkman has derived autoreactive CTL clones (16). A histological study by Guillen (18) indicated that large granular leukocytes (LGL) appeared in acute MiHA-GVHD, and the investigators suggested that they might be natural killer (NK) cells. Our laboratory has persistently failed to find NK activity in the B10.D2 → BALB/c model (33), and we point out that NS cells (which we do find) also have the phenotype of LGL (33).

D. Cytokines and MiHA-GVHD

The role of various cytokines in the progression and pathogenesis of MiHA-GVHD is just now being explored. IFN-β has been implicated (23,24) as has IFN-γ (22-24,32). IFNs, at least indirectly, may be responsible for decreased IL-2 production (19). It is generally agreed that experimental chronic GVHD tends to wane with time if the animal survives. Although this has not been studied in great detail, the lymphocyte depletion in the tissues would tend to decrease the T-cell "signals" (i.e., cytokines) which drive GVHD, and gradually the autoreactive processes should cool down. This subject will be touched upon later in this chapter in Sec. IV.

III. IMMUNOLOGICAL ASPECTS OF A MiHA GVHD

A. GVHD Protocol

In our laboratory, we have utilized a murine model of chronic GVHD which closely resembles the clinical situation in BM transplantation (20,33). We use B10.D2 mice as donors and BALB/c (600r) as recipients. These two strains of mice are identical at both the MHC (H-2^d) and mls locus (mls^b), and, therefore, there is no primary in vitro MLR between these two strains of mice. As mentioned before this is similar to human BM transplantation where the donor and recipient are usually HLA-matched and MLR non-reactive in vitro.

The usual protocol that we use to induce chronic GVHD is to inject 5×10^7 B10.D2 spleen cells into BALB/c recipients that have received 600 rads of irradiation. Control mice include BALB/c (600r) that have received syngeneic BALB/c spleen cells or no spleen cells at all. The B10.D2 → BALB/c (600r) mice develop chronic GVHD that is characterized by weight loss (20), sclerodermatous-like cutaneous changes (20), liver pathology (34,35), and immunodeficiency (36). These conditions are also seen in human chronic GVHD following BM transplantation (37). At various times postinduction of GVHD, the spleen cells from these mice are removed and assayed in vitro for their ability to respond in various mitogen or MLR assays, and for their ability to suppress mitogen or MLR responses of normal spleen cells.

B. Immunodeficiency and Immunosuppression in MiHA GVHD

Table 2 shows that GVHD spleen cells are not able to respond to either the T-cell mitogen Con A or the B-cell mitogen LPS (36). The results in this table also show that the GVHD spleen cells contain potent suppressor activity. This was assayed by their ability to inhibit the Con A or LPS proliferative response of normal spleen cells. In contrast, the spleen cells from the control mice are able to respond to the mitogens (albeit at less than normal levels) and display very little ability to suppress normal spleen cell mitogen responses. Similar results are obtained in MLR and CTL assays utilizing the GVHD spleen cells as either responders or suppressors (38). Thus, spleen cells from mice undergoing GVHD are both immunologically unresponsive and contain potent suppressors of immune reactions (36).

Table 2 10-Day GVHD Spleen Cells Are Both Unresponsive to Mitogens and Suppress the Mitogen Response of Normal Spleen Cells[a]

	CPM $\times 10^{-3}$			
	Prolif. activity[b]		Supp. activity[c]	
Source of spleen cells	Con A prolif.	LPS prolif.	Supp. of Con A (% Cntrl)	Supp. of LPS (% Cntrl)
Normal BALB/c	325	111	356 (110)	117(105)
B10.D2 → BALB/c (600r)	1	1	5 (2)	4 (4)
BALB/c → BALB/c (600r)	143	29	348 (107)	96 (86)
None → BALB/c (600r)	98	4	333 (102)	90 (81)

[a]BALB/c (600r) mice were injected on day 0 and their spleen cells assayed 10 days later.

[b]2.5×10^5 spleen cells/well + either Con A or LPS.

[c]1×10^5 GVHD spleen cells were added to 2.5×10^5 normal BALB/c spleen cells + either Con A or LPS. Percent control is versus 2.5×10^5 normal BABL/c spleen cells + the appropriate mitogen.

C. GVHD Spleen Cells Suppress in a Genetically Unrestricted Manner

Table 3 shows that 10-day GVHD spleen cells can suppress the mitogen responses of spleen cells from MHC-disparate mouse strains (21). It should be noted that the GVHD spleen cells show their weakest suppression against the B10.D2 LPS response (B10.D2 is syngeneic to donor). The reason for this will be explained later in this section. GVHD spleen cells also suppress both MLR and CTL cultures in a genetically unrestricted manner (38).

Table 3 10-Day GVHD Spleen Cells Suppress Mitogen-Induced Proliferation in a Genetically Unrestricted Manner

		Spleen cells added[b]		
Resp. spleen cells[a]	Mitogen	None (CPM $\times 10^{-3}$)	GVHD (CPM $\times 10^{-3}$)	% Control response[c]
BALB/c	Con A	333	8	3
B10.D2	″	205	2	1
(BALB/c $\times$ B10.D2)F$_1$	″	262	5	2
C57BL/6	″	209	2	1
C3H/HeN	″	324	2	1
BALB/c	LPS	115	4	3
B10.D2	″	62	10	16
(BALB/c $\times$ B10.D2)F$_1$	″	71	5	7
C57BL/6	″	131	8	6
C3H/HeN	″	122	4	3

[a]2.5×10^5 normal responder spleen cells were cultured with the indicated mitogen.

[b]2.0×10^5 10-day GVHD spleen cells were added to the indicated cultures.

[c]Percent control is versus 2.5×10^5 normal spleen cells + mitogen.

Table 4 Characteristics of GVHD Splenic Suppressor Cells

Thy 1.2⁻
Ig⁻
Plastic nonadherent
Enriched in light density   →   Therefore, Natural Suppressors (NS)
Percoll fractions
NK 1.1⁻
Do not kill YAC-1

D. Characterization of GVHD Splenic Suppressor Cells

Table 4 summarizes some of the more important characteristics of the suppressor cells found in the B10.D2 → BALB/c GVHD spleens (21). If the GVHD spleen cells are treated with anti-Thy 1.2 + C′ to remove T cells, the majority of the suppressor activity is left intact. If the GVHD spleen cells are panned on anti-Ig coated plates to remove B cells, again the suppressor activity is left intact. When plastic-adherent, esterase-positive macrophages were removed from GVHD spleen cells, the suppression is also untouched. These and other data indicate that the suppressor cells found in GVHD spleen are not mature T cells, B cells, or macrophages.

The suppressor activity present in GVHD spleen can be enriched in light-density Percoll fractions (22). All the above characteristics—Thy⁻, Ig⁻, plastic nonadherence, and enrichment in light-density Percoll fractions—are found with NK cells. However, the suppressor cells found in GVHD spleen are not eliminated by anti-NK 1.1 + C′ treatment, and they do not lyse the NK-sensitive target YAC-1. Thus, these suppressor cells found in chronic GVHD have been called natural suppressor (NS) cells (21,39), because of their similarities to NK cells and their inhibitory activity.

E. Cellular Requirements for the In Vivo Induction of GVHD NS Cell Activity

Donor T cells are required and sufficient for the induction of lethal GVHD (7), so we investigated whether T cells alone are sufficient to induce GVHD immunoincompetence and suppression in our system (40). Table 5 shows that when untreated B10.D2 spleen cells were given to BALB/c (600r) recipients, the recipient spleen cells were unresponsive to Con A and also suppressive of a normal Con A response. However, if the donor spleen cells were treated with anti-Thy 1.2 + C′ to remove T cells, the resulting unresponsiveness and suppression were much less evident. Donor nylon wool-nonadherent lymph node (NW-NA LN) cells, as an enriched source of T cells, induced only modest unresponsiveness and suppressor activity. However, mixtures of T-depleted spleen and T-cell-enriched NW-NA LN cells produced significant unresponsiveness and also induced potent suppression. As few as 5% LN T cells added to 95% T-depleted spleen cells produced more unresponsiveness and suppression than could be expected from the sum of their separate abilities. Thus, it seems that although T cells are required (but not sufficient) for in vivo induction of GVHD suppression, only a relatively small number of them are sufficient for maximum induction if non-T cells are coinjected.

Table 5 T and non-T Cells Are Required for the In Vivo Induction of Maximum NS Activity

Cell type and No. injected[a]			CPM × 10^{-3}	
Untreated spleen	Anti-Thy + C' spleen	NW-NA LNC	Con A response[b]	Supp. of Con A (% Supp.)[c]
Normal BALB/c:			311	356 (−14)
Experimental:				
B10.D2:				
4 × 10^7	−	−	0	35 (89)
−	4 × 10^7	−	39	320 (−3)
−	−	4 × 10^7	18	254 (18)
−	2 × 10^7	2 × 10^7	0	85 (73)
−	3.3 × 10^7	6.7 × 10^6	0	67 (78)
−	3.8 × 10^7	2.2 × 10^6	1	83 (73)
−	−	−	149	346 (−11)

[a]B10.D2 cells of the indicated type were injected into BALB/c (600r) hosts on day 0. Normal BALB/c are mice neither irradiated nor injected. The cell types injected were either untreated spleen cells, or anti-Thy 1.2 + complement-treated spleen cells (i.e., T-cell-depleted), or nylon wool-nonadherent (NW-NA) lymph node cells (i.e., T-cell-enriched) or a mixture of the later two. The GVHD spleen cells were assayed 10 days later.

[b]2.5 × 10^5 spleen cells/well + Con A (4 μg/ml).

[c]1 × 10^5 GVHD spleen cells were added to 2.5 × 10^5 normal BALB/c spleen cells + either Con A or LPS. Percent control response is versus 2.5 × 10^5 normal BALB/c spleen cells + the appropriate mitogen.

Since NS cells do not bear phenotypic markers of mature T cells, we believe that NS cells arise from the non-T-cell population (probably the stem cells). We hypothesize that the development of maximum NS cell activity from the non-T-cell population requires T-cell "signals" which, in this system, are generated from donor T cells reacting against recipient minor histocompatibility antigens.

F. NS-Cell Activity Requires T-Cell "Signals" In Vitro

From the above it is apparent that T cells are required for the in vivo *induction* of NS-cell activity in this model of chronic GVHD. This led us to explore the role of T cells in the *expression* of NS activity in vitro.

Figure 1 shows that GVHD-induced NS cell activity is long lasting but does wane slowly (21,33). As time goes on post-GVHD induction, it becomes relatively more difficult for the GVHD splenic NS cells to suppress an LPS response compared to a Con A response.

We think this relative inability to suppress an LPS response versus a Con A response is because NS cells are stimulated by activated T cells (probably via lymphokines) and can therefore suppress any in vitro response where activated T cells are present. This would be especially apparent when GVHD NS cells are become quiescent late in GVHD (i.e., >40 days). Thus, late GVHD spleen cells cannot suppress an LPS response because very few if any T cells are activated by this B-cell mitogen. This is especially apparent using indicator spleen cells that are syngeneic to the NS cells, as this eliminates

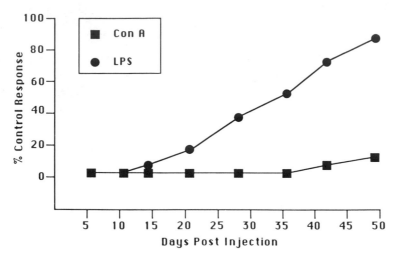

Figure 1 GVHD spleen cells lose the ability to suppress the LPS response of B10.D2 cells with time. BALB/c (600r) recipients were injected on day 0 with 5×10^7 B10.D2 spleen cells. At various times subsequently, 2×10^7 GVHD spleen cells were cocultured with 2.5×10^7 normal B10.D2 spleen cells plus either Con A or LPS. Percent control response is versus 2.5×10^7 normal B10.D2 spleen cells plus the appropriate mitogen.

any MLR-type reactions which may also activate T cells. On the other hand, these same late GVHD spleen cells can suppress a Con A response because this mitogen stimulates large numbers of T cells.

If the above is correct, one should be able to activate the NS cells in the LPS suppressor assay by the addition of activated T cell "signals" (lymphokines) (22,40). Figure 2 (A) shows that Con A supernate (CAS) as a source of activated T-cell signals can stimulate NS activity in an LPS suppressor assay to almost 100% suppression. Note that the CAS has little effect on the responder population alone. Therefore, GVHD NS cells can be activated by T-cell signals.

We wanted to know what component of the CAS was activating the NS cells. Figure 2 (B and C) also shows that two molecules, recombinant IFN-gamma (rIFN-γ) and recombinant IL-2 (rIL-2), were found to mimic CAS enhancement of GVHD NS activity in vitro.

Note the relatively small amounts of IFN-γ and the large amounts of rIL-2 required for NS stimulation. This and other data led us to the idea that the IL-2 was not directly stimulating the NS activity, but was doing so by stimulating the production of IFN-γ, which was then activating NS cells. We used anti-IFN-γ antibody to see if this was the case (41). If IL-2 was working indirectly by stimulating the production of IFN-γ, then anti-IFN-γ should inhibit IL-2 enhancement of GVHD NS activity. Figure 3 (A) shows that this is indeed the case. Figure 3B also shows that the anti-IFN-γ inhibits the GVHD spleen cell suppression of a Con A response. Therefore, the activated T-cell signal that NS cells respond to is IFN-γ, and IL-2 acts indirectly by its ability to stimulate IFN-γ synthesis.

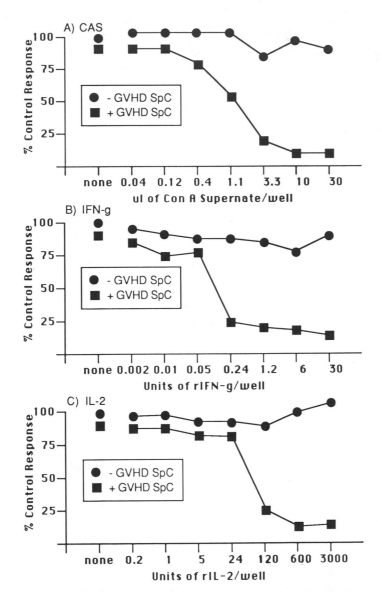

Figure 2 48-day GVHD spleen cell suppression of a B10.D2 LPS response is greatly enhanced by the addition of T-cell lymphokines. 48-day GVHD spleen cells (2×10^5) were added to 2.5×10^5 normal B10.D2 spleen cells + LPS. These assays were performed with or without the addition of various concentrations of (A) Con A supernate (CAS), (B) recombinant IFN-gamma (rIFN-g), or (C) recombinant IL-2 (rIL-2). Percent control response is versus 2.5×10^5 B10.D2 spleen cells + LPS.

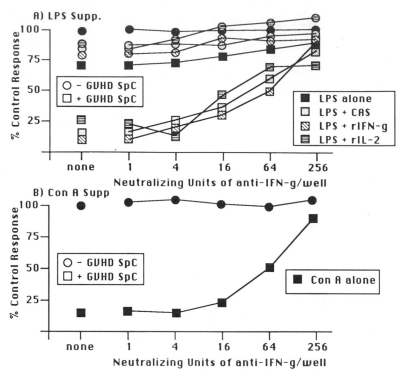

Figure 3 Addition of anti-IFN-g antibody removes the ability of 48-day GVHD spleen cells to suppress, and also removes the ability of CAS, rIFN-g, and rIL-2 to enhance suppression. 48-day GVHD spleen cells (2×10^5) were added to 2.5×10^5 normal B10.D2 spleen cells + LPS alone, LPS + CAS (15 ul), LPS + rIFN-g (7 U), or LPS + rIL-2 (70 U) in panel A, and Con A in panel B. The mitogen responses of the indicator cells without GVHD spleen cells is shown in circles; the response of the indicator cells plus GVHD spleen cells is shown in squares. The suppressor assays were done with or without various amounts of anti-IFN-g antibody, which is depicted as the amount of IFN-g it can neutralize. Percent control is versus 2.5×10^5 B10.D2 spleen cells + LPS for panel A, and + Con A for panel B.

G. Exogenous IL-2 Does Not Remove Suppressor Activity Caused by GVHD Spleen Cells

As mentioned before, GVHD splenic NS cells can inhibit MLR and CTL responses just as they do mitogen assays. It is possible that the suppression of MLR and CTL cultures by the NS cells is due to their consumption of interleukin-2 (IL-2) produced during the assay. To test this and an alternative possibility that the suppression is due to an induced overridable defect in IL-2 production, exogenous recombinant IL-2 was added to MLR cultures used to show GVHD NS cell suppression of CTL generation (38). Table 6 shows that the addition of up to 1000 U/ml of IL-2 has little effect on the CTL generated in an BALB/c anti-C57BL/6 MLR. Moreover, the added IL-2 (10 and 100 U/ml) has little effect on the suppression mediated by 5×10^6 or 1×10^6 GVHD spleen cells whereas 1000 U/ml of IL-2 resulted in a tendency toward enhanced suppression. These data show that IL-2 is not the limiting factor in the cultures where NS cell suppression is taking place.

Table 6 Suppression by GVHD Spleen Cells Is Not Reversed with Exogenous IL-2[a]

| | | GVHD SpC | | % Lysis of EL-4 | |
| | | added $\times$ 10^{-6} | | 6:1 | 50:1 |
Stimulator	Responder		IL-2(U/ml)		
C57BL/6	BALB/c	—	—	31	60
C57BL/6	BALB/c	—	10	34	59
C57BL/6	BALB/c	—	100	40	62
C57BL/6	BALB/c	—	1000	45	63
C57BL/6	BALB/c	5	—	0	4
C57BL/6	BALB/c	5	10	2	4
C57BL/6	BALB/c	5	100	1	4
C57BL/6	BALB/c	5	1000	−2	−2
C57BL/6	BALB/c	1	—	3	15
C57BL/6	BALB/c	1	10	5	17
C57BL/6	BALB/c	1	100	6	16
C57BL/6	BALB/c	1	1000	−1	7

[a]Stimulator cells (5×10^6) and 5×10^6 responder cells ± irradiated, day 12 GVHD spleen cells were cultured for 5 days with or without added IL-2. Cells were assayed for cytotoxicity in standard 4-hr ^{51}Cr-release assay using EL-4 as targets.

H. Direct Cell Contact Is Not Required for GVHD Splenic Suppression

To examine the possibility that GVHD splenic NS cells might mediate their suppressive activity via soluble factor(s), experiments were done with culture well inserts which separate cell populations by a microporous membrane (38). Table 7 shows some of this work. The simple presence of the chambers has no significant effect on the generation of BALB/c anti-C57BL/6 CTL (first line). This table shows the suppressive effect of GVHD spleen cells added into the chambers on the generation of CTL on the outside (lines 4 and 5 versus lines 2 and 3). Here it can be seen that while some of the suppression is lost, a significant amount remains. These results indicate that conjugate formation between suppressors and effectors is not required for suppression; however, close cell contact does appear to allow for more efficient suppression. The results suggest further that the suppression may be mediated at least in part by soluble factor(s).

I. Suppression by GVHD Spleen Cells Is Partially Removed by Indomethacin

Since some prostaglandins are known to be inhibitory of many immune functions, indomethacin, an inhibitor of prostaglandin synthesis, was added to the MLR used to generate CTL (38). The presence of 5×10^{-6} and 5×10^{-5} M indomethacin in the cultures had little effect on the generation of BALB/c anti-C57BL/6 CTL, as shown in the first three lines of Table 8. In lines 4-6, 5×10^6 GVHD spleen cells were added to the MLR cultures with or without indomethacin. It is seen here that some of the suppression is reversed. This reversal of suppression by indomethacin, although still incomplete, is more apparent when fewer GVHD spleen cells (2×10^6) are cocultured. These results suggest that prostaglandins are involved in the suppression mediated by GVHD spleen cells.

Table 7 Direct Cell Contact is Not Required for GVHD Splenic NS Suppressor activity[a]

	Location			% Lysis of EL-4 by cells from the outer chamber	
Resp. + Stim.		GVHD SpC			
outside	inside	outside	inside	12:1	50:1
+	−	−	−	25	49
+	−	5×10^6	−	−3	−5
+	−	2×10^6	−	−1	19
+	−	−	5×10^6	5	24
+	−	−	2×10^6	21	36

[a]Chambers with a microporous membrane were inserted into culture wells. BALB/c responders (5×10^6) and C57BL/6 stimulators (5×10^6) were cultured in wells outside chambers, and the CTL activity of these outside chambers was assayed 5 days later. Irradiated 10-day GVHD spleen cells (2×10^6 or 5×10^6) were added to either the inside or outside of the chambers.

Table 8 Suppression by GVHD Spleen Cells is Partially Removed by Indomethacin[a]

Stimulator	Responder	GVHD SpC Added $\times 10^{-6}$	Indomethacin concentration	% Lysis of EL-4	
				6:1	50:1
C57BL/6	BALB/c	−	−	23	68
C57BL/6	BALB/c	−	5×10^{-6}	23	62
C57BL/6	BALB/c	−	5×10^{-5}	28	72
C57BL/6	BALB/c	5×10^6	−	−2	−3
C57BL/6	BALB/c	5×10^6	5×10^{-6}	−1	9
C57BL/6	BALB/c	5×10^6	5×10^{-5}	−2	17
C57BL/6	BALB/c	2×10^6	−	6	27
C57BL/6	BALB/c	2×10^6	5×10^{-6}	12	47
C57BL/6	BALB/c	2×10^6	5×10^{-5}	12	56

[a]Stimulator cells (5×10^6) and 5×10^6 responder cells ± irradiated, day-10 GVHD spleen cells were cultured for 5 days with or without added indomethacin. Cells were assayed for cytotoxicity in standard 4-hr ^{51}Cr-release assay using EL-4 as targets.

However, these data do not indicate if they are the final suppressor effector molecules produced by GVHD NS cells or if they may be involved in a more proximal step in a cascade of events leading to suppression.

J. Model of Immunological Aspects Seen in This Murine GVHD System

Figure 4 depicts a simple model of what we think may be occurring in this MiHA-GVHD system to induce such potent immunodeficiency and immunosuppression. T cells from the B10.D2 spleen cell inoculum react with BALB/c MiHA in the recipient. These activated T cells, among other things, release various cytokines. Included among these cytokines are growth factors which can influence stem cell proliferation and differentiation. Therefore, in this model there is rapid proliferation of B10.D2 stem cells in the irradiated BALB/c host. Associated with this stem cell proliferation is the development of NS cell activity. (NS cell activity is associated with environments of rapid stem cell proliferation [39].) Finally, these NS cells, which are themselves very responsive to T-cell cytokines, become highly activated by other cytokines (e.g., IFN-γ) produced by the BALB/c reactive B10.D2 T cells. Thus, the final outcome is the induction of a highly suppressive environment in these animals undergoing chronic GVHD.

K. Summary and Conclusions of NS Cell Activity in Mice Undergoing Chronic GVHD Across MiHA

In summary, the immunologic findings concerning the immunodeficiency associated with chronic GVHD in this model are as follows:

- The spleen cells of mice undergoing chronic GVHD are immunologically unresponsive in vitro.

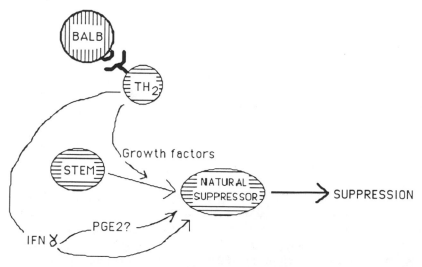

Figure 4 A schematic representation of the development of natural suppressors in chronic GVHD. Growth factors may include IL-3, IL-4, heparin-binding growth factors, etc.

●The spleen cells of GVHD mice are very suppressive of normal mitogen, MLR, and
  CTL responses.
●This suppression is genetically unrestricted.
●The cells responsible for this suppression are plastic nonadherent, Ig⁻, Thy⁻, and NK
  1.1⁻, and can be enriched in light density Percoll fractions.

Therefore, *GVHD suppression is caused by natural suppressor (NS) cells.*

●NS-cell activity develops rapidly in the spleens of GVHD mice, is maximal about 2
  weeks, and slowly wanes with time.
●GVHD NS cells suppress a Con A response more easily than an LPS response.
●However, the NS suppressive ability towards an LPS response can be enhanced by CAS,
  rIFN-γ, or rIL-2.
●Anti-IFN-γ antibody removes the ability of rIL-2 as well as the rIFN-γ and CAS to ac-
  tivate the NS cells, and thus it appears that the IL-2 is working via the stimulation
  of IFN-γ production.
●Anti-IFN-γ antibody also removes the ability of the GVHD NS cells to suppress a Con
  A response.

Therefore, *GVHD NS cells are responsive to T-cell signals (IFN-γ).*

●The suppression by NS cells is not due to their consumption of or interference with the
  production of IL-2.
●The suppression by NS cells can be partially overcome by indomethacin.
●The suppression by NS cells is at least partially mediated by a soluble factor(s).

Finally, we have extended these findings to NS-cell activity found in other loca-
tions, including normal BM and after the cytoreductive/immunosuppressive protocol of
high dose cyclophosphamide (21,41,42). Thus, an increased understanding of NS cells
and their activity is especially important in bone marrow transplantation, where the cyto-
reductive/immunosuppressive pretransplantation regimen, the bone marrow inoculum,
and the frequent development of GVHD all have NS-cell activity associated with them.

IV. MINOR HISTOCOMPATIBILITY GVHD AS A MODEL FOR AUTOIMMUNE DISEASES

As mentioned in the beginning of this chapter, MiHA-GVHD is of great interest because
the clinical picture resembles several autoimmune syndromes. These same syndromes also
occur in human MiHA-GVHD, but these situations are obviously less manipulable than
laboratory models.

A. Histology of Chronic GVHD

An early description came from Stastny et al., who described GVHD (then called "homologous disease") in rats, where the histological picture was reminiscent of systemic lupus
erythematosus and scleroderma (43). A more complete histological description was provided by Halle-Pannenko and her group, using the B10.D2 → (B10.D2 × DBA/2) model
(2). They described both acute and chronic GVHD. As mentioned before, we have explored the B10.D2 → BALB/c (600r) model because it closely resembles the clinical situation in which BM donors and recipients differ only at loci for MiHA and whose cells were
unreactive in the MLR (33). Not only did we find activation of the NS system, but there

was extensive evidence of scleroderma-like changes in the skin (20). These changes included: (1) increased collagen deposition and cutaneous fibrosis, (2) a mononuclear cell infiltrate containing T helpers, T suppressors, and macrophages but no B cells, (3) loss of dermal fat and appendages, (4) increased MHC class II (Ia) antigens on the epidermal cells and the dermal fibroblasts (44).

B. Mast Cell Changes in MiHA-GVHD

A most unexpected finding was the inability to find mast cells in the skin of MiHA-GVHD mice (45). Another group had independently noted the same cutaneous mast cell "dropout" (25). We then devised a double fluorescent technique to detect granulated and degranulated mast cells (46), which allowed us to follow up these observations. These studies led us to the conclusion that mast cells were indeed present in normal numbers in the skin of MiHA-GVHD mice but were degranulated and were therefore not seen with standard toluidine blue stains. This is because toluidine blue stains mast cell granules and not mast cell membranes. We called these degranulated cells "phantom mast cells" (amid some opposition to the term). Of even more significance was the demonstration by electron microscopy that "phantom mast cells" were not only degranulated, but were also activated to become secretory rather than resting storage cells (47). We do not know what they are secreting, but it is our opinion that the activated mast cell is causally related to the fibrotic process (48,49), possibly through the mediation of heparin-binding growth factors, as shown in Figure 5 (see below).

C. Application of These Findings to Scleroderma

We have been anxious to see if these mast cell changes also occur in human idiopathic scleroderma. Certainly patients with this disease show cutaneous changes similar to those seen in chronic experimental MiHA-GVHD, namely, cutaneous fibrosis and mononuclear cell inflammation, loss of dermal fat and appendages, and increased dermal expression of class II MHC antigens (50). So far, our results indicate that patients with scleroderma also have increased mast cell numbers (51) and increased mast cell reactivity to histamine liberators (52). There are preliminary findings that "phantom" (degranulated) mast cells are more common in scleroderma than in normal skin (53). Whether these changes are causative or epiphenomena with regard to chronic fibrosis remains to be seen.

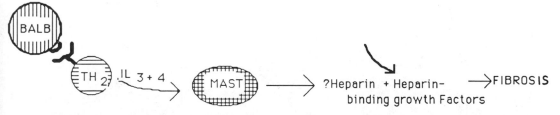

Figure 5 A schematic representation of mast-cell-dependent fibrosis. Mast cells are activated by TH$_2$ products such as IL-3 and IL-4. Heparin is released from activated mast cells and acts in concert with heparin-binding growth factors (from a variety of cells, including T cells, endothelial cells and macrophages).

V. UNIFICATION OF SUPPRESSIVE AND
IMMUNOPATHOGENIC ASPECTS OF CHRONIC GVHD

It may be useful to try to integrate the two main thrusts of this chapter, namely the *inflammatory and fibrotic changes* of chronic GVHD induced across minor histocompatibility barriers and *natural suppression.*

The basic mechanism starts with alloreactive donor T cells recognizing and reacting against the foreign MiHA in the recipient. Why this is so difficult to demonstrate in vitro in a primary MLR is difficult to understand. The rapid rejection of skin grafts across MiHA barriers suggests that it is not due merely to a paucity of precursor donor T cells. During this GVH reaction, various T-cell lymphokines are undoubtedly generated and liberated (23,24), and an inflammatory process is initiated, which is most marked in the skin (44) although other organs may be involved (2,34,35).

We may be biased because of all the work we have done on activated mast cells in chronic GVHD, but it is possible to explain several apparently unrelated phenomena using the mast cell as a link.

The possible role of activated mast cells in fibrosis has been raised primarily because of pathological findings showing that fibrotic conditions have increased numbers of mast cells (48,49). More recent work on the nature of various growth factors, including endothelial cell-derived growth factor (ECGF), and angiogensis factors, and both acidic and basic fibroblast growth factors has shown that these comprise a class of "heparin-binding growth factors" (HBGF) (54). Indeed, these factors are best purified on heparin columns. We propose that mast cell activation leads to heparin release and the potentiation of HBGF with resulting fibrosis. The details of this hypothesis are unknown, but the general schema is shown in Figure 5.

The possible relation of mast cells to natural suppressor activity is also of interest. We believe that natural suppression is probably not a function of a single cell type, but a function that might be carried out by a number of cells of different lineages. Our discussion earlier in this chapter mentioned that NS activity is highest at times when hemato-

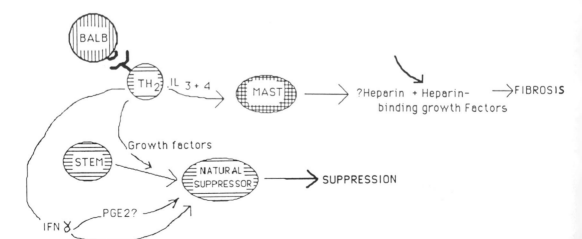

Figure 6 A schematic representation of natural suppressor cell development and the activation of mast-cell-dependent fibrotic pathways.

poietic stem cells are proliferative, a point emphasized by Strober (55) and us (39). Therefore, we see NS activity in GVHD models, in the context of hematopoietic stem cell activity, initiated by donor stem cells (usually in an irradiated environment) and abetted by T-cell signals favoring hematopoiesis, such as colony-stimulating factors (CSFs). Some of these cytokines, such as IL-3 and IL-4, are active on mast cells and their precursors. Active mast cells are probably involved in fibrosis (see above) and, in addition natural suppressor cells derived from newborn mice have been shown to have NS activity and to respond to IL-3 (56). Although a cell that responds to IL-3 is not necessarily a mast cell precursor, the latter is one of the prime targets of IL-3. We speculate that the GVHD environment includes sufficient T-cell signals to activate NS cells derived from the inoculum (and which may be of the mast cell lineage) and to activate resident host mast cells to become involved in the fibrotic process. This schema is outlined in Figure 6, which combines the schema of Figures 4 and 5.

ACKNOWLEDGMENTS

We thank Drs. Bruce Jaffee, James Holda, Ken Lee Choi, Ralph Giorno, Richard A. F. Clark, and Clark Huff for their scientific contributions, Mrs. Roberta Fairchild for her excellent technical assistance, and Miss Kathryn Utschinski for her secretarial skills.

Supported in part by The Arthritis Foundation, The Leukemia Society of America, The Medical Research Council of Ontario, NIH grants AR-31220 and CA-47657, and RGK Foundation, and the Rocky Mountain Chapter of The Arthritis Foundation.

REFERENCES

1. Cantrell JL, and Hildemann WH: Characteristics of disparate histocompatibility barriers in congenic strains of mice. I. Graft-versus-host reactions. Transplantation 1972;14:761-770.
2. Rappaport H, Khalil A, Halle-Pannenko O, Pritchard L, Dantchev D, Mathe G: Histopathologic sequence of events in adult mice undergoing lethal graft-versus-host reaction developed across H-2 and/or non-H-2 histocompatibility barriers. Am J Path 1979;96:121-142.
3. Halle-Pannenko O, Pritchard LL, Mathe G: Immunobiology of minor histocompatibility antigens in the lethal graft-versus-host reaction induced in adult mice. In *Immunobiology of Bone Marrow Transplantations*, edited by Thierfelder S, Rodt H, Kolb HJ. Springer-Verlag, Berlin, Heidelberg, New York, 1980; pp. 75-91.
4. Halle-Pannenko O, Pritchard LL, Motta R et al.: Lethal graft-versus-host reaction to minor histocompatibility antigens is decreased by donor immunization against H-2 and varies as a function of the H-2 haplotype. Transplant Proc 1979;XI:652-656.
5. Halle-Pannenko O, Pritchard LL, Rappaport H: Alloimmunization-activated suppressor cells. I. Abrogation of lethal graft-versus-host reaction directed against non-H-2 antigens. Transplantation 1983;36:60-68.
6. Pritchard LL, Halle-Pannenko O: Interactions of major and minor histocompatibility antigens in the graft-versus-host reaction. Transplantation 1981;31:257-261.
7. Korngold R, Sprent J: Lethal graft-versus-host disease after bone marrow transplantation across minor histocompatibility barriers in mice: Prevention by removing mature T cells from marrow. J Exp Med 1978;148:1687-1698.
8. Sprent J and Korngold R: Immunogenetics of graft-versus-host reactions to minor histocompatibility antigens. Immunol Today 1981;10:189-195.

9. Korngold R, Sprent J: Variable capacity of L3T4$^+$ T cells to cause lethal graft-versus-host disease across minor histocompatibility barriers in mice. J Exp Med 1987;165:1552-1564.

10. Korngold R, Sprent J: Surface markers of T cells causing lethal graft-vs-host disease in class I vs Class II H-2 differences. J Immunol 1985;135:3004-3010.

11. Hamilton BL: Absence of correlation between cytolytic T lymphocytes and lethal murine graft-versus-host disease in response to minor histocompatibility antigens. Transplantation 1984;38:357-360.

12. Hamilton BL, Parkman R: Kinetics of the anti-recipient cytotoxic cell response of mice with minor histocompatibility antigen graft-vs-host disease. J Immunol 1982;128:376-379.

13. Hamilton BL: L3T4-positive T cells participate in the induction of graft-vs-host disease in response to minor histocompatibility antigens. J Immunol 1987;139:2511-2515.

14. Hamilton BL, Bevan MJ, Parkman R: Anti-recipient cytotoxic T lymphocyte precursors are present in the spleens of mice with acute graft-versus-host disease due to minor histocompatibility antigens. J Immunol 1981;126:621-625.

15. Hamilton BL, Parkman R: Acute and chronic graft-versus-host disease induced by minor histocompatibility antigens in mice. Transplantation 1983;36:150-155.

16. Parkman R: Clonal analysis of murine graft-vs-host disease. I. Phenotypic and functional analysis of T lymphocyte clones. J Immunol 1986;136:3543-3548.

17. Bril H, Molendijk-Lok BD, Hussaarts-Odijk LM, Benner R: Synergism of T lymphocyte subsets in the response to mls-locus coded antigens during graft-versus-host reaction. Cell Immunol 1984;83:370-378.

18. Guillen FJ, Ferrara J, Hancock WW, Messadi D, Fonferko E, Burakoff SJ, Murphy GF: Acute cutaneous graft-versus-host disease to minor histocompatibility antigens in a murine model: Evidence that large granular lymphocytes are effector cells in the immune response. Lab Invest 1986;55:35-42.

19. Ferrara JLM, Daley JP, Burakoff SJ, Miller RA: Functional T cell deficits after bone marrow transplantation across minor histocompatibility barriers: Effects of graft-vs-host disease on precursor frequency of reactive cells. J Immunol 1987;138:3598-3603.

20. Jaffee BD, Claman HN: Chronic graft-versus-host disease (GVHD) as a model for scleroderma. I. Description of model systems. Cell Immunol 1983;77:1-12.

21. Maier T, Holda JH, Claman HN: Graft-versus-host reactions (GVHR) across minor murine histocompatibility barriers. II. Development of natural suppressor cell activity. J Immunol 1985;135:1644-1651.

22. Holda JH, Maier T, Claman HN: Natural suppressor activity in graft-vs-host spleen and normal bone marrow is augmented by IL-2 and interferon-γ. J Immunol 1986;137:3538-3543.

23. Cleveland MG, Lane RG, Klimpel GR: Spontaneous IFN-β production: A common feature of natural suppressor systems. J Immunol 1988;141:2043-2049.

24. Cleveland MG, Annable CR, Klimpel GR: In vivo and in vitro production of IFN-β and IFN-γ during graft vs host disease. J Immunol 1988;141:3349-3356.

25. Charley MR, Bangert JL, Hamilton BL, Gilliam JN, Sontheimer RD: Murine graft-versus-host skin disease: A chronologic and quantitative analysis of two histologic patterns. J Invest Derm 1983;81:412-417.

26. Salaman MH, Wedderburn N, Festenstein H, Huber B. Detection of a graft-versus-host reaction between mice compatible at the H-2 locus. Transplantation 1973;16:29-31.

27. Claman HN, Jaffee BD: Minor antigen graft-versus-host reactions revealed in irradiated spleen and popliteal lymph node assays. Transplantation 1984;38:392-395.

28. Lilliehook B, Blomgren H: Weak graft-versus-host response of CBA lymphocytes against the H-2 identical strain, C3H. Scand J Immunol 1974;3:637-644.
29. Bellgrau D, Smilek D, Wilson DB: Induced tolerance in F_1 rats to anti-major histocompatibility complex receptors on parental cells. J Exp Med 1981;153:1660-1665.
30. Korngold R, Sprent J: Lethal GVHD across minor histocompatibility barriers: Nature of the effector cells and role of the H-2 complex. Immunol Rev 1983;71: 5-29.
31. Okunewick JP, Buffo MJ, Kociban DL: Evidence for two distinct mechanisms in acute fatal graft-versus-host reaction across minor histocompatibility barriers. Exp Hematol 1987;15:365-372.
32. Wall DA, Hamberg SD, Reynolds DS, Burakoff SJ, Abbas AK, Ferrara JLM: Immunodeficiency in graft-versus-host disease. I. Mechanism of immune suppression. J Immunol 1988;140:2970-2976.
33. Holda JH, Maier T, Claman HN: Murine graft-versus-host disease across minor barriers: Immunosuppressive aspects of natural suppressor cells. Immunol Rev 1985; 88:87-105.
34. Vierling JM, Ruderman WB, Jaffee BD, Fennell RH Jr, Claman HN: Hepatic lesions in murine chronic graft-versus-host disease to minor histocompatibility antigens: A reproducible model of non suppurative destructive cholangitis. Transplantation 1900;48:717-718.
35. Ruderman WB, Jaffee BD, Fennell RH Jr, Claman HN, Vierling JM: Evolution of hepatic lesions in murine chronic graft-versus-host disease to minor histocompati-unpublished observations.
36. Holda JH, Maier T, Claman HN: Graft-versus-host reactions (GVHR) across minor histocompatibility barriers. I. Impairment of mitogen responses and suppressor phenomena. J Immunol 1985;134:1397-1402.
37. Press DW, Schaller RT, Thomas ED: Bone marrow transplant complications. In *Complications of Organ Transplantation*, edited by Toledo-Pereyra LH. Marcel Dekker, New York, 1987; pp. 399-424.
38. Lee Choi K, Maier T, Holda JH, Claman HN: Suppression of alloreactive cytotoxic T cell generation by natural suppressor cells from mice with graft-vs-host disease. Cell Immunol 1988;112:271-278.
39. Maier T, Holda JH, Claman HN: Natural suppressor (NS) cells: Member of the LGL regulatory family. Immunol Today 1986;7:312-315.
40. Maier T, Holda JH, Claman HN: Synergism between T and non-T cells in the in vivo induction and in vitro expression of graft-versus-host disease induced natural suppressor cells. J Exp Med 1985;162:979-992.
41. Holda JH, Maier T, Claman HN: IFN-gamma is responsible for natural suppressor activity in GVHD spleen and normal bone marrow. Transplantation 1988;45:772-777.
42. Maier T, Holda JH, Claman HN: Murine natural suppressor (NS) cells in newborn, in bone marrow, and after cyclophosphamide: Genetic variations is dependent on IFN-γ. J Immunol 1989;143:491-498.
43. Stastny P, Stembridge VA, Ziff M: Homologous disease in the adult rat, a model for autoimmune disease. I. General features and cutaneous lesions. J Exp Med 1963; 118:635-648.
44. Giorno R, Lee Choi K, Katz HR, Claman HN: Monoclonal antibody analysis of skin in chronic murine graft-vs.-host disease produced across minor histocompatibility barriers. Cell Immunol 1987;106:76-87.
45. Claman HN, Jaffee BD, Huff JC, Clark RAF: Chronic graft-versus-host disease (GVHD) as a model for scleroderma. II. Mast cell depletion with deposition of immunoglobulins in the skin and fibrosis. Cell Immunol 1985;94:73-84.

46. Giorno R, Lee Choi K, Claman HN: Simultaneous in situ detectors of IgE receptors and cytoplasmic granules in murine cutaneous mast cells. J Immunol Meth 1987; 99:163-166.

47. Claman HN, Lee Choi K, Sujansky W, Vatter AE: Mast cell "disappearance" in chronic murine graft-vs-host disease (GVHD)-ultrastructural demonstration of "phantom mast cells." J Immunol 1986;137:2009-2013.

48. Lee Choi K, Claman HN: Mast cells, fibroblasts, and fibrosis: New clues to the riddle of mast cells. Immunol Res 1987;6:145-152.

49. Claman HN: Mast cells, T cells and abnormal fibrosis. Immunol Today 1985;6: 192-195.

50. Silver RM, LeRoy EC: Systemic sclerosis (scleroderma). In *Immunologic Diseases*, edited by Samter, M. 4th ed., Little, Brown & Co., Boston, 1988; pp. 1417-1436.

51. Hawkins RA, Claman HN, Clark RAF, Steigerwald JC: Increased dermal mast cell populations in progressive systemic sclerosis: A link in chronic fibrosis? Ann Int Med 1985;102:182-186.

52. Pearson ME, Huff JC, Giorno RC, Panicheewa S, Claman HN, Steigerwald JC: Immunologic dysfunction in scleroderma: Evidence for increased mast cell releasability and HLA-DR positivity in the dermis. Arth Rheum 1988;31:672-677.

53. Giorno RC, Seibold JR, Claman HN: unpublished results.

54. Lobb RR: Clinical applications of heparin-binding growth factors. Eur J Clin Invest 1988;18:321-336.

55. Strober S: Natural suppressor (NS) cells, neonatal tolerance and total lymphoid irradiation: Exploring obscure relationships. Ann Rev Immunol 1984;2:219-243.

56. Jadus MR, Parkman R: The selective growth of murine newborn-derived suppressor cells and their probable mode of action. J Immunol 1986;136:783-792.

6

Syngeneic Graft-vs.-Host Disease

Allan D. Hess

The Johns Hopkins University School of Medicine
Baltimore, Maryland

I. INTRODUCTION

Graft-vs.Host Disease (GVHD) occurs after allogeneic bone marrow transplantation (BMT) and is classically thought to be the response of donor lymphocytes to foreign major and/or minor histocompatibility antigens of the recipient (1). However, several reports have indicated that, in man, a GVHD-like syndrome can occur after marrow transplantation performed between identical twins (syngeneic) or after autologous marrow transplantation (2-4). In fact, a recent review has estimated that 10-15% of autologous or syngeneic BMT recipients exhibit this GVHD-like syndrome (5). These early reports were met with great skepticism since they challenged the universal concept that histocompatibility differences between donor and host are absolute requirements for the induction of GVHD as once postulated by Billingham (6). Moreover, the occurrence of autologous or syngeneic GVHD also raised fundamental questions regarding our understanding of the immunobiology of GVHD, the antigens which induce this reaction, and the mechanisms accounting for donor to host and for self-tolerance in the lymphohematopoietic chimera. Certainly, the developing immune system after BMT is subject to chemical (drug) and environmental insults that may result in perturbation of the immune system leading to a dysregulation of self: non-self-discrimination and autoimmunity.

Recent studies have indicated that limited treatment of rats after syngeneic BMT with the immunosuppressive drug cyclosporine (CsA) results in the induction of this auto-aggressive syndrome upon discontinuation of therapy (7). These results were indeed surprising and paradoxical since CsA is used therapeutically to prevent GVHD after allogeneic BMT. However, the induction of syngeneic GVHD appears to be related to the ability of CsA to affect thymic function, thus perturbing the development of the immune system after BMT. Nevertheless, the development of this animal model of syngeneic GVHD has strengthened the concept that histocompatibility differences are not absolute requirements for GVHD but that GVHD may include a failure of the mechanisms responsible for the maintenance of self-tolerance. In addition, this animal model has allowed for the dissection of the immunological mechansms in GVHD and in self: non-self-discrimination.

The present review will discuss the immunobiological mechanisms associated with syngeneic GVHD as discerned primarily from studies in this animal model. Although some of the salient features and mechanisms of syngeneic GVHD have been elucidated, current studies suggest that this autoimmune syndrome is complex and that many questions remain to be resolved.

II. BASIC MODEL OF SYNGENEIC GVHD AND ELEMENTAL REQUIREMENTS

The experimental induction of autoimmune GVHD after autologous or syngeneic BMT was first reported by Glazier et al. (7). Lethally irradiated rats that were reconstituted with syngeneic bone marrow and treated with CsA for 40 days developed a severe autoaggression syndrome 14 to 28 days after discontinuation of CsA therapy. In contrast, non-CsA-treated syngeneic marrow recipients recovered normally. The affected recipients with this augoaggressive disease exhibited erythroderma of the ears, dermatitis, and hair loss—classic clinical signs of GVHD. Histologic evaluation revealed lesions characteristic of GVHD in the skin, tongue, and liver. Of particular interest was the presence of lymphocytic exocytosis, vacuolar changes in the basal layer, epidermal destruction, and dyskeratosis in the skin. The observed histologic damage in this autoaggression syndrome was virtually indistinguishable from the damage observed in GVHD after allogeneic BMT and included similar target organs (8). More recent studies have indicated that there is a rapid progression of the disease to a more chronic type of GVHD with its relevant histological features (9). Based on these findings, the autoaggression syndrome after syngeneic BMT and CsA therapy was termed syngeneic GVHD (7). Of additional importance in this initial report was the observation that syngeneic GVHD could be induced in animals undergoing autologous marrow reconstitution after receiving total body irradiation but with lead shielding of the tibia. The induction of syngeneic GVHD after autologous recovery ruled out minor antigen differences due to genetic drift among syngeneic rats as the target antigens responsible for initiating this autoaggressive syndrome. This single observation also reversed a landmark concept that histocompatibility differences were absolute requirements for induction of GVHD (6,7). These findings implicated the aberrant recognition of self antigens in syngeneic GVHD.

Glazier et al. (7,8) also reported two important findings; (1) this disorder could only be adoptively transferred by T lymphocytes to irradiated secondary recipients and (2) syngeneic GVHD only occurred in syngeneic BMT recipients that were treated with CsA. These findings suggested that CsA was a necessary requirement for the induction of syngeneic GVHD and that it allowed for or caused the development of self-reactive T lymphocytes, observations confirmed by Sorokin et al. (10). Two other important factors required for the induction of syngeneic GVHD have been clearly identified. One essential requirement is irradiation. Cheney and Sprent (11) and Glazier et al. (8) reported that normal, nontransplanted animals treated with CsA do not develop this autoaggression syndrome even if treated with very high doses of CsA or for prolonged periods of time. This is in contrast to the routine induction of syngeneic GVHD after whole body irradiation and syngeneic BMT. Further studies by Glazier et al. (8) have indicated that the field of irradiation include the thymus since shielding of the thymus during total body irradiation results in the failure to induce this syndrome. These findings indicate that radiation and the thymus play essential roles in the pathogenesis of autologous and syngeneic GVHD. Sorokin et al. (11) provided compelling evidence that the thymus plays a pivotal role since syngeneic GVHD could not be induced in thymectomized animals but required that an intact thymus be present (the role of the thymus in syngeneic GVHD will be further discussed below).

Taken together, these findings suggest that there are three basic elements necessary for the induction of self-reactive lymphocytes and syngeneic GVHD. They include (1) CsA treatment, (2) whole body irradiation, and (3) an intact thymus. Even though these elements were clearly identified as critical requirements for the successful induction of syngeneic GVHD, the basic concept of this autoaggression syndrome was still received with skepticism. This was primarily due to the failure to consistently induce syngeneic GVHD in mice and in rats in different laboratories (12). Because of these difficulties, an endogenous virus was proposed as the etiologic agent of syngeneic GVHD even though viral-free animals were used in the original experiments (12). More recent studies may clarify this issue. Studies by Fischer et al. (13) in a rat model demonstrated that there is a correlation of age with the successful induction of syngeneic GVHD. Virtually a 100% incidence of syngeneic GVHD was observed if the animals were transplanted and treated with CsA prior to 6 weeks of age. Thereafter, the incidence of syngeneic GVHD decreased dramatically with the increasing age of the animals: A variable incidence (10-30%) was observed if animals were used at 8-12 weeks of age approaching 0% if the animals used were 6 months old at the time of transplant. Of particular importance in these studies was the finding that not only the age of the recipient was a significant variable, but the age of the marrow donor had the greatest effect. Syngeneic GVHD could be consistently induced in older animals if the marrow was derived from animals under the age of 6 weeks. Although the effect of the age of the receipient appears to be related to thymic function (14) and the effect of CsA (see below), it is unclear what immunological mechanisms are imparted by using marrow from young donors. Several possibilities exist including the presence of regulatory cells (i.e., natural suppressor cells) in the marrow obtained from older animals (15) which may modify the induction of syngeneic GVHD or an increased frequency of cells capable of repopulating the thymus in the marrow derived from very young animals. Certainly, these issues remain to be resolved but, nevertheless, these studies demonstrate that age of both the recipient and the donor are critical variables for the induction of syngeneic GVHD. This may explain some of the reported difficulties in inducing this autoaggression syndrome after autologous and/or syngeneic BMT.

III. THE PIVOTAL ROLE OF THE THYMUS IN SYNGENEIC GVHD

Current evidence strongly suggests that the thymus plays a central role in syngeneic GVHD as indicated above. Secondarily, the primary effect of CsA in the induction of this autoaggressive syndrome after syngeneic BMT appears to be primarily related to the ability of this drug to alter thymic function and/or T-cell differentiation in the thymus.

The importance of the thymus in syngeneic GVHD was first suggested by the observation of Glazier et al. (8), in which thymic shielding during irradiation prevented the development of autoaggression in this animal model. However, the key observations were reported by Sorokin et al. (10). Syngeneic GVHD could not be induced in rats that were thymectomized prior to irradiation, bone marrow reconstitution and CsA therapy. However, this autoaggression syndrome could be induced provided that thymic lobes were implanted in thymectomized rats prior to CsA therapy. The failure of a single cell suspension of thymocytes to replace the intact thymic lobe suggested that an intact thymic element (epithelial cells? see below) was essential for the successful induction of syngeneic GVHD. Further studies by Sorokin et al. (10) demonstrated that thymectomy was only effective in preventing syngeneic GVHD if performed prior to transplant. In contrast, thymectomy performed 2 weeks or later after syngeneic marrow transplant (CsA therapy was maintained for 6 weeks starting from the day of transplant) was ineffective at preventing the development of this autoaggressive syndrome. These data implied that the CsA-induced autoimmune cell population originated in the thymus, and these cells exit the thymus during the course of CsA treatment. The hypothesis that CsA treatment leads to the origin of the autoimmune cell population responsible for syngeneic GVHD is supported by the observation of Beschorner et al. (16). Adoptive transfer of thymocytes from irradiated, syngeneic bone marrow-reconstituted animals that were maintained on CsA into secondary irradiated recipients results in the successful transfer of syngeneic GVHD in the secondary hosts. On the other hand, transfer of thymocytes from non-CsA-treated animals failed to induce this disease. Taken together, these data demonstrate the thymic origin of the cells responsible for the induction of syngeneic GVHD and the apparent role of CsA in allowing the generation of these autoreactive cells.

The mechanism whereby CsA allows for the generation of the cells responsible for mediating syngeneic GVHD remains unknown. However, a number of studies have now demonstrated that CsA does have remarkable effects on the thymus. Some of the first observations on the effects of CsA on the thymus were made in normal (nonirradiated) animals. CsA treatment of both rats and mice with pharmacologic doses of this immunosuppressive drug induces a rapid ablation of the thymic medulla (17,18). This was found to be associated with a loss of medullary but not cortical epithelium (18). In addition, expression of class II major histocompatibility antigens (Ia) was markedly reduced owing much, in part, to the reduction of medullary epithelial cells (11,18). In contrast, Ia expression in cortical areas showed little change due to CsA treatment. The changes observed in the CsA-treated animal were rapidly reversible if the animals were not irradiated (17,18), however, these changes were prolonged or permanent in the irradiated recipient (14). Further studies by Beschorner et al. (14) indicated that there was an age-related variable on the effects of CsA on the thymus in rats receiving mediastinal irradiation. Pronounced changes of medullary ablation, reduction of Ia antigen expression, and reduction of medullary epithelial cells incluing Hassall's corpuscles were observed in young animals (5-6 weeks of age). In contrast, treatment of older rats (48-60 weeks of age) that received mediastinal irradiation and CsA treatment did not result in significant medullary involution. Although the Hassall's corpuscles were absent, fusiform epithelium, dendritic cells, and Ia antigen expression was still observed despite CsA treatment. The mechanism of resistance of the thymus from older animals to the effects of CsA remains unclear. It appears likely that this thymic resistance may account for the resistance to induction of syngeneic GVHD in older animals as discussed above.

The above studies clearly demonstrate a marked affect of CsA on thymic architecture with elimination of thymocytes and epithelial cells and a reduction in Ia antigen expression in the thymic medulla while sparing the cortex. It is also likely that these

significant change in the thymic microenvironment leading to altered T-
n with the generation of autoreactive T cells or a failure to eliminate
data have indicated that the thymic microenvironment, including the
lls and Ia antigen expression, play a critical role in triggering appro-
tiation and clonal deletion of autoreactive clones (19). Cheney and
ent (11) and Hess et al. (20) have postulated that these thymic changes induced by
CsA, particularly the reduction of medullary Ia antigen expression, would lead to a failure
of T-lymphocyte maturation and/or a failure to eliminate Ia-autoreactive clones, an hypothesis supported by the finding of Ia-reactive cytotoxic T cells in syngeneic GVHD
(20). Experimental evidence to date support the concept that CsA alters T-cell differentiation in the thymus.

To fully appreciate the effects of CsA on T-lymphocyte differentiation in the thymus, a brief discussion about the events in this differentiative process in the normal animal is warranted. The more classic approach to assess T-cell differentiation has been
monitoring the phenotypic expression of the CD4 and CD8 cell surface determinants,
determinants which mark distinct T-cell functions restricted by class I (via CD8) and
class II (via CD4) MHC antigens (21). The basic process can be summarized as follows:
(1) cells which express neither the CD4 and CD8 determinants are considered the most
immature cells and constitute a very small percentage (1-5%) of the population; (2)
progression of T-cell maturation is marked by expression of both determinants (double
positives) and is the dominant population in thymus (60-80%); and (3) the final stage
of maturation occurs with expression of either the CD4 or CD8 determinant (single positives) and makes up the remaining percentage of the thymocyte population. The single
positive cells are mature T lymphocytes and exit the thymus. Along with phenotype expression in the maturation process is the progressive rearrangement of the T-cell receptor
(TCR) gene segments leading to surface expression of either a TCR gamma delta or a TCR
alpha beta (21-24). Thymocytes that productively rearrange and express TCR gamma
delta maintain a $CD4^-8^-$ phenotype and appear to represent a stable distinct lineage from
TCR alpha beta bearing thymocytes. Cells that fail to productively rearrange their
gamma or delta genes probably continue to rearrange their alpha and beta genes and also
initiate expression of CD4 and CD8, resulting in a $CD4^+8^+TCR^-$ alpha beta (low density)
intermediate stage thymocyte. Current evidence indicates that deletion of potentially
self-reactive T cells occurs at this stage (25). A small subset of $CD4^+8^+$ thymocytes
undergoes a subsequent differentiation step characterized by an increase in surface TCR
density and down-regulation of either the CD4 or CD8 accessory molecules resulting in
the single positive TCR alpha beta (high density) of mature T cells.

The effect of CsA on T-cell differentiation in the thymus has been assessed. Recent
studies by Hess et al. (26) and Beschorner et al. (18) demonstrated that CsA markedly
altered T-cell differentiation as determined by phenotype expression of the CD4 and CD8
determinants. Thymocytes from CsA-treated bone marrow-reconstituted animals demonstrated a virtual absence of CD4 single positives and a slight reduction of CD8 single
positive thymocytes. In contrast, double negatives and double positives were significantly increased. In addition, the thymocytes from the CsA-treated animals were refrac-
tive to stimulation (Con A, IL 2) compared to the vigorous proliferative response of
thymocytes from control animals. These data suggested a CsA-induced maturational
arrest of CD4 single positive T cells, lymphocytes associated with helper cell function.
Further studies suggested that the incompletely differentiated T cells were released into
the peripheral blood since cells with early thymocyte differentiation antigens (OX 7) and

expression of both CD4 and CD8 determinants could be detected in the peripheral circulation (26). Based on these findings, it appeared reasonable to assume that the ongoing selection and elimination of autoreactive cells in the thymus was ablated by CsA treatment. However, the most informative information with regards to the effect of CsA on T-cell differentiation was recently reported by Jenkins et al. (27). CsA treatment mediated two striking effects on T-cell maturation. The development of mature single positive cells (CD4$^+$8$^-$, CD4$^-$8$^+$) expressing the B chains of the T-cell receptor were markedly inhibited without discernibly affecting the development of CD4$^-$8$^-$ cells expressing the gamma delta T-cell receptor. More importantly, Jenkins et al. (27) showed that among the small number of single positive thymocytes that do develop, a high percentage (10-20%) of these cells expressed the T-cell receptor for self-determinants as determined by expression of the VB-17a gene. This marker delineates T-cell receptors which have a high degree of anti I-E reactivity. In contrast, a very small number (0.6%) of single positive thymocytes from control non-CsA treated animals expressed this marker leading to the conclusion that CsA interferes with the clonal deletion of autoreactive cells.

Taken together, these data strongly suggest that CsA interferes or alters the T-cell differentiation process and abrogates normal clonal deletion mechanisms. The mechanism of action of CsA in mediating these specific affects remains unknown. It appears likely however, that the microenvironment of the thymus responsible for controlling the events of thymic differentiation is significantly altered by CsA and that the abrogation of clonal deletion mechanisms may be secondary to a reduction in Ia antigen expression in the medulla thought to be critical for tolerance induction (19). Certainly further studies on CsA and thymic function will be highly informative.

IV. EFFECTOR MECHANISMS IN SYNGENEIC GVHD

Initial studies in the syngeneic GVHD model demonstrated that this autoaggression syndrome could be specifically transferred to secondary recipients with splenic T lymphocytes. However, these early studies offered no indication of the complexity of the effector mechanisms, identification of the T-cell subsets involved or the target antigens involved in syngeneic GVHD. Because of the prominent effect of CsA on the reduction of Ia antigen expression in the thymus such that the developing T cells would fail to recognize this antigen as self, it seemed reasonable to assume that the Ia molecule may be one of the target antigens involved in syngeneic GVHD. The experimental data to date strongly support this hypothesis.

Recent studies by Hess et al. (20) have demonstrated that the induction of syngeneic GVHD is associated with the development of autoreactive CD8$^+$ cytotoxic T cells. These cells can be detected in the spleens of animals at the onset of syngeneic GVHD. Furthermore, the cytotoxic T cells associated with this autoaggression syndrome recognize a public determinant of Ia antigens since, in addition to self, the effector cells were capable of lysing PHA blast cells from several different strains of rats which differed for antigen determinants of the major histocompatibility complex. The lysis of the blast cells could only be effectively blocked with monoclonal antibodies recognizing a public determinant on the Ia molecule. In contrast, anit-MHC class I-specific antibodies were ineffective. The apparent public recognition by the effector cells from animals with syngeneic GVHD was rather perplexing and still remains unresolved if this is due to cross-reactivity or if, indeed, the effector cells are recognizing a common determinant on the Ia molecule. It must be noted that similar observations have been reported in man (28).

Patients undergoing autologous marrow transplant and induction of autologous GVHD with CsA to provide an antitumor effect for end-stage lymphoma exhibit Ia-specific cytotoxic T cells that appear with the onset of disease. After resolution of syngeneic GVHD, the cytotoxic T cells could no longer be detected. Another surprising finding in the rat model was the expression of the CD8 marker by the Ia-specific effector cell associated with syngeneic GVHD. Previous studies from cloning experiments have suggested that the majority of the cytotoxic T cells recognizing the Ia molecule express the CD4 determinant. However, in support of the observations of the specificity and phenotype of the effector cell in the peripheral compartment of the rat are the results from Jenkins et al. (27) demonstrating the presence of CD8[+] lymphocytes with a T-cell receptor for self I-E in thymi from CsA-treated mice as described above.

In view of these observations, it seems likely that the effector cell specific for Ia antigens arises in the thymus due to a maturational failure or was not eliminated by clonal deletion mechanisms and is subsequently transported to the periphery where it is now capable of mediating tissue destruction.

Although the demonstration of Ia-specific, autoreactive cytotoxic cells that appeared with the onset of syngeneic GVHD could simply explain the pathogenesis of this autoaggression syndrome, there were a few reported observations which suggested that syngeneic GVHD was more complex than just the generation of this autoreactive cell. These observations included the findings that (1) CsA must be withdrawn to allow development of the disease (7) even though the CD8[+] effector cells developed despite the presence of CsA (27), (2) the onset of syngeneic GVHD was associated with the reappearance of CD4[+] cells in the peripheral blood (29) and (3) the disease could be effectively transferred with the CD4[+] subset of T cells from animals with active syngeneic GVHD (10).

These findings indicated that the generation of the CD8[+] Ia-specific autocytotoxic cells was not singularly responsible for the development of syngeneic GVHD but that the CD4[+] T helper cell subset was required. On the one hand, it seemed likely that the T helper cell subset provided a maturation and/or amplification signal (i.e., IL-2, IL-4) for CD8[+] autocytotoxic cells allowing subsequent clonal expansion and development of autoaggression. This hypothesis is consistent with the observation that CsA profoundly affects IL-2 production (30) such that IL-2 production would only occur after withdrawal of CsA therapy. However, the development of the disease usually occurs 10-14 days after CsA therapy has been stopped, a much greater time period than needed for adequate CsA clearance allowing for the production of IL-2. Secondly, CD4[+] T helper cells appear to primarily develop in the thymus with subsequent transport to the peripheral lymphoid compartments only after CsA therapy has been withdrawn. These data would suggest that, on the other hand, the CD4[+] T helper cell may also participate in the histological effects observed in syngeneic GVHD. However, it is possible and rather likely that both mechanisms (IL-2 producton, CD4[+]-mediated tissue damage) work in concert in the development of this autoaggression syndrome. One major caveat is that if the T helper cells play an important role, they must develop autorecognition capabilities in the thymus in the absence of CsA. This woud suggest that the development of autoreactivity in the thymus and the inhibition of T helper cell formation are independent effects of CsA. This question remains unresolved.

It is of interest that the cell-mediated immune events histologically are a reflection of the events in the peripheral lymphoid compartments with respect to the development of CD8[+] and CD4[+] T-lymphocyte subsets (20,26,27,29). At the onset of syngeneic

GVHD, histological evaluation revealed changes primarily consistent with acute type GVHD (dyskeratosis, lymphocytic infiltrates were in intimate contact with injured epithelial cells). Immunoperoxidase studies demonstrated that the majority of the infiltrating lymphocytes (mucosa of the tongue) were $CD8^+$, $CD4^-$ T lymphocytes (9). A large percentage of lymphocytes in the submucosa and lamina propria appeared to express both cell surface determinants. The presence of the $CD8^+$ cytotoxic subset is consistent with the epithelial cell destruction observed histologically (31). Within 2 weeks after the onset of the autoaggression syndrome, histological evaluation revealed a rapid progression to a chronic-type GVHD with prominent fibrosis; the majority of the infiltrating lymphocytes had the $CD8^-$, $CD4^+$ phenotype or T helper cells. A number of cells also demonstrated coexpression of both the CD4 and CD8 markers. The predominance of the $CD4^+$ T helper cell subset in the chronic GVHD phase is similar to that observed in allogeneic chronic GVHD and in delayed-type hypersensitivity reactions (32). It is thought that release of lymphokines such as IL-4 leads to the fibrosis due to stimulation of fibroblasts (33). Of interest in these studies was that the expression of class II MHC antigen increased over time, suggesting that Ia antigen expression could be important in the pathogenesis of the peripheral tissue manifestations.

The time sequential histological evaluation of syngeneic GVHD has provided evidence that this autoaggression undergoes an evolution from acute to chronic type of GVHD. The progression of the disease is also characterized by distinct changes in the type of cells infiltrating the tissue and reflects the putative development of $CD8^+$ and $CD4^+$ autoreactive cells in the thymus and their transport to peripheral lymphoid tissues. It remains unknown if the acute and chronic phases of the disease is a natural, interrelated and interdependent progression of this autoimmune syndrome or if they are distinct entities separately mediated by functionally different autoreactive T-cell subsets. Further studies adoptively transferring distinct subsets of T lymphocytes should resolve this issue.

V. AUTOREGULATION AND SYNGENEIC GVHD

The majority of the studies with syngeneic GVHD have focused on identifying cell-mediated effector mechanisms, assessing the specificity of these effector cells, and defining the role of the thymus and CsA. Little attention has been paid to an apparently key mechanism in controlling the development of this autoaggressive syndrome, the role of autoregulation.

In some of the initial studies, experimental evidence was provided supporting the presence of an autoregulatory system which modified the action of the autoaggressive T cells mediating syngeneic GVHD. Studies by Glazier et al. (7,8) demonstrated that syngeneic GVHD could only be adoptively transferred into irradiated secondary recipients. On the other hand, infusion of spleen cells from animals with active disease into normal animals was ineffective in transferring autoaggression due to some resident regulatory system which negated the activity of the effector cells. Other support for a regulatory system was provided by the studies of Cheney and Sprent (11), which showed that CsA treatment of normal animals did not induce the syngeneic GVHD syndrome but that adoptive transfer of these spleen cells into irradiated secondary recipients resulted in the induction of syngeneic GVHD. The interpretation of these findings is that the effector cells were generated in the primary host but could only mediate disease after removal of a radiation-sensitive, regulatory component. Since these initial reports, further evidence has been provided clearly documenting autoregulatory cells which modulate the activity of the effector cells mediating syngeneic GVHD.

The approach taken to document and characterize this autoregulatory system was the adoptive transfer of effector splenocytes from animals with active disease into secondary recipients that were differentially pretreated with radiation or cytotoxic drugs. The premise in these experiments was that radiation and/or chemotherapy would perturb the autoregulatory system, thus allowing for the successful adoptive transfer of syngeneic GVHD (34,35). Successful transfer of syngeneic GVHD only occurred if the secondary Lewis recipients were total and/or upper body irradiated with 750R, or treated with 100 mg/kg of cyclophosphamide. Secondary syngeneic GVHD was routinely observed 10-20 days after adoptive transfer. In contrast, syngeneic GVHD could not be transferred into secondary recipients either left untreated or prepared with low-dose total body irradiation (500R), lower body irradiation with 1050R or treatment with busulfan. These results suggest that the autoregulatory system is sensitive to irradiation (750R) and cyclophosphamide but resistant to lower doses of irradiation (500R) and busulfan. The finding that upper body irradiation but not the lower body irradiation allowed for the successful transfer of syngeneic GVHD suggested that this autoregulatory system was thymic dependent. Further direct support for an autoregulatory system was provided by Fischer et al. (36) and Hess et al. (37) by the adoptive transfer of regulatory cells. Adoptive transfer of nylon wool nonadherent splenic T cells from normal animals along with spleen cells from animals with active syngeneic GVHD into irradiated secondary recipients prevented the transfer of the disease. This suppressive effect of the T cells which expressed OX19 (a specific marker of T lymphocytes) from normal animals was dose dependent relative to the number of spleen cells used from animals with active disease. Further characterization of the autoregulatory cell system revealed that both CD4$^+$ and CD8$^+$ T lymphocytes were required to mediate effective regulation or suppression of syngeneic GVHD as studied in the adoptive transfer model. The CD8$^+$ lymphocytes from normal animals were slightly more effective than the CD4$^+$ T cell subset in regulating the activity of the effector cells of syngeneic GVHD. These results suggested that the CD8$^+$ T-cell subset maybe the effector cell of autoregulation while the CD4$^+$ subset may supply an amplification or induction signal for the CD8$^+$ regulatory cells. However, the mechanism of suppression of these autoregulatory cell has not been defined, and a veto process cannot be excluded (38).

The importance of these autoregulatory cells and their role in the induction of syngeneic GVHD can only be inferred from comparing the requirements for induction of syngeneic GVHD versus the adoptive transfer of the disease into differentially prepared recipients. Fischer et al. (36) demonstrated that irradiation dose responses could separate subtle differences between induction versus adoptive transfer of syngeneic GVHD. Irradiation of the recipients with 750R allowed for the successful adoptive transfer of syngeneic GVHD in 100% of the aimals. In contrast, this dose was minimally effective in allowing the primary induction of syngeneic GVHD with CsA treatment. Cyclophosphamide treatment of the recipients only allowed for the adoptive transfer of this autoaggression syndrome. In addition to these findings, Fischer et al. (36) described the critical period—post-BMT reconstitution—in which to initiate CsA therapy in the inductive phase and to demonstrate the critical period of reconstitution of a regulatory system. Delay of the initiation of CsA therapy for one week following syngeneic BMT dramatically reduced the incidence in the induction of this autoaggression syndrome. In comparison, the results of the adoptive transfer of disease only occurred if the effector splenocytes from animals with active disease were infused within the first week after irradiation and BMT reconstitution; thereafter, infusion of effector splenocytes was remarkably ineffective in transferring disease.

These data, taken together, clearly suggest that the autoregulatory system must first be eliminated in order to induce syngeneic GVHD. Secondarily, it follows that CsA treatment must also prevent the development of this autoregulatory system but permits the generation of the autoreactive effector cells. This imbalance between autoreactive and autoregulatory cells appears to be essential to allow for the development of syngeneic GVHD.

VI. SYNTHESIS AND CONCLUSIONS

The occurrence of syngeneic GVHD certainly challenges our previously held concepts that minor or major antigen differences between donor and host are responsible for the induction of GVHD. However, this autoaggression syndrome reflects a much more fundamental process in which the developing immune system in the lymphohemato-poietic chimera is perturbed with a disruption of the mechanisms responsible for establishing tolerance to self major histocompatibility antigens, a fundamental tenet of immunology. Implicit in this concept of tolerance is the ability of the immune system to discern and discriminate between self and nonself. To account for tolerance to self MHC antigens, Burnet put forth the concept of clonal selection whereby self-reactive clones are deleted during the ontogeny of the immune system in the neonate and during reconstitution after BMT (39). The concept of clonal deletion has recently received strong experimental support at the molecular level (21,25). Nevertheless, clonal deletion is not complete with a small percentage of autoreactive cells leaving the thymus. Therefore, a peripheral autoregulatory system is required to modulate the activity of these autoreactive cells. Perturbation of the developing immune system by interfering with clonal deletion mechansims and/or elimination of autoregulatory mechanisms would alter the immunologic homeostasis accounting for self:nonself discrimination leading to autoaggression. Such a dysregulation of the immune system appears to be the cause for CsA-induced syngeneic GVHD. Although the precise mechanism of action of CsA remains to be elucidated, several important concepts have been established which lead to the induction of syngeneic GVHD. They include: (1) elimination of a peripheral autoregulatory mechanism by total body irradiation, (2) elimination or alteration of clonal deletion mechanisms in the thymus by CsA treatment, and (3) the failure to regenerate the autoregulatory system apparently due to the action of CsA. These three key elements appear to alter the delicate balance of autoregulatory and autoreactive cells in the periphery leading to the manifestation of autoaggression.

It is of interest that these three elements necessary for induction of syngeneic GVHD are present not only after syngeneic BMT but also after allogeneic BMT and therefore questions the relationship of allogneic and syngeneic GVHD. In general, CsA therapy is inadequate to completely suppress GVHD after allogeneic BMT and often recurs once CsA therapy is stopped. It may be that a "syngeneic" GVHD occurs after allogeneic BMT, a concept supported by recent studies in a rat model (40). On the other hand, results from clinical allogeneic BMT have suggested that the incidence of chronic GVHD has not decreased despite the use of CsA and may actually be increased (1). Since autoreactive cells play a dominant role in chronic GVHD (33) and syngeneic and chronic GVHD are histologically similar (16), it may be that chronic GVHD represents an autoimmune disease that occurs either after acute GVHD (damaging the thymus, elimination of autoregulatory mechanisms) or after CsA therapy alters autoregulatory/autoreactive homeostasis. Furthermore, understanding the principles involved in establishing self tolerance with the ability to alter these mechanisms may allow us to mobilize this autoimmune response to eliminate tumor cells which express the antigens (Ia) recognized by the effector cells. This latter concept is being evaluated in man (28).

In conclusion, although some of the mechanisms have been identified, many problems remain unresolved regarding syngeneic GVHD. In any case, this model at least will allow us to probe into the mechanisms accounting for self:nonself discrimination. It may also change our concepts of the immunobiology of GVHD occurring after allogeneic BMT.

ACKNOWLEDGMENT

Supported in part by grants from the U.S. Department of Health and Human Services (CA 15396, AI 24319).

REFERENCES

1. Santos GW, Hess AD, Vogelsang GB: Graft-versus-host reactions and disease. Immunol Rev 1985;88:169.
2. Gluckman E, Devergie A, Sohier J, Sauret JH: Graft-versus-host disease in recipients of syngeneic bone marrow. Lancet 1980;1:253.
3. Rappeport J, Reinherz E, Mihm M, Lopanski, S, Parkman R: Acute graft-versus-host disease in recipients of bone marrow transplantation from identical twin donors. Lancet 1979,2:717.
4. Thien SW, Goldman JM, Galton DG: Acute "graft-versus-host disease" after autografting for chronic granulocytic leukemia in transplantation. Ann Intern Med 1981; 94:210.
5. Hood AF, Vogelsang GB, Black LP, Farmer ER, Santos GW: Acute graft-versus-host disease. Development following autologous and syngeneic bone marrow transplantation. Arch Derm 1987;123:745.
6. Billingham RE. The biology of graft-versus-host reactions. Harvey Lectures (1966-1967,62:21.
7. Glazier A, Tutschka PJ, Farmer ER, Santos GW: Graft-versus-host disease in cyclosporin A treated rats after syngeneic and autologous bone marrow reconstitution. J Exp Med 1983;158:1.
8. Glazier A, Tutschka PH, Farmer ER: Studies on the immunobiology of syngeneic and autologous graft-versus-host disease in cyclosporine treated rats. Transplant Proc 1983,15:3035.
9. Beschorner WE, Shinn CA, Fischer AC, Santos GW, Hess AD: Cyclosporine-induced pseudo-graft-versus-host disease in the early post-cyclosporine period. Transplantation 1988;46(Suppl):1125.
10. Sorokin R, Kimura H, Schroder K, Wilson DH, Wilson DB: Cyclosporine-induced autoimmunity. Conditions for expressing disease, requirement for intact thymus, and potency estimates of autoimmune lymphocytes in drug-treated rats. J Exp Med 1986,164:1615.
11. Cheney RT, Sprent J: Capacity of cyclosporine to induce autograft-versus-host disease and impair intrathymic T cell differentiation. Trans Proc 1985;17:528.
12. Chow LH, Mosbach-Ozmen L, Ryffel B, Borel JF: Syngeneic graft-versus-host disease induced by Cyclosprone-A reappraisal. Transplantation 1988;46(Suppl):1075.

13. Fischer AC, Beschorner WE, Hess AD: Age related factors in the induction of syngeneic GVHD. Trans Proc 1989;21:3033.

14. Beschorner WE, Gennaro K, Hess AD, Santos GW: Cyclosporine and the thymus: influence of irradiation and age on thymic immunopathology and recovery. Cell Immunol 1987;110:350.

15. Noga SJ, Wagner JE, Horwitz LR, Donnenberg AD, Santos GW, Hess AD: Characterization of the natural suppressor cell population in adult rat bone marrow. J Leuk Biol 1988,43:279.

16. Beschorner WE, Hess AD, Shinn CA, Santos GW: Transfer of cyclosporin A associated syngeneic graft-versus-host disease (GVHD) by thymocytes: resemblance to chronic GVHD. Transplantation 1988;45:209.

17. Ryffel B, Deyssenroth A, Borel JF: Cyclosporin A: Effects on the mouse thymus. Agents Actions 1981,11:373.

18. Beschorner WE, Namnoum, JD, Hess AD, Shinn CA, Santos GW: Cyclosporin A and the thymus: Immunopathology. Amer J Path 1987;126:487.

19. Ready AR, Jenkinson EJ, Kingston R, Owen JJ: Successful transplantation across major histocompatibility barrier of deoxyguanosine-treated embryonic thymus expressing class II antigens. Nature 1984;310:231.

20. Hess AD, Horwitz L, Beschorner WE, Santos GW: Development of graft-versus-host disease-like syndrome in cyclosporine treated rats after syngeneic bone marrow transplantation I. Development of cytotoxic T lymphocytes with apparent polyclonal anti-Ia specific including autoreactivity. J Exp Med 1985;161:718.

21. von Boehmer H: The developmental biology of T lymphocytes. Ann Rev Immunol 1988,6:309.

22. Pardoll DM, Kruisbeek AM, Fowlkes BJ, Coligan JE, Schwartz RH: The unfolding story of T cell receptor gamma. FASEB Journal 1987;1:103.

23. Lew AM, Pardoll DM, Maloy WL, Fowlkes BJ, Kruisbeek A, Cheng SF, Germain RN, Bluestone JA, Schwartz RH, Coligan JE: Characterization of T cell receptor gamma chain expression in a subset of murine thymocytes. Science 1986;234:1401.

24. Pardoll DM, Fowlkes BJ, Bluestone JA, Kruisbeek A, Maloy WL, Coligan JE, Schwartz RH: Differential expression of two distinct T-cell receptors during thymocyte development. Nature 1987;326:79.

25. Fowlkes BJ, Schwartz RH, Pardoll DM: Deletion of self-reactive thymocytes occurs at a $CD4^+8^+$ precursor stage. Nature 1988;334:620.

26. Hess AD, Volgelsang GB, Heyd J, Beschorner WE: Cyclosporine induced syngeneic graft-versus-host disease: Assessment of T-cell differentiation. Trans Proc 1987;19:2683.

27. Jenkins MK, Schwartz RN, Pardoll DM: Effects of cyclosporine A on T cell development and clonal deletion. Science 1988;241:1655.

28. Vogelsang GB, Jones RJ, Hess AD, Geller R, Schucter L, Santos GW: Induction of autologous graft-versus-host disease. Trans Proc 1989;21:2997.

29. Bos GMJ, Majoor GD, Vander Gaar MJ, van Breda Vriesman PJC: Autoimmune reactivity after syngeneic bone marrow transplantation and cyclosporine treatment is associated with repopulation on the T helper cell subset. FASEB Journal 1988;2:a3578.

30. Hess AD, Colombani PM, Esa AH: Cyclosporine and the immuno response: Basic aspects. Crit Rev Immunol 1986;6:123.

31. Beschorner WE, Tutschka PJ, Santos GW: Sequential morphology of graft-versushost disease in the rat radiation chimera. Clin Immuno Immunopathol 1982;22:203.

32. Beschorner WE, Tutschka PJ, Santos GW: Characterization of T lymphocyte subsets in target tissues with acute and chronic graft-versus-host disease (GVHD). Fed Proc 1982;41:620A.

33. Parkman R: Clonal analysis of murine graft-versus-host disease: 1. Phenotypic and functional analysis of T lymphocyte clones. J Immunol 1985;136:3543.
34. Hess AD, Fischer AC, Vogelsang GB, Beschorner WE, Santos GW: Syngeneic graft-versus-host disease: Failure of self:non-self discrimination. In: Recent Advances and Future Directions in Bone Marrow Transplantation, edited by Baum SJ, Santos GW, Takaku F. Experimental Hematology Today 1987; pp. 12-17.
35. Fischer AC, Beschorner WE, Hess AD: Syngeneic graft-versus-host disease: Failure of autoregulation in self:non-self discrimination. Trans Proc 1988;20(Suppl 3):493.
36. Fischer AC, Beschorner WE, Hess AD: Requirements for the induction of adoptive transfer of syngeneic GVHD. J Exp Med 1989;169:1031.
37. Hess AD, Fischer AC, Beschorner WE: Regulation of syngeneic graft-vs-host disease by autosuppressor mechanisms. Trans Proc 1989;21:3013.
38. Fink PJ. Veto Cells. Ann Rev Immunol 1988;6:115.
39. Burnet F. The clonal selection theory of acquired immunity. Cambridge University Press, Cambridge. 1959.
40. Hess AD, Vogelsang GB, Silanskis M, Friedman KA, Beschorner WE, Santos GW: Syngeneic graft-versus-host disease (GVHD) after allogeneic bone marrow transplantation and cyclosprone treatment. Trans Proc 1988;20(Suppl 3):487.

7

Histologic Correlates of Immune Functional Deficits in Graft-vs.-Host Disease

Tariq Ghayur
Dana-Farber Cancer Institute
Harvard Medical School
Boston, Massachusetts

Thomas A. Seemayer
The Montreal Children's Hospital
McGill University Faculty of Medicine
Montreal, Quebec, Canada

Wayne S. Lapp
McGill University
Montreal, Quebec, Canada

I. INTRODUCTION

Animal models have contributed vastly to our understanding of the mechanisms contributing to the development of Graft-vs.-Host Disease (GVHD) and have provided insights into the ontogeny and organization of a functional immune system in an adult animal. The two most commonly employed murine models of GVHD are: (1) the radiation model and (2) the parent → F_1 hybrid (P → F_1) model. In the radiation model, the recipient's marrow stem cells and the immune system are destroyed prior to donor stem cell transplantation. This GVHD model takes into consideration the effects of radiation on recipient tissues and is therefore considered to be closer to the clinical setting. This model is also considered as the only system to study the development of a functional immune system in an adult animal. In contrast to the radiation model, in the P → F_1 GVHD model, mature parental lymphoid cells (spleen and/or lymph node cells) (PLC) are injected into adult non-X-irradiated F_1 mice that possess a normal immune system. The parental lymphoid cells recognize alloantigens of the other parent on F_1 tissues as foreign and initiate an immunological attack against the F_1 tissues. The P → F_1 model is employed to study the effects of GVH reaction per se without the complications of radiation effects (structural/functional) on host tissues. This model has thus far not been employed to study the development of a functional immune system in an adult animal.

Several different assay systems are employed to determine the induction and intensity of GVH reaction. In the radiation model, weight loss and mortality are the main assays used (1,2). However, development of histopathological lesions in the lymphoid and nonlymphoid organs has also been employed to determine the severity of GVH reactions (3). It has been suggested that one of the reasons for both weight loss and mortality is the development of histopathological lesions in the gut which leads to diarrhea, malabsorption, and malnutrition (4-6). On the other hand, in the $P \to F_1$ model, the main assays employed to determine the induction and severity of GVH reactions are: (1) spleen index, which determines the degree of splenomegaly (7), (2) development of histopathological lesions in the lymphoid and nonlymphoid organs (8,9), and (3) immunosuppression (8-10). Splenomegaly, the most commonly used parameter (assay) in the $P \to F_1$ model, reflects donor cell-induced recruitment of host cells, mainly of myeloid and erythroid (11-14) lineages. The type and specificity of tissue lesions observed in the lymphoid and nonlymphoid organs during early acute GVH (aGVH) reactions in the two experimental models are almost identical, the only exception being the skin lesions which have not been detected or thoroughly investigated in the $P \to F_1$ model, but which are observed in the radiation model. Immunosuppression is used as an assay in $P \to F_1$ model since the F_1 immune system is intact prior to GVH induction. In contrast, in the radiation model, immune functional assays are employed to determine the rate and status of immune functional reconstitution which may reflect, directly or indirectly, immunosuppressive mechanism(s).

In the $P \to F_1$ model, no systematic studies are available on the relationship between splenomegaly, immune functional, and histopathological changes observed during the early acute GVHD (aGVHD), i.e., the first 4 weeks following GVH reaction induction. It is not clear whether a single effector mechanism or multiple mechanisms are responsible for inducing all of the changes observed during the early aGVHD. Furthermore, although it is clear from our previous studies (8) that both splenomegaly and histopathology (in particular, the thymic dysplasia) play a role in causing immunosuppression following GVHD induction, the contribution of each of these GVHD-associated changes in determining the severity and duration of immunosuppression is not clear.

In this chapter, we shall describe some of our studies in the GVH reaction using the $P \to F_1$ hybrid model. We shall address three topics: (1) The relationship between splenomegaly, immune functional and histopathological changes observed during the first 4 weeks following GVHD induction, including the nature of effector cells responsible for these changes. (2) The relationship between the initial severity of thymic dysplasia and the duration of T-cell immunodeficiency. (3) The process of thymic architectural regeneration and immune functional recovery in long-term survivors of $P \to F_1$ GVH reactions.

II. EXPERIMENTAL DESIGN

The basic experimental protocol consisted of a single intravenous injection of pooled parental spleen and lymph node cells (parental lymphoid cells or PLC) into adult (8-12 weeks) non-X-irradiated F_1 hybrid mice. In all experiments, as described below, the T-, B-, and NK-cell functions of the donor mice and/or the donor inoculum were determined prior to GVH induction. Following GVH induction, spleen index or splenomegaly was determined by the method of Simonsen (7). Immunosuppression was determined by the T- and B-cell mitogen responses, the plaque forming cell (PFC) response to sheep red blood cells (SRBC) (which determines the T-cell dependent B-cell responses), and natural killer (NK) cell activity (15,16). In the studies reported here, NK/NK-like activity is defined on a functional basis, i.e., killing of YAC-1 tumor targets in vitro.

Histopathological alterations were determined by light microscopy. Different intensities of histopathological alterations in the thymus (17) and nonlymphoid organs (15) have been described in detail previously. Splenomegaly, immune functions, and the intensity of histopathological alterations were determined in each GVH-reactive animal.

III. RELATIONSHIP BETWEEN SPLENOMEGALY, IMMUNE FUNCTIONS, AND HISTOPATHOLOGICAL ALTERATIONS FOLLOWING GVH INDUCTION: THE NATURE OF EFFECTOR MECHANISMS

Detailed studies on the relationship between different GVH-associated changes were undertaken following our initial observations on the relationship between the various immune functions and the development of tissue damage. In these initial studies, GVH reactions of various intensities were induced in $(C57BL/6 \times A)F_1$ $(B6AF_1)$ mice by injecting different doses $(10, 20, \text{or } 30 \times 10^6)$ of either A or C57BL/6 (B6) PLC (15,17). On different days after GVHD induction, 3-4 animals were randomly picked from each group and sacrificed. Complete autopsy was performed on each animal and splenic T-, B-, and NK-cell functions were determined for each group. Briefly, the results from these studies showed that: (1) The aGVHD-associated tissue alterations first appeared at a time when NK cell activity was at its peak and T- and B-cell functions were severely suppressed, (2) the time of peak NK-cell activity, rather than the overall augmented NK-cell activity, correlated with the severity of tissue damage following GVH induction; and (3) severe suppression of T-cell functions was observed only in those groups of GVH mice that developed thymic medullary alterations whereas only partial transient suppression of T-cell functions was observed in groups of F_1 mice in which no visible thymic alterations were observed (17). These studies suggested that NK cells and T cells may have different thresholds for activation and/or suppression and that the two cell types may play different roles (affect different changes) during the GVH reaction. We proposed that the initial activation of donor T cells would recruit donor NK cells (present in the inoculum), which would then cause tissue alterations (15).

A. The Role of Donor T Cells and NK Cells During aGVHD

To test the proposals that donor T cells and NK cells may play different roles during GVH reaction and that NK cells of donor origin may play a crucial role in the development of aGVHD-associated tissue damage, different $P \to F_1$ GVH combinations of beige/beige (bg/bg) mutant (deficient NK cytotoxic function) (18,19), and +/beige (+/bg) (normal NK cytotoxic function) mice were employed (16).

Prior to GVHD induction, T-cell functions of donor B6 bg/bg and B6 +/bg mice were assessed by skin graft rejection, the PFC response to SRBC and Con A and PHA induced proliferative responses, whereas NK cell functions were assessed by YAC tumor cell killing. Although the B6 bg/bg donor mice were severely deficient in NK cycotoxic functions, the T-cell functions of B6 bg/bg donor mice were the same as those of B6 +/bg donor mice (16). Thus, if donor T cells and NK cells play different roles during aGVHD, then the different $P \to F_1$ GVHD combinations of bg/bg and +/bg mice should allow us to dissect the role of these two donor cell populations following GVHD induction.

In these experiments, 50×10^6 B6 bg/bg or +/bg PLC were injected into (B6 × C3H/HeJ bg/bg)F_1 (bg/bg F_1) and (B6 × C3H/HeJ +/bg)F_1 (+/bg F_1) mice thus creat-

Table 1 Summary of the Relationship Between Splenomegaly, Development of Tissue Lesions, and Immune Functions in bg/bg F_1 and +/bg F_1 Mice that Received B6 bg/bg or B6 +/bg PLC

GVH combinations		Splenomegaly	Tissue damage	NK activity	PFC response to SRBC	Mitogen response
Parent	F_1					
bg/bg	bg/bg	++++	−	+	−	++
bg/bg	+/bg	++++	−	+++	−	++
+/bg	bg/bg	++++	++++	+++	−	−
+/bg	+/bg	++++	+++	++++	−	−
Control bg/bg F_1		−	−	−	++++	++++

50×10^6 B6 bg/bg or B6 +/bg PLC were injected into bg/bg F_1 and +/bg F_1 mice to induce GVHD.

ing four experimental groups (Table 1) (16). Following GVHD induction, F_1 mice were sacrificed on different days, and splenomegaly, T- and B-cell function, NK-cell activity, and the severity of tissue damage in the lymphoid and nonlymphoid organs was determined in each animal. The results from these experiments showed that bg/bg donor PLC possessed the capacity to induce splenomegaly, yet failed to cause significant aGVHD-associated tissue damage. GVH reactions activated NK/NK-like activity of both the host and donor origin, but the development of aGVHD-associated tissue damage correlated with the activation of NK/NK-like cells of donor (B6 +/bg PLC → bg/bg F_1) origin, but not host (B6 bg/bg PLC → +/bg F_1) origin (Table 1) (16). The fact that splenomegaly could be induced, without the development of tissue damage in both bg/bg F_1 and +/bg F_1 mice that received B6 bg/bg PLC, suggested that splenomegaly and tissue damage are two independent symptoms of the P → F_1 GVHD. Each symptom is mediated by a distinct effector mechanism; we proposed that splenomegaly is caused by the activation of donor T cells, whereas tissue damage is mediated by an activated NK cell of donor origin. From these results, we further suggested that splenomegaly may not be useful for predicting the eventual fate of animals experiencing a GVH reaction (16).

An analysis of the immune-functional status of bg/bg F_1 and +/bg F_1 mice that received either the B6 bg/bg or B6 +/bg PLC showed that the PFC response to SRBC, i.e., a T-cell dependent B-cell response, was more sensitive to the suppressive effects of GVHD than the T-cell mitogen induced prolfierative response (Table 1). In bg/bg F_1 and +/bg F_1 mice that received B6 bg/bg PLC, complete to severe suppression of the PFC response to SRBC, but only partial suppression of T-cell mitogen responses, was observed. These groups of F_1 mice displayed significant splenomegaly but did not develop tissue damage. On the other hand, severe and persistent suppression of both the PFC response to SRBC and T-cell mitogen responses was observed in bg/bg F_1 and +/bg F_1 mice that received B6 ÷/bg PLC. These groups of F_1 mice developed tissue damage as well as splenomegaly (16).

We have previously demonstrated two distinct phases of immunosuppression during GVHD, namely, an early phase and a late phase, each caused by a distinct mechanism (8). During the early phase, a quantitative increase in splenic macrophages (the principal cause of splenomegaly) was observed (13,14). These splenic macrophages produced copious amounts of prostaglandins of the E series which suppressed T helper cell functions (20). In contrast, the late phase of immunosuppression was found to be due to T helper cell maturational arrest resulting from GVH-induced thymic dysplasia (21-23). Thus, collectively our results employing the different P → F_1 GVHD combinations of bg/bg and +/bg mice strongly suggested that following GVHD induction, activation of donor NK/NK-like cells would cause tissue damage, in particular, thymic dysplasia, which would then lead to severe prolonged immunosuppression.

B. Induction and Elimination of Donor ASGM1$^+$ Cells with NK Activity that Cause Tissue Damage

In contrast to our studies showing that NK/NK-like cells of donor origin may be effectors of aGVHD-associated tissue damage, several workers had suggested that NK/NK-like cells of host origin may be responsible for tissue damage following GVH induction (24-27). The proposal that host NK cells are essential for aGVHD-associated tissue damage was based upon studies showing that anti-asialo-GM1 antibodies (anti-ASGM1), which eliminate NK cells (28) when given to recipients prior to and during the first few days after GVH induction prevented GVHD-associated mortality and skin lesions (24,25).

In contrast, treatment of donor mice or the donor inoculum with anti-ASGM1 prior to GVH induction had no effect (24). To resolve the controversy concerning the origin (host vs. donor) of ASGM1$^+$ cells with NK activity that appear to play a crucial role in the development of aGVHD-associated tissue damage, we reasoned that treatment of recipient mice with anti-ASGM1 prior to and a few days after GVH induction would eliminate ASGM1$^+$ NK/NK-like cells of host origin as well as the NK/NK-like cells of donor origin that are activated/recruited following transplanation.

To test this proposal, attempts were made to deplete the donor inoculum of both the endogenous and inducible ASGM1$^+$ cells with NK activity prior to GVH induction. The protocol employed to eliminate both the endogenous and inducible ASGM1$^+$ cells with NK activity from the donor inoculum has been described in detail previously (29). Briefly, donor B6 mice were treated in vivo with anti-ASGM1 to eliminate endogenous ASGM1$^+$ cells with NK activity. ASGM1$^+$ cells with NK activity were also induced in B6 mice by treating the B6 animals with 15×10^6 recipient (B6AF$_1$) lymphoid cells for 44-48 hr. The induced ASGM1$^+$ cells with NK activity were eliminated by in vivo treatment with anti-ASGM1. Anti-ASGM1 treatment did not affect T-cell functions but almost completely abrogated both the endogenous and the induced NK activity as assessed by YAC tumor cell killing in vitro (29).

The results from these experiments demonstrated that lymphoid cells depleted of either only the endogenous or both the endogenous and inducible ASGM1$^+$ cells with NK activity caused the same degree of splenomegaly (Table 2). Lymphoid inoculum depleted of both the endogenous and inducible ASGM1$^+$ cells with NK activity failed to cause any detectable tissue damage in F$_1$ mice, whereas moderate to severe tissue damage was observed in all F$_1$ mice that received lymphoid cells depleted of only the endogenous ASGM1$^+$ cells with NK activity (Table 2). These studies also confirmed our earlier results (16, and as desribed above), showing that the PFC response to SRBC is more sensitive to the suppressive effects of GVH reaction than the T- and B-cell mitogen responses. Furthermore, severe prolonged immunosuppression of both the PFC response to SRBC and T-cell mitogen response was associated with thymic medullary alterations. Collectively, these results again demonstrated that splenomegaly and aGVHD-associated tissue damage are two separate symptoms of the GVH reaction mediated by distinct mechanisms. Tissue lesions are initiated by an induced/activated ASGM1$^+$ cell of donor origin that exhibits NK activity, whereas splenomegaly is mediated by donor T cells.

C.   The Induction Requirements and Specificity of Donor ASGM1$^+$ Cells with NK Activity that Cause Tissue Damage

To investigate the induction requirements and specificity of GVH-effector cells, the ASGM1$^+$ cells with NK activity were induced in B6 donor mice by either B6AF$_1$ cells (specific B6-anti-B6AF$_1$ induction) (29) or by poly I:C, a nonspecific inducer of interferon (nonspecific induction) (30). These induced cells were then eliminated by anti-ASGM1 as described previously (29,30). Donor B6 lymphoid cells depleted of either the specifically or nonspecifically induced ASGM1$^+$ cells with NK activity were used to initiate GVHD in B6AF$_1$ and B6C3HF$_1$ mice. These two strains share the H-2K and H-2I regions, but differ at the H-2D region of the H-2 complex. It should be pointed out that the donor B6 lymphoid cells depleted of the specifically induced ASGM1$^+$ cells with NK activity retained the capacity to proliferate and generate specific CTL responses against both the B6AF$_1$ and B6C3HF$_1$ alloantigens in vitro.

Table 2 Effect of Eliminating the Endogenous or Both the Endogenous and Induced ASGM1[+] Cells with NK Activity from the Donor Inoculum in Influencing Various GVHD-Associated Parameters

Donor treatment[a]		Splenomegaly	Tissue damage	PFC response to SRBC	Mitogen response
B6AF$_1$ cells	α-ASGM1				
−	−	++++	++++	−	−
+	−	+++	++++	−	−
−	+	+++	++++	−	−
+	+	+++	−	+	++++
Control B6AF$_1$		−	−	++++	++++

[a]Donor B6 mice were sacrificed 44–48 hr after various treatments. 50×10^6 donor cells were injected into B6AF$_1$ mice to induce GVHD.

[b]The different GVHD-associated parameters were studied on day 22 after GVHD induction.

The results from these studies showed that B6 lymphoid cells depleted of specifically induced B6-anti-B6AF$_1$ ASGM1$^+$ cells with NK activity failed to cause thymic dysplasia and severe prolonged immunosuppression in B6AF$_1$ mice but still induced severe lesions and immunosuppression in B6C3HF$_1$ mice. Splenomegaly was evident in both F$_1$ strains. In contrast, lymphoid cells depleted of the nonspecifically induced ASGM1$^+$ cells with NK activity caused splenomegaly, severe lesions, and immunosuppression in both B6AF$_1$ and B6C3HF$_1$ mice. These results suggested that the ASGM1$^+$ GVH-effector cells of donor origin that exert NK activity are induced following specific stimulation and that the specificity of these effector cells may be directed toward the H-2D (or a closely related) region of the H-2 complex (Table 3).

The results described above suggest that depending upon the stimulus, two ASGM1$^+$ cell populations that exert NK activity can be induced in the donor inoculum. However, only the allo-induced, but not poly I:C-induced ASGM1$^+$ cells with NK activity appear to be crucial in the development of aGVHD-associated tissue damage. The precise nature of, or the relationship between, these two ASGM1$^+$ cells with NK activity is not clear at the moment. Recent studies have, however, shown that the poly I:C-induced NK cells do not express functional transcripts of α-β- or γ-chain genes of the T cell receptor (31). Whereas the allo-induced ASGM1$^+$ cells with NK activity express functional transcripts of $\gamma\delta$ chain genes of the T-cell receptor (32-37). We (8,29) and several other workers (38,39) have previously suggested that the NK cells of donor origin that play an important role in the development of tissue damage may belong to the T-cell lineage. If the allo-induced ASGM1$^+$ cells with NK activity belong to the T-cell population that bear the $\gamma\delta$ T-cell receptor (T3-$\gamma\delta$ cells), then one can explain both the specificity of the ASGM1$^+$ cells with NK activity (as discussed above) as well as our earlier observations showing that NK cell activity of donor, but not host, origin correlates with the development of aGVHD-associated tissue damage.

D.   The Role of Donor ASGM1$^+$ Cells with NK Activity in aGVHD and Early Graft Rejection

We have previously reported that a proportion of B6 lymphoid cells is rapidly rejected (within 48 hours) by B6AF$_1$ hybrids via the phenomenon of hybrid resistance (30,46), which is mediated by F$_1$ hybrid NK cells (40-42). Thus, we have proposed that a critical number of donor lymphoid cells must survive the F$_1$ NK-mediated rejection mechanism for the aGVHD-associated lesions and immunosuppression to develop (15). To investigate whether the B6 donor lymphoid cells depleted of the specifically induced ASGM1$^+$ cells are rapidly rejected by the F$_1$ NK-mediated rejection mechanism and therefore fail to cause tissue damage and immunosuppression, the following experiments were performed. Lymphoid cells from: (1) normal B6 mice, (b) B6 mice treated with B6AF$_1$ cells alone (cells containing the endogenous and induced ASGM1$^+$ cells) and (3) B6 mice treated with B6AF$_1$ cells and anti-ASGM1 (cells depleted of the endogenous and induced ASGM1$^+$ cells) were labeled with fluoresceinisothiocyanate (FITC) (30). These FITC-labeled donor cells were injected into either normal B6AF$_1$ mice, B6AF$_1$ mice treated with hydrocortisone (HC) to transiently suppress host NK cell activity (43), or B6AF$_1$ mice treated with poly I:C to boost host NK cell activity (30,44,45). Three to five F$_1$ mice were sacrificed 48 hr later and the number of FITC-labeled donor cells was determined in their spleens (30). The remaining mice were sacrificed on days 18-22, and the severity of tissue damage and immunosuppression was assessed.

Table 3 Degree of Splenomegaly and Tissue Damage Observed in B6AF$_1$ and B6C3HF$_1$ Mice Injected with Lymphoid Cells from B6 Mice Treated with Either B6AF$_1$ Cells and/or α-ASGM1 or Poly I:C and/or α-ASGM1

Donor treatment[a]			Degree of splenomegaly and tissue damage observed in different F$_1$ mice			
B6AF$_1$ cells	poly I:C	α-ASGM1	B6AF$_1$		B6C3HF$_1$	
			Splenomegaly	Tissue damage	Splenomegaly	Tissue damage
−	−	−	++++	+++	++++	+++
+	−	−	+++	+++	+++	+++
+	−	+	+++	−	+++	+++
−	+	−	+++	+++	+++	+++
−	+	+	+++	+++	+++	+++

[a]Donor B6 mice were treated with 15 × 10^6 B6AF$_1$ cells (i.v.) and/or 100 μl α-ASGM1 (i.v.) or with 100 μg poly I:c (i.p.) and/or 100 μ α-ASGM1 (i.v.). 44-48 hr after the above treatments, animals were sacrificed and their spleen and lympho node cells were used to induce GVHD in F$_1$ mice.

[b]60 × 10^6 B6 lymphoid cells were injected into B6AF$_1$ and B6C3HF$_1$ mice. F$_1$ mice were sacrificed on day 22 after GVHD induction.

Table 4 Recovery of FITC-Labeled B6 Cells Either Containing the Induced ASGM1[+] Cells or Depleted of the Induced ASGM1 Cells from the Spleens of Nontreated B6AF$_1$ Mice, HC-Treated B6AF$_1$ Mice, and Poly I.C-Treated B6AF$_1$ Mice

Donor treatment[a]		Recovery of FITC-labeled cells[b,c]		
B6AF$_1$ cells	α-ASGM1	Nontreated B6AF$_1$ mice	HC-treated B6AF$_1$	poly I:C treated B6AF$_1$ mice
−	−	+++	+++++	+
+	−	++	+++++	+
+	+	++++	+++++	+

[a]Donor B6 mice were treated with 15×10^6 B6AF$_1$ cells (i.v.) and/or 100 μl α-ASGM1 (i.v.). 44-48 hr after the above treatments, animals were sacrificed and their spleen and lymph node cells were labeled with FITC.

[b]Different doses ($30, 45, 60 \times 10^6$) of FITC-labeled donor cells were injected into F$_1$ mice.

[c]B6AF$_1$ mice were treated with either 2.5 mg HC (i.p.) or 100 μg poly I:C (i.p.), 36-40 hr prior to the injection of FITC-labeled donor cells.

The results from these studies demonstrated that a much lower proportion of B6 lymphoid cells containing the induced ASGM1[+] cells was recovered (high rejection) from the spleens of normal F$_1$ mice than compared to normal FITC-labeled B6 cells (46). Therefore, a higher number of lymphoid cells ($50-60 \times 10^6$) containing the induced ASGM1[+] cells was required to cause the moderate to severe tissue damage and immunosuppression that was caused by a lower number of normal B6 cells (30×10^6). In contrast, a higher proportion of B6 lymphoid cells depleted of both endogenous and induced ASGM1[+] cells was recovered from the spleens of normal F$_1$ mice (no rejection) than compared with normal FITC-labeled B6 donor cells (Table 5) (46), but as outlined above no aGVHD-associated pathological lesions were observed.

The suppression of the F$_1$ hybrid NK-mediated rejection mechanism by HC treatment allowed a larger proportion of donor cells to survive (than observed in normal F$_1$ mice) and also enhanced the susceptibility of HC-treated F$_1$ mice to GVHD by normal B6 cells and B6 cells containing the induced ASGM1[+] cells, but not to B6 cells depleted of the induced ASGM1[+] cells. On the other hand, augmentation of F$_1$ hybrid NK-mediated rejection mechanism by poly I.C resulted in a lower recovery of donor cells regardless of the prior donor treatment (46) (Table 4). Treatment of F$_1$ mice with poly I:C prior to GVH induction enhances their resistance to GVHD (47). The above observations collectively suggest that it is not the number of donor cells per se that survive the initial rejection that would determine the intensity of tissue damage, but a critical number of a specific population (probably the induced ASGM1[+] cells) of donor B6 cells must survive rejection in order to cause tissue damage and severe immunosuppression. These results further suggest that the presence of the induced ASGM1[+] cells in the donor inoculum activates the F_1 NK-mediated rejection mechanism and that these induced cells themselves become the target of rejection (46).

IV. RELATIONSHIP BETWEEN THE INITIAL SEVERITY OF THYMIC DYSPLASIA AND THE DURATION OF T-CELL FUNCTIONAL DEFICIENCY

Previous studies have shown that thymic medullary dysplasia prevents the acquisition by T-helper (Th) cells of both the IL-2-producing capacity (48,49) and hydrocortisone resistance (50) but does not prevent the acquisition of the surface marker, L3T4 (CD4) (50). Moreover, thymic medullary dysplasia does not affect the production of IL-2 responsive Lyt-2$^+$ (CD8$^+$) T-cytotoxic/suppressor cells (48,49). Since the IL-2-producing Th cells play a pivotal role during the initiation of the immune response, the absence of these cells renders GVH mice immune-deficient. If thymic medullary dysplasia is indeed the cause of severe prolonged T-cell deficiency, then it would appear that T-cell functions should reappear when, and if, the GVH-dysplastic thymuses recover and regain a normal architecture. In fact, we have recently reported that, with time and proper conditions after GVH induction, the GVH-dysplastic thymuses do indeed regenerate and regain a normal architecture (51) (also see below). More importantly, the recovery of T-cell functions was observed only after the thymic medulla had regenerated and displayed near-normal/normal morphology (51).

To investigate the role of thymic medullary alterations in determining the duration of T-cell immunodeficiency, the following protocol was employed. Different intensities of thymic medullary alterations (mild, moderate, or severe) (Table 5) were induced in large groups of B6AF$_1$ mice by manipulating the dose and genotype of the donor inoculum, as described previously (17). On different days after GVH induction, six to ten animals were sacrificed and thymic histology and immune functions were determined in each animal. The results of these studies showed that the initial severity of thymic dysplasia (on day 16) determined both the time required by the thymuses to regain a normal architecture as well as the recovery of the T-cell functions. Recovery of the thymic medulla and the PFC response to SRBC was observed first in the group that developed mild lesions, then, in the group that displayed moderate lesions and finally, in the groups that displayed severe lesions. In all instances, regardless of the initial severity of the thymic dysplasia, the recovery of the PFC response was observed only after the thymic medulla had regained a normal architecture (51, Ghayur et al., manuscript in preparation).

The initial severity of thymic dysplasia could be clearly characterized on day 16 after GVH induction, however, by day 30, the moderately and severely dysplastic thymuses could not be distinguished morphologically from one another, yet significant differences were observed in the time required for complete medullary regeneration and thereby the recovery of the PFC response. One of the reasons for the lack of morphologically distinguishing features in moderately and severely dysplastic thymuses on day 30 could be the drastic involution and extreme hypocellularity of the organ. The differences observed between the time required by moderately and severely dysplastic thymuses to regenerate may be due to the differences in intensities of effector mechanism(s) generated early after GVH induction that may maintain the lesions (52).

Table 5 Summary of Characteristics of Various Degrees of Thymic Changes Observed in B6AF$_1$ Mice Undergoing GVH Reactions of Different Intensities

Degree of thymic lesions	Thymic size	Cortical depletion	Cortico-medullary demarcation	Medullary Changes			
				Epithelial cells		Hassall's corpuslces	Degree of lymphocytic infiltrates
				Individual	Clusters		
Normal	++++	None	+	+	+	+	–
Mild	+++	Partial	+	±	–	–	–
Moderate	++	Severe	–	–	–	–	–
Severe	+	Severe	–	–	–	–	+

The various degrees of thymic changes were charactered on day 16 after GVH induction. The various degrees of thymic changes are illustrated and described in detail previously (17). GVH reactions of different intensities were induced in B6AF$_1$ mice by injecting the following PLC doses: 10×10^6 PLC → B6AF$_1$, mild GVH; 30×10^6 B6 PLC → B6AF$_1$, moderate GVH; and 20×10^6 A PLC → B6AF$_1$ severe GVH (for details see Refs. 15, 17). (+) = present; (–) = absent.

Table 6 Summary of the Characteristics of Various Stages of Thymic Regeneration

Stages of thymic regeneration	Characteristic features of each stage
Stage 1	- increase in thymic size - repopulation of cortex - reappearance of corticomedullary demarcation - medulla contains a large number of lymphocytes - medulla devoid of pale individual epithelial cells, pale epithelial cell clusters, and Hassall's corpuscles
Stage 2	- medulla contains a large number of lymphocytes - reappearance of numerous small dark irregular-shaped individual epithelial cells - rare pale individual epithelial cells observed in localized areas of the medulla - no visible Hassall's bodies
Stage 3	- reduction in the numbers of medullary lymphocytes - abundant pale individual epithelial cells and pale epithelial cell clusters observed throughout the medulla - no visible Hassall's bodies
Stage 4	- normal medulla with abundant pale individual epithelial cells, pale epithelial cell clusters, and Hassall's bodies

The various stages of thymic regeneration were illustrated and described in detail previously (51). GVH reactions were induced in B6AF$_1$ mice by injecting 20 × 10^6 A PLC (51).

V. THE KINETICS OF THYMIC REGENERATION AND IMMUNE FUNCTIONAL RECOVERY IN LONG-TERM SURVIVORS OF THE GVH REACTIONS

A. Kinetics of Thymic Structural Regeneration

In the groups of GVH mice that display moderate to severe lesions, the thymic regeneration occurs in the following sequence: cortical regeneration followed by medullary regeneration (Table 6) (51). During medullary regeneration, morphologically distinct epithelial cells appear in a definite sequence: individual small dark epithelial cells, individual pale epithelial cells, pale epithelial cell clusters, and finally Hassall's bodies (51). Whether these epithelial cells represent different populations or are different stages of maturation/differentiation is not clear. However, the sequence with which these medullary epithelial cells reappear during regeneration resembles the sequence observed during thymic ontogeny in humans as described by Haynes (53).

Moreover, as long as the pale epithelial cell clusters do not reappear, the medulla contains a large number of lymphocytes, which is unlike a normal medulla. With the reappearance of pale epithelial cell clusters and a decline in the numbers of medullary lymphocytes, the medulla regains a near-normal morphology (51). These observations suggest that the pale epithelial cells may also play an important role in regulating the numbers of medullary lymphocytes besides the cortico-medullary demarcation in an adult animal. During the process of thymic regeneration, a longer time interval is needed for complete medullary regeneration after cortical repopulation (approximately 3 months) than the time interval needed for cortical regeneration after moderate to severe dysplasia (approximately 1½ months). It is of interest to note that the initiation of thymic regeneration (cortical repopulation) coincided with the spontaneous complete repopulation of the bone marrow, following its severe depletion (54,55), suggesting that the limiting factor in the initiation of thymic regeneration might be the spontaneous complete repopulation of the bone marrow.

B. Kinetics of Immune Functional Recovery

The immune functional studies on the animals in which the thymic regeneration was studied (as described above) showed that the recovery of the PFC response to SRBC is observed only when the thymus had regained a normal architecture. During the course of these studies (51), we recognized that although all the animals sacrificed on day 150-160 after GVH induction displayed normal thymic architecture, not all animals responded to SRBC. Furthermore various degrees of Con A response (% of normal response) as well as different numbers of PFC to SRBC were noted in the spleens of mice that did respond. Animals sacrificed on day 180 gave a higher Con A response than observed on day 150-160 after GVH induction, and all animals responded to SRBC in the PFC assay at that time. Variations in the numbers of the PFC to SRBC in the spleens of these mice were also observed. The precise reasons for the presence of a "lag phase" between the thymic architectural regeneration and the recovery of the PFC response (day 150-160), the variations in the numbers of PFC in the spleens of mice during the immune functional recovery, and the gradual increase in the Con A responses (day 150-160 vs. day 180) are not clear (51). Two possibilities were considered: (1) Since the PFC response to SRBC is a T-cell-dependent B-cell response, the "lag phase" during the immune functional recovery may be due to a lack in the functional potential of T and/or B cells, and (2) although the thymus recovers structurally from the GVH-induced dysplasia, it probably requires a longer time to regain function, i.e., hormone production.

To understand the reasons for the lag period as well as the variations observed in the numbers of PFC to SRBC during the immune functional recovery, we investigated the sequence and kinetics of B-cell and T-cell functions and their relation to the PFC response in each animal. The results from these studies showed that LPS-induced B-cell proliferative responses recovered to almost normal levels by day 60-80 after GVH induction. At this time, the thymuses displayed only cortical regeneration and the T-cell functions (proliferative and IL-2 production) were severely deficient (55). The T-cell functions started to recover gradually at a time when the thymic medulla displayed near-normal/normal architecture (day 150-160). The Con A-induced proliferative responses and IL-2 production following Con A stimulation recovered more rapidly than the PHA-induced functions (55). Furthermore, when the T- and B-cell proliferative responses were plotted as a function of the PFC/spleen response to SRBC, the results showed that (1) animals with only 1-2% of the normal PFC response showed up to 50-60% of Con A response, 30-45% of PHA response, and 90 to above 150% of LPS response and (2) after the initial recovery of T-cell proliferative function (about 90% for Con A and 70% for PHA), further increase in T-cell functions were less dramatic but the increase in the recovery of the PFC response was very obvious. These results suggested that (1) the B- and T-cell proliferative functions recover at different rates, independent of each other, (2) perhaps after the recovery of the proliferative functions, the regenerating immune system requires further maturation to acquire the capability to elicit T-B cell cooperative responses, and (3) the T-cell functional recovery may be gradual and depend upon the gradual thymic functional regeneration following its architectural regeneration.

C. Does Thymic Structural Recovery Precede Thymic Hormone Production (i.e., Functional Recovery)?

To test the proposal that the thymic functional recovery may also be gradual and would require more time after thymic architectural recovery, the following protocol was employed: GVH reactions were induced in large groups of F_1 mice and 6-10 animals were sacrificed at different stages of thymic regeneration. Their thymuses were examined histologically and the numbers of PFC to SRBC determined in their spleens. Splenocytes of animals with no PFC to SRBC (such mice are deficient in Con A and PHA mitogen responses) were pooled and then aliquoted. Aliquots were treated with either medium alone, or a thymic hormone (Thymosin), or agents that mimic the effect of thymic hormones, for example, prostaglandins of the E-series (PGE_1 and PGE_2) (56-58), and then tested for Con A- and PHA-induced proliferation responses.

The results from these studies demonstrated that thymosin, PGE_1, or PGE_2 pretreatment of GVH-splenocytes dramatically enhanced the T-cell proliferative functions only at the time when the thymic medulla had regenerated a near-normal morphology (10-20% of normal response of media-treated GVH splenocytes vs. 60-80% of normal response of thymosin or PGE_1- or E_2-treated GVH splenocytes). As long as the pale medullary epithelial cell clusters did not reappear in the thymic medulla, neither thymosin nor PGE_1 nor PGE_2 pretreatment had any significant effect on the proliferative responses of GVH-splenocytes. These observations suggest that the T-cells that could be induced to undergo at least the proliferative functions are present in the spleens of mice that display normal thymic medullary architecture, but these T-cells cannot yet respond to mitogens by themselves. It has been suggested that complete T-cell maturation requires both the physical contact with the thymic epithelial cells as well as thymic factor(s) elaborated by thymic epithelial cells (59,60). Thus, our observations would suggest that the inducible GVH T cells might have received the first signal, i.e., physical contact, and therefore encounter with the second signal in vitro, i.e., thymic factors or agents that mimic the effects of thymic factors, induces function in these T cells. Our observations, as described above, provide some evidence for the notion that the gradual recovery of T-cell functions after thymic architectural recovery may reflect the gradual functional recovery of the thymus (Ghayur et al., manuscript in preparation). These observations may also provide information for designing protocol(s) to enhance immune functions in immune-deficient patients.

Interestingly, even when thymic medullary dysplasia is evident, $L3T4^+$ ($CD4^+$) and $Lyt-2^+$ ($CD8^+$) cells are present in the GVHD dysplastic thymus and spleen (50). However, only the $Lyt-2^+$ but not the $L3T4^+$ cells acquire hydrocortisone resistance (50). Furthermore, GVHD-splenocytes can proliferate in the presence of IL-2 and PHA, but lack the ability to produce IL-2 following Con A or PHA stimulation and to initiate a proliferative response (48,49,55). These observations suggest that the $Lyt-2^+$ cells can acquire both phenotypic and "functional" maturity, whereas the $L3T4^+$ cells acquire only phenotypic maturity in the absence of a thymic medulla. The fact that the GVHD splenocytes can be induced to proliferate following thymosin, PGE1, or PGE2 pretreatment only at a time when the thymic medulla has regained normal architecture, suggests that acquisition of surface marker and functional capabilities might be two discrete events during the maturation of CD4$^+$ T cells. It is possible that the thymic environment, other than the medulla, is sufficient to induce phenotypic maturation, however, functional maturation of CD4$^+$ T cells may be dependent upon the presence of thymic medullary epithelial cells and thymic factors.

In brief, the studies described here concerning the thymic architectural (and functional) regeneration and immune functional recovery in long-term survivors of GVH reactions effectively suggest that the P → F$_1$ model of the GVHD can be employed to study the ontogeny of the immune system in an adult animal.

VI. CONCLUSIONS

The results described here demonstrate the significance of multiparameter kinetic studies in determining those early events that may provide an understanding of not only the eventual outcome of the GVHD, but also an understanding of the possible immune functional abnormalities during the ontogeny of the immune system in an adult animal. Our studies suggest that the initial severity of thymic dysplasia determines both the time needed for complete thymic regeneration as well as the duration of T-cell immune deficiency. It would therefore appear that the primary event that would determine the eventual outcome of the GVHD may be activation of effector mechanism(s) that initiates aGVHD-associated tissue lesions. Our studies suggest that the effector cell that plays a crucial role in the initiation of aGVHD-associated tissue damage is a specifically induced ASGM1$^+$ cell of donor origin that exhibits NK-cell activity. Further evidence that ASGM1$^+$ cells (with NK phenotype) of donor origin may cause tissue lesions is provided by Ferrara et al. (61).

Although we (8,29) and several other workers (38,39) have previously suggested that the NK/NK-like cell that plays a crucial role in the development of aGVHD-associated tissue damage may belong to T-cell lineage, the precise nature of this induced ASGM1$^+$ cell with NK activity is not clear at the moment. However, we have observed that either the elimination of this induced ASGM1$^+$ cell that exerts NK activity or an inherent deficiency in the cytotoxic function of NK cells does not affect the functions attributed to the classical T cells, i.e., T cells bearing the alpha/beta receptors (T3-$\alpha\beta$ cells). For instance, lymphoid cells depleted of this induced ASGM1$^+$ cell with NK activity or lymphoid cells deficient in NK cytotoxic function (bg/bg mutant mice) retain the ability to reject skin grafts, respond to SRBC antigens in the PFC assay, respond to T-cell mitogens (Con A and PHA), produce IL-2 following Con A and PHA stimulation in vitro, proliferate in response to alloantigens (including host antigens) in vitro, generate specific allo-CTL (including anti-host CTL) in vitro, and induce splenomegaly in F$_1$ mice. Moreover, the ASGM1$^+$ NK activity that is crucial for the development of tissue damage is induced within 44-48 hr following alloantigen (specific) but not poly I:C (nonspecific) stimulation. These observations and the studies described above collectively suggest that the induced ASGM1$^+$ cell that exerts NK activity may be distinct from the classical T cells (T3-$\alpha\beta$ cells) as well as the poly I.C-induced "classical NK cells" that do not express functional transcripts of α, β, or γ chain genes of the T-cell receptor (31). We suggest that this induced ASGM1$^+$ cell with NK activity may belong to the class of newly described T cells which bear the gamma/delta T-cell receptor (T3-$\gamma\delta$ cells).

Since our studies (16,29) have demonstrated that splenomegaly and tissue damage are two separate symptoms of the P → F$_1$ GVHD, and since it is now believed that the T3-$\alpha\beta$ T cells and the T3-$\gamma\delta$ T cells exhibit distinct lineages, homing patterns, and perhaps distinct functions (32), it becomes important to make a distinction between the roles of T3-$\alpha\beta$ and T3-$\gamma\delta$ cells during GVHD. We propose that the activation of T3-$\alpha\beta$ cells would play a major role in causing splenomegaly, whereas activation of T3-$\gamma\delta$ cells would play a major role in initiating aGVHD-associated tissue damage. Our suggestion that the effector cell for the aGVHD-associated tissue damage may belong to the T3-$\gamma\delta$ lineage is based upon observations showing that these T3-$\gamma\delta$ cells: (1) are induced following allo-stimulation (33,34), but not following poly I:C stimulation (31), (2) are ASGM1$^+$ (35) and exert NK cell-like cytotoxic activity (36,37), and (3) show specificity toward the H-2D (or a closely related) region of the H-2 complex (33). These features of the T3-$\gamma\delta$ cells are in agreement with the characteristics of the induced ASGM1$^+$ cell with NK activity described in this study. It has been recently suggested that the main function of the T3-$\gamma\delta$ cell may be surveillance of epithelial cells (32), and epithelial cells represent one of the prime targets of aGVHD (8). Furthermore, it is possible that besides the epithelia, the induced ASGM1$^+$ (T3-$\gamma\delta$) cells may also play a role in the surveillance of all rapidly proliferating cells as well as the various stem cell populations; both the rapidly proliferating cells and stem cells are also the prime targets of aGVHD (62).

If the induced ASGM1$^+$ cells that display NK activity (T3-$\gamma\delta$) initiate aGVHD-associated tissue lesions, then what is the role of the classical T (T3-$\alpha\beta$) cells in GVHD? Experimental studies have clearly demonstrated that depleting T cells (a procedure that might not necessarily deplete the induced ASGM1$^+$ cells) from the donor inoculum prevents GVH-associated mortality (64). Furthermore, mortality was related to the number of T cells added back to the T-cell-depleted graft (64). Similarly, in clinical settings, depletion of T cells from the graft prior to transplantation has reduced to varying degrees both the incidence and severity of observable aGVHD (65,66). Although T-cell depletion of the graft has decreased the incidence and severity of GVHD, the procedure has dramatically increased the incidence of graft rejection/graft failure (65-67). Thus, it is becoming apparent that depending upon the presence or absence of T cells in the inoculum, the transplanted cells can either cause GVHD or facilitate graft rejection/graft failure. It therefore appears that the classical T cells do play a critical role following transplantation. However, the observations concerning the presence or absence of T cells in the graft raise an important issue, that is, whether the classical T cells are the only effector cells involved in both the GVHD and graft rejection/graft failure processes or the classical T cells interact with a second cell population which also plays a crucial role in both GVHD and graft rejection/graft failure processes.

Studies from animal models of GVHD do, in fact, suggest that two donor cell populations interact to bring about the various symptoms of the GVHD (16,29.68,69). Furthermore, since our studies show that the induced ASGM1$^+$ cell with NK activity also plays a crucial role following GVHD induction, we suggest that the classical T cells may interact directly or indirectly with the induced ASGM1$^+$ cells, and thus these two cell populations would determine the outcome of the transplant. One can envision at least two forms of interaction between the classical T cells and the induced ASGM1$^+$ cell with NK activity; (1) the induction/recruitment of the ASGM1$^+$ effector cell is dependent upon the initial activation of T cells (15,29,79), and (2) the activation/induction of ASGM1$^+$ cells may be independent of T-cell activation, however, release of lymphokines by activated T cells may enhance recruitment and/or boost the functions of the induced ASGM1$^+$ cells (29). Regardless of the nature of interactions between the classical T (T3-$\alpha\beta$) cells and the induced ASGM1$^+$ cells with NK activity (T3-$\gamma\delta$), it is possible that both these cell populations may determine the eventual outcome of the transplant.

If two donor cell populations do determine the fate of the graft, then what might be the possible explanation for the increased incidence of graft rejection/graft failure of T-cell-depleted grafts? We suggest that if the T-cell depletion procedure(s) is not effective in eliminating the induced ASGM1$^+$ cells from the donor inoculum, then at least two additional possibilities should be considered, besides those already proposed (65-67), to explain the increased incidence of T-depleted graft rejection/graft failure: (1) the activation/induction of the ASGM1$^+$ aGVHD—effector cell would activate the host NK-mediated rejection mechanism (as discussed above) which would affect the stem cell numbers in the graft, i.e., perhaps only a few, if any, "stem" cells would survive. It should be pointed out that the NK-mediated rejection mechanism is highly effective in eliminating not only the marrow cells (70,71), but, once activated, other cell types as well (30; Ghayur et al., manuscript in preparation). (2) The activation/induction of ASGM1$^+$ cell that exerts NK activity might cause damage to the marrow stroma. The damaged marrow stroma may not be able to support the growth of the grafted stem cells. We have reported that GVHD induces severe reduction of bone marrow cellularity and a complete cessation of B-cell genesis (54,55). These observed changes in the bone marrow may be associated with the GVHD-associated bone marrow structural alterations (72,73). Our recent studies have demonstrated that depletion of the specifically induced ASGM1$^+$ cells with NK activity from the donor inoculum prevents both the aGVHD-associated decline of marrow cellularity as well as the cessation of B-cell genesis (78). Since our results in the P → F$_1$ GVHD model suggest that the specifically induced ASGM1$^+$ cell plays a crucial role in both the aGVHD and early graft rejection processes, we propose that complete depletion of this induced ASGM1$^+$ cell population that exerts NK activity from the inoculum (with or without depleting the classical T cells) might be beneficial for "stable" engraftment.

The P → F$_1$ GVHD model has thus far not been employed to study the regeneration of the immune system in an adult animal. Studies from our laboratory as well as by other workers have shown that both the thymic (9,17) and marrow (72,73) stroma are affected by the GVH reaction and both organs become extremely hypocellular. These stromal alterations of the primary lymphoid organs result in the cessation of production and/or maturation of T cells, particularly of the helper lineage (21-23), and B cells (54,55). We have also shown that with time after GVH induction, spontaneous complete repopulation of bone marrow and B-cell genesis is observed (54,55), followed by thymic structural (and functional) regeneration and then T-cell functional recovery (51). Thus, the initial (structural and/or functional) injury to, followed by spontaneous regeneration of the primary lymphoid organs provide not only a model to study the ontogency of the immune system in an adult animal, but may also provide insight into the immune functional abnormalities that may arise during immune functional regeneration in an adult animal.

An analysis of the kinetics of immune functional recovery in the P → F$_1$ hybrid GVHD model shows that the B-cell proliferative responses recover earlier than the T-cell functions (55). In fact, we have observed that in some animals that were severely deficient for T-cell functions, as well as NK-cell functions (74), the B cells were hyperresponsive to LPS. Thus, it appears that for a certain period of time during the immune recovery phase of the GVH reaction, the B cells may be the only "competent" cell type present in the spleens of GVH mice. These B cells may not be under the regulatory influences of either the T cells or NK cells. It is therefore possible that the differences in the rate of recovery of functionally competent B cells and T cells (as well as the functional status of NK cells) may be one of the reasons for B-cell "functional abnormalities." B cells in the absence of regulatory influences may give uncontrolled proliferation and may be susceptible to transformation, i.e., B-cell lymphomas (75-77).

The studies described here, as well as those reported previously (51), also demonstrate that the thymic medulla may require up to 3 months for complete regeneration. The significance of this long process of medullary regeneration in an adult animal is not clear. However, it has been suggested that thymic medullary epithelial cells may play a crucial role in T-cell education, i.e., class II restriction and self tolerance. Since during the initial stages of thymic regeneration the medulla lacks (pale) epithelial cells, it is possible that the T cells processed and released by such thymuses (lacking the restriction elements) may not learn self-nonself discrimination and may thus possess autoimmune potential. Such autoreactive T cells may contribute to the development of chronic GVHD, which is regarded as an autoimmune phenomenon. Moreover, T cells not properly educated (autoreactive) may activate B cells "abnormally," giving rise, again, to B-cell "functional abnormalities," e.g., auto-antibodies and related complications.

Our recent studies ((51) and as described above) have shown that the recovery of the T-cell functions in long-term survivors of the GVHD is observed only after the thymic medulla has regained a normal architecture. Thus, it would appear that factors that would determine the rate of thymic regeneration would also determine the rate of immune functional recovery. We have suggested that at least four factors may be crucial in determining the time required for thymic architectural and functional regeneration (51). These factors are: (1) the genetic disparity between the host (thymic stroma) and donor (transplanted cells); (2) the donor:host stem cell ratio repopulating the system, i.e., the degree of chimerism; (3) the intrinsic regeneration capacity of the host thymus which may be a function of the recipient's age, (4) the intensity of the effector mechanism(s) generated during the initial aGVHD that maintain lesions; one such radiosensitive mechanism has been described previously (52). Since the thymic structural (and probably functional) regeneration occurs in a definite sequence, i.e., different epithelial cells appear during different stages of medullary regeneration (51), it is important to recognize that a delay and/or block at a particular stage of thymic regeneration may prolong the period of time required for complete thymic structural (and functional) regeneration. We suspect that the longer the time required for thymic structural and functional regeneration, the greater might be the risk of developing both immune functional abnormalities and chronic GVHD.

In summary, the results described here suggest that the primary event that would determine the eventual fate of the animal undergoing a GVH reaction may be the initial severity of tissue damage, in particular the magnitude of injury to the primary lymphoid organs. The effector cell that plays a crucial role in initiating tissue damage and early graft rejection is a specifically induced $ASGM1^+$ (perhaps T3-$\gamma\delta$ cell) cell of donor origin that exerts NK activity. However, both the immune functional "abnormalities" and the development of chronic GVHD that are observed later following transplantation might reflect complications of regeneration of the immune system in an adult animal, i.e., recapitulation of ontogeny in a postnatal environment. Furthermore, the sequential structural (and functional) regeneration of the thymus of an adult animal may provide a powerful tool to study the role of thymic elements in the maturation of T cells or in the generation of stable chimeras, as well as provide insight into the role of various thymic epithelial elements at different stages of T-cell ontogeny.

ACKNOWLEDGMENTS

This work was supported by the Medical Research Council of Canada and the National Cancer Institute of Canada. We thank Ailsa Lee Loy, Rosemarie Siegrist-Johnstone, and Letti Pegorari for careful technical assistance and Carolyn Gregory for preparing the manuscript.

REFERENCES

1. Grebe SC, Streilein WJ: Graft-versus-host reactions: a review. Adv. Immunol. 1976; 23:120.
2. McBridge RA: Graft-versus-host reaction in lymphoid proliferation. Cancer Res 1966;26:1135.
3. Rappaport H, Khalil A, Halle-Pannenko O, Pritchard L, Dautchev D, Mattie G: Histologic sequence of events in adult mice undergoing lethal graft-versus-host reaction developed across H-2 and/or non-H-2 histocompatibility barriers. Am J Pathol 1979;96:1.
4. Hedberg CA, Reiser S, Reilly RW: Intestinal phase of the runting syndrome in mice. II. Observations on the nutrient absorption and disaccharidase abnormalities. Transplant 1968;6:104.
5. Van Bekkum DW, Roodenberg J, Heidt PJ et al.: Mitigation of secondary disease of allogeneic mouse radiation chimeras by modification of the intenstinal microflora. J Natl Cancer Inst 1974;52:401.
6. Van Bekkum DW, Knnau S: Brief communication: Role of bacterial microflora in development of intestinal lesions from graft-versus-host reaction. J Natl Cancer Inst 1977;52:401.
7. Simonsen M: Graft-versus-host reactions: Their natural history and applicability as tools of research. Progr Allergy 1962;6:349.
8. Lapp WS, Ghayur T, Mendez M, Seddik M, Seemayer TA: The functional and histological basis for graft-versus-host-induced immunosuppression. Immunol Rev. 1985; 88:107.
9. Seemayer TA, Lapp WS, Bolande RP: Thymic epithelial injury in graft-versus-host reactions following adrenalectomy. Am J Pathol 1978;93:325.
10. Shearer GM, Pollisson RP: Suppression of immune potential of F1 hybrid mice by parental T-lymphocytes: I. Genetic and mechanistic parameters associated with abrogation of T cell mediated cytotoxicity. J Exp Med 1980;151:20.
11. Howard JG, Michie D, Simonsen M: Splenomegaly as a host response in graft-versus-host disease. Brit J Exp Pathol 1961;42:476.
12. Fox M: Cytological estimation of proliferating donor cells during graft-versus-host disease in F1 hybrid mice injected with parental lymphoid cells. Immunol 1962;5:489.
13. Elie R, Lapp WS: Graft-versus-host induced immunosuppression. Depressed T cell helper functions in vitro. Cell Immunol 1976;21:31.
14. Elie R, Lapp WS: Graft-versus-host induced immunosuppression. Mechanism of depressed T helper cell function in vitro. Cell Immunol 1977;34:38.
15. Ghayur, T, Seemayer TA, Lapp WS: Kinetics of natural killer (NK) cell cytotoxicity during the graft-versus-host reaction. Relationship between NK cell activity, T and B

cell activity and development of histopathological alterations. Transplant 1987;44: 254.

16. Ghayur T, Seemayer TA, Kongshawn PAL, Gartner JS, Lapp WS: Graft-versus-host (GVH) reactions in the beige mouse: An investigation of the role of host and donor natural killer cells in the pathogenesis of GVH disease. Transplant 1987;44:261.

17. Ghayur, T, Seemayer TA, Lapp WS: Association between the degree of thymic dysplasia and the kinetics of thymic NK cell activity during the graft-versus-host reaction. Clin Immunol Immunopathol 1988;48:19.

18. Roder JC: The beige mutation in the mouse. I. A stem cell predetermined impairment in natural killer cell function. J Immunol 1979;123:2168.

19. Roder JC, Duwe A: The beige mutation in the mouse selectively impairs natural killer cell function. Nature 1979;278:451.

20. Lapp WS, Mendes M, Kirchner H, Gemsa D: Prostaglandin synthesis by lymphoid tissue of mice experiencing a graft-versus-host reaction: relationship to immunosuppression. Cell Immunol 1980;50:271.

21. Seddik M, Seemayer TA, Kongshaun PAL, Lapp WS: Thymic epithelial functional deficit in chronic graft-versus-host reactions. Transplant Proc 1979;11:967.

22. Seddik M, Seemayer TA, Lapp WS: T cell functional defect associated with thymic epithelial cell injury induced by a graft-versus-host reaction (1980).

23. Seddik, M, Seemayer TA, Lapp WS: The graft-versus-host reaction and immune function. I. T helper cell immuno-deficiency associated with graft-versus-host induced thymic epithelial cell damage. Transplant 1984;37:286.

24. Charley MR, Mikheal A, Bennett M, Gillam JM, Southeimer RD: Prevention of lethal, minor-determinate graft-versus-host disease in mice by the in vivo administration of anti-asialo GM1. J Immunol 1983;131:2101.

25. Varkila K, Hurme M: Acute graft-versus-host disease mortality in murine parent vs. F1 model can be prevented by treatment of the recipient mice with anti-asialo GM1 antibody. J Leukocyte Biol 1985;38:124.

26. Varkila K: Depletion of asialo-GM1[+] cells from the F1 recipient mice prior to irradiation and transfusion of parental spleen cells prevents mortality to acute graft-versus-host disease and indution of anti-host specific cytotoxic T cells. Clin Exp Immunol 1987,69:652.

27. Guillen F, Ferrara J, Hancock W, Messadi D, Fonferko E, Burakoff S, Murphy G: Acute cutaneous graft-versus-host disease to minor histocompatibility antigens in a murine model II. Evidence that large granular lymphocytes are effector cells in the immune response. Lab Invest 1986;55:35.

28. Kasai M, Yoneda T, Habu S, Maruyama Y, Okumura K, Tokunaga T. In vivo effect of anti-asialo GM1 antibody on natural killer cell activity. Nature 1981;291:5813.

29. Ghayur, T, Seemayer TA, Lapp WS: Prevention of murine graft-versus-host disease by inducing and eliminating ASGM1[+] cells of donor origin. Transplant 1988;45:586.

30. Peres A, Nestel FP, Seemayer TA, Lapp WS: The effects of polyionsinic:polycytidylic acid (pI:C) on the graft-versus-host reaction. II. An NK-mediated rejection of C57BL/6 lymphocytes by (C57BL/6 × A) F1 mice. J Immunol 1986;137:3420.

31. Tutt M, Kuziel WA, Hackett J, Bennett M, Kumar V: Murine natural killer cells do not express functional transcripts of the alpha-beta or gamma-chain genes of the T cell receptor. J Immunol 1986;137:2998.

32. Janeway CA, Jones B, Hayday A: Specificity and function of T cells bearing the γδ receptor. Immunol Today 1988;9:74.

33. Matis LA, Cross R, Bluestone JA: Major histocompatibility complex-linked specificity of γδ receptor bearing T lymphocytes. Nature 1987;330:262.

34. Macda K, Nakanishi N, Roger BL, Haser WG, Shitara K, Yoshida H, Takagaki Y, Augustin AA, Tonegawa S: Expression of the T cell receptor γ chain gene products

on the surface of peripheral T cells and T cell blasts generated by allogeneic mixed lymphocyte reaction. Proc Natl Acad Sci USA 1987;84:6534.

35. Romani N, Stingle G, Tschachler E, Witmer WD, Steinman RN, Shevach EM, Schuler G: The Thyl bearing cell of murine epidermis. J Exp Med 1985;161:1368.

36. Alarcon B, Devries J, Pettery C, Boyston A, Yssel H, Terhorst C, Spits H: The T cell receptor γ chain-CD3 complex: Implication in the cytotoxic activity of a CD3$^+$ CD4$^-$ CD8$^-$ human natural killer clone. Proc Natl Acad Sci USA 1987;84:3861.

37. Moingeon P, Titsukawa S, Fauve F, Troalen F, Tribel F, Graziani M, Forestier F, Bellet D, Bohuom C, Herchaud TA: γ Chain complex forms a functional receptor on cloned human lymphocytes with natural killer-like activity. Nature 1987;325: 723.

38. Dokhelar M, Wiels J, Lipinski M, Tetaude C, Devergie A, Gluckman E, Tursz T: Natural killer cell activity in human bone marrow recipients. Early appearance of peripheral natural killer activity in graft-versus-host disease. Transplant 1981;31:61.

39. Clancy J, Mauser L, Chapman AL: Level and temporal pattern of naturally cytolytic cells during actue graft-versus-host disease (GVHD) in the rat. Cell Immunol 1983; 79:1.

40. Waterfall M, Rayfield LS, Brent L: The role of natural killer cells in resistance to allogeneic and parental hybrid resistance. Transplant 1987;43:312.

41. Warner JF, Dennert G: Effects of cloned cell line with NK activity on bone marrow transplants, tumor development and metastasis in vivo. Nature 1982;300:31.

42. Waterfall M, Rayfield LS, Brent L: Abrogation of resistance to bone marrow transplantation by induction of specific tolerance in natural killer cells? Nature 1984; 311:663.

43. Cudowicz G, Hochman PS: Do natural killer cells engage in regulated reactions against self to ensure homeostasis? Immunol Rev 1979;44:13.

44. Gidlund M, Orn A, Wigzell H, Senik A, Gresser I: Enhanced NK cell activity in mice infected with interferon and interferon inducers. Nature 1978;223:259.

45. Herberman RB, Djeu JY, Kay MD, Ortaldo JR, Riccardi C, Bonnard GD, Holden HT, Fagnani R, Santoni A, Pucceli R: Natural killer cells: Characteristics and regulation of activity. Immunol Rev 1979;44:43.

46. Ghayur T, Agopian I, Xenocostas A, Lapp WS: Relationship between hybrid resistance and graft versus host reaction. Fed Proc 1988;

47. Peres A, Seemayer TA, Lapp WS: The effects of polyinosinic:polycytidylic (pI.C) on the graft-versus-host reaction: Immunopathological observations. Clin Immunol Immunopathol 1986;39:102.

48. Mendez M, Rode H, Lapp WS: Murine graft-versus-host disease associated with interleukin-1 and interleukin-2 defects. Transplant Prod 1985;17:541.

49. Mendez ML, Rode H, Peres A, Kongshaun PAL, Lapp WS: Interleukin-1 and interleukin-2 defects associated with murine graft-versus-host induced immunodeficiency. Transplant 1985;39:418.

50. Kornbluth M, Seemayer TA, Lapp WS: The effects of GVH-induced thymic dysplasia on thymocyte differentiation. Fed Proc 1987;45:1358.

51. Ghayur, T, Seemayer TA, Xenocostas A, Lapp WS: Complete sequential regeneration of graft-versus-host (GVH) induced severely dysplastic thymuses. Implications for the pathogenesis of chronic GVH disease. Am J Pathol 1988;133:39.

52. Seddik M, Seemayer TA, Lapp WS: The graft-versus-host reaction and immune function. II. Recruitment of pre-T cells in vivo by graft-versus-host induced dysplastic thymuses following irradiation and bone marrow treatment. Transplant 1984;37: 286.

53. Haynes BF. The human thymic microenvironment. Adv Immunol 1984;36:87.

54. Xenocostas A, Lapp WS, Osmond DG: Suppression of B lymphocyte genesis in the bone marrow by systemic graft-versus-host reactions. Transplant 1987;43:549.

55. Ghayur, T, Xenocostas A, Seemayer TA, Lapp WS: Kinetics of recovery of NK and immune functions of graft-versus-host immunosuppressed mice. Fed Proc 1986,45:268.

56. Bach MA, Bach JF: In: Robinson HJ and Vane JR, eds. Prostaglandin synthesis inhibitors. Raven Press, New York, p. 241.

57. Garaci CR, Favalli C, Gobbo VD, Garaci E, Jaffe BM: Is thymosin action mediated by prostaglandin release? Science 1983;220:1163.

58. Garaci E, Garaci CR, Gobbo VD, Favalli C, Santoro MG, Jaffe BM: A synthetic analogue of PGE2 is able to induce in vivo theta antigens on spleen cells of adult thymectomized mice. Cell Immunol 1981;62:8.

59. Stutman O: Intrathymic and extrathymic T cell maturation. Immunol Rev 1978; 42:138.

60. Zinkernagel RM: Thymus and lympho-hemopoietic cells: Their role in T cell maturation, in selection of T cells' H-2 restriction specificity and in H-2 linked Ir gene control. Immunol Rev 1978;42:224.

61. Ferrara JLM, Guillen FJ, van Dijken PJ, Marion A, Murphy GF, Burakoff SJ: Evidence that large granular lymphocytes of donor origin mediate acute graft-versus-host disease. Transplant (in press).

62. Snover D: Acute and chronic graft-versus-host disease: histopathological evidence for two distinct pathogenetic mechanisms. Human Pathol 1983;15:202.

63. Lafferty KJ, Walker KZ, Scollary RG, Killby VAA: Allogeneic interactions provide evidence for a novel class of immunological reactivity. Transplant Rev 1972; 12:198.

64. Korngold R, Sprent J: Lethal GVHD across minor histocompatibility barriers: Nature of the effector cells and role of the H-2 complex. Immuno Rev 1983;71:5.

65. Martin PJ, Hansen JA, Storb R, Thomas ED: Human marrow transplantation: An immunological perspective. Adv Immunol 1987;40:379.

66. Gale RP, Reisner Y: Graft rejection and graft-versus-host disease: Mirror images. Lancet 1986;1:1468.

67. Kernan NA, Flomenberg N, Dupont B, O'Reilly RJ: Graft rejection in recipients of T cell-depleted HLA-nonidentical marrow transplants for leukemia: Identification of host-derived anti-donor allocytotoxic T lymphocytes. Transplant 1987;43: 842.

68. Cantor H, Asofsky R: Synergy among lymphoid cells mediating the GVH response. II. Synergy in GVHR produced by Balb/c lymphoid cells of differing anatomic origin. J Exp Med 1970;131:235.

69. Cantor H, Asofsky R: Synergy among lymphoid cells mediating the graft-versus-host response. III. Evidence for interaction between two types of thymus dependent cells. J Exp Med 1972;135:764.

70. Harmon RC, Clark EA, O'Toole C, Wicker LS: Resistance to H-2 heterozygous mice to parental tumors. I. Hybrid resistance and natural cytotoxicity to EL-4 are controlled by the H-2D-Hh-1 region. Immunogenet 1977;4:601.

71. Cudhowicz G, Bennett M: Peculiar immunobiology of bone marrow allografts. II. Rejection of parental grafts by resistant F1 hybrid mice. J Exp Med 1971;134:1513.

72. Hirabayashi N: Studies on GVHRs. I. Impairment of hemopoietic stroma in mice suffering from GVHD. Exp Hematol 1981;9:101.

73. Ishihara K, Shimaninie T. Structural changes of murine bone marrow in GVHR. Pathol Res Pract 1980;169:84.

74. Roy C, Ghayur, T, Kongshaun PAL, Lapp WS: Natural killer cell activity by spleen, lymph node, and thymus cells during the graft-versus-host reaction. Transplant 1982,34:144.

75. Armstrong MYK, Gleichmann E, Gleichmann H, Beldotti L, Andre-Schwartz J,

Schwartz RS: Chronic allogeneic disease. II. Development of lymphomas. J Exp Med 1970;132:417.

76. Cornelius EA: Induction of both host and donor type tumors as a result of graft-versus-host reaction. Transplant 1972,13:589.

77. Gleichmann E, Gleichmann H, Wilke W: Autoimmunization and lymphomagenesis in parent into F1 combinations differing at the major histocompatibility complex: model for spontaneous disease caused by altered self-antigens. Immunol Rev 1988; 31:156.

78. Xenocostas A, Ghayur T, Osmond DG, Lapp WS: Elimination of asialo-GM1 positive cells prevents graft-versus-host induced depression of primary B cell production in mouse bone marrow. FASEB J 1988;2:1024.

79. Ferrara J, Marion A, Murphy G, Burakoff S: Acute graft-versus-host disease: Pathogenesis and prevention with a monoclonal antibody in vivo. Transplant Proc 1987; 19:2662.

8

Immunologic and Hematopoietic Deficiencies of Graft-vs.-Host Disease

Frances T. Hakim and Gene M. Shearer
National Cancer Institute
National Institutes of Health
Bethesda, Maryland

The multiple effects of graft-vs.-host disease on host tissues have been studied in a variety of murine models. All of these models are based upon the effect of injected allogeneic or semiallogeneic lymphocytes on hosts which are not competent to react against the donor inoculum. Host immune incompetence toward the donor lymphocytes may be due to (1) depletion in irradiated hosts, (2) immaturity in neonatal hosts, or (3) tolerance in F_1 offspring of the donor and another strain. This review of GVH will concentrate on the results of work done on the last of these three model systems.

In these "parent into F_1" (P-into-F_1) studies, the F_1 host is tolerant of the donor antigens and cannot reject donor cells (with the exceptions discussed below). The donor cells, however, are stimulated by the alloantigens expressed on the F_1 host cells. When large numbers of donor cells (greater than 100×10^6) are injected into F_1 hosts, the resulting disease bears a strong resemblance to GVHD in irradiated hosts. Mice exhibit severe wasting, diarrhea, skin lesions, and early death. When fewer donor cells are injected ($20\text{-}60 \times 10^6$), the resulting graft vs. host disorder (GVHD) rarely is fatal in the short term. Although some weight loss is common, severe wasting or skin lesions occur rarely, if at all. At these threshold doses, the main target of the GVHD in unirradiated F_1 hosts is the lymphohematopoietic system, and the main effects measurable in these mice are immune dysfunctions. In order to describe the current state of information on these immune changes and their mechanisms of induction, this review will concentrate on the GVHD produced by threshold levels of donor lymphocytes.

The form of the graft vs. host induced immune dysfunction is dependent upon the genetic disparity between the donor and the host (1-6). When the disparity involves both class I and class II major histocompatibility (MHC) antigens, the result is an acute, suppressive GVHD. This form of GVHD is characterized by a profound immune deficiency (GVHID) of all T- and B-cell functions, the direct attack of donor cells on lymphohematopoietic tissues and the reconstitution of the host lymphohematopoietic system with donor-derived cells (5,7-11). When the disparity involves only a difference in class II (Ia antigen) loci, then a chronic "stimulatory" form of GVHD develops, characterized by only a limited engraftment of donor cells within the host lymphohematopoietic system, by a limited T-cell functional deficiency, and by polyclonal B-cell activation and production of autoantibodies (1,3,5-7,12). Class I disparities alone are rarely sufficient to produce a GVHD in the unirradiated P-into-F_1 model (3-5); in association with disparities at minor histocompatibility loci or with certain viral infections, these disparities can generate an immune deficit comparable to that engendered by a full MHC disparity GVHD (13-15). Disparities only at minor histocompability loci do not generate GVHID in unirradiated hosts. Each of these forms of GVHD will be examined in this chapter, emphasizing donor lymphohematopoietic engraftment, immune dysfunction, immune suppressive mechanisms, and thymic alterations.

I. IMMUNOLOGIC AND HEMATOPOIETIC CHANGES IN CLASS I + II GVHD

A. Development of Donor/Host Lymphohematopoietic Chimerism

GVHD induced across a disparity in both class I and class II MHC antigens produces a direct cell-mediated attack on host lymphohematopoietic populations, resulting in the reconstitution of the host with cells derived from the donor (5,7,10,11,16,17). Replacement of as much as 70% of splenic cells with donor-derived cells may occur as early as 6-8 weeks after induction of GVHD (Hakim and Shearer, in preparation). The process of replacement occurs in three phases. During the first phase, both donor and host cells proliferate. One of the earliest observable alterations in GVHD is a marked splenomegaly; within a week the spleen may as much as triple in size. In the second phase, there is a drastic decrease in splenic cell populations, both donor and host. In the third phase, donor cells increase in number once more, repopulating and numerically dominating the lymphohematopoietic system. Similar sequences of events occur in several combinations of donor and host strains examined; the data below was generated by injecting 50×10^6 C57Bl/10 spleen cells into (B10 X B10.BR)F_1 hosts. Different strain combinations may vary in terms of the degree of long-term donor engraftment, but not in the initial events.

The early increase in spleen size is produced in part by an influx of donor T-cell populations, but the majority of the increase is due to host non-T cells (Fig. 1). By 2 weeks after induction of GVHD, T-cell populations predominate, constituting almost 50% of the total cells in the enlarged spleen. Both host and donor T cells have increased and are about equal in number. Both the L3T4$^+$ (CD4$^+$) and Lyt-2$^+$ (CD8$^+$) T subsets have increased, but the Lyt-2$^+$ T cells have increased disproportionately in both host and donor T populations, outnumbering the L3T4$^+$ population. Donor B cells have also appeared in the spleen by this point. During weeks 3-4, the majority of both donor and host splenic cells die. Large numbers of dead cells are found in the spleen. Although macrophage numbers are increased as early as the first week of GVHD, only in this period do macrophage lineage (Mac-1$^+$) cells become a major population in the spleen. Also present in significant numbers at weeks 3-4 are null cells which do not express T-, B-, or macrophage cell markers. After this period of cell death, more than half the cells in the spleen are of donor origin. At 6 weeks post-GVHD, a few donor B cells are found. At 8-10 weeks, B-cell levels recover; these cells are predominantly of donor origin. T-cell levels

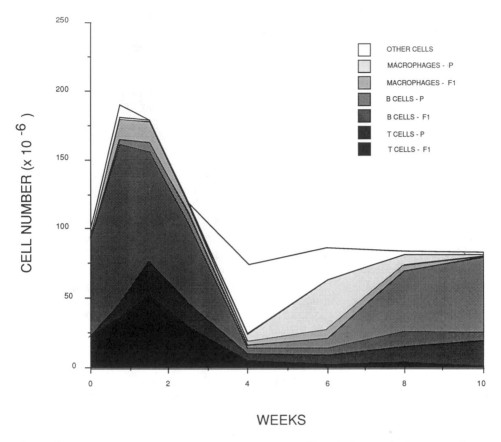

Figure 1 Timecourse of changes in parental and host F_1 splenic populations over the first 10 weeks of acute, suppressive GVHD. $(B10 \times B10.BR)F_1$ mice were injected with 50×10^6 C57Bl/10 parental spleen cells at periods ranging from 5 days to 10 weeks prior to colletion of host spleens, counting of nucleated cells, and analysis of cell populations by two-color FACS analysis. Different splenic populations were identified by surface expression of macrophage (Mac-1), B-cell (surface IgM), and T-cell (CD3) markers. Host cells were distinguished from parental donor cells by expression of H-2K^k (36.7.5). The category "other" cells could include NK cells, null cells and differentiating myeloid and erythroid lineage cells, all of which are common in the spleen at 3-6 weeks of GVHD.

recover more slowly, requiring 15-20 weeks to return to normal levels of L3T4$^+$ and Lyt-2$^+$ cells. These are entirely donor in origin as well.

Examination of bone marrow populations reveals a similar timecourse. Total marrow cells increase during the first 2 weeks of GVH. At 3-4 weeks the marrow is drastically depleted, reduced to as little as 10% of normal cell numbers, and appears white due to depletion of erythroid precursors. Erythropoiesis, as measured by ^{59}Fe incorporation into marrow cells, is markedly decreased, as is the peripheral blood hematocrit (9). T-cell populations, particularly Lyt-2$^+$ T cells, increase disproportionately in the bone marrow, increasing from 3-4% in normal marrow to 6-16% during weeks 3-4 (Hakim and Shearer, in preparation). Cell numbers and T-cell frequencies return to normal by 6-8 weeks. Assessment of the degree of bone marrow reconstitution by donor cells is difficult to measure directly because of the weak expression of class I antigens on many marrow cells. Indirectly, the reconstitution of the spleen with donor-derived cells after the period of general destruction (weeks 3-4) suggests that the marrow populatons have been replaced by donor-derived stem cells. Furthermore, if GVHD is induced by injection of donor populations which lack stem cells, such as parental lymph node cells, then the GVHD is invariably fatal by 5 weeks. After the injection of lymph node cells, spleen and bone marrow never show the burst in stem cell numbers found after induction of GVHD by injection of donor spleen cells (104). This evidence is consistent with a dependence upon donor precursor populations to reconstitute the depleted lymphohematopoietic system of the host.

The stability of the donor/host chimeras over the long term varies depending on the strain combination involved in the GVHD. Two systems were examined in which $H-2^b$ spleen cells were injected into $(H-2^b \times H-2^k)$ F_1 hosts (Hakim and Shearer, in preparation). In $(B10 \times B10.BR)F_1$ mice injected with $50\text{-}60 \times 10^6$ C57Bl/10 (B10) spleen cells, spleens contained predominantly donor cells after 6-8 weeks of GVHD, as noted above. As late as 18 months after induction of GVHD, spleens of 10 out of 12 mice examined were still composed of greater than 90% donor cells. One mouse had significant populations of host non-T cells, but only donor T cells. One mouse had predominantly host T and non-T populations, with only $L3T4^+$ donor T cells remaining. Injection of similar doses of C57Bl/6 spleen cells into $(C57Bl/6 \times C3H/HeN)F_1$ $(B6C3F_1)$ results in spleens containing primarily donor cells at 6 weeks of GVHD. Repopulation by autologous cells is much greater in this strain than in $(B10 \times B10.BR)F_1$, however. After only 10-12 months, spleens of 2 of 9 mice tested had reverted completely to host phenotype; 4 had mostly host T and non-T cells with only $L3T4^+$ T cells of donor origin remaining; 1 had mixed origin T cell populations but predominantly host non-T cells; only 2 were predominantly donor in phenotype. The pattern of recovery of host phenotype cells appears, therefore, to be first the non-T populations and subsequently the T-cell populations. The $L3T4^+$ donor T cells are apparently the last cells to be eliminated.

This long-term instability is not found in other murine hematopoietic reconstitution /GVHD models. In irradiated mice injected with marrow grafts disparate from the host at major histocompatibility loci, mixed donor host chimerism is common, particularly at lower radiation doses or donor marrow inoculums. In these systems, however, the degree of lymphoid and erythroid chimerism is stable between 3 and 12 months (18,19). Similarly in antibody facilitated bone marrow chimeras, involving injection of allogeneic and semiallogeneic cells into unirradiated hosts, chimerism is stable in both lymphoid and erythroid populations for over 16 months (20,21). In clinical bone marrow transplantation studies, in contrast, mixed chimerism has been considered to be a transient and unstable state, heralding graft rejection and repopulation by cells of host origin (22).

The mechanisms involved in this long-term recovery of the host phenotype are unknown. Possibly, remaining host stem cells have a positive advantage and eventually proliferate more extensively than donor cells. The disparity in donor/host chimerism in the two murine class I + II GVHD systems studied could then be due to the degree to which host stem cells were eliminated during the period of donor attack on host cells early in GVHD. Another possibility is that remaining host stem cell populations are able to generate effectors which actively eliminated donor stem cells. In the two strain combinations studied, there is a strong element of host hybrid resistance to the stem cells of the parental donor strain. Hybrid resistance refers to the ability of F_1 hosts of these strains to reject tumor or hematopoietic stem cells of the H-2^b parent (23-25). This rejection is mediated by NK cells and is based on detection of the hybrid histocompatibility antigen Hh-1, expressed only on homozygous H-2^b cells and not on F_1 cells (25-28). Hybrid resistance may contribute to an increased threshold of H-2^b parental cells required for the initial induction of GVHD, as compared with that necessary in the non-H-2^b parent (16, 29-31); for example, 30 × 10^6 B10.BR (H-2^k) spleen cells reliably induce an acute suppressive GVHD in (B10 × B10.BR)F_1 hosts, while 50 × 10^6 B10 (H-2^b) spleen cells are required. Host hybrid resistance is apparently lost early in GVHD (see below) (11,32). If host stem cell precursors for NK cells survived, it is possible that hybrid resistance could again become effective. The reappearance of hybrid resistance in long-term chimeric GVH mice has not been assessed, however.

B. Immune Deficiency in GVHD

Beginning shortly after induction of GVHD, a profound immune deficiency develops in vivo, resulting in increased susceptibility to bacterial infections and reduced capacity to reject skin grafts (33,34). This deficiency is evident in vitro in assays of T-cell proliferative response to mitogens (such as Concanavalin A), and proliferation and generation of cytolytic T lymphocytes (CTL) in response to modified syngeneic and allogeneic stimulators (4,16,35-38). B-cell functions such as proliferative response to LPS and generation of anti-sRBC plaque forming cells (PFC) are also markedly depressed (3,39-41). Host NK cell functions are rapidly lost as well.

The functions of all subsets of host T cells are affected by GVHD (Fig. 2). Concanavalin A is a broadly acting T-cell mitogen, affecting the entire population of T cells. In acute, suppressive GVHD in the C57Bl/10-into-(B10 × B10.BR)F_1 system, Concanavalin A proliferative responses are depressed at 1 week, reach their lowest point at 3-4 weeks, and begin to recover after 8 weeks, returning to normal by 10 weeks. Primary CTL responses are more sensitive, in part because only a limited portion of the T-cell repertoire is involved. CTL generation to allogeneic stimulators decreases to baseline levels during the first week of GVHD and remains depressed for several weeks, returning to normal by 15-20 weeks. CTL generation to TNP-modified syngeneic stimulators (TNP-self) is similarly depressed, but eventual recovery of this function varies depending upon the strain combination used in GVHD.

CTL generation to TNP-modified syngeneic stimulators has been demonstrated to require L3T4$^+$ T_H cells, which provide help for Lyt-2$^+$ precursor CTL (pCTL) (42,43). CTL generation to allogeneic stimuli is a broader response, involving both L3T4$^+$ T_H and Lyt-2$^+$ T_H, as well as Lyt-2$^+$ pCTL (42-44). T helper function in both the L3T4$^+$ and the Lyt-2$^+$ T_H subsets is compromised by GVHD, as assessed by a decrease in IL-2 production in response to either TNP-modified syngeneic or allogeneic stimulators (6). Furthermore, differentiation of pCTL is affected, because supplementing the primary CTL culture media with T-cell growth factors (a Concanavalin A-stimulated supernatant of normal spleen cells) does not promote the differentiation of CTL (7,36).

On the other hand, mature CTL may be less susceptible to the immune defects of GVHD. If host mice have been repeatedly primed against allogeneic cells, prior to the induction of GVHD, an alloantigen-specific response is retained after GVHD. Thus, if a sufficient population of primed T helper and effector cells have previously been generated, then the immune deficiency engendered by GVHD does not affect their activity (45).

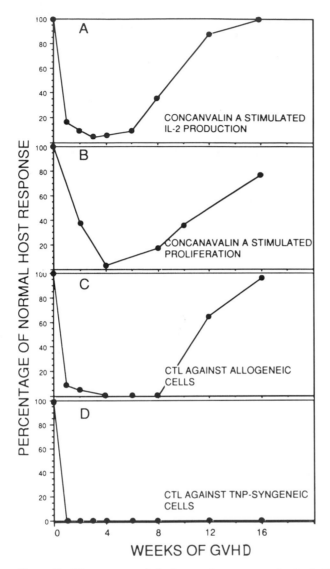

Figure 2 Timecourse of the loss and recovery of splenic T-cell functions over the first 16 weeks of GVHD. $(B10 \times B10.BR)F_1$ mice were injected with 50×10^6 C57Bl/10 spleen cells at periods ranging from 1 to 16 weeks prior to the experiment. (A) Splenic cells were cultured for 24 hours with Concanavalin A to generate IL-2-containing supernatants, which were assayed on an IL-2-dependent cell line (CTLL). (B) Splenic cells were cultured for 72 hours with Concanavalin A to measure proliferation by ^{3}H-thymidine incorporation during the final 18 hours. (C) Splenic cells were cultured for 5 days with irradiated allogeneic stimulators (B10.D2) and then assayed for CTL generation in a 4-hour ^{51}Cr release assay on allogeneic (Concanavalin A-stimulated) lymphoblasts. (D) Splenic cells were cultured for 5 days with irradiated, TNP-modified C57Bl/10 spleen cells (TNP–self) and assayed for CTL generation in a 4-hour ^{51}Cr release assay on TNP-modified C57Bl/10 lymphoblasts. All data is expressed as a percentage of normal $(B10 \times B10.BR)F_1$ response.

At different time points in acute GVHD, several factors may contribute to the immune deficits measured. During weeks 3-6, there is an absolute numerical deficit in T-cell populations (7) (Fig. 1). This may contribute to the low point in immune functions reached during these weeks. Certainly immune functions do not recover until significant splenic repopulation by donor cells has occurred. But numerical deficits are not the only factor, because functional deficits occur during the first 2 weeks of GVHD, a period of normal or increased T cell frequency.

Another important factor in early GVHD may be a decrease in the production of interleukin 2 (IL-2) and in the expression of the IL-2 receptor. Since T-cell proliferation and differentiation of CTL from precursor cells are both dependent upon IL-2, a decline in IL-2 production would decrease these responses. IL-2 production in Concanavalin A generated splenic supernatants is depressed at 1 week in acute suppressive GVHD, reaches a low point at 3-4 weeks, and begins to recover after 6 weeks. Normal levels are reached by 10 weeks. IL-2 receptor expression (in Concanavalin A-stimulated spleen cells) is also markedly decreased at 2 weeks of acute GVHD (46). This decrease in IL-2 receptors could contribute to failure of T-cell growth factors to restore function in CTL cultures. Thus, a deficit in IL-2 production and responsiveness could be partly responsible for the early immune deficit in GVHD.

Primary B-cell responses are also defective during GVHD. LPS response is decreased as early as 8 days after induction of GVHD (39). Decreases in plaque forming cell (PFC) response to sheep red blood cells (sRBC) have been found as early as 4 days of GVHD in some strain combinations (39) and remain depressed for several weeks (3, 40,47). During the course of acute GVHD, deficits in B-cell numbers in the spleen and in pre-B cells in the bone marrow have been found (9,48,49) (Fig. 1). The deficit in B-cell function, however, precedes the numerical loss of B cells (48). As was the case with primed CTL, primed B-cell responses may be resistant to the effects of GVHD (45). Responses to pathogens such as cytomegalovirus (CMV) can be retained after induction of GVHD in mice that have been previously primed against CMV. Without prior immunization against CMV, little or no antibody against CMV is generated in mice undergoing GVHD, and the infection is lethal even in normally resistant strains. If CMV-primed mice undergoing GVHD are challenged with CMV, however, all mice survive the infective challenge. The resistance to CMV may involve expanded populations of primed T cells, primed B cells, or merely protective levels of circulating antibody. Nonetheless, as with allogeneic priming, virus-primed lymphoid populations appear able to function after GVHD, while primary responses have ceased.

A third aspect of immune function which is adversely affected by GVHD is host resistance to tumors and to marrow grafts (11,32,50). As noted above, irradiated F_1 hosts demonstrate a "hybrid resistance" to the engraftment of tumor lines or normal hematopoietic stem cells from parents bearing certain hybrid histocompatibility (Hh) antigens (23-25,51). In the classic case, irradiated F_1 mice heterozygous for Hh-1, mapping near H-2D^b, reject marrow grafts from H-2^b parents. This host resistance is mediated by NK effectors, following activation by interferon secreted by host macrophages (3,52). Treatments which enhance NK activity, such as interferon inducers like poly-[I,C], increase host resistance (52); treatments which deplete NK cells decrease host resistance (26,28). Finally, hybrid resistance can be overcome by competitive inhibition with large numbers of H-2^b stem cells or tumor cells that exhaust the capacity of hybrid resistance effector cells (51,53).

F_1 hybrid resistance is rapidly abrogated by the GVHD. That is, if F_1 host mice, injected with H-2^b parental spleen cells to induce GVHD, are subsequently irradiated and injected with H-2^b marrow, the normal F_1 resistance to marrow engraftment is rapidly lost. Initially, the decrease in hybrid resistance in GVHD may be due to a competitive inhibition of host resistance to injected marrow; the large number of hematopoietic stem cells in the original donor inoculum may numerically overwhelm and exhaust host resistance to H-2D^b bearing cells in the test marrow graft. Such a decrease in host resistance would be dependent upon injection of H-2D$^{b/b}$ hemopoietic cells in GVHD donor spleen inoculum (53) and could occur independently of GVHID in hosts receiving T-depleted or class I MHC disparate donor grafts (32). The complete loss of hybrid resistance that occurs after the first week of GVH, however, is dependent on GVHD-induced immune deficiency, not merely competitive inhibition by H-2^b stem cells in the GVHD-inducing inoculum. This loss of hybrid resistance parallels the depression in host immune functions including CTL generation, MLR proliferation, and anti-sRBC PFC response (11,32). Both the immune deficiencies in T- and B-cell functions and the loss of hybrid resistance are dependent on injection of T cells (11,32). Furthermore, the loss of host resistance has been demonstrated in strain combinations in which the GVHD-inducing inoculum was heterozygous for Hh antigens, hence could not competitively inhibit host resistance to Hh-1$^+$ marrow grafts (e.g., (B10 × B10.A(5R)F_1-into-(B10 × B10.A)F_1) (32). Furthermore, injection of donor spleen cells which are capable of competitively inhibiting hybrid resistance (i.e., H-2D$^{b/b}$), but which are unable to induce a GVHD immune deficiency in the host, produces no significant decrease in host resistance by the second week of GVHD (B10.A(2R)-into-(B10.A(2R) × B10.A)F_1) (32). Recently, a Thy 1.2$^+$, Lyt-1$^+$2$^-$ T cell has been reported to be involved in the initial recognition of H-2^b stem cells, triggering the effectors of hybrid resistance (54). Given the profound depression in all T-cell functions that has been observed in GVHD, possibly this T cell is affected as well.

The loss in host resistance has also been correlated with a loss of host NK function. NK activity, including both host- and donor-derived NK cells, increases in the first week of acute GVHD (37,39) and then decreases to baseline levels. NK activity present after the first week is primarily donor derived (11,37,39) and may be due in part to asialo-GM1$^+$, Lyt-2$^+$ T cells (10).

The GVHD-induced loss of host resistance may play a significant role in allowing the engraftment of bone marrow transplants. In both murine and human studies of marrow grafts, an inverse correlation has been noted between the occurrence of GVHD and the successful engraftment of donor cells; depletion of donor marrow T cells has reduced the incidence of GVHD, but significantly increased the frequency of engraftment failure (55,56).

C. Immune Suppression in GVHD

During the early weeks of GVHD, immune responses are not only deficient but are actively suppressed. When spleen cells from GVHD spleens are cocultured with spleens from normal host (F_1) or donor strain mice, the immune responses of the normal cells are suppressed. Generation of CTL against allogeneic or TNP-modified syngeneic stimulators are suppressed as early as the first week of GVHD (57). Suppression of CTL generation in cocultures continues for the first 6 weeks of GVHD (7,58) (Fig. 3). IL-2 generation in response to allogeneic stimulators is suppressed over a similar timecourse. Even stronger responses, such as Concanavalin A-stimulated IL-2 production, are suppressed during weeks 3-5 of GVHD. Indeed, even the Concanavalin A responses of third-party (neither host nor donor) spleen cells are suppressed by GVHD spleen cells during weeks 3-5 (Fig. 3) (104).

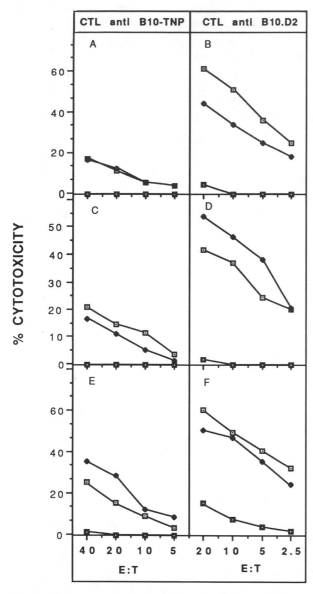

Figure 3 Suppression of both donor and host CTL generation against both TNP-self and allogeneic targets by coculture with GVHD spleen cells. Spleen cells were cultured for 5 days with irradiated TNP-self (C57Bl/10) (panels A, C. E) or allogeneic (B10.D2) (panels B, D, F) stimulators and then assayed in a 4-hour ^{51}Cr release assay on TNP-modified syngeneic or allogenic lymphoblasts at four effector:target ratios. In the first row (panels A, B), CTL generation by C57Bl/10 (□), (B10 X B10.BR)F$_1$ (◆) and [C57Bl/10 → (B10 X B10.BR)F$_1$] GVHD (■) responders is shown. In the second row (panels C, D), the responses of normal (B10 X B10.BR)F$_1$ spleen cells cocultured with C57Bl/10, additional F$_1$ or GVHD spleen cells are shown. In the third row (panels E, F), the responses of normal C57Bl/10 spleen cells cocultured with additional C57Bl/10, F$_1$ or GVHD spleen cells are shown.

One possible mechanism responsible for GVHD-induced suppression is the generation of anti-F_1 suppressor/cytotoxic cells. Donor-anti-host effectors could specifically eliminate cocultured normal F_1 cells during the multiday culture periods involved in immune bioassays, hence reducing the final readout of immune function. Donor strain cytotoxic T cells specific for F_1 host alloantigens have been identified in several strain combinations in GVHD (7,11). As noted above, Lyt-2$^+$ T cells predominate during weeks 2-6 of GVHD. A population of asGM1$^+$, Lyt-2$^+$, NK1.1$^-$ T cells, constituting as much as 1/5 of total spleen cells by 2 weeks, has been found to have strong anti-host cytotoxic activity (10). Furthermore, suppression of CTL generation in cocultured F1 cells has been shown to be dependent upon the presence of parental-derived Lyt-2$^+$ T cells; depletion of Lyt-2$^+$ cells from GVHD spleens prior to setting up cocultures with F_1 cells eliminates the suppression (57).

Yet nonspecific suppressor cells or factors are also involved in GVHD. As noted above, IL-2 production by parental donor strain or even by third-party strain spleen cells is inhibited by GVHD spleen cells. Production of prostaglandins by macrophages has been suggested as a mechanism of suppression in early GVHD (59). Splenic macrophages are relatively increased at weeks 3-4 or GVHD, and prostaglandins have been shown to inhibit production of IL-2. Allo-suppressive Lyt-2$^+$ T cells (as opposed to allo-killer T cells) have been found to predominate in some strain combinations in acute GVHD (3, 8, 40). Such allo-suppressors might function by elaboration of lymphokines such as γ-interferon. In models of GVHD in irradiated mice, γ-interferon has been found to be involved in suppression—either as a direct inhibitor of cell function or as an activator of natural suppressor cells (60,61). Indeed, the presence of a significant population of null cells (lacking T, B, or macrophage markers) during weeks 3-4 of GVHD is consistent with the presence of natural suppressor cells, similar to those that have been described in GVHD spleens in irradiated hosts (61-63).

D.   Deficiencies in Stem Cells and Colony Stimulating Factor Production

During acute suppressive GVHD, the host lymphohematopoietic populations are decimated (9,64) (Fig. 1). Not only are mature T and B cells lost, but host stem cell populations are also affected. At 6 weeks of GVHD in the B6-into-B6C3F$_1$ system, the hematopoietic stem cell populations in the bone marrow are significantly decreased. GVHD marrow transplanted to irradiated hosts has fewer colony forming units than normal marrow, as measured by 7th day splenic colony forming units or by 5th day in vivo splenic proliferation (^{125}I-IUdR incorporation) (49). While these assays primarily assess erythroid colony forming units, a deficit in pre-B and pre-T cells in GVHD marrow can also be demonstrated by a delay in the recovery of mitogen stimulated proliferation and plaque forming cell function (PFC) in irradiated hosts transplanted with GVHD bone marrow (14,49). The decrease in the numbers of pre-B cells in the bone marrow has been directly demonstrated as early as the second week of GVHD, in the severe A-into-B6AF$_1$ system by double immunofluorescence labeling for surface and cytoplasmic Ig (48). When myeloid stem cells are assessed by colony forming unit assays in soft agar, myeloid progenitors are found to decrease 20-fold in the bone marrow at 3 weeks of GVHD (Fig. 4) (64). The levels of myeloid stem cells recover only in mice injected with a source of stem cells. When no parental stem cells are injected, as when GVHD is induced by injection of lymph node rather than spleen cells, myeloid stem cell levels continue to decline and GVHD is fatal.

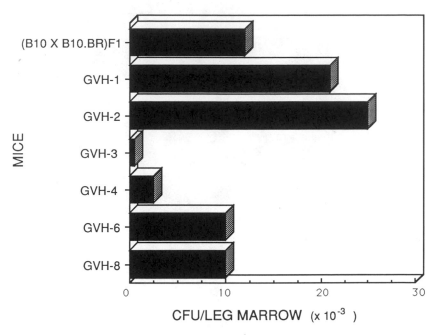

Figure 4 Timecourse of myeloid progenitors in hind leg marrow over the first 8 weeks of acute suppressive GVHD. GVHD was induced in $(B10 \times B10.BR)F_1$ hosts by the injection of 50×10^6 C57Bl/10 spleen cells at periods of 1 to 8 weeks prior to the experiment. The number of myeloid progenitors per 10^5 marrow cells was determined by measuring myeloid colony formation in 7-day soft agar cultures supplemented with G and GM-CSF. The total myeloid CFU found in the hind leg marrow was then calculated from the total numbers of bone marrow cells recoverable from tibias and femurs.

Several factors may contribute to the decrease in stem cells. One possibility is an alteration in the host stem cell microenvironment. If such a change occurs, it is short-lived, for parental stem cells readily engraft in the GVHD host spleen and bone marrow. Furthermore, even following lethal (850 rad) irradiation, GVHD hosts readily accept grafts of parental (donor) marrow (49).

A second possibility is a direct attack on host stem cells. When bone marrow is cultured with granulocyte and granulocyte/macrophage colony stimulating factors (G and GM-CSF) in microtiter wells, myeloid progenitors proliferate and incorporate ^{3}H-thymidine, providing the basis for an assay of GVHD inhibition of stem cell growth. Consistent with data from soft agar cultures of myeloid colony forming units, bone marrow from GVHD mice (weeks 3-5) proliferated less than normal F_1 host marrow in these microtiter cultures. GVHD and normal F_1 marrow was then irradiated (to block proliferation) and cocultured with normal F_1 marrow plus CSF. When compared with cocultures with normal F_1 host marrow, GVHD bone marrow produced a decrease in F_1 marrow proliferation. Thus, cells present in the GVHD bone marrow, or factors generated by these cells, suppress bone marrow growth (Fig. 5).

During weeks 3-5 of GVHD, the greatest decrease in bone marrow stem cell populations occurs. During this period, an increased percentage of T cells, particularly Lyt-2$^+$ (CD8) T cells, is found in the bone marrow. These Lyt-2$^+$ cells may be cytotoxic T cells

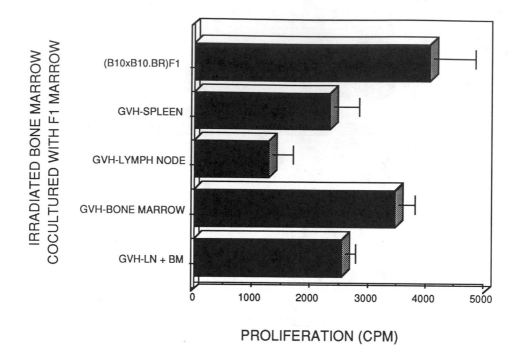

Figure 5 Suppression of host marrow proliferation in cocultures with GVHD bone marrow cells. Acute suppressive GVHD was induced in $(B10 \times B10.BR)F_1$ hosts by the injection of 50×10^6 spleen, 30×10^6 lymph node or 30×10^6 lymph node plus 10×10^6 bone marrow cells from C57Bl/10 donors. Injection of 50×10^6 bone marrow cells alone did not produce GVHD, as assessed by chimerism or immune function, and serves as a control for the effect of the injection of donor stem cells on host marrow function. Bone marrow cells from normal $(B10 \times B10.BR)F_1$ mice were cocultured with (1000 rad) irradiated normal F_1 or GVHD marrow cells in GM-CSF–supplemented media in a 4-day proliferation assay. Bone marrow cells from spleen-, lymph node-, or lymph node plus bone marrow-induced GVHD mice significantly suppress normal marrow proliferation in response to CSF.

which could attack host marrow cells. As noted above, T cells with specificity for host alloantigens have been identified in GVHD spleens (7,11). Furthermore, a population of $CD3^+, CD8^+$ T cells has been identified in recipients of allogeneic bone marrow transplants which inhibit marrow proliferation (CFU-GM and BFU-E) in an MHC-restricted manner (65,66). Alternatively, macrophages may be involved in inhibition of stem cell growth in GVHD. Macrophages increase during early GVHD and have also been shown to inhibit stem cell growth in recipients of allogeneic bone marrow grafts (66). Finally, NK cells may contribute to the loss of host stem cells in GVHD (66). Donor NK cells increase in early GVHD in mice (39,67) and have been implicated in much of the GVHD tissue damage in both lymphoid (68) and nonlymphoid tissues (39,69,70). NK cells are particularly good candidates for a role in marrow attack, for they have been linked to stem cell death in several systems, involving both syngeneic and allogeneic marrows (71-73).

These cells may have direct (presumably cytolytic) effects upon the bone marrow. In addition, a variety of factors produced by activated lymphocytes, NK cells, and macrophages have been shown to inhibit stem cell proliferation. Both lymphotoxic and tumor necrosis factor have been shown to inhibit stem cell colony formation in vitro (74). γ-interferon has been shown to act synergistically with these cytokines in inhibiting marrow growth (74). Activated T cells may produce lymphotoxin and γ-interferon; activated macrophages and NK cells secrete TNF. Although tumor necrosis factor (TNF) has not been detected in the serum of mice undergoing GVHD (75) (Ploznik, personal communication), treatment of GVH mice with antibodies against TNF reduces the cytotoxic effects of GVH on skin and gut cells (75). Thus the cytokines produced by donor cells activated during the course of the immune response against host antigens may play a part in the decrease in bone marrow proliferative response.

The final mechanism by which GVHD may affect bone marrow proliferation is linked back to the immunosuppressive effect of GVHD on T-cell functions. T cells produce interleukin 3 (IL-3), the colony stimulating factor with the broadest effect on stem cell populations, as well as GM-CSF, a factor which broadly promotes myeloid proliferation and differentiation. If the production of T-cell-derived growth factors were altered, the normal proliferation of marrow stem cells might be affected. During the first 2 weeks of GVHD, colony stimulating factors are produced spontaneously, such that CSF activity is measurable in serum samples and in supernatants from unstimulated splenic cultures (75, 105). During this same period, spleen size increases dramatically, bone marrow cellularity increases, and increased numbers of promyeloblasts are found in the spleen (76). Similar results have been found by in vivo treatment with murine recombinant IL-3 (77). During weeks 2-6 of GVHD, concomitant with the development of T-cell immune deficiency, both spontaneous and Concanavalin A-stimulated production of colony stimulating factors decreases (64, 105). At the lowest period, during weeks 3-4 of GVHD, Concanavalin A-stimulated splenic production of CSF is less than 5% of normal. This low period in CSF production capacity corresponds to the lowest point in bone marrow stem cell levels. While stimulating T-cell production of CSF is an artificial measure of CSF production capacity, if the GVHD T cells cannot respond to Concanavalin A, it is likely that normal homeostatic feedback mechanisms for CSF production are also inoperative. The capacity to produce CSF recovers beginning at 6-8 weeks of GVHD. This period corresponds to the period of reconstitution of the bone marrow by donor stem cells. The GVHD-induced deficiency in CSF production may therefore contribute to the decrease in stem cell populations during the cytolytic period of GVHD; the recovery in CSF production capacity may likewise contribute to the rapid engraftment of parental donor stem cells.

E. GVHD-Induced Defect in Thymic Function

The acute suppressive GVHD induced by injection of parental cells into F_1 hosts has been shown to have dramatic effects on F_1 immune function. In the short term in GVHD, a profound immunosuppression limits primary responses to new antigens or pathogens. Over the long term, the lymphohematopoietic system may be reconstituted with parental cells, but deficits in some immune functions may remain. The GVHD-induced effects on lymphoid organs may not be limited to these short-term effects on host lymphoid populations, but may also affect the immune functional potential of the donor (and eventually host) cells which repopulate the mouse. One mechanism producing a long-term effect on host immune function would be reduction in the stem cell content of the marrow. As noted above, however, erythroid, myeloid, and B-cell lineage stem cell numbers are only transiently reduced during acute GVHD. Another target of donor attack in GVHD is the thymus. Alterations in the thymus could temporarily or permanently compromise the ability of the thymus to educate new T cells. During the first weeks of GVHD, the host thymuses undergo marked histological changes including a marked decrease in size, loss of thymic epithelium, and Hassell's corpuscles (37,67,68). Intrathymic L3T4$^+$ and Lyt-2$^+$ cells are severely reduced, and Ly6$^+$ cells are dramatically increased (78). GVHD also induces thymic hormonal dysfunction (79). These results all indicate that GVHD affects immunologically relevant cells in the thymus. The question is whether these alterations in cell populations are temporary, as in the marrow, or whether permanent effects remain.

To test for possible GVHD-induced changes in thymic function, F_1 mice that had been injected with parental spleen cells 30 days earlier were irradiated and transplanted with T-cell-depleted F_1 bone marrow (GVHD-BMT). Over a period of 14 to 33 weeks, spleen cells from these marrow-reconstituted GVHD-BMT mice were tested for their ability to generate in vitro CTL and IL-2 responses to TNP-self and H-2 alloantigens. Depending on the parent and F_1 strain combinations used, spleen cells from GVHD-BMT mice either failed to respond to both stimuli (80) or were selectively deficient in response to TNP-self (81). GVHD-BMT mice in which GVHD was induced by B10.A-into-(C57Bl/10 × B10.A)F_1 mice resulted in failure of all T-cell responses (80), whereas C57Bl/6-into-B6C3F$_1$ resulted in a selective failure to develop TNP-self but not allogeneic (ALLO) CTL activity. The reason for this difference in CTL responses in these two models my be due to the fact that the former parent-F_1 combination induces a stronger GVHD than the latter, as measured by threshold dose of donor cells required to produce immune deficiency.

To further elucidate the defect, spleen cells from GVHD-BMT mice were stimulated with TNP-self in cultures to which either T helper factors or L3T4-enriched cells from normal mice had been added. In both cases CTL function was restored, which indicated that T effector function for TNP-self was not deficient (81). The fact that IL-2 production to TNP-self was also reduced indicated that these mice had lost T helper cell (T_H) function (81). To test whether the deficiency was due to a GVHD-induced defect in thymic maturation of T cells, GVHD mice were grafted with thymic lobes from neonatal donor (parental) strain mice one week before bone marrow transplantation. Thymic grafting resulted in restoration of T_H function for TNP-self (81).

Taken together, these results indicate that GVHD followed by irradiation and bone marrow transplantation induces a defect in T_H but not in T effector function. The observation that the defect was selective for TNP-self, but not for responses to H-2 alloantigens, is of particular interest, because it suggests that GVHD may affect not a specific portion of the T_H repertoire, but rather a subset of T helper cells. It has previously been demonstrated that the CTL response of murine spleen cells to TNP-self is strictly dependent upon MHC class II self-restricted L3T4$^+$ (CD4) T helper cells (42,43). The CTL response to H-2 alloantigens, however, can utilize any of three different T_H pathways: an L3T4$^+$, self-restricted T_H pathway (responding to alloantigens in the context of self class II antigens); an L3T4$^+$, allo-restricted T_H pathway (responding to allogeneic class II antigens); and a Lyt-2$^+$, allo-restricted T_H pathway (responding to allogeneic class I antigens) (42-44). Thus, if the GVHD induced a selective defect in the development of L3T4$^+$ T_H, but not in Lyt-2$^+$ T_H function, then one would expect a selective defect in the TNP-self, but not in the ALLO response. This selective defect was demonstrated by completely abrogating the ALLO response in GVHD-BMT mice through depleting the allogeneic antigen presenting cells (needed for Lyt-2^+ T_H function) (81). In normal BMT mice this depletion only slightly decreases CTL formation, because L3T4$^+$ helper pathways are still operative. Thus, it appears that the defect in the C3H-into-B6C3F$_1$ GVHD-BMT mice involves a GVHD-induced selective thymic defect in ability to generate L3T4$^+$ self-restricted T_H, but not Lyt-2^+, allo-restricted T_H nor T effector functions. We do not presently know whether this defect includes L3T4$^+$, allo-restricted T_H function. It is noteworthy that this selective defect was shown not to involve a defect in syngeneic APC function, and was not due to suppressor cells (81). Furthermore, adequate numbers of L3T4$^+$ cells were present in the spleens of the GVHD-BMT mice, despite the fact that these mice exhibited L3T4$^+$-mediated T_H dysfunction.

This defect in L3T4 T_H function can be detected not only in GVHD-BMT mice, but can also be found in some strain combinations following long-term GVHD alone. As noted above, the alterations in immune function in GVHD mice consists of three functional phases: initial suppression of T-cell function; depletion of all T-cell populations, and recovery of most T-cell functions by the engrafted donor T cells. During the recovery period the broadest-based responses, such as Concanavalin A-stimulated proliferation or lymphokine production, reappear first followed by lymphokine generation and CTL responses to allogeneic stimulators (see Fig. 2). In some strain combinations, such as C3H-into-B6C3F$_1$, the CTL response to TNP-modified syngeneic cells reappears, although always well after the allogeneic response. In other strains (such as C57Bl/6-into-B6C3F$_1$ and C57Bl/10-into-(B10 X B10.BR)F$_1$) the response does not reappear after as many as 18 months, although L3T4$^+$ cells reach normal proportions. The reason that the GVHD-induced thymic defect is not seen in all strain combinations may be that the thymic lesion is masked by surviving host lymphocytes and by the mature donor T cells introduced in the GVHD inoculum. Alternatively, only the most severe GVHD attack on the thymus, or a second "hit" in the form of lethal irradiation, may be necessary for the defect in thymic education of L3T4 cells to occur.

The GVHD-BMT model summarized in this section may be of value for investigating the role of the thymus in T-cell development and MHC restriction. Furthermore, it provides a method for preparing mice that are selectively deficient in CD4-mediated T_H function without depleting CD4$^+$ cells, and could be a useful model for studying the immunological changes that occur in T-cell immunodeficiencies. For example, this model is similar with respect to immune functional changes (but not etiology) to the immune dysregulation observed in symptomatic HIV seropositive individuals who exhibit a selective loss in CD4-mediated T_H function without a critical loss in CD4$^+$ cell numbers (82, 106). Finally, the GVHD-BMT model could have implications for the clinical observations that bone marrow transplant patients who have undergone a chronic GVHD frequently exhibit a long delay in recovery of immune function (83,84). If the thymus of marrow-transplanted humans is involved in reconstitution of T_H function, a GVHD might interfere with T-cell maturation.

F. Cell Populations Required to Induce Acute Suppressive GVH

Induction of acute, immune-suppressive GVHD in unirradiated mice has two primary requirements: a sufficient number of alloreactive donor T cells and a full class I + II MHC disparity between donor and host. Injection of spleen cells from T deficient nu/nu donors or from spleens depleted of T cells by treatment with anti-Thy 1 antibody fails to produce any of the symptoms of GVHD, such as splenomegaly, donor/host chimerism, histopathological changes in organs or immune dysfunction (5,10,32). Furthermore, both donor L3T4[+] and Lyt-2[+] T-cell subsets are required for complete development of host immune deficiency (3,5,8,40,57,85). Depletion of either T subset prevents the development of full immune-suppressive GVH (5). Early in GVHD, a Lyt-1[+],2[-] (presumably L3T4[+]) population is activated, perhaps contributing to the transient lympho-proliferation of the first weeks of GVHD (3). Subsequently, Lyt-2[+] allo-suppressor/killer cells predominate (10,40,57).

The involvement of donor NK cells in the pathological changes in GVHD is still a subject of dispute. An increase in NK activity (i.e., killing of YAC-1 tumor targets) early in GVHD has been correlated with the development of histopathological lesions in lymphoid and nonlymphoid organs (39,68). When NK-deficient bg/bg mutant mice are used as the GVHD donors, this early increase in NK activity does not occur, but host mice nonetheless develop splenomegaly, donor/host chimerism and deficiency in the sensitive B-cell anti-sRBC PFC assay (10,37). Severely suppressed T- and B-cell responses to mitogens, anti-host cytotoxic effectors, and histopathological lesions fail to develop, however (10,37). Similarly, in vivo depletion of an activated population of donor asialo-GM1[+] (ASGM1) cells with NK activity precludes development of severe immune deficiency, anti-host cytotoxicity, and tissue lesions (10,69). These activated donor cells have been depleted by two different protocols: a) in vivo anti-ASGM1 trestment of donors that have been pretreated with poly [IC] to induce ASGM1 expression (39) and b) in vivo anti-ASGM1 treatment of host mice during the course of GVHD (10). Depletion of GVHD spleen cells in vitro with ASGM1 or in vivo depletion of donors abolishes the GVHD-induced increase in NK cell activity (39). The question remains whether the early GVHD cytotoxic cells with activity on NK targets are classic NK cells or T cells activated by the lymphokines released in GVHD. A significant percentage of anti-YAC-1 cytotoxic activity in C57Bl/6-into-B6D2F1 GVHD is lost by depeltion with anti-Lyt-2 sera and a population of ASGM1[+], Thy 1.2[+], Lyt-2[+] T cells constitutes as much as 19% of donor cells in the GVHD spleen at 12 days (10).

In addition to T-cell populations, a source of donor stem cells are required in order to prolong survival beyond the first weeks of GVHD and to repopulate the host lympho-hematopoietic system. Splenic populations contain large numbers of stem cells, fully 1/10 to 1/5 as many as an equal number of marrow cells. Induction of suppressive GVHD with injection of donor spleen cells produces a severe anemia and rapid depletion of marrow stem cells (9). Injection of parental donor populations lacking in stem cells, such as lymph node cells, fails to repopulate the hematopoietic system and produces a lethal GVHD. Injection of as many as 50×10^6 parental bone marrow cells, however, cannot induce GVHD, due to the paucity of mature T cells. Injection of both lymph node and as few as 10×10^6 bone marrow cells produces a immune suppressive GVHD with donor/host chimerism comparable to that in donor spleen-induced GVHD (Hakim and Sheater, in preparation).

II. IMMUNE DYSREGULATION INDUCED BY A CLASS II GVHD

Thus far this overview of murine GVHD-induced immune abnormalities has been concerned with the acute suppressive immune dysfunction induced by injection of parental T lymphocytes into F_1 hosts in which: a) the donor inoculum contains both L3T4[+]

(CD4$^+$) and Lyt-2$^+$ (CD8$^+$) T cells; and b) the donor T lymphocytes recognize both class I and class II MHC products of the host as foreign. In this form of the GVHD, the host is immune-deficient for both CD4$^-$ and CD8-mediated T$_H$ function, as well as T effector (T$_E$) and B-cell function (3,4,35,39). Furthermore, suppressor cells can be detected which abrogate all of these functions in coculture with spleen cells from normal syngeneic mice (7,57). Anemia, hypogammaglobulinema, increased mortality, and extensive donor repopulation of host lymphohematopoietic tissues are common (7,8).

If only donor L3T4$^+$ T cells are involved in GVHD, and/or if the donor T cells recognize only a disparity in class II MHC determinants in the host, a chronic immunostimulatory or autoimmune type of GVHD develops that resembles the condition that develops in MRL/Mpj *lpr/lpr* mice and in human systemic lupus erythematosus (2,3,5,7, 85). The hosts develop marked splenomegaly and hypergammaglobulinemia; a variety of autoantibodies are produced and hosts may eventually die of immune complex glomerulonephritis (1,3,12,85-90). Compared with the acute suppressive GVHD, the degree of T-cell immune dysfunction and donor engraftment is markedly limited, affecting primarily L3T4$^+$ cells (5-7). Suppressor cells affect primarily L3T4 T-cell function, as well (6,7). These differences are summarized in Table 1.

This form of autoimmune or stimulatory GVHD can be generated by three different methods: a) selection of parental and host strain combinations involving a genetic disparity at class II MHC only (class II GVHD) as in C57Bl/6-into-(C57Bl/6 × B6.C.H.2^{bm12})F$_1$, (3,6,12,91); b) depletion of donor Lyt-2$^+$ T cells prior to injection into a class I + II disparate F$_1$ host (5,7,85); and c) injection of DBA/2-into-B6D2F$_1$ mice (2,7,9,12,87,92). All of these combinations result in chronic stimulatory GVHD as assessed by autoantibody production and selective T-cell defects (3,6,7,12,85,93). In examples a) and b) donor cells are limited to recognition of class II MHC, either by virtue of a class II MHC disparity only (example a), or by a severe reduction in donor Lyt-2$^+$ cells (that would have recognized primarily class I alloantigens). Although the reason for a stimulatory GVHD in the DBA/2-into-B6D2F$_1$ combination (genetically a class I + II GVHD) was not initially understood, it has been recently found that DBA/2 spleens exhibit a twofold reduction in Lyt-2$^+$ T-cell number and a ninefold reduction in pCTL frequency to B6D2F$_1$, compared to the other parent, C57Bl/6 (which induces a typical class I + II GVH) (7). Thus, upon close examination, the DBA/2-into-B6D2F$_1$ GVHD behaves as a class II GVHD because of a natural deficiency in pCTL for the C57Bl/6 parent, comparable to the effect of depletion of donor Lyt-2 T cells.

The T-cell defect in class II or stimulatory GVHD was originally described as the development of allohelper T cells which responded to the class II disparity and polyclonally stimulated the host B cell populations to generate a variety of autoantibodies (2,3, 12). In vitro assays, however, reveal a defect in the ability of host T and B cells to respond to new antigens (6,94). Furthermore, the T helper defect is selective for L3T4-(CD4)-mediated T$_H$ function, but not for Lyt-2(CD8)-mediated T$_H$ or T$_E$ function (5,6). The evidence for a selective defect is similar to that described above, for GVHD-BMT mice. IL-2 is produced and CTL cells are generated in response to allogeneic stimulators, for Lyt-2$^+$ T$_H$ and T$_E$ can contribute to the allogeneic response. Il-2 is not generated, however, in response to TNP-self stimulators (6,7), for this response is dependent on L3T4$^+$ T$_H$ (42,43). While no CTL are generated against TNP-self stimulators, addition of T-cell growth factors results in CTL generation (6,7). Thus, the defect in the TNP-self response is limited to the L3T4$^+$ T$_H$ cells. This finding contrasts with the class I + II GVHD defect, in which all detectable L3T4$^-$ and Lyt-2-mediated T$_H$ and T$_E$ function is

Table 1 Effect of Graft vs. Host Reaction Across Different Genetic Disparities on Lymphohematopoietic Cells and Functions

MHC antigen Disparity	Donor chimerism	CTL function		F1 coculture (suppression)		B-cell function		Serum Auto-AB	Stem cell	Thymic function	Hybrid resistance
		TNP	ALLO	TNP	ALLO	PFC	LPS				
I + II	ALL	↓	↓	↓	↓	↓	↓	N	↓	↓	↓
II	L3T4	↓	N	↓	N	↓	?	↑	?	N	↓
I	LYT 2	↓	N	?	?	N	?	N	?	N	?
I + minor	ALL	?	?	?	?	↓	↓	↑	↓	↓	?

↓/↑ = Decreased/increased function or level.

N = Normal function or level.

? = Not tested in this mode.

abolished and cannot be recovered by addition of T-cell growth factors (see above). Finally, the selective L3T4 T_H defect in class II GVHD is associated with activation of a suppressor cell which selectively suppresses L3T4-mediated T_H function of spleen cells from normal syngeneic mice, but does not inhibit Lyt-2 T_H function (6,7). The suppressor cells in class I + II GVHD, in contrast, suppressed all T- and B-cell function. In this regard, the class II GVHD system is also distinct from the GVHD-BMT mice, in which no suppressors are found.

The final distinction between class I + II and class II only GVHD involves a difference in the degree of donor engraftment and in the donor T-cell requirement for induction of GVHD. The main population which engrafts in class II GVHD is donor L3T4$^+$ T cells (5,7). T-cell chimerism in class II disparate GVH has been traced by the injection of C56Bl/6.PL-Thy-1^a lymphocytes, which express the Thy 1.1 allele, into (C57Bl/6 × B6.C.H.2^{bm12})F$_1$ hosts. In this combination, mainly donor L3T4$^+$ cells and a smaller component of donor Lyt-2$^+$ cells engraft, but significant levels of host T cells remain (5). Similar results have been observed in DBA/2-into-B6D2F$_1$ GVH (7). Unlike class I + II GVHD, no wholesale repopulation of the host lymphohematopoietic system occurs. Furthermore, only the L3T4$^+$ T-cell population is required for induction of stimulatory GVHD; depletion of Lyt-2$^+$ T cells does not prevent the development of class II GVHD as defined by chimerism or T-cell functional assays (5).

III. IMMUNE DYSFUNCTION ASSOCIATED WITH CLASS I GVHD

Injection of parental spleen cells into F$_1$ mice in which the donor T lymphocytes only recognize host class I antigens as allogeneic does not produce as clear-cut a result as class II disparity GVHD. In some strain combinations, injection of class I disparate donor cells has no observable effect. For example, if (B10.A × B10.A[2R])F$_1$ mice are injected with spleen cells from either parent (which recognize only H-2D as allogeneic), no effect on host immune function is observed (4). In contrast, if C57Bl/6 or B6.C-H-2^{bm1} donor spleen cells are injected into (C57Bl/6 × B6.C-H-2^{bm1})F$_1$ mice, (a GVHD involving recognition of the bm1 mutation), a selective defect in L3T4 T_H function is often observed (5). Alternatively, if L3T4$^+$ T cells are depleted from the donor inoculum in strain combinations involving a full class I + II antigenic disparity, no observable GVHID or engraftment of donor cells results in most strain combinations. If, however, there is a strong class I antigenic disparity between donor and host, then the Lyt-2$^+$ T_H will generate a class I disparity GVHD. An example of the latter is the injection of L3T4 T-cell-depleted B6 spleen cells into a (B6.C-H-2^{bm1} × B6.C-H-2^{bm12})F$_1$ mouse (5). These characteristics are summarized in Table 1.

Thus, two different results have been observed in a class I GVHD; a) no detectable effect on immune function in F$_1$ hosts when the donor cells recognize H-2D (4); and b) a selective defect in L3T4 T_H function when GVHD involves recognition of the bm1 mutation (5). This latter result may be due to the fact that the bm1 mutation elicits a very strong T-cell response by C57Bl/6 responding cells. It is noteworthy that irrespective of whether GVHD is induced by recognition of class I or class II mutations, the GVHD results in a selective loss of L3T4 T_H function.

Although no immune abnormality was observed in the class I GVHD that involved recognition of H-2D alloantigens, this example of parent-into-F$_1$ is not completely inert, because infection with murine cytomegalovirus can synergize with the class I disparities to result in acute suppressive GVH (see below).

Class I disparity GVHD associated with minor histocompatibility antigens may also produce a severe GVHD. For several years Lapp and coworkers have studied the GVHD produced by injection of A strain donor cells into (CBA × A)F_1 hosts. This donor/host combination differs not only at H-2D, but also at a variety of minor loci, including Mls. This form of GVHD is characterized by T- and B-cell functional defects, including depressed Concanavalin A-induced proliferation and IL-2 production and depressed LPS-induced proliferation and sRBC PFC responses (13-15,95) (Table 1). As in the acute, suppressive GVHD induced by a class I + II disparity, there is an attack on host stem cell populations, particularly B cells (14). Furthermore, the host thymus is severely affected early in the course of the disorder and subsequently fails to produce functional T cells (13,95).

IV. SYNERGISTIC EFFECTS BETWEEN GVHD AND MURINE CYTOMEGALOVIRUS

Cytomegalovirus (CMV) infection is a major cause of mortality in allogeneic bone marrow recipients (96). These patients frequently die of CMV-induced interstitial pneumonitis, a condition which is most often seen in patients undergoing a GVHD (97,98). To determine whether synergistic effects could be demonstrated between CMV and GVHD in the parent-into-F_1 model of GVHD, experiments have been performed in which F_1 mice were injected with parental lymphocytes and a nonlethal dose of murine cytomegalovirus (MCMV). Two basic approaches have been used to study the possible synergistic effects of GVHD and MCMV. First, mice were injected with doses of parental spleen cells that were below the threshold for induction of GVHID. Thus, whereas injection of 20×10^6 parental cells into an F_1 host-induced GVHID, 2×10^6 cells did not. However, the combined effects of MCMV infection of the F_1 host plus the low dose of parental cells induced GVHID (99,100), and this combination of insults also induced interstitial pneumonitis (99,101). Furthermore, the pneumonitis induced by GVHD ± MCMV was associated with infiltration of donor T lymphocytes into the lungs of the mice, whereas the lungs of F_1 mice that had been injected with only parental cells did not contain detectable numbers of donor T cells (101). Thus, by using a suboptimal dose of donor lymphocytes, a synergistic effect can be demonstrated between GVHD and MCMV both for GVHID as well as for interstitial pneumonitis.

The second approach used to demonstrate this synergy takes advantage of the observation that a class I + II GVHD, affects both CD4 and CD8 T-cell function, a class II GVHD selectively abrogates only CD4 function, and a class I GVHD (that does not involve the bm1 mutation) does not induce any detectable defect in T-cell function. Therefore, this approach might permit us to determine whether MCMV provides a "class II-like" or a "class I-like" signal in the synergy with GVHD. The results of such experiments indicate that MCMV synergized with the class I GVHD signal, but did not synergize with the class II GVHD signal (Via and Shearer, in preparation). Thus MCMV + class I GVHD abrogated both CD4 and CD8 T-cell function in the host, whereas MCMV + class II GVHD had no detectable effect on T-cell function of the host beyond that induced by the class II GVHD alone (i.e., abrogation of L3T4 T_H function). It appears, therefore, that MCMV was able to provide a class II-like signal, but not a class I-like signal in synergy with a GVHD. Experimental models of this type may be useful for elucidating the mechanistic aspects of the suspected synergy between CMV and GVHD in bone marrow transplant patients.

V. POTENTIAL RELEVANCE OF THESE EXPERIMENTAL OBSERVATIONS TO CLINICAL EXPERIENCE

This brief review of the immunologic and hematopoietic deficiencies that can occur as a result of Graft- vs. Host Disease could be relevant to several human disorders. The observation that a pCTL deficit contributes to the development of the DBA/2 autoimmune GVHD has led to a model of the mechanism of SLE in humans (102). It is postulated that the initial defect that results in antibody-mediated autoimmunity is not due to excessive T helper activity (although excessive T_H is the immediate cause), but rather is due to a lack of effector cells which normally function to clear antigen (102). This failure to clear antigen results in continuous T_H activation, which eventually results in polyclonal B-cell activation and autoantibody production (102).

Some of the observations made in the P-into-F_1 murine GVHD model may also provide insights into the clinical problems of immune reconstitution following bone marrow transplantation. For example, the observation that mice with GVHD fail to develop normal T-cell function, particularly in $CD4^+$ T cells (see above), may be relevant for the clinical observations that marrow grafted patients who have had chronic GVHD frequently exhibit a delay in recovery of immune function or, in some cases, do not regenerate immune function (83).

If the thymus of hematopoietic-reconstituting humans is important for development of T-lymphocyte function, then the GVHD could have damaged the potential for this organ to regenerate T-cell function. It would be important to know whether this is the case, because therapy of such immunodeficient patients might include protocols that would take such knowledge into consideration.

Another example in which this experimental model of GVHD is relevant to the clinical experience is the finding that GVHD can abolish natural resistance to marrow grafts (11,32). The correlation between improved depletion of T lymphocytes from human bone marrow and increased frequency of graft failure (103) raises the possibility that GVHR in bone marrow transplant patients may abolish host natural resistance that can interfere with engraftment. The demonstration that a clinically asymptomatic GVHD induced in the murine parent-into-F_1 GVHD model abolished hybrid resistance to a parental marrow graft (32) supports this interpretation of the human experience.

Finally, it should be noted that GVHD can occur (at least in some of the murine models summarized above) which would not be detectable by the more traditional symptoms. That is, a GVHD is not necessarily always associated with weight loss, skin lesions, and/or diarrhea. Such a GVHD may only be detectable by measurements of immune functions, yet may still affect the differentiation and the function of T cells, and may synergize with viral pathogens. It may therefore be worthwhile to consider more sensitive diagnostic assays to test for more subtle forms of GVHD, such as increases in class II MHC antigen expression or changes in T-cell-mediated immune function.

REFERENCES

1. Gleichmann E, Gleichmann H: Pathogenesis of graft-versus-host reactions (GVHR) and GVH-like diseases. J Invest Dermatol 1985;85(1 suppl):115s-120s.
2. Gleichmann E, Pals ST, Rolink AG, Radaszkiewicz T, Gleichmann H: Graft-vs-host reactions: clues to the etiopathology of a spectrum of immunological diseases. Immunol Today 1984;5:324-332.

3. Rolink AG, Pals ST, Gleichmann E: Allosuppressor and allohelper T cells in acute and chronic graft-vs.-host disease. II. F1 recipients carrying mutations at H-2K and/or I-A. J Exp Med 1983;157:755-771.

4. Shearer GM, Levy RB: Graft-vs.-host-associated immune suppression is activated by recognition of allogeneic murine I-A antigens. J Exp Med 1983;157:936-946.

5. Moser M, Sharrow SO, Shearer GM: Role of L3T4$^+$ and Lyt-2$^+$ donor cells in graft-versus-host immune deficiency induced across a class I, class II, or whole H-2 difference. J Immunol 1988;140:2600-2608.

6. Moser M, Mizuochi T, Sharrow SO, Singer A, Shearer GM: Graft-vs-host reaction limited to a class II MHC difference results in a selective deficiency in L3T4$^+$ but not in Lyt-2$^+$ T helper cell function. J Immunol 1987;138:1355-1362.

7. Via CS, Sharrow SO, Shearer GM: Role of cytotoxic T lymphocytes in the prevention of lupus-like disease occurring in a murine model of graft-vs-host disease. J Immunol 1987;139:1840-1849.

8. Rolink AG, Radaszkiewicz T, Pals ST, van der Meer WG, Gleichmann E: Allosuppressor and allohelper T cells in acute and chronic graft-vs-host disease. I. Alloreactive suppressor cells rather than killer T cells appear to be the decisive effector cells in lethal graft-vs.-host disease. J Exp Med 1982;155:1501-1522.

9. Van Elven EH, Rolink AG, Van der veen F, Gleichmann E: Capacity of genetically different T lymphocytes to induce lethal graft-versus-host disease correlates with their capacity to generate suppression but not with their capacity to generate anti-F1 killer cells. A non-H-2 locus determines the inability to induce lethal graft-versus-host disease. J Exp Med 1981;153:1474-1488.

10. Knobloch C, Dennert G: Asialo-GM1-positive T killer cells are generated in F1 mice injected with parental spleen cells. J Immunol 1988;140:744-749.

11. Knobloch C, Dennert G: Loss of F1 hybrid resistance to bone marrow grafts after injection of parental lymphocytes. Transplantation 1988;45:175-183.

12. van Rappard-van der Veen FM, Rolink AG, Gleichmann E: Diseases caused by reactions of T lymphocytes towards incompatible structures of the major histocompatibility complex. VI. Autoantibodies characteristic of systemic lupus erythematosus induced by abnormal T-B cell cooperation across I-E. J Exp Med 1982;155:1555-1560.

13. Seddik M, Seemayer TA, Lapp WS: The graft-versus-host reaction and immune function. I. T helper cell immunodeficiency associated with graft-versus-host-induced thymic epithelial cell damage. Transplantation 1984;37:281-286.

14. Seddik M, Seemayer TA, Lapp WS: The graft-versus-host reaction and immune function. IV. B cell functional defect associated with a depletion of splenic colony-forming units in marrow of graft-versus-host-reactive mice. Transplantation 1986;41:242-247.

15. Seddik M, Seemayer TA, Lapp WS: The graft-versus-host reaction and immune function. III. Functional pre-T cells in the bone marrow of graft-versus-host-reactive mice displaying T cell immunodeficiency. Transplantation 1986;41:238-242.

16. Ishikawa H, Kubota E, Wilkinson NM, Saito K: Modulation of F1 cytotoxic potentials by GvHR: suppression of cytotoxic T cell responses of F1 mice correlates with F1 inability to resist the proliferation of GvHR-inducing parental T lymphocytes. J Immunol 1982;129:1181-1188.

17. van Rappard-van der Veen FM, Radaszkiewicz T, Terraneo L, Gleichmann E: Attempts at standardization of lupus-like graft-vs-host disease: inadvertent repopulation by DBA/2 spleen cells of H-2-different nonirradiated F1 mice. J Immunol 1983;130:2693-2701.

18. Ferrara JLM, Michaelson J, Burakoff SJ, Mauch P: Engraftment following T cell-depleted bone marrow transplantation. III. Differential effects of increased total-

body irradiation on semiallogeneic and allogeneic recipients. Transplantation 1988; 45:948-952.

19. Ferrara JLM, Mauch P, McINtyre J, Michaelson J, Burakoff SJ: Engraftment following T cell depleted bone marrow transplantation. II. Stability of mixed chimerism in semisyngeneic recipients after total body irradiation. Transplantation 1987;44:495-499.

20. McCarthy SA, Griffith IJ, Gambel P, Francescutti JH, Wegmann TG: Characterization of host lymphoid cells in antibody-facilitated bone marrow chimeras. Transplantation 1985;40:12-17.

21. Francescutti LH, Gambel P, Wegmann TG: Characterization of hemopoietic stem cell chimerism in antibody-facilitated bone marrow chimeras. Transplantation 1985; 40:7-11.

22. Hill RS, Petersen FB, Storb R: Mixed hematologic chimerism after allogeneic marrow transplantation for severe aplastic anemia is associated with higher risk of graft rejection and a lessened incidence of acute graft-versus-host disease. Blood 1986; 67:811-816.

23. Bennett M: Biology and genetics of hybrid resistance. Adv Immunol 1987;41:333-445.

24. Cudkowicz G, Nakamura I: Genetics of the murine hemopoietic-histocompatibility system. Transplant Proc 1983;15:2058-2063.

25. Cudkowicz G, Bennett M: Peculiar immunobiology of bone marrow allografts. II. Rejection of parental grafts by resistant F1 hybrid mice. J Exp Med 1971;134:1513-1528.

26. Daley JP, Wroblewski JM, Kaminsky SG, Nakamura I: Genetic control of the target structure recognized in hybrid resistance. Immunogenetics 1987;26:21-30.

27. Kiessling R, Hochman PS, Haller O, Shearer GM, Wigzell H, Cudkowicz G: Evidence for a similar or common mechanism for natural killer cell activity and resistance to hemopoietic grafts. Eur J Immunol 1977;7:655-663.

28. Waterfall M, Rayfield LS, Brent L: The role of natural killer cells in resistance to allogeneic and parental hybrid resistance. Transplantation 1987;43:312-314.

29. Shearer GM, Polisson RP: Mutual recognition of parental and F lymphocytes. III. Parental determinants recognized by F host mice in resistance to graft-vs-host-associated immunosuppression map to H-2D^b. J Immunol 1981;126:545-547.

30. Peres A, Nestel FP, Seemayer TA, Lapp WS: The effects of polyinosinic:polycytidylic acid (pl:C) on the graft-vs-host (GVH) reaction. II. Increased NK-mediated rejection on C57BL/6 lymphocytes by (C57BL/6 X A)F1 mice. J Immunol 1986; 137:3420-3427.

31. Peres A, Seemayer TA, Lapp WS: The effects of polyinosinic:polycytidylic acid (pl: C) on the GVH reaction: immunopathological observations. Clin Immunol Immunopathol 1986;39:102-111.

32. Hakim FT, Shearer GM: Abrogation of hybrid resistance to bone marrow engraftment by graft-vs-host-induced immune deficiency. J Immunol 1986;137:3109-3116.

33. Howard JG, Woodruff MFA: Effect of the graft-versus-host reaction on immunological responsiveness of the mouse. Proc R Soc Lond B Biol Sci 1961;154:532.

34. Lapp WS, Moller G: Prolonged survival of H-2 incompatible skin allografts on F1 animals treated with parental lymphoid cells. Immunology 1969;17:339-344.

35. Shearer GM, Polisson RP: Mutual recognition of parental and F1 lymphocytes. Selective abrogation of cytotoxic potential of F1 lymphocytes by parental lymphocytes. J Exp Med 1980;151:20-31.

36. Langlade Demoyen P, Larsson EL: Development of a model system for analyzing graft-versus-host-mediated immune suppression. Scand J Immunol 1986;24:119-125.

37. Ghayur T, Seemayer TA, Kongshavn PA, Gartner JG, Lapp WS: Graft-versus-host reactions in the beige mouse. An investigation of the role of host and donor natural killer cells in the pathogenesis of graft-versus-host disease. Transplantation 1987;44: 261–267.

38. Ishikawa H, Kubota E, Saito K: Modulation of F1 cytotoxic potentials by GvHR: role and mode of action of non-MHC genes that determine the hybrid resistance to GvHR-associated suppression of F1 cytotoxic potential. J Immunol 1984;132:2218–2225.

39. Ghayur T, Seemayer TA, Lapp WS: Kinetics of natural killer cell cytotoxicity during the graft-versus-host reaction. Relationship between natural killer cell activity, T and B cell activity, and development of histopathological alterations. Transplantation 1987;44:254–260.

40. Pals ST, Radaszkiewicz T, Gleichmann E: Allosuppressor- and allohelper-T cells in acute and chronic graft-vs-host disease. IV. Activation of donor allosuppressor cells is confined to acute GVHD. J Immunol 1984;132:1669–1678.

41. Moller G: Suppressive effect of graft-versus-host reaction on immune response to heterologous red cells. Immunology 1971;20:597–609.

42. Singer A, Kruisbeek A, Andrysiak PM: T cell-accessory cell interaction that initiate allospecific cytotoxic T lymphocyte responses. Existence of both Ia-restricted and Ia-unrestricted cellular interation pathways. J Immunol 1984;142:2199–2209.

43. Mizuochi T, Golding H, Rosenberg AS, Glimcher LH, Malek TR, Singer A: Both L3T4$^+$ and Lyt2$^+$ helper T cells initiate cytotoxic T lymphocyte responses against allogeneic major histocompatibility antigens but not against trinitrophenyl-modified self. J Exp Med 1985;162:427–443.

44. Guimezanes A, Schmitt-Verhulst AM: Inhibition of helper function with anti-Lyt-2 or anti-L3T4 monoclonal antibodies depending on stimulating antigens. Eur J Immunol 1985;15:1187–1191.

45. Iwasaki T, Hallam JA, Joseph LJ, Shearer GM: Antigen-specific protection against graft-vs-host induced immune deficiency. J Immunol 1987;138:3604–3610.

46. Joseph LJ, Iwasaki T, Malek TR, Shearer GM: Interleukin 2 receptor dysfunction in mice undergoing a graft-vs-host reaction. J Immunol 1985;135:1846–1850.

47. Pals ST, Gleichmann H, Gleichmann E: Allosuppressor and allohelper T cells in acute and chronic graft-vs-host disease. V. F1 mice with secondary chronic GVHD contain F1-reactive allohelper but no allosuppressor T cells. J Exp Med 1984;159: 508–523.

48. Xenocostas A, Lapp WS, Osmond DG: Suppression of B lymphocyte genesis in the bone marrow by systemic graft-versus-host reactions. Transplantation 1987;43:549–555.

49. Iwasaki T, Fujiwara H, Shearer GM: Loss of proliferative capacity and T cell immune development potential by bone marrow from mice undergoing a graft-vs-host reaction. J Immunol 1986;137:3100–3108.

50. Pals ST, Zijstra M, Radaszkiewicz T, Quint W, Cuypers HT, Schoenmakers HJ, Melief CJ, Berns A, Gleichmann E: Immunologic induction of malignant lymphoma: graft-vs-host reaction-induced B cell lymphomas contain integrations of predominantly ecotropic murine leukemia proviruses. J Immunol 1986;136:331–339.

51. Cudkowicz G, Stimpfling JH: Induction of immunity and of unresponsiveness to parental marrow grafts in adult F1 hybrid mice. Nature 1964;204:450–453.

52. Affifi MS, Kumar V, Bennett M: Stimulation of genetic resistance to marrow grafts in mice by interferon alpha/beta. J Immunol 1985;134:3739–3745.

53. Daley JP, Nakamura I: Natural resistance of lethally irradiated F1 hybrid mice to parental marrow grafts is a function of H-2/Hh-restricted effectors. J Exp Med 1984; 159:1132–1148.

54. Kosmatopoulos K, Bravo-Cuellar A, Wachowiak J, Orbach-Arbouys S: Inhibition of hybrid resistance by 5-fluorouracil. Destruction of a Thy-1$^+$ Lyt-1$^+$2$^-$ spleen cell implicated in the expression of hybrid resistance. Transplantation 1987;44:202–208.

55. Soderling CC, Song CW, Blazar BR, Vallera DA: A correlation between conditioning and engraftment in recipients of MHC-mismatched T cell-depleted murine bone marrow transplants. J Immunol 1985;135:941–946.

56. Vallera DA, Soderling CC, Carlson GJ, Kersey JH: Bone marrow transplantation across major histocompatibility barriers in mice. II. T cell requirement for engraftment in total lymphoid irradiation-conditioned recipients. Transplantation 1982; 33:243-248.

57. Hurtenbach U, Shearer GM: Analysis of murine T lymphocyte markers during the early phases of GvH-associated suppression of cytotoxic T lymphocyte responses. J Immunol 1983;130:1561-1566.

58. Polisson RP, Shearer GM: Mutual recognition of parental and F1 lymphocytes. II. Analysis of graft-vs-host-induced suppressor cell activity for T cell-mediated lympholysis to trinitrophenyl self and alloantigens. J Immunol 1980;125:1865-2861.

59. Lapp WS, Mendes M, Kirchner H, Gemsa D: Prostaglandin synthesis by lymphoid tissue of mice experiencing a graft-versus-host reaction: relationship to immunosuppression. Cell Immunol 1980;50:271-281.

60. Wall DA, Hamberg SD, Reynolds DS, Burakoff SJ, Abbas AK, Ferrara JL: Immunodeficiency in graft-versus-host disease. I. Mechanism of immune suppression. J Immunol 1988;140:2970-2976.

61. Holda JH, Maier T, Claman HN: Evidence that IFN-gamma is responsible for natural suppressor activity in GVHD spleen and normal bone marrow. Transplantation 1988;45:772-777.

62. Holda JH, Maier T, Claman HN: Natural suppressor activity in graft-vs-host spleen and normal bone marrow is augmented by IL 2 and interferon-gamma. J Immunol 1986;137:3538-3543.

63. Maier T, Holda JH, Claman HN: Graft-vs-host reactions (GVHR) across minor murine histocompatibility barriers. II. Development of natural suppressor cell activity. J Immunol 1985;135:1644-1651.

64. Hakim FT, Pluznik DH, Shearer GM: Reduction of bone marrow myeloid progenitors and colony stimulating factor production in graft-vs-host reaction. J Cell Bioch 1988;Suppl 12c:107.

65. Vinci G, Vernant JP, Cordonnier C, Bracq C, Rochant H, Breton-Gorius J, Vainchenker W: HLA-DR restriction on suppression of hematopoiesis by T cells from allogeneic bone marrow transplants. J Immunol 1986;136:3225-3230.

66. Vinci G, Vernant JP, Cordonnier C, Henri A, Breton-Gorius J, Rochant H, Vainchenker W: In vitro inhibition of hematopoiesis by HNK1,DR-positive T cells and monocytes after allogeneic bone marrow transplantation. Exp Hematol 1987;15: 54-64.

67. Roy C, Ghayur T, Kongshavn PA, Lapp WS: Natural killer activity by spleen, lymph node, and thymus cells during the graft-versus-host reaction. Transplantation 1982; 34:144-146.

68. Ghayur T, Seemayer TA, Lapp WS: Association between the degree of thymic dysplasia and the kinetics of thymic NK cell activity during the graft-versus-host reaction. Clin Immunol Immunopathol 1988;48:19-30.

69. Ghayur T, Seemayer TA, Lapp WS: Prevention of murine graft-versus-host disease by inducing and eliminating ASGM1$^+$ cells of donor origin. Transplantation 1988;45: 586-590.

70. Seemayer TA, Gartner JG, Colle E, Lapp WS: Acute graft-versus-host reaction in the pancreas. Transplantation 1983;35:72-77.

71. Bordignon C, Daley JP, Nakamura I: Hematopoietic histoincompatibility reactions by NK cells in vitro: model for genetic resistance to marrow grafts. Science 1985; 230:1398-1401.

72. Holmberg LA, Miller BA, Ault KA: The effect of natural killer cells on the development of syngeneic hematopoietic progenitors. J Immunol 1984;133:2933-2939.

73. Degliantoni G, Perussia B, Mangoni L, Trinchieri G: Inhibition of bone marrow colony formation by human natural killer cells and by natural killer cell-derived colony-inhibiting activity. J Exp Med 1985;161:1152-1168.

74. Barber KE, Crosier PS, Watson JD: The differential inhibition of hemopoietic growth factor activity by cytotoxins and interferon-gamma. J Immunol 1987;139: 1108-1112.

75. Piguet PF, Grau GE, Allet B, Vassalli P: Tumor necrosis factor/cachectin is an effector of skin and gut lesions of the acute phase of graft-vs.-host disease. J Exp Med 1987;166:1280-1289.

76. Crapper RM, Schrader JW: Evidence for the in vivo production and release into the serum of a T-cell lymphokine, persisting-cell stimulating factor (PSF), during graft-versus-host reactions. Immunology 1986;57:553-558.

77. Kindler V, Thorens B, Vassalli P: In vivo effect of murine recombinant interleukin 3 on early hemopoietic progenitors. Eur J Immunol 1987;17:1511-1514.

78. Levy RB, Cotterell AH, Jones M, Malek TR: Graft-versus-host reaction-induced immune modulation. I. Donor-recipient genetic disparity and the differential expression of Lyt-2, L3T4, and Ly-6 during acute reactions in the host thymus. J Immunol 1988;140:1717-1725.

79. Lang P, Dardenne M, Savino W, Moritz S, Shearer G: Cytotoxic T cell response and thymic hormonal dysfunction in graft-vs-host mice. J Immunol 1986;136:1999-2004.

80. Lang P, Miller MW, Shearer GM: Failure of bone marrow cells to reconstitute T cell immunity in graft-vs-host mice. J Immunol 1985;134:2050-2052.

81. Fukuzawa M, Via CS, Shearer GM: Defective thymic education of L3T4$^+$ T helper cell function in graft-vs-host mice. J Immunol 1988;141:430-439.

82. Shearer GM, Bernstein DC, Tung KS, Via CS, Redfield R, Salahuddin SZ, Gallo RC: A model for the selective loss of major histocompatibility complex self-restricted T cell immune responses during the development of acquired immune deficiency syndrome (AIDS). J Immunol 1986;137:2514-2521.

83. Brkic S, Tsoi M-S, Mori T, Lachman L, Gillis S, Thomas SD, Storb R: Cellular interactions in marrow-grafted patients. III. Normal interleukin 1 and defective interleukin 2 production in short-term patients and in those with chronic graft-versus-host disease. Transplantation 1985;39:30-35.

84. Lum LG, Seigneuret MC, Storb R, Witherspoon RP, Thomas ED: In vitro regulation of immunoglobin synthesis after marrow transplantation. I. T-cell and B-cell deficiencies in patients with and without chronic graft-versus-host disease. Blood 1981; 58:431-439.

85. Rolink AG, Gleichmann E: Allosuppressor- and allohelper-T cells in acute and chronic graft-vs.-host (GVH) disease. III. Different Lyt subsets of donor T cells induce different pathological syndromes. J Exp Med 1983;158:546-558.

86. Rolink AG, Gleichmann H, Gleichmann E: Diseases caused by reactions of T lymphocytes to incompatible structures of the major histocompatibility complex. VII. Immune-complex glomerulonephritis. J Immunol 1983;130:209-215.

87. van der Veen FM, Rolink AG, Gleichmann E: Autoimmune disease strongly resembling systemic lupus erythematosus (SLE) in F1 mice undergoing graft-versus-host reaction (GVHR). Adv Exp Med Biol 1982;149:669-677.

88. van der Veen F, Rolink AG, Gleichmann E: Diseases caused by reactions of T

lymphocytes to incompatible structures of the major histocompatibility complex. IV. Autoantibodies to nuclear antigens. Clin Exp Immunol 1981;46:589-596

89. Van Elven EH, van der Veen FM, Rolink AG, Issa P, Duin TM, Gleichmann E: Diseases caused by reactions of T lymphocytes to incompatible structures of the major histocompatibility complex. V. High titers of IgG autoantibodies to double-stranded DNA. J Immunol 1981;127:2435-2438.

90. van der Veen JP, Rolink AG, Gleichmann E: Diseases caused by reactions of T lymphocytes to incompatible structures of the major histocompatibility complex. III. Autoantibodies to thymocytes. J Immunol 1981;127:1281-1286.

91. Kimura M, van Rappard-van der Veen FM, Gleichmann E: Requirement of H-2-subregion differences for graft-versus-host autoimmunity in mice: superiority of the differences at class-II H-2 antigens (I-A/I-E). Clin Exp Immunol 1986;65: 542-552.

92. Portanova JP, Kotzin BL: Lupus-like autoimmunity in murine graft-versus-host disease. Concepts Immunopathol 1988;6:119-140.

93. Portanova JP, Claman HN, Kotzin BL: Autoimmunization in murine graft-vs-host disease. I. Selective production of antibodies to histones and DNA. J Immunol 1985;135:3850-3856.

94. Kimura M, Gleichmann E: Depressed antibody responses to exogenous antigens in mice with lupus-like graft-versus-host disease. Clin Immunol Immunopathol 1987; 43:97-109.

95. Mendes ML, Rode H, Peres A, Kongshavn PA, Lapp WS: Interleukin-1 and inter-leukin-2 defects associated with murine graft-versus-host-induced immunodeficiency. Transplantation 1985;39:418-424.

96. Neiman PE, Reeves W, Ray G: A prospective analysis of interstitial pneumonia and opportunistic viral infection among recipients of allogeneic bone marrow grafts. J Infec Dis 1975;136:754-767.

97. Meyers JD, Spencer HC, Watts JC: Cytomegalovirus pneumonia after human bone marrow transplantation. Ann Intern Med 1975;82:181-188.

98. Meyers JD, Glournoy N, Thomas ED: Nonbacterial pneumonia after allogeneic marrow transplantation: a review of ten years' experience. Rev Infect Dis 1982; 4:1119-1132.

99. Grundy JE, Shanley JD, Shearer GM: Augmentation of graft-versus-host reaction by cytomegalovirus infection resulting in interstitial pneumonitis. Transplantation 1985;39:548-553.

100. Via CS, Shanley JD, Weatherly BR, Lang P, Shearer GM: Altered threshold for the induction of graft-versus-host immunodeficiency following murine cytomegalovirus infection. Transplantation 1988;46:298-302.

101. Shanley JD, Via CS, Sharrow SO, Shearer GM: Interstitial pneumonitis during murine cytomegalovirus infection and graft-versus-host reaction. Characterization of bronchoalveolar lavage cells. Transplantation 1987;44:658-662.

102. Via CS, Shearer GM: T-cell interactions in autoimmunity: insights from a murine model of graft-versus-host disease. Immunol Today 1988;9:207-213.

103. Martin PJ, Hansen JA, Buckner CD, Sanders JE, Deeg HJ, Stewart P, Appelbaum FR, Clift R, Fefer A, Witherspoon RP, Kennedy MS, Sullivan KM, Flournoy N, Storb R, Thomas ED: Effects of in vitro depletion of T cells in HLA-identical allogeneic marrow grafts. Blood 1985;66:664-672.

104. Hakim FT, Pluznik DH, Shearer GM: Multiple factors contribute to the decrease in Concanavalin A induced colony stimulating factors in acute suppressive graft-versus-host disorder. Transplantation 1990;in press.

105. Hakim FT, Pluznik DH, Shearer GM: Alteration in T cell derived colony stimulating factors associated with GVH induced immune deficiency. Transplantation 1990;in press.

106. Clerici M, Stocks NI, Zajac RA, Boswell RN, Lucey DR, Via CS, Shearer GM: Detection of three distinct patterns of T helper cell dysfunction in asymptomatic, HIV-seropositive patients. Independence of CD4[+] cell numbers and clinical staging. J Clin Invest 1989;84:in press.

9

Autoimmune Diseases Induced by Graft-vs.-Host Disease

Antonius G. Rolink, Andreas Strasser,* and Fritz Melchers
Basel Institute for Immunology
Basel, Switzerland

I. INTRODUCTION

Heterozygous F_1 mice are tolerant towards lymphocytes and tissue of both parents. One parental strain is, however, not tolerant to the other, genetically different parent. Therefore injection of T cells of one parent into F_1 recipients will lead to an alloreaction of these T cells against the foreign antigens encoded by the other parental strain in the F_1 mice. The major antigens recognized in a graft-versus-host response in F_1 hosts with a fully competent hemolymphopoietic system are the MHC antigens encoded by the major histocompatibility complex (1-4). The outcome of this alloreaction depends on the histocompatibility antigens recognized by the parental T cells, and/or the functions of the subset of parental T cells injected (1-4). Thus, a class II MHC difference between donor and host leads to a hyperplastic syndrome with many features of systemic lupus erythematosus (SLE) and other collagen vascular diseases (1,3,4). The parental T cells responsible for this syndrome are $CD4^+$ MHC class II reactive alloreactive T helper (T_H) cells (1-3,5). If the two parents of an F_1 mouse with an intact hemolymphopoietic system differ only in class I MHC antigens, no significant pathological alterations are observed when parental T cells are injected into the F_1 animals (1). On the other hand, a hypoplastic GVH syndrome is observed in cases where parental T cells are transferred into F_1 combinations that differ in both class I and class II MHC antigens (1-3,6-9). Both alloreactive $CD4^+$ class II MHC reactive parental T_H cells and $CD8^+$ class I MHC reactive parental cytotoxic/suppressor T ($T_{c/s}$) cells are required for the induction of the hypoplastic GVH syndrome (1-3, 5-8). Removal of the $CD8^+$ T cell population from the parental donor cell inoculum abolishes the capacity of the donor cells to induce

---

Present affiliation: The Walter and Eliza Hall Institute of Medical Research, Melbourne, Victoria, Australia

the hypoplastic GVH syndrome. By contrast, the $CD8^+$-depleted cells now induce SLE-like GVHD, indicating once more that $CD4^+$ alloreactive T_H cells are responsible for the induction of the SLE-like GVHD (2-3). When parental T cells deprived of $CD4^+$ cells are injected into F_1 recipients, different in class I and class II MHC, no significant GVHD is observed (2,3).

Not all parent F_1 combinations which differ at class I and class II MHC genes give rise to a hypoplastic GVH syndrome. The best studied combination of this kind is the injection of unseparated T cells of strain DBA/2 into (C57BL/6 X DBA/2)F_1 (BDF$_1$) recipients. For unknown reasons the injection of DBA/2 T cells into BDF$_1$ mice preferentially triggers $CD4^+$ alloreactive T helper cells leading to an SLE-like GVHD (3,6,7,9-14). The pathological and clinical abnormalities of the two basic forms of GVHD are summarized in Table 1.

The hyperplastic syndrome has many features of SLE and other collagen vascular diseases. The B-cell compartment is strongly activated resulting in increased levels of Ig (especially IgG) in the circulation. Many SLE-like autoantibodies are present in these mice, such as antibodies against nuclear antigens, ds DNA, erythrocytes, thymocytes, mitochondria, cytoskeleton proteins, kidney tubular brush border proteins, and proteins encoded by genes from endogenous murine leukemia viruses (1-4,9-12). Probably as a consequence of this autoantibody formation, the GVH F_1 mice often develop immune complex glomerulonephritis (ICGN) which can become so severe that the animals develop ascites and finally die (13). Thus far, antibodies against nuclear antigens, proteins encoded by genes from endogenous murine leukemia viruses and kidney tubular brush border proteins could be eluted from kidneys with ICGN, indicating that these autoantibodies might be involved in the progression of the disease (12,13).

The SLE-like stimulatory GVHD is often accompanied by symptoms characteristic of other collagen vascular diseases like arteritis, polyarthritis, Sjögren and scleroderma-like lesions (3,9,14,15).

The second form of GVHD in unirradiated F_1 mice is characterized by hypoplastic pathological symptoms (Table 1). In the initial phase of the disease, these mice show stimulation of the lymphohemopoietic system, particularly a strong B-cell activation. This then is followed by severe hypoplasia of the lymphohemopoietic system resulting in aplastic anemia and decreased levels of Ig in the circulation (1-3,6-9). This hypoplastic GVH syndrome seems to result from a sequential activation of, first, class II-MHC reactive $CD4^+$ donor T_H cells, and, then, class I-MHC reactive $CD8^+$ $T_{c/s}$ cells (1-3,5-9). The $CD4^+$ donor T_H cells seem to be responsible for the stimulation of the lymphohemo-poietic system observed early in these GVHD mice and probably also enable optimal induction of $CD8^+$ donor $T_{c/s}$ effector cells. These $CD8^+$ donor $T_{c/s}$ then cause the cellular depletion of the lymphohematopoietic system of the host resulting in a state of

Table 1 Spectrum of Pathological Alterations Found in Nonirradiated F_1 Mice with GVHD

Hyperplastic (SLE-like) syndrome	Hypoplastic syndrome
Hyper-γ-globulinemia	Hypo-γ-globulinemia
SLE-like autoantibodies and ICGN	Thymic hypoplasia
Scleroderma-like lesions	Pancytopenia
Lymphocyte infiltrations in multiple organs	

severe immunodeficiency (1-3,6-9). Under conventional housing conditions these animals then die from infections (8,16). Under pathogen-free conditions these animals might survive the immunodeficiency disease. Cells in the lymphohematopoietic system of the mice surviving this type of GVHD are of donor origin (6). This indicates that the few stem cells present in the donor cell inoculum have repopulated the F_1 host.

The T-cell compartment in these chimeras is only partially tolerant to the F_1 host. Thus, T cells reactive to class I MHC of the F_1 mice are absent, while T cells reactive to class II MHC are readily detectable in these chimeras (6). A possible explanation for this split tolerance might be that the donor $CD8^+$ $T_{c/s}$ cells have deleted all the class II positive cells from the F_1 host, consequently new donor T cells arising from stem cells in the donor cell inoculum do not encounter this antigen in the thymus of the F_1 host and do not get tolerized against it.

In the following we will concentrate on the SLE-like GVHD. It should be noted that this disease can only be induced in an F_1 host with an intact lymphohemopoietic system. In F_1 hosts devoid of hemolymphopoietic cells the GVHD is normally lethal. One thousand-fold fewer parental T cells directed against minor transplantation antigens are also sufficient to induce this lethal GVHD (17,18).

II. NEW INSIGHTS INTO THE INITIATION AND PROGRESSION OF SLE-LIKE GVHD

A. Alloreactive T_H-cell Clones

The SLE-like GVHD is induced by $CD4^+$ alloreactive parental T_H cells triggered by foreign class II MHC antigens in the F_1 hosts (1-5). The question arises whether alloreactive T_H-cell clones can induce a similar disease. Therefore alloreactive T_H-cell clones directed against class II MHC antigens, or T_H-cell clones specific for the male specific antigen H-Y were prepared. Either type of T-cell clone in vitro induced specifically polyclonal B-cell stimulation, indicating that they indeed belonged to the helper T-cell subset. In vivo however, none of these T-cell clones induced the SLE-like GVHD in the relevant recipients. In contrast, quite a large number of different class II MHC specific as well as H-Y specific T_H cell clones induced acute death (2-3 days after injection) in adult, nonirradiated recipient mice expressing the antigens recognized by the injected T-cell clones (19). Histological examination of these mice revealed that death was caused by a systemic DTH-like reaction in the liver and lung. Mice not expressing the specific antigen injected with these T-cell clones did not show any histological alterations. It is noteworthy that *unprimed* female T cells do not cause significant GVHD in unirradiated as well as irradiated syngeneic male mice (17).

The result with uncloned, primary T cells might suggest that low doses of those T-cell clones which, at high doses, induce death, as well as any doses of those T-cell clones which do not induce death, could induce SLE-like GVHD. This, however, is not the case. A possible explanation might be that the homing capability of these T-cell clones is impaired (20). They may not migrate to the proper sites (i.e., spleen and lymph nodes) where primary uncloned T cells go. Another (and not mutually exclusive) explanation might be that these T-cell clones only induce a polyclonal IgM production (as they do in vitro) and do not cause switching to IgG production which, as will be discussed below, is an important feature of the SLE-like GVHD.

B. Autoreactive B-Cell Repertoires in Mice with SLE-like GVHD Are Largely Indistinguishable From Those of Normal Mice

Antibodies to a variety of self antigens have been found in the sera of normal individuals (21). Cells producing these antibodies have been cloned as murine hybridomas from fetal, newborn, and adult normal mice and as EBV-transformed B cells or as hybridomas from normal human individuals (22-26). These findings have implied that the normal immune system includes autoreactive B cells.

We have now investigated the question whether the autoreactive B-cell repertoire triggered by parental alloreactive T_H cells in F_1 recipients is different from that found in normal (nonautoimmune) mice. Therefore, collections of hybridomas were made from mice with SLE-like GVHD at different stages of disease as well as from normal mice, mice injected with the polyclonal B cell stimulator lipopolysaccharide and mice injected with the antigen sheep red blood cells. All hybridomas were tested for the production of antibodies capable of binding to a panel of self antigens. A summary of these results can be found in Table 2.

The hybridomas were tested for the production of autoantibodies binding to mouse kidney cryosections, to DNA, and to the cell surface of a panel of cells including B cells, T cells, macrophages, and fibroblasts. Between 9.6 and 17.7% of the hybridomas produced antibodies that bound to any of the tested autoantigens. The data in Table 2 also indicates that the frequencies of hybridomas producing these autoantibodies are not significantly different between those derived from GVHD mice and those from normal mice. Moreover, the predominant part of the repertoire of hybridomas producing these autoantibodies does not change with time after injection of alloreactive prenatal T helper cells. This appears to suggest that the development of ICGN at later times after induction is not simply due to an increased number of activated splenic B cells producing autoantibodies of different specificities.

Altogether, these results argue for a polyclonal activation of the B-cell compartment by the alloreactive parental T cells. The frequencies of hybridomas producing autoantibodies to cell surface antigens contribute a higher portion of the total in the group of GVH hybridomas compared with those derived from normal mice. The specificities of these antibodies will be discussed. However, monoclonal autoantibodies binding to T and B cells are also found in normal mice.

C. Autoantibodies Found Only in Mice with GVHD, but Not in Normal Mice

Thus far, differences have been found between the autoreactive B-cell repertoires of normal and GVHD mice in the class of Ig produced and in some specificities for self antigens (11,27). These differences are summarized in Table 3. First, only autoantibodies of the IgM class are found in normal animals, whereas the majority of the autoantibodies derived from GVHD mice are of the IgG class (11). This might indicate that normally the system does not allow switching of self antigen reactive B cells to IgG. On the other hand, a signal from the alloreactive parental T_H cell, recognizing the foreign class II MHC antigen on the F_1 cells lets B cells switch to IgG production. T_H cells are also claimed, to induce processes in B cells leading to Ig-variable gene hypermutations (28). Alloreactive T_H cells in the GVHD might, therefore, also induce somatic hypermutations in self antigen reactive B cell clones.

Table 2 Frequencies and Specificities of Autoantibody-Producing B-Cell Hybridomas Derived from Spleen Cells of Mice with SLE-like GVHD and Normal Mice

Hybridomas made from spleen cells of	Number of hybridomas	Number of hybridomas producing autoantibodies (%)	Autoantibodies binding to		
			Kidney-cryosections	DNA	Cell surface determinants
Normal mice	112	18 (16.1)	17	1	3
SRBC-injected mice	211	24 (11.4)	23	1	1
LPS-injected mice	181	32 (17.7)	28	4	2
GVHD mice (wk1)	22	3 (13.6)	2	–	1
GVHD mice (wk2)	311	30 (9.6)	21	10	17
GVHD mice (wk5)	129	17 (13.2)	11	2	7
GVHD mice (wk8)	122	21 (17.12)	11	2	12

Spleen cells of normal (BDF_1) mice, of BDF_1 mice twice injected with SRBC (on day 4 after 2nd injection) of BDF_1 mice 3 days prior to injected i.v. with 100 μg LPS and of BDF_1, mice at week 1, 2, 5, and 8 after injection of 2×10^7 DBA/2 splenic T cells (GVHD mice) were fused with the non-secreting, azaguanine-resistant hybridoma cell line SP2/0 as described (11).

The fused cells were plated into microtiter plates under limiting dilution conditions. Autoanitbody production was measured from those cultures that showed positive growth and, according to Poisson's distribution, had a >98% probability of being a hybridoma clone. Fusion frequencies obtained with spleen cells from SRBC-injected mice, LPS-injected mice, and GVHD mice were about identical (1 in 10^5 to 1 in 5×10^5 spleen cells) whereas the fusion frequencies obtained with spleen cells of normal mice were 1 in 10^7 spleen cells. All hybridomas were tested in an indirect immuno-fluorescence test for production of autoantibodies binding kidney cryosections and to cell surface determinants of a panel of cells, including B cells, T cells, macrophages, and fibroblasts. Autoantibodies to DNA tested in an ELISA as described (11).

Two types of autoantibodies have been found only in GVHD animals but not in the normal repertoires. The first type is monoclonal antibodies directed against a 160 kD glycoprotein present in the microvilli of kidney brush borders. Such autoantibodies could also be eluted from the glomerulae of mice with ICGN. This suggests an involvement of the autoantibodies in this disease (11,12). However, transfer of these autoantibodies to native recipients so far has not led to ICGN (12).

The second type of autoantibodies found only in GVHD animals are directed against a 70 kD glycoprotein (gp 70) encoded by genes which are found in endogenous murine leukemia viruses (27). These antibodies were characterized by their binding to a panel of cells expressing gp70 of known retroviruses. Immunoprecipitations revealed that the GVH-derived hybridomas produce antibodies which recognize a known form of the MulV envelope glycoprotein gp70 on the surface of some of the tested cells. The percentage of hybridomas producing these anti-gp70 antibodies can be as high as 15% of the total hybridoma repertoire of a single GVHD mouse. By now we have made 169 hybridomas derived from GVHD mice that produce anti-gp70 antibodies. Based on bind-

Table 3 IgM/IgG Class Distribution of All Monoclonal Autoantibodies and Frequencies of Autoantibodies Reactive to Kidney Tubular Brush Border and gp70 Envelope Glycoprotein of Murine Leukemia Viruses

Hybridomas made from spleen cells of	Number of hybridomas	Number of hybridomas producing autoantibodies	Autoantibody-secreting hybridomas producing		Autoantibodies binding to	
			IgM (%)	IgG (%)	Brush border	gp70
Normal mice	112	18	100	0	0	0
SRBC-injected mice	211	24	100	0	0	0
LPS-injected mice	181	32	100	0	0	0
GVHD mice (wk1)	22	3	0	100	0	0
GVHD mice (wk2)	311	30	8	92	2	2
GVHD mice (wk5)	129	17	15	85	5	1
GVHD mice (wk8)	122	21	19	81	2	9

Production of hybridomas as in Table 2. IgM/IgG class distribution was determined with an ELISA as described (11). Autoantibodies binding to brush border antigens were determined with indirect immunofluorescence on kidney cryosections and to gp70 by indirect immunofluorescence on a panel of cells expressing gp70 on the surface and by immunoprecipitation (27).

ing assays with the fibroblast cell line Ltk⁻, the T cell hybridoma K62, the macrophage cell line P388D$_1$, and LPS-activated splenic B cells, we were able to divide these 169 anti-gp70 producing hybridomas into at least three groups. The vast majority (≈80%) of these hybridomas bind to P388D$_1$ macrophages and LPS-activated splenic B cells, and not, or only weakly, to Ltk⁻ and K62 cells. About 10% bind to all four cell types tested, whereas the other 10% bind only to Ltk⁻ cells and the T-cell hybridoma K62 and not to P388D$_1$ and LPS-activated B-cell blasts. This indicates that within GVHD mice, activated B cells produce antibodies to different gp70 molecules specifically and/or preferentially expressed in cells of different lineages (macrophages and B cells versus T cells and fibroblasts).

D. The Role of Antigens Capable of Crosslinking Ig-Receptors on B Cells in SLE-like GVHD

Gleichmann et al. (3,10) have proposed a model of abnormal T-B-cell cooperation as being responsible for the SLE-like GVHD. In this model, the injected alloreactive parental T$_H$ cells triggered by the foreign class II MHC antigens of the F$_1$ host are expected not to induce a polyclonal B stimulation but to lead to a preferential activation and clonal expansion of those B cells (including autoreactive B cells) that have their Ig-receptors crosslinked by antigen. This model was based on the findings that autoantibodies were found in the serum of mice with SLE-like GVHD, only to self antigens that have the potential of crosslinking the Ig-receptors by repetitive antigenic determinants on the respective B cells, like DNA and cell surface antigens. Autoantibodies to mouse thyroglobulin and insulin (self antigens which do not possess the capacity to crosslink the Ig-receptors on the respective B cells), on the other hand, appear conspicuously absent. Moreover, no increased levels of antibodies to foreign antigens are found in the serum of these mice (29).

In agreement with the model outlined above, it has also been found that foreign antigens with a potential to crosslink Ig-receptors evoked much stronger B-cell responses when injected in F$_1$ mice together with parental T cells than those with no crosslinking capacity. No differences in antibody responses were observed using normal proteins as antigens (29-33). Moreover, haptenated mouse red blood cells, which are tolerogens when injected into normal mice, turned out to be potent antigens when injected into F$_1$ mice together with parental T cells (34,35). In disagreement with these results are our findings of a polyclonal activation of the B-cell compartment by the alloreactive parental T$_H$ cells. In this activation the role of surface Ig in B-cell triggering seems to be circumvented, although it remains unclear how. We will discuss this in more detail below.

E. Alloreactive T Cells Convert a Tolerogen into an Immunogen

The role of antigens capable of crosslinking the Ig-receptors on B cells in SLE-like GVHD was studied in more detail using mouse red blood cells coupled with the hapten 4-hydroxy-3-iodo-5 nitrophenyl (NIP-MRBC) as a model antigen. Two GVH combinations which commonly yield strong SLE-like GVHD (namely C57BL/6 T cells injected into (C57BL/6 × B6-C-H-2^{bm12})F$_1$ ((B6 × BM12)F$_1$)) mice and DBA/2 cells injected into BDF$_1$ recipients were used throughout these studies. These F$_1$ mice were injected with parental T cells and NIP-MRBC, and the anti-NIP antibody titer in the serum of these mice was monitored at different times after injection. Both GVH combinations gave similar results. An example of the anti-NIP response in (B6 × BM12)F$_1$ mice is shown in Fig.

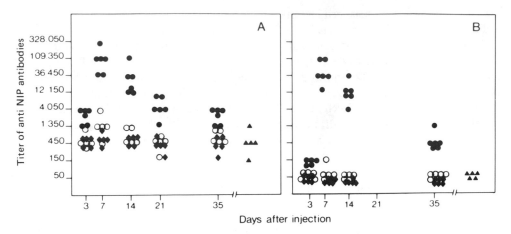

Figure 1   (B6 × BM12)F$_1$ (●) mice were injected with 2 × 10^7 B6 splenic T cells together with a 2 × 10^9 NIP-MRBC. NIP coupling was performed as described (34,35).
At regular times after injection the anti-NIP titer was determined in an ELISA system
using NIP coupled to bovine serum albumin. (B6 × BM12)F$_1$ mice not injected (▲),
injected with 2 × 10^7 B6 splenic T cells (○), or only with 2 × 10^9 NIP-MRBC (♦) served
as controls. Panel A represents the titer of IgM and IgG anti-NIP antibodies in the serum
of individual mice out of these groups, whereas panel B represents the IgG compartment
of the anti-NIP response.

1. The anti-NIP antibody response peaks at day 7 after injection of T$_H$ cells and antigen
and is mainly of the IgG class (Fig. 1B). No anti-NIP response is observed in F$_1$ mice
injected only with NIP-MRBC, or only with parental T cells. Thus, the class II reactive
parental T$_H$ cells can activate and clonally expand F$_1$ B cells that have their Ig-receptors
crosslinked by antigen.

    We also monitored the quality of the anti-NIP response. B-cell hybridomas were
prepared from (B6 × BM12)F$_1$ mice on day 7 after injection of B6 splenic T cells and
NIP-MRBC and from normal (B6 × BM12)F$_1$ mice injected with NIP coupled to the
protein carrier ovalbumin (NIP-OVA). One characteristic of a primary anti-NIP response
in B6 mice is the high incidence of λ light chain in NIP-specific antibodies (36). From
the 107 anti-NIP antibody-producing hybridomas derived from (B6 × BM12)F$_1$ mice
injected with B6 T cells and NIP-MRBC, 43 had λ light chains, indicating a similar light
chain usage with this type of immunization protocol. Also, the affinities of the monoclonal anti-NIP antibodies derived from the GVH mice were comparable to those derived
from the F$_1$ mice injected with NIP-OVA. As shown in Figure 2, the affinities of anti-
NIP antibodies derived from GVH F$_1$ mice ranged from 5 × 10^{-5} mole/1 to 3 × 10^{-8}
mole/1, and those derived from NIP-OVA injected mice ranged from 10^{-5} mole/1 to
10^{-7} mole/1. Similar affinities of 32 monoclonals derived from GVH mice, compared
to 12 monoclonals derived from a normal immunization protocol, might indicate that
somatic hypermutations followed by selection through self antigen which give rise to
antibodies of higher affinity are rare under GVH conditions. (They are also rare in normal primary responses.) We then sequenced the λ light chains of some of these NIP-
specific monoclonal antibodies of GVHD mice. Only one nonsilent point mutation was

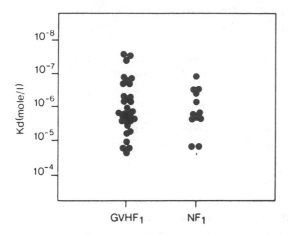

Figure 2   Monoclonal anti-NIP antibodies derived from (B6 X BM12)F_1 mice injected with 2 X 10^7 B6 splenic T cells and 2 X 10^9 NIP-MRBC (GVHF$_1$) and from (B6 X BM12)F_1 mice injected with 100 μg of NIP-OVA in complete Freunds adjuvant were affinity purified on a sepharose column coupled with NIP. Affinity for NIP was determined by equilibrium dialysis as described (37) using N^{125}IP-caproic acid as antigen.

found in seven λ light chain variable regions of GVH induced anti-NIP antibodies. Thus, somatic hypermutations appear not to be frequent in these antibodies.

F. Suppression of Secondary Alloreactions

The anti-NIP response disappears at about 4-5 weeks after primary induction (Fig. 1). Surprisingly, the anti-NIP-response in these mice cannot be rescued by repeated injections of NIP-MRBC and/or T cell of either parental strain.

   The GVHR appears not to delete the NIP-specific B cells from the system. Limiting dilution analysis using the polyclonal B cell stimulator LPS revealed similar frequencies of anti-NIP antibody producing B cells in mice with GVHD (1 in 900 spleen cells) and normal mice (1 in 800 spleen cells). GVHD mice injected with the type II T-cell-independent antigen NIP-Ficoll showed normal anti-NIP responses while GVHD mice injected with the T-dependent antigen NIP-OVA showed half the normal response. We conclude that the failure to induce a secondary anti-NIP response with NIP-MRBC is not due to a depletion of functional B cells.

   The finding that a second injection of NIP-MRBC alone did not elicit a secondary response was not surprising since parental T cells can no longer be detected in F_1 hosts 4 weeks or later after injection. It was, however, more surprising that coinjection of NIP-MRBC and parental T cells did not either lead to a secondary anti-NIP-response. This might indicate that animals once undergone a GVHR are insensitive (resistant) to a secondary GVHR. This unresponsiveness seems to be long lasting. As long as 4 months after induction of a primary GVHR no secondary GVHR could be induced, as measured by levels of polyclonally stimulated IgM- and IgG-producing B cells. Thus, it seems likely that GVH F_1 mice build up immunity against the parental cells. This immunity might either consist of a suppression or a direct elimination of all parental T cells injected in a secondary challenge. Transfer experiments are planned, which might help us to identify a possible cellular basis of this GVH resistance.

In summary, our data indicate that only in the initial phase of the GVHR can the alloreactive parental T_H cells trigger those B cells that have their Ig-receptors crosslinked by antigen. This mode of B-cell triggering, however, does not seem to set the stage for high rate of somatic hypermutations. In later stages of the GVHR, and when the SLE-like disease manifests itself, antigens capable of crosslinking the Ig-receptors on B cells do not appear to play an important role in the pathogenesis of SLE-like GVHD.

III. POSSIBLE MECHANISMS CONTRIBUTING TO THE INDUCTION AND PROGRESSION OF SLE-LIKE GVHD

The findings that alloreactive parental T cells cannot be detected in the F_1 host after 4 weeks and thereafter, and that a long-lasting state of unresponsiveness to a secondary challenge with alloreactive parental T cells of *either* parent is induced by the primary T-cell injection argues against a continuous helper action of these alloreactive cells in the F_1 host. It argues for their action in induction, but against an action in the progression of the disease. We, therefore, are looking for mechanisms which could operate on a "hit-and-run" basis. Alloreactive parental T_H cells would provide the "hit."

There are various possibilities by which the host could contribute to a progression of GVHD by a change in its immune system. It has been shown recently by several authors that B cells responsible for type 2 T-cell-independent immune responses, as well as Ly-1 B cells which, at least partly, are involved in these responses, have long life spans (38-40). Ly-1 B cells are known to contribute a large part of the production of the naturally occurring IgM autoantibodies (38,41). Under GVH stimulation one could imagine autoantibody producing Ly-1 B cells to switch to IgG production. In fact, it has been shown that the IgG part of the antibody responses to type 2 T-cell-independent antigens is increased under GVH conditions (33). In analogy to the GVH-induced NIP-MRBC responses, the injection of parental alloreactive T_H cells may also lead to the clonal expansion of those autoreactive Ly-1 B cells that have their Ig-receptors crosslinked by antigen. Although the NIP-MRBC antibodies induced by GVH stimulation do not show somatic mutations, the possible long life span of GVH-induced autoreactive Ly-1 B cells might contribute to the SLE-like GVHD.

A second possibility for progression of the autoimmune disease can be envisaged to reside in the activation of endogenous *env* genes encoding retroviral gp70 by the activation of cells via alloreactive parental T_H cells (42-47). The finding that up to 15% of the B-cell hybridomas derived from mice with SLE-like GVHD produce antibodies that are specific for the envelope glycoprotein gp70 of murine leukemia viruses, whereas none of the hybridomas derived from normal mice, or from mice injected with SRBC or the polyclonal B-cell stimulator LPS produce these types of antibodies, supports this general idea.

Moreover, the absence of these types of hybridomas in the hybridoma repertoire derived from polyclonal stimulated B cells indicates that the production of the anti-gp70 antibodies in GVHD mice is under control of T cells. Since donor T cells cannot be found anymore from week 4 onwards after induction of the GVHR, the anti-gp70 antibody response might be under control of F_1 host T cells. If the gp70 determinants have not previously been expressed then the immune system should not be tolerant to them. As a consequence, host T_H cells restricted to F_1 MHC class II antigens and specific for these "foreign" gp70 determinants would be activated. If the cells which express these gp70 molecules can also process and present them to the host T_H, a continuous stimulation of gp70-specific T_H cells would certainly result in a continuous activation of gp70-specific B cells (which might or might not produce gp70 themselves), and consequently to a preferential outgrowth of gp70-specific B-cell clones. The gp70-specific antibodies would then attack, via complement or opsonized macrophages, all cells of the body expressing native, but not necessarily processed gp70. In this mechanism the "hit" would be delivered by the parental alloreactive T_H cells, the "run" would be propagated by F_1 host-derived T_H cells recognizing the activated gp70.

Another possibility would be that a foreign gp70 T cell determinant is generated by mutation of one or recombination of two endogenous *env* genes either belonging to *defective* or *competent* retroviruses (42,48,49). Experiments using a panel of cells infected with known types of murine leukemia virus and thus expressing known gp70 molecules on the surface have indicated that at least some of anti-gp70 antibodies are specific for recombinant gp70. This might suggest that during the GVHR recombination of viral genes takes place, resulting in the expression of recombinant viruses and/or recombinant viral proteins. Pals et al. (42) have shown that in many of the GVHR-induced B-cell lymphomas, recombination of murine leukemia virus genes has taken place. If the *env* genes belonged to defective viruses, the spread of the recombinant gene(s) would be restricted to the clonal progeny of cells, in which the genetic change happened. It is likely that this would not suffice to induce a neodeterminant-gp70-specific host T_H cell response. If the *env* genes belonged to competent infectious retroviruses a genetic change could spread by infection. Moreover, the host range of infection could be controlled (and altered) by a variation in the tropism of virus, and consequently determine the pathological action of gp70 specific attacks of the immune system and, thereby, ultimately determine the tissue type of autoimmune disease, including SLE-like GVHD and maybe autoimmune diseases in general.

A third possible mechanism that might be involved in SLE-like GVHD comes from the finding that the thymus is affected by the induction of the GVHR (14,50,51). The thymus might now malfunction so that autoreactive T cells (i.e., T cells with high affinity receptors for self MHC determinants and self antigens) are not eliminated anymore. A similar mechanism had been suggested as being responsible for the autoimmune disease observed in irradiated, syngeneic bone marrow reconstituted and cyclosporin A-treated CBA/N mice (52), a disease which has features of that observed in GVHD mice.

How could the F_1 host remain nontolerized to endogenous gp70, before the onset of the GVHR? For one, the *env* genes could belong to endogenous defective retroviruses in which the *env* gene in question would be under the control of differentiation, i.e., lymphocyte-activation-specific promoters, and may be enhancers. As an example, the *env* genes could be under the control of regulators which turn on genes after activation of mature B cells. In normal immune responses the total contribution of this activation would be too low to activate gp70-specific T_H cells efficiently. Only in allo-reactions, where 100-1000-fold more cells are activated might the amount of gp70 expressed suffice to activate host T_H cells with specificity for these processed gp70 determinants.

Another puzzling feature of the GVH-triggered immune system in the F_1 host is the long-lasting polyclonal activation of IgG-secreting B cells. Here we come back to the question of whether B-cell activation can lead to proliferation and maturation to Ig-secreting cells even though surface Ig might not be occupied. The continued B-cell response of 5-15% of all activated B cells to gp70 might well be affected by the continued presence of the antigen and, thus, by the occupance of the specific surface Ig. For the rest of the activated B cells we do not know whether surface Ig is occupied by an antigen. To explain the polyclonal B-cell activation we might suggest that B cells are sites of expression and/or targets of infection for viruses which get expressed during the GVHR as suggested above. Like Epstein-Barr virus with human B cells (53,54) these viruses might polyclonally activate B cells by being mitogens (like LPS) or by transforming B cells. In this way of activation, T cells would not be needed. Athymic nu/nu mice and thymectomized, irradiated, bone-marrow-reconstituted mice should be polyclonally activatable in this way by a "hit" of the parental alloreactive T_H cells.

Another way to explain polyclonal B-cell activation would be to imply F_1 host T_H cells specific for the activated gp70. If B cells in the GVH-induced mice express gp70 these mutated or recombinant gp70 molecules might then combine with class II MHC molecules, giving rise to an altered self structure on the surface of B cells in GVHD F_1 mice. This then might trigger F_1 host T_H cells recognizing these gp70/altered self MHC structures. At the same time one would have to postulate that such T_H cells could activate B cells polyclonally, i.e., under the circumvention of any antigen binding to surface Ig, independent of their specificity. This, then, would contradict the ideas quoted above (3,10) which assume a critical role of crosslinking of surface Ig by repetitive determinants of self antigens in the induction and progression of SLE-like GVHD.

The original "hit" by alloreactive parental T_H cells induces polyclonal switching to IgG production and secretion. The various autoantibodies, therefore, are no longer of the IgM class which, as the cells producing them, are short-lived in the system. They are now, as the cells produce them, long-lived. While IgG repertoires of normal mice are devoid of autoantibodies (and probably reflect the experience of the host with foreign antigens), IgG repertoires of GVH-induced F_1 mice begin to accumulate long-lived IgG autoantibodies. They should then be capable of opsonizing macrophages and granulocytes and direct effector functions, which normally fight foreign invaders, against self structures.

It is evident that no single event can account for the full induction and progression of GVH-induced SLE-like autoimmune disease. The scenarios and mechanisms which we have discussed are all likely candidates in a cascade of reactions leading to a full manifestation of the disease.

ACKNOWLEDGMENTS

We thank Dr. T. Radaszkiewicz (Department of Pathologie, University of Vienna, Austria) for his help in characterizing the monoclonal autoantibodies. We thank Mrs. Annick Peter, Hannie Rolink-van Eis, and Denise Richterich for able technical assistance and Nicole Schoepflin for typing the manuscript.

The Basel Institute for Immunology was founded and is supported by F. Hoffmann-La Roche Ltd., Basel, Switzerland.

REFERENCES

1.   Rolink AG, Pals ST, Gleichmann E: Allosuppressor and allohelper T cells in acute and chronic graft-vs.-host disease. II. F_1 recipients carrying mutations of H-2K and/or I-A. J Exp Med 1983;157:755-768.
2.   Rolink AG and Gleichmann E: Allosuppressor and T cells in acute and chronic graft-vs.-host (GVH) disease. III. Different Lyt subsets of donor T cells induce different pathological syndromes. J Exp Med 1983;158:546-558.

3. Gleichmann E, Pals ST, Rolink AG, Radaszkiewicz T, Gleichmann H: Graft-versus-host reactions: clues to the etiopathology of a spectrum of immunological diseases. Immunol Today 1984;5:324-332.

4. Rappard-van der Veen FM, Rolink AG, Gleichmann E: Diseases caused by reactions of T lymphocytes towards incompatible structures of the major histocompatibility complex. VI. Autoantibodies characteristic of systemic lupus erythematosus induced by abnormal T-B cell cooperation across I-E. J Exp Med 1982;155:1555-1560.

5. Rolink, AG, van der Meer W, Melief GJM, Gleichmann E: Itrra-H-2 requirements for the induction of maximal positive and negative allogenic effects in vitro. Eur J Immunol 1983;13:191-201.

6. Pals ST, Gleichmann H, Gleichamnn E: Allosuppressor and allohelper T cells in acute and chronic graft-vs.-host disease. V. F_1 mice with secondary chronic GVHD contain F_1-reactive allohelper but no allosuppressor T cells. J Exp Med 1984;159:508-520.

7. Elven EH van, Rolink AG, van der Veen F, Gleichmann E: Capacity of genetically different T lymphocytes to induce lethal graft-versus-host disease correlates with their capacity to generate suppression but not with their capacity to generate anti-F_1 killer cells. A non-H-2 locus determines the inability to induce lethal graft-versus-host disease. J Exp Med 1981;153:1474-1490.

8. Rolink AG, Radaszkiewicz T, Pals ST, van der Meer WGJ, Gleichmann E: Allosuppressor- and allohelper-T cells in acute and chronic graft-versus-host disease. I. Alloreactive suppressor cells rather than killer-T cells appear to be the decisive effector cells in lethal graft-versus-host disease. J Exp Med 1982;155:1501-1520.

9. Pals ST, Radasziewicz T, Gleichmann E: Allosuppressor- and allohelper-T cells in acute and chronic graft-vs.-host disease. IV. Activation of donor allosuppressor cells is confined to acute GVHD. J Immunol 1984;132:1669-1676.

10. Gleichmann E, van Elven EH, van der Veen JPW: A systemic lupus erythematosus-like disease in mice induced by abnormal T-B cell cooperation. Preferential formation of autoantibodies characteristic of SLE. Eur Exp Med 1982;12:152-168.

11. Rolink AG, Radaszkiewicz T, Melchers F: The autoantigen binding B cell repertoires of normal and of chronically graft-versus-host diseases mice. J Exp Med 1987;165:1675-1687.

12. Rolink AG, Radaszkiewicz T, Melchers F: Monoclonal autoantibodies specific for kidney tubular brush border from mice with experimentally induced chronic graft-versus-host disease. Scan J Immunol 1988;28:29-41.

13. Rolink AG, Gleichmann H, Gleichmann E: Diseases caused by the reaction of T lymphocytes to incompatible structures of the major histocompatibility complex. VII. Immune-complex glomerulonephritis. J Immunol 1983;130:209-221.

14. Rappard-van der Veen FM van, Radaszkiewicz T, Terraneo L, Gleichmann E: Attempts at standardization of lupus-like GVHD: Inadvertant repopulation be DBA/2 spleen cells of H-2-different nonirradiated F_1 mice. J Immunol 1983;130:2693-2701.

15. Pals ST, Radaszkiewicz T, Roozendaal L, Gleichmann E: Chronic progressive polyarthritis and other symptoms of collagen vascular disease induced by GVHR. J Immunol 1985;134:1475-1482.

16. Bekkum DW van, Roodenburg J, Heidt PJ, van der Waaij D: Mitigation of secondary diseases of allogeneic mouse radiation chimeras by modification of the intestinal microflora. J Natl Cancer Inst 1975;52:401-415.

17. Korngold R, Sprent J: Lethal graft-versus-host disease after bone-marrow transplantation across minor histocompatibility barriers in mice. Prevention by removing mature T cells from marrow. J Exp Med 1978;148:1687-1699.

18. Korngold R, Sprent J: T cell subsets and graft-versus-host disease. Transplantation 1987;44:335-339.

19. Schreier MH, Tees R, Radaszkiewicz T, Rolink AG: The in vivo effects of antigen-specific and I-A restricted T cell clones. In *T Cell Clones*, edited by von Boehmer H, Haas W, Eelsevier, 1985; pp. 173-182.

20. Dailey MO, Fathman G, Butcher EC, Pillemer E, Weissman I: Abnormal migration of T lymphocyte clones. J Immunol 1982;128:2134-2136.

21. Guilbert B, Dighiero G, Avrameas S: Naturally occurring antibodies against nine common antigens in normal humans. I. Detection, isolation and characterization. J Immunol 1982;128:2779-2788.

22. Dighiero G, Lymberi P, Bazié J, Rouyre S, Butler-Browne GS, Whalen RG, Avrameas S: Murine hybridomas secreting natural monoclonal antibodies reacting with self antigens. J Immunol 1983;131:2267-2275.

23. Dighiero G, Lymberi P, Holmberg D, Lundquist I, Coutinho A, Avrameas S: High frequency of natural autoantibodies in normal newborn mice. J Immunol 1985; 134:765-773.

24. Prabhakar BS, Saeguza J, Onodera T, Notkins AB: Lymphocytes capable of making monoclonal autoantibodies that react with multiple organs are a common feature of the normal B cell repertoire. J Immunol 1984;133:2815-2820.

25. Vakil M, Kearney JF: Functional characterization of monoclonal autoanti-idiotype antibodies isolated from the early B cell repertoire. Eur J Immunol 1986; 16:1151-1160.

26. Garselli C, Taib FE, Schaff JE, Prabhakar BS, Ginsberg-Fellner F, Notkins AL: Epstein-Barr virus-transformed lymphocytes produce monoclonal autoantibodies that react with antigens in multiple organs. J Virol 1984;52:722-730.

27. Strasser A: Analysis of the repertoire of autoreactive hematopoietic cell-specific B cells in normal and graft-versus-host induced autoimmune mice. Ph.D. thesis, University of Basel, Basel, Switzerland; 1988.

28. Clark SH, Huppi K, Ruezinsky D, Staudt L, Gerhard W, Weigert M: Inter- and intraclonal diversity in the antibody response to influenza hemagglutinin. J Exp Med 1985;161:687-704.

29. Rappard-van der Veen FM, Landegent J, Kiesel U, Melief CJM, Terraneo L, Poels L, Schuler W, Gleichmann E: Further evidence against polyclonal antibody formation in mice with lupus-like graft-versus-host disease. J Immunol 1984;132: 1814-1824.

30. McCullagh PJ: The abrogation of sheep erythrocyte tolerance in rats by means of the transfer of allogeneic lymphocytes. J Exp Med 1970;132:916-922.

31. Klaus GGB, McMichael AJ: The immunological properties of haptens coupled to thymus-independent carrier molecules. II. The influence of the graft-versus-host reaction on primary antibody responses to hapten-coupled polysaccharides and proteins. Eur J Immunol 1974;4:505-515.

32. Katz DH. In *Lymphocyte Differentiation, Recognition, and Regulation*. Academic Press 1977; p. 482.

33. Golding H, Rittenberg MB: In vitro and in vivo allogenic effects: Differential modulation of B cell subpopulations. J Immunol 1982;128:1625-1630.

34. Hamilton JA, Miller JFAP: Hapten-specific tolerance: unresponsiveness in T cell-depleted populations. Eur J Immunol 1973;3:457-460.

35. Hamilton JA, Miller JFAP: Induction of a primary antihapten response in vivo by a GVHR. J Exp Med 1983;138:1009-1014.

36. Reth M, Imanishi-Kari T, Rajewsky K: Analysis of the anti-NP antibodies in C57Bl/6 mice by cell fusion. II. Characterization of idiotypes by monoclonal anti-idiotype antibodies. Eur J Immunol 1979;9:1004-1011.

37. Kabat EA, Mayer MM: Experimental Immunochemistry (2nd edition). C. C. Thomas Publisher, 1967; pp. 715-719.
38. Möller G (Ed). B cell lineages. Immunol Rev 1986;93:5-169.
39. Förster I, Gu H, Rajewsky K: Germline antibody V regions as determinants of clonal persistence and malignant growth in the B cell compartment. EMBO J 1988; in press.
40. Udhayakumar V, Goud SV, Subbarao B: Physiology of murine B lymphocytes. I. Life-spans of anti-μ and hapenated Ficoll-reactive B cells. Eur J Immunol 1988; 18:1593-1599.
41. Hayakawa K, Hardy RR, Honda M, Herzenberg LA, Steinberg AD, Herezenberg LA: Ly-1 B cells: Functionally distinct lymphocytes that secrete IgM autoantibodies. Proc Natl Acad Sci USA 1984;81:2494-2498.
42. Pals ST, Zylstra M, Radaszkiewicz T, Quint W, Cuypers HT, Schienmakers HJ, Melief CJM, Berns A, Gleichmann E: Immunologic induction of malignant lymphoma: GVHR-induced B cell lymphomas contain integrations of predominantly ecotropic murine leukemia proviruses. J Immunol 1986;136:331-339.
43. Hays EF: Graft-versus-host reactions and the viral induction of mouse lymphoma. Cancer Res 1972;32:270-275.
44. Levy JA, Datta SK, Schwartz RS: Recovery of xenotropic but not ecotropic virus during graft-versus-host reaction in mice. Clin Immunol Immunopathol 1977;7: 262-275.
45. Varet B, Cannat A, Feingold N, Wechsler J, Levy JP: Enhancement of virus-induced leukemias and sarcomas in F_1 hybrid mice inoculated with parental spleen cells. Cancer Res 1973;33:759-765.
46. Greenberger JS, Philips SM, Stephenson JR, Aaronson SA: Induction of mouse c-type virus by lipopolysaccharide. J Immunol 1975;115:317-322.
47. Armstrong MYK, Weiniger RB, Binder D, Himsel CA, Richards F: Role of endogenous murine leukemia virus in immunologically triggered lymphoreticular tumors. II. Isolation of B-tropic mink-cell focus-inducing (MCF) murine leukemia virus. Virology 1980;104:173-182.
48. Herr W, Gilbert W: Somatically acquired recombinant murine leukemia proviruses in thymic leukemias of AKR/J mice. J Virol 1983;46:70-80.
49. Van der Putten H, Quint W, van Raay J, Robanus-Maandag E, Berns A: M-MuLV-induced leukemogenesis: integration and structure of recombinant provirus in tumors. Cell 1981;24:729-740.
50. Seemayer TA, Lapp WS, Bolande RP: Thymic involution in murine graft-versus-host reaction: epithelial injury mimicking human thymic dysplasia. Am J Pathol 1977;88:119-125.
51. Lapp WS, Ghayur T, Mendes M, Seddik M, Seemayer TA: The functional and histological basis for graft-versus-host-induced immunosuppression. Immunol Rev 1985;88:107-133.
52. Marcos MAR, De La Hera A, Gaspar ML, Marquez C, Bellas C, Mampaso F, Toribio ML, Martinez C: Modification of emerging repertoires by immunosuppression in immunodeficient mice results in autoimmunity. Immunol Rev 1986;94:51-74.
53. Bird GA, Britton S, Ernberg I, Nilsson K: Characteristics of Epstein-Barr virus activation in human B lymphocytes. J Exp Med 1981;154:832-839.
54. Tosato G, Blaese MR: Epstein-Barr virus infection and immunoregulation in man. Adv Immunol 1985;37:99-149.

10

Graft-vs.-Leukemia Effect

Robert L. Truitt, Ann V. LeFever, Charles C.-Y. Shih,
Jan M. Jeske, and Tammy M. Martin
Medical College of Wisconsin
Milwaukee, Wisconsin

I. INTRODUCTION

Bone marrow transplantation has become an accepted treatment for certain leukemias that are resistant to conventional therapeutic approaches (1,2). The primary strategy of bone marrow transplantation is to use supralethal doses of drugs and radiation in the hope of curing the tumor-bearing host, followed by "rescue" of the host from therapy-induced hematopoietic failure by adoptive transfer of marrow stem cells from a normal donor. Transplanted marrow cells or their immunocompetent progeny may contribute to elimination of leukemia, but the importance of the immunologic component is widely debated (3). This chapter will focus on experimental models used to study the antileukemic or "graft-versus-leukemia" (GVL) effect of allogeneic bone marrow transplantation and its relationship to Graft-vs.-Host Disease (GVHD).

Indirect evidence in humans for an immunologic mechanism which contributes to leukemia cure after marrow transplantation is based on (a) occurrences of remission during episodes of acute GVHD (4), (b) the inverse association between GVHD and leukemia recurrence found in retrospective statistical analyses of allogeneic transplants (5-7), (c) comparison of relapse rates in recipients of marrow from monozygotic twins versus allogeneic, HLA-identical siblings (2,8), and (d) higher relapse rates following autologous marrow transplantation (2). Collectively, these observations support the hypothesis that an antileukemic or GVL effect may derive from alloreactivity that is manifested clinically as GVHD.

The possibility that allogeneic bone marrow transplantation would eliminate leukemia was first tested experimentally by Barnes et al. (9) in the late 1950s. These investigators hypothesized that when leukemia was not eliminated by pretransplant therapy, allogeneic but not syngeneic bone marrow might provide an immunologic reaction capable of eradicating residual tumor. They also recognized that such an immune reaction might "destroy" the host. Although the concept of an antileukemic or GVL effect of allogeneic marrow transplantation dates to the earliest days of transplantation research, experimental as well as clinical efforts to understand and manipulate the immulologic reaction continues to the present time. Of particular interest is whether the GVL effect is distinct from or a manifestation of GVHD.

GVHD is the major complication of clinical marrow transplantation; however, substantial progress has been made in methods to deplete mature T cells from donor marrow prior to transplantation in order to avoid GVHD (10-12). If T cells which cause GVHD also mediate or contribute to any antitumor effect, then T-cell depletion of marrow given to leukemia patients could lead to an increase in relapse rates and loss of survival benefit gained by avoiding GVHD disease. Recent reports from several transplant teams (13-16) and data from the International Bone Marrow Transplant Registry (17,18) confirm this prediction. Increased leukemia relapse following transplantation of T-cell-depleted bone marrow provides direct, but circumstantial, evidence for a contributing role of T cells to "cure" of neoplastic patients; the level of antileukemia reactivity may be modest in comparison to that provided by chemoradio-therapy (18).

We (19,20) and others (21) have shown in murine models that GVH reactivity can be successfully manipulated to obtain antileukemic and survival benefits. However, earlier studies by Bortin and colleagues (22,23) using a murine T-cell leukemia suggested that there might be a GVL effect of allogeneic bone marrow transplantation that is independent of GVHD. This conclusion was based primarily on the observation that the level of GVH reactivity caused by immunocompetent cells from various strains of mice did not always correlate with their ability to eliminate leukemia in vivo. Most notably, the GVH mortality associated with transplantation of cells from some H-2-compatible strains was comparable to that seen with H-2-incompatible cells; however, H-2-compatible cells were not able to readily eradicate leukemia from the host. GVH reactivity alone did not guarantee a curative GVL reaction, but the GVL effect was never observed in the absence of GVHD. These experimental studies are similar to the clinical observations reported by Sullivan et al. (24), who found that intentionally increasing GVHD in high-risk leukemia patients did not guarantee a beneficial GVL effect following transplantation of HLA-matched marrow. It is clear that, in addition to a better understanding of the nature of cells involved in the GVL and GVH reactions, strategies which would allow for enhancement of the GVL effect without fatal GVHD are needed.

In this chapter, we review our previous studies and present additional data on the nature of GVL effector cells following transplantation of MHC-compatible cells in mice, placing particular emphasis on their role in GVHD. The tumor model used in these studies was the acute T-cell leukemia/lymphoma which develops spontaneously in AKR (H-2^k) mice at approximately 8 months of age (25). This tumor was selected, in part, because the host's immune response to autochthonous tumor is minimal except under highly artificial experimental conditions.

II. INDUCTION OF GVL REACTIVITY BY ALLOIMMUNIZATION

In 1979, Bortin et al. (26) reported that in vivo priming of donor mice with lymphoid cells from allogeneic strains induced a population of cells that resulted in a curative GVL reaction when adoptively transferred into leukemic mice. More importantly, the GVL

Table 1 Evaluation of Immunocompetent Cells from H-2^k Donor Mice for GVL Reactivity in Leukemic AKR (H-2^k) Mice and for GVH Reactivity in Nonleukemic AKR Mice

H-2^k donor	Survival of AKR hosts given cells from H-2^k donor mice alloimmunized[a] with:						
	—	AKR(k)	CBA/J(k)	B10.BR(k)	C3H/He(k)	BALB/c(d)	C57BL/10(b)
GVL Reactivity[b]							
CBA/J	1/192 (0.5%)	44/44 (100%)	—	97/101 (96%)	74/99 (75%)	43/55 (78%)	17/23 (74%)
B10.BR	0/12 (0%)	8/8 (100%)	9/9 (100%)	—	17/23 (74%)	0/20 (0%)	1/12 (0%)
C3H/He	0/13 (0%)	9/9 (100%)	6/11 (55%)	14/17 (82%)	—	12/16 (75%)	14/15 (93%)
GVH Reactivity[c]							
CBA/J	113/158 (72%)	35/95 (37%)	11/12 (92%)	48/72 (67%)	47/50 (94%)	12/12 (100%)	12/12 (100%)
B10.BR	4/53 (8%)	3/36 (8%)	1/30 (3%)	0/18 (0%)	6/36 (17%)	2/35 (6%)	ND
C3H/He	0/13 (0%)	ND	ND	ND	ND	ND	ND

[a]Donor mice (H-2^k) received 2-6 weekly immunizations i.p. with 1×10^7 lymphoid cells from the indicated strains; the H-2 haplotype of the immunizing strain is in parentheses. Mice were used as donors 1-2 weeks after the last immunization.

[b]GVL reactivity was measured in a bioassay system described in detail elsewhere (26,30). Briefly, young, irradiated AKR hosts were given 1×10^5 leukemia cells obtained by pooling the spleens of aged AKR mice that had spontaneously developed acute T-cell leukemia/lymphoma. One day later, the leukemic AKR "primary" hosts were given spleen cells (20×10^6) or bone marrow (10×10^6) plus lymph node (10×10^6) cells i.v. from H-2^k donors to be tested. Six days later, all spleen cells from each individual AKR primary host were transferred i.p. to healthy individual AKR "secondary" hosts. The secondary hosts were observed for survival for 90 days; all deaths were due to leukemia transferred from the AKR primary hosts as confirmed in separate experiments by flow cytometric analysis. GVL reactivity of test cells is expressed as the proportion of leukemia-free AKR primary hosts as evidenced by 90-day survival of the AKR secondary hosts. Combined representative data from multiple experiments over several years are shown; additional data can be found elsewhere (26-29,51).

[c]GVH reactivity was measured in lethally irradiated (8-9 Gy) AKR hosts given 20×10^6 spleen or 10×10^6 bone marrow plus 10×10^6 lymph node cells i.v. from the H-2^k donors to be tested. GVH reactivity is expressed as the proportion of mice surviving 90 days after transplantation. Combined data from multiple experiments over several years are shown; additional data can be found elsewhere (26,51). ND = not done.

reactivity induced by alloimmunization was not accompanied by augmentation of GVH disease as measured in immunosuppressed nonleukemic mice (26). This alloimmunization-induced GVL phenomenon subsequently was demonstrated in a variety of donors that were H-2-compatible with the leukemic host (AKR mice, H-2^k) (27). Representative examples from these experiments are shown in Table 1. The level of GVL reactivity induced by alloimmunization was highly variable and was dependent on both the H-2^k strain being immunized and the strain from which the immunizing cells were obtained (27). In all cases, H-2-compatible donor cells from unimmunized mice failed to mount a significant GVL reaction. Specific immunization of the donor against host antigens (on normal or neoplastic cells) induced a curative GVL effect; however, the beneficial GVL reaction developed concurrently with an increase in GVH reactivity (Table 1). In contrast, alloimmunization did not increase GVH reactivity even in H-2-compatible donors that were strongly reactive against AKR (e.g., B10.BR) (Table 1). Exceptions occurred only in those few combinations in which cells from the immunizing strain (e.g., RF) shared significant non-H-2-alloantigens with AKR (28).

The possibility that a beneficial GVL reaction could be induced by alloimmunization of the donor prior to transplant without increasing the risk of GVHD led us to examine the immunogenetics and effector mechanisms involved in this phenomenon. The central questions examined were whether distinct (and therefore separable) GVL and GVH effector cells were involved, or whether identical cells with differing thresholds of activity mediated the reaction. As a result of these studies, we have gained significant insight into the cells that mediate a GVL reaction and their relationship to GVHD, and we have developed strategies to manipulate these immunologic reactions in favor of the leukemia-bearing host.

A. Role of Non-H-2-Encoded Antigens in Alloimmunization-Induced GVL Reactivity

The role of non-H-2-encoded antigens in the induction of GVL reactivity following allo-immunization was established through histogenetic procedures using F_1-hybrid and congenic strains of mice (27,29). Alloimmunization with lymphoid cells from H-2 mismatched congenic strains that were identical for non-H-2-encoded antigens failed to induce GVL reactivity (e.g., B10.BR anti-B10 in Table 1 and C3H/He anti-C3H.B10 and others cited in Ref. 29). Except as noted below, significant GVL reactivity was induced only when the strains differed in non-H-2-encoded alloantigens (e.g., B10.BR anti-CBA/J and C3H/He anti-B10 in Table 1). The level of GVL reactivity induced by immunizing against non-H-2 antigens was diminished if the alloimmunogen also was H-2-incompatible (29 and unpublished data).

In some mice, cells reactive against the AKR leukemia could not be induced by alloimmunization. For example, cells from CBA/J mice alloimmunized with tissues from the H-2^d strain BALB/c exerted a GVL reaction, but B10.BR mice immunized with BALB/c cells did not, even though cells from B10.BR anti-BALB/c mice had significantly stronger GVH reactivity against AKR (Table 1). Introduction of B10.BR antigens onto CBA/J (in F_1-hybrids) abolished the ability of CBA mice to mount a GVL reaction after alloimmunization with BALB/c tissues (29). Similarly, (CBA × BALB/c)F_1 mice failed to generate a GVL reaction after alloimmunization with B10.BR tissues (29) to which the parental CBA strain responded (CBA anti-B10.BR in Table 1). Both (CBA × B10.BR)F_1 and (CBA × BALB/c)F_1 hybrid mice generated a vigorous GVL response after specific immunization with AKR tissues. Thus, some combinations of donor and alloimmunogen (e.g., B10.BR anti-BALB/c) may not be disparate at a sufficient number of non-H-2-encoded antigens, shared by the alloimmunogen and target (BALB/c and AKR leukemia, respectively), to induce an effective GVL response. This suggests the existence of an "immunogenetic threshold" that is necessary for induction of a GVL response in this model.

Alloimmunization of H-2^k donor mice with cells from some strains (e.g., DBA/1, DBA/2, SJL/J) consistently induced lower levels of GVL reactivity in all donors tested (26,27). Dose-response studies (Fig. 1) showed that a "high" or "low" level of GVL reactivity after transfer of cells from these donor-immunogen combinations was directly related to the dose of cells transplanted. Increasing the dose of alloimmune spleen cells adoptively transferred from a "low" donor-immunogen combination (e.g., CBA anti-DBA/1 in Fig. 1) into leukemic AKR hosts resulted in an effective GVL reaction. Thus, there were quantitative differences in the level of response following alloimmunization.

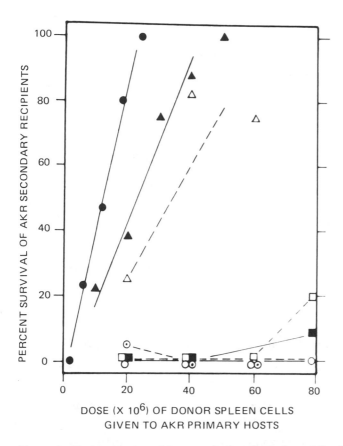

Figure 1 Dose response of donor spleen cells evaluated for GVL reactivity in vivo. Graded doses of spleen cells from unimmunized or alloimmunized H-2^k donor mice were given to irradiated, leukemic AKR primary hosts. The dose of leukemia (1 X 10^5) and the length of the GVL reaction (6 days) were kept constant. Each point represents at least seven mice (ave. = 11 mice). Spleen cell donors were ■, unimmunized CBA/J (n = 36); □, unimmunized B10.BR (n = 47); ⊙, B10.BR anti-B10.K (n = 36); ○, B10.BR anti-B10 (n = 43); △, B10.BR anti-CBA/H (n = 23); ▲, CBA/J anti-DBA/1 (n = 66); and ●, CBA/J anti-B10 (n = 75).

However, spleen cells from unimmunized donors or from mice immunized with lymphoid cells identical at non-H-2-encoded antigens failed to eliminate the leukemia at all cell doses evaluated (Fig. 1).

B. Effector Cells in the Alloimmunization-Induced GVL Reaction

We have examined the nature of the cells responsible for the GVL reaction in vivo and compared them to cytolytic cells detected in vitro (30). Spleen cells from alloimmunized CBA/J (H-2^k) mice were selectively depleted of various subpopulations by treatment with antibody and complement, then evaluated in vivo for GVL reactivity. Cell suspensions depleted of Thy 1.2, Lyt-1, or Lyt-2 lymphocytes had no significant GVL reactivity in vivo, whereas suspensions depleted of NK 1.2 cells retained a level of GVL reactivity comparable to that of untreated cells (30). The GVL-reactive cells persisted in the alloimmunized mice at least 56 days after their last immunization (30). These results suggested that the GVL reaction involved a T-cell-mediated mechanism.

Lymphocytes that lysed AKR leukemia cells in vitro could be detected in the spleens of alloimmunized mice following expansion of the cells in IL-2 (30). Negative selection experiments with monoclonal antibodies and complement revealed that the cytolytic cells were Lyt-1^+2^+ (30). Limiting dilution analysis (LDA) of cytotoxicity was used to estimate the frequency of in vitro leukemia-reactive CTL from spleens of alloimmune donors which had high, low or no GVL reactivity based on in vivo bioassays (Table 2) (28,30, and unpublished data). The results showed a direct correlation ($r^2 = 0.99$) between the frequency of leukemia-reactive CTL detected in vitro and the GVL efficacy of the cells in vivo. Furthermore, when leukemia-bearing AKR hosts were given graded doses of spleen cells from a single donor, the average number of CTL present in the host spleens correlated with the dose of CTL injected ($r^2 = 0.8$ for all doses; 0.99 for 5 to 20 X 10^6) (Table 3). Adjusting the concentration of injected cells from "low" GVL-reactive donor-immunogen combinations (such as CBA anti-DBA/1) to a level equivalent to the CTL concentration found in cell inoculums from "high" GVL-reactive combinations (such as CBA anti-B10) resulted in comparable levels of antileukemic reactivity in vivo (30). Thus, the level of GVL reactivity in vivo correlated with the magnitude of the clonal CTL response to alloimmunization of the donor. As shown in Figure 1 and Table

Table 2 Frequency of Antileukemic CTL in Spleens of Donor Mice Correlated with Level of GVL Reactivity In Vivo

		GVL reactivity[b]
Spleen cell donor	Average CTL frequency (range)[a]	N leukemia-free mice at 90 days/N mice tested (%)
Normal CBA/J	1/26,800 (13,700-56,400)	0/12 (0%)
CBA/J anti-DBA/1	1/12,800 (10,600-15,200)	3/12 (25%)
CBA/J anti-B10	1/5,500 (3,400-8,800)	10/12 (83%)

[a]Frequency of CTL against AKR leukemia cells was measured by LDA as described in (30). Average of three LDA assays is shown.

[b]See footnotes to Table 1 for details on the GVL bioassay and alloimmunization procedures. 20 X 10^6 donor spleen cells were injected into the leukemic AKR hosts.

Table 3 Number of Leukemia-Reactive CTL Present in Spleens of Leukemic AKR Hosts Given Immunocompetent Cells from an Alloimmune Donor Correlated with the Number of CTL Injected

CBA anti-B10.BR → AKR_x + Leukemia[a]					
Pretransplant			Posttransplant		
Spleen cell dose	CTL frequency	No. CTL injected	Spleen cells per mouse[b]	Average CTL frequency	Average CTL per spleen
5×10^6	1/2,290	2,183	18×10^6	1/6,700	2,687
10×10^6	1/2,290	4,367	5×10^6	1/300	16,580
20×10^6	1/2,290	8,734	7.5×10^6	1/170	43,605
40×10^6	1/2,290	17,467	11×10^6	1/220	49,500

[a]Various numbers of spleen cells from alloimmune CBA anti-B10.BR donors (pretransplant) were injected into irradiated (AKR_x) leukemic hosts. Six days later (posttransplant), the spleens of treated mice were used as responders in LDA microcytotoxicity assays to estimate the CTL frequency.

[b]Average of two mice at each dose.

2, adoptive transfer of cells from unimmunized donors, which contained only naive (precursor) CTL, did not eliminate leukemia in vivo at any of the doses evaluated.

To further identify the cells involved in alloimmunization-induced GVL reactivity we used flow cytometry to positively select Lyt-2[+] (CD8) lymphocytes from the spleens of alloimmunized donors (unpublished data). Quantitative LDA cytotoxicity assays were done before and after adoptive transfer of the cells to leukemic AKR mice. Results from one experiment are shown in Table 4. Transfer of 2×10^6 splenocytes, enriched to 80-90% for Lyt-2 expression (1,470 CTL transplanted), resulted in the apperance of cytolytic cells in the spleens of leukemic AKR hosts (CTL frequency = 1 per 2,930 spleen cells). In contrast, the spleens of mice given 5×10^6 splenocytes depleted of Lyt-2[+] cells by treatment with allele-specific antibody and complement (98 CTL transplanted) contained no detectable CTL after transplant. There was no enhanced accumulation of CTL in the spleens of mice given a mixture of Lyt-2-enriched (positive selection by FACS) and Lyt-1-enriched (negative selection with anti-Lyt-2 antibody and complement) cell populations. That is, all of the cytolytic reactivity resided in the adoptively transferred Lyt-2[+] population.

Collectively, these data indicte that Lyt-2[+] CTL from H-2-compatible donor mice immunized against non-H-2-encoded antigens play a significant role in the alloimmunization-induced GVL reaction. However, participation of other cells including radio-resistant host cells as well as natural killer (NK) cells, lymphokine-activated killer (LAK) cells or naive donor T-cells activated posttransplant cannot be ruled out. Naive cells from unimmunized H-2-compatible donors become sensitized against AKR antigens after transfer into the leukemic host (unpublished data); however, these cells cannot expand rapidly enough to eliminate the leukemia cells, thereby allowing the leukemia to gain a growth advantage. Leukemia-free survival, under these conditions, is dependent on the balance between tumor burden at the time of transplant and the rate of tumor growth in relation to the pace and magnitude of the immune response. While specific immunization against host (AKR) antigens strengthened and accelerated the pace of the immune response (and/or activated additional GVL effector mechanisms), it also increased the risk of un-

Table 4 Lytic Activity in the Alloimmune Donor Spleen Resided Exclusively in the Lyt-2$^+$ (CD8) Subset

| | | | | CBA anti-B10.BR → AKR$_x$ + Leukemia | | | |
| | Pretransplant | | | | Posttransplant | | |
Injected cells[a]	Number	CTL frequency[b]	CTL injected	Average spleen size	Average CTL frequency	Average CTL per spleen	CTL ratio[c]
Unsorted	11 × 10^6	1/1,500	7,338	4 × 10^6	1/830	4,850	1.5:1
Lyt-1	5 × 10^6	1/50,880	98	36 × 10^6	None	None	—
Lyt-2	2 × 10^6	1/1,360	1,470	1 × 10^6	1/2,930	362	4.1:1
Lyt-1 + Lyt-2	12 × 10^6	1/7,200	1,660	2 × 10^6	1/1,370	1,012	1.6:1

[a]Spleen cells from alloimmune CBA anti-B10.BR donors, passed over nylon wool, were labeled with FITC-anti-Lyt-2 antibody (Becton/Dickinson), then sorted using a FACS IV ("Lyt-2") or labeled and used without sorting ("unsorted"). "Lyt-1" indicates alloimmune spleen cells depleted of Lyt-2$^+$ cells by two treatment cycles with allele-specific anti-Lyt-2 antibody and complement; this suspension contained other cells in addition to Lyt-1 lymphocytes.

[b]At the time of transplant into irradiated leukemic hosts (AKR$_x$ + leukemia), aliquots of unsorted Lyt-1 and Lyt-2 cell suspensions were tested in LDA microcytotoxicity assays (30). The number of CTL in the mixture of Lyt-1 + Lyt-2 cells was calculated from frequencies of the individual populations. Similar LDA assays were done 6 days later using the spleens of treated, leukemic AKR mice as responders. The large number of cells in the spleens of mice given Lyt-1 cells was due to leukemia progression; all other mice were leukemia-free. Average of two mice is shown.

[c]Ratio of CTL injected to CTL recovered.

acceptable GVHD (Table 1). In contrast, alloimmunization against a limited number of host non-H-2-encoded antigens induced an effective GVL reaction without increasing GVH-related mortality.

C. Clonal Basis for the GVL Effect Induced by Alloimmunization

Using LDA techniques, we were able to show that CTL in the spleens of alloimmunized donor mice prior to transplant had heterogeneous cytotoxic specificities (30). That is, some of the CTL preferentially lysed leukemia targets while others lysed only nonleukemic AKR target cells or both leukemic and nonleukemic targets in vitro. Competitive inhibition experiments using spleen cells from alloimmune donors, expanded in the presence of alloantigenic stimulators and interleukin-2 (IL-2), revealed that the majority of CTL were H-2-restricted and specific for non-H-2 antigens shared by the AKR leukemia and alloimmunizing cells (30).

These studies were subsequently repeated using spleen cells from transplanted, leukemia-cured AKR mice as responding and effector cells (Fig. 2). Under the conditions of limiting dilution assays, the spleens of leukemic AKR mice, given cells from alloimmune CBA donors 6 days earlier, were found to contain a significant population of killer cells that lysed cultured AKR leukemia cells but not nonleukemic AKR lymphoblasts (upper left quadrant of Figure 2) in addition to cells that recognized both normal and leukemic AKR cells (upper right quandrant). Very few cells recognized the nonleukemic T-cell targets exclusively (lower right quadrant). Cells that had low, but detectable, lytic activity against nonleukemic AKR targets usually showed significant reactivity after further expansion in IL-2-conditioned medium; however, we were not successful in maintaining continuous cultures of the leukemia-"specific" cells that had no detectable lytic activity against normal AKR cells.

Additional evidence for functional heterogeneity of lytic effector cells in the spleens of leukemia-cured AKR mice was obtained from cold target inhibition studies (Fig. 3). Unlabeled ("cold") AKR leukemia cells inhibited the lytic activity of splenic effector cells taken from leukemic AKR mice given CBA anti-B10 donor cells 7 days earlier (>70% inhibition at cold:hot target cell ratios as low as 10:1). These effector cells were not cultured but used in direct CML assays against ^{51}Cr-labeled ("hot") AKR leukemia cells. Only a portion of the lytic activity could be inhibited by Con A-activated (nonleukemic) lymphoblasts of AKR, B10.BR, or B10 origin or by a mixture of AKR and B10.BR cells (Fig. 3). Although the level of lytic activity without expansion of the cells in vitro was low (10-30% in different experiments at E:T = 50:1), the pattern of cold target inhibition was consistent. This pattern was in contrast to the inhibition pattern seen when IL-2-expanded donor cells were evaluated prior to transplant, in which nonleukemic AKR and B10.BR cells inhibited all lytic activity (30). These data support the hypothesis that additional GVL effector populations are activated after transplantation.

Using allele-specific antibodies, we found (in four out of five experiments) that lytic cells in the spleens of leukemic AKR mice that had been given CBA anti-B10 alloimmune donor cells were predominantly Lyt-1$^+$2$^-$ donor cells (Table 5). In contrast, in three of three experiments, lytic cells in the spleens of mice given CBA anti-B10.BR alloimmune donor cells contained lytic cells that were predominantly Lyt-1$^+$2$^+$ (Table 5). Thus, although these alloimmune donors both manifested a significant GVL reaction in vivo (Table 1), phenotypically distinct subpopulations of lytic T cells were detected

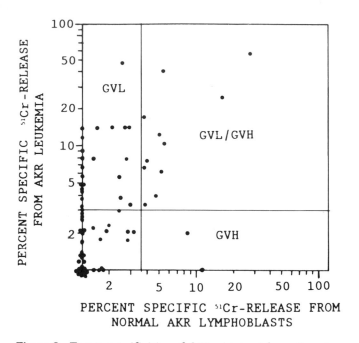

Figure 2 Target specificities of CTL obtained from the spleens of leukemia-cured AKR hosts given alloimmune H-2^k donor cells 6 days earlier. The cellular contents of individual microwells from limiting dilution cytotoxicity assays were split and evaluated simultaneously against chromium-labeled cultured AKR leukemia cells (y-axis) and nonleukemic AKR target cells (Con A-activated lymphoblasts) (x-axis). The vertical and horizontal lines delineate the levels of lysis (three standard deviations above background) considered to be positive against nonleukemic and leukemic targets, respectively. Each point represents lytic activity of cells in individual microwells with a high probability of being a clonal population based on Poisson statistics and the CTL frequency estimate. GVL and GVH refer to quadrants containing cells from individual microwells that lysed only leukemic or nonleukemic targets, respectively, or lysed both (GVL/GVH) in vitro.

in the spleens of the leukemia-cured animals. Our previous studies had consistently shown that lytic cells in the spleens of both CBA anti-B10 (30) and CBA anti-B10.BR (Table 4) donor mice were Lyt-2$^+$; Lyt-2$^-$ cells had no lytic activity prior to adoptive transfer. These results suggest the activation or recruitment of a distinct Lyt-2$^-$ killer cell population de novo in the AKR hosts after transplantation. These Lyt-2$^-$ killer cells were either Lyt-1$^+$ or they were dependent on the presence of Lyt-1$^+$ donor cells for expression of their lytic activity, even in the presence of IL-2-conditioned medium. Donor origin of the cells was confirmed by expression of the Lyt-1 allele of CBA (Lyt-1.1) and not AKR (Lyt-1.2) (Table 5). They also were susceptible to lysis with antibodies to Thy 1.2 (CBA) and resistant to anti-Thy 1.1 (AKR) (data not shown).

Collectively, the above results demonstrate the presence of multiple lytic effector cell populations. Some of these cells were specific for target antigens expressed on both leukemic and nonleukemic host (AKR) T lymphoblasts, while others appeared to be leukemia-"specific." The former appear to be antigen-specific Thy 1.2$^+$ CTL, while the

Scholtens Wristers

academische boekhandel

Guldenstraat 20
9712 CE Groningen

Vestiging AZG
Oostersingel 59
9713 EZ Groningen

Postbus 1
9700 AA Groningen
Nederland

Telefoon
(050) 13 97 88
Telefax
(050) 13 82 49

Gekocht 23/9/92

1 x   Graft - vs. - Host disease

ƒ 390,60

*) Onderdeel van Boekhandels Groep Nederland

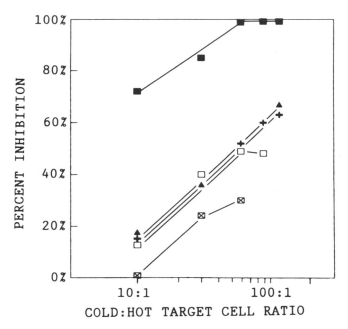

Figure 3 Cold target inhibition of lytic cells obtained from the spleens of leukemia-cured AKR mice given alloimmune CBA anti-B10.BR cells 6 days earlier. Splenic effector cells were used directly in standard chromium-release cytotoxicity assays (i.e., without culture) against a labeled AKR leukemia cell line ("hot" targets) at an E:T ratio of 50:1. Unlabeled AKR leukemia (■) or Con A-activated lymphoblasts from AKR (□), B10.BR (▲), or B10 (⊠) mice were added individually or as a 1:1 mixture of AKR and B10.BR blasts (+) as competitive inhibitors ("cold" targets) at the cold:hot target cell ratios shown along the X-axis (2,500 "hot" leukemia targets/well). Data are presented as percent inhibition of specific lysis in the presence of unlabeled, syngeneic CBA lymphoblasts added at similar ratios (ave. = 10.2% lysis at a 50:1 E:T ratio).

Table 5 Phenotypically Distinct Lytic Cells Found in Leukemic AKR Hosts After Transplantation of Spleen Cells from H-2-Matched CBA/J Donors Alloimmunized with Cells from Either B10($H\text{-}2^b$) or B10.BR($H\text{-}2^k$) Mice

Cell treatment	Cell recovery (specific lysis)[a]	CTL frequency[b]	CTL per 1×10^6 cells treated[b]	Percent specific reduction[c]
CBA anti-B10 → AKR$_x$ + Leukemia				
None	42% (−)	1/2,010	209	−
C′ Only	41% (−)	1/1,625	252	−
anti-Lyt 1.1 + C′	14% (66%)	1/40,180	3	−99%
anti-Lyt 2.1 + C′	42% (0%)	1/1,530	275	+ 9%
CBA anti-B10.BR → AKR$_x$ + Leukemia				
None	55% (−)	1/870	632	−
C′ Only	28% (−)	1/480	583	−
anti-Lyt 1.1 + C′	5% (82%)	1/2,390	21	−96%
anti-Lyt 2.1 + C′	28% (0%)	1/2,870	98	−83%

[a]Spleen cells from irradiated leukemic AKR (Lyt-1.2) hosts (AKR$_x$ + leukemia) given alloimmune CBA/J (Lyt-1.1) donor cells 6-7 days earlier were treated with allele-specific antibodies plus complement (C′), C′ only or used untreated. Specific lysis was calculated in comparison to cells treated with C′ only. Data from two of six experiments are shown.

[b]Treated or untreated spleen cells were evaluated for lytic activity against cultured AKR leukemia cells in limiting dilution assays. The frequency of CTL per 1×10^6 cells treated was calculated using the formula: (cell recovery) × (CTL frequency) × (1×10^6).

[c]Reduction in CTL was calculated using the formula: $100 \times$ (CTL per 10^6 cells treated with C′ only− CTL per 10^6 cells treated with antibody plus C′)/(CTL per 10^6 cells treated with C′ only).

latter are Thy 1.2^+, Lyt-2^- LAK-like killer cells activated de novo after transplantation. Activation of the Lyt-2^- killer cells is dependent on the presence of antigen primed Lyt-2^+ donor T cells, since depletion of Lyt-2^+ cells abrogated the GVL reaction (30 and Table 4).

In the remainder of this chapter we will describe the results of our recent studies evaluating GVL/GVH reactions mediated by antigen-specific CTL that were cloned from the spleens of alloimmunized donor mice and by lymphokine-activated killer (LAK) cells.

III. CLONAL ANALYSIS OF GVL EFFECTOR CELLS AND THEIR RELATIONSHIP TO GVHD

Cloned CTL, specific for non-H-2-encoded histocompatibility antigens present on both leukemic and nonleukemic AKR cells, were derived according to the method of Glasebrook et al. (31) from a variety of effector cell sources, including fresh or MLC-expanded spleen cells from alloimmunized mice and from leukemia-cured AKR mice previously transplanted with alloimmune spleen cells for immunotherapy. Most of the lytic cells were found to be specific for non-H-2-encoded antigens present on both leukemic and nonleukemic AKR lymphoblasts; some recognized class I molecules encoded in the T1a/

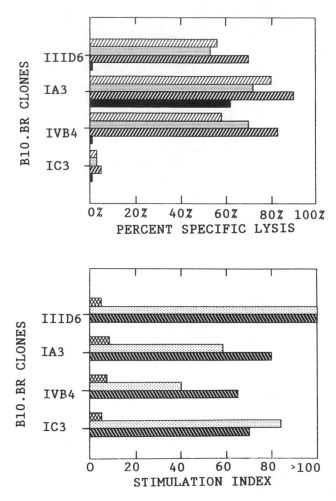

Figure 4 Upper panel—Lytic activity of T-cell clones derived from alloimmune B10.BR anti-CBA mice and grown in IL-2-conditioned medium. Standard chromium release cytotoxicity assays were done at E:T ratios of approximately 5:1. Target cells were AKR-Leukemia (▨) and EL-4 (■) tumor cell lines or Con A-activated nonleukemic lymphoblasts from AKR/J (▦) and CBA/J (▨) mice. Lower panel—Proliferation of the same B10.BR-derived T-cell clones 48 hr after stimulation with alloantigen (irradiated CBA cells) (▦), IL-2 (▦), or both antigen and IL-2 (▨). Proliferation data are presented as stimulation indices calculated by dividing the CPM of ^{3}H-thymidine incorporation in the presence of CBA_x and/or IL-2 by the CPM of ^{3}H-thymidine incorporation in medium alone (ave. background = 100 CPM). All values are significantly higher than background.

Qa region. Shown in Figure 4 are examples of alloactivated clones derived from the high GVH-reactive B10.BR (H-2^k) strain. Preliminary characterization of these cells involved measuring their lytic activity against both cultured AKR (H-2^k) leukemia cells and an H-2-disparate cultured leukemia (EL4, H-2^b) (upper panel, Fig. 4). EL4 targets were included in order to detect H-2-unrestricted CTL specific for T1a/Qa-encoded antigens (31,52). After an initial screening, the CTL clones which lysed AKR leukemia were tested against Con A-activated lymphoblasts from AKR as well as from the relevant mouse strain (alloimmunogen) used to induce the alloreactive clones (e.g., against CBA/J lymphoblasts when B10.BR anti-CBA mice were used). Clones with lytic activity were expanded in culture and tested for antigen-driven proliferation in the presence or absence of exogenous IL-2 (lower panel, Fig. 4). All of the B10.BR-derived clones, shown in Figure 4, proliferated extensively in response to IL-2-conditioned medium with or without alloantigen present. They had a low, but statistically significant, proliferative response to alloantigen in the absence of exogenous IL-2 (range in stimulation indices was 5.0 to 8.5). The nonlytic T-cell clone IC3 is included in Figure 4 for comparison.

A. GVH Reactivity of Cloned CTL That Lyse AKR Leukemia In Vitro

We sought to determine whether B10.BR-derived CTL clones that lysed AKR leukemia in vitro (Figure 4) caused (or contributed to) GVHD (Table 6). GVHD was assessed in irradiated AKR hosts (young, nonleukemic mice) given bone marrow syngenic to the clone followed by one to three i.v. or i.p. injections of the T-cell clone to be evaluated. The donor bone marrow was not depleted of T cells prior to transplant. Among the B10.BR(H-2^k)-derived clones used were a Qa-1-specific CTL (IA3), two minor histocompatibility antigen(miHA)-specific CTLs (IVB4 and IIID6) and a nonlytic, antigen-specific clone (IC3). All of these clones exhibited weak antigen-driven proliferation (lower panel, Fig. 4). The precise miHA recognized by these CTL clones is not known, but in studies not shown here, we found that the target antigen was encoded outside the MHC, was H-2-restricted, and was expressed on both normal and leukemic AKR cells (50).

B10.BR-derived clones showed significant variation in their effects on marrow transplanted nonleukemic AKR hosts (Table 6). Clone IA3 (anti-Qa-1) caused marked weight loss (up to 41% below that of the BM controls) after two i.v. injections, and all mice were dead by day 28. The clinical appearance of the mice was similar to that seen in mice undergoing a polyclonal GVH reaction characterized by diarrhea, ruffled and dull fur, hunching, dyspnea, and a general wasted appearance with loss of body weight. Using LDA microcytotoxicity assays, we found a high frequency of cytolytic cells (one per 250 mononuclear cells recovered) on day 13 in the lungs of a mouse given clone IA3 i.v. (unpublished data). The wasting syndrome was less intense when IA3 cells were given i.p. Two of six mice given IA3 cells i.p. survived beyond 35 days (Table 6), and their clinical appearance improved after the first 2 weeks.

The miHA-specific B10.BR clone IVB4 also produced a distinctive GVH-like clinical pattern when injected in vivo. A single injection of relatively low numbers of IVB4 cells (less than 4×10^6) i.v. caused only minimal changes in the body weight and clinical appearance of marrow-transplanted mice; however, injection of large numbers of IVB4 cells (12×10^6 or greater) i.v. resulted in death within 48-96 hours (data not shown). Histologic examination of the lungs revealed a marked lymphocyte infiltration as compared to normal lungs; however, the alveoli were not obstructed (A. V. LeFever, unpublished data). Early mortality in AKR mice given a large dose of IVB4 cells was antigen-specific since injection of the same cells into irradiated C57BL/10 (H-2^b) mice, which lacked the appropriate target antigen, had no effect. As shown in Table 6, multiple

Table 6 Effect of B10.BR T-Cell Clones on Survival and Body Weight of B10.BR → AKR Allogeneic Bone Marrow Chimeras

Clone	Dose ×10⁶	Day given	Route	Days 10-13			Days 17-20			Days 32-35			Days 60-63		
				N alive/ N injected	Avg. b. wt.	% change	N alive	Avg. b. wt.	% change	N alive	Avg. b. wt.	% change	N alive	Avg. b. wt.	% change
IA3	4,4	0,4	i.v.	3/5	17.0	-31%	3	15.8	-41%	0	—	—	—	—	—
IA3	8	0	i.p.	3/6	20.9	-15%	2	24.8	- 7%	2	19.7	-21%	1	23.1	-10%
IVB4	4,4,4	0,4,7	i.v.	5/5	21.7	-12%	5	19.4	-27%	5	15.7	-37%	0	—	—
IVB4	8,8,8	0,4,7	i.p.	4/5	20.9	-15%	4	23.5	-12%	4	22.6	-10%	4	21.3	-17%
IIID6	4,4,1	0,4,7	i.v.	5/5	25.5	+ 3%	5	26.7	0%	5	25.0	0%	5	27.1	+ 5%
IIID6	8,8	0,4	i.p.	5/5	24.3	- 2%	5	26.8	0%	5	24.6	- 2%	5	26.3	+ 2%
IC3	8,4	0,4	i.v.	5/5	23.5	- 4%	5	25.0	- 6%	5	23.9	- 4%	5	25.3	- 2%
IC3	16,8	0,4	i.p.	4/4	25.4	+ 3%	4	27.1	+ 1%	4	24.1	- 4%	2[b]	27.8	+ 8%
None (BM only)			—	14/14	24.6	—	14	26.7	—	14	25.0	—	14	25.8	—
None (TBR only)			—	6/12	23.9	- 3%	0	—	—	—	—	—	—	—	—
None (Age-matched AKR mice)			—	10	30.2	+23%	10	29.9	+12%	ND[c]	—	—	ND	—	—

[a]Irradiated AKR mice (9 Gy) were given 1×10^7 B10.BR bone marrow (BM) i.v. alone or followed by B10.BR clones in the doses indicated on the days shown. AKR mice given total body radiation (TBR) only, as well as untreated age-matched AKR mice, are shown for comparison. Percent change in body weight (b. wt.) was calculated relative to mice given BM only for each time point.

[b]Two mice were sacrificed between 35 and 53 days.

[c]ND = not determined.

injections of clone IVB4 i.v. at lower cell doses (three injections totaling 12×10^6 cells) resulted in chronic weight loss and eventual death; the first death occurred after 48 days, and all mice were dead by day 59. In contrast, immunosuppressed, marrow-transplanted AKR mice given IVB4 cells i.p. (total of 24×10^6 cells) sustained their body weight for two months, although at a level 10-17% below that of mice given B10.BR marrow alone (Table 6). The clinical manifestations of this clonal GVH-like disease was moderate in comparison with clone IA3.

In contrast to mice given IA3 or IVB4 cells, mice given the miHA-specific cyto-toxic clone IIID6 or the nonlytic clone IC3 showed no adverse effects. Their clinical appearance was not different from that of the bone marrow controls (i.e., sleek, nonruf-fled fur, normal levels of activity, and no diarrhea) and average body weights were within ±8% of the control group.

The presence of injected cytolytic cells in the lungs and peritoneal cavity of mice given cloned IVB4 or IIID6 cells i.v. or i.p. 2 weeks earlier was confirmed in LDA micro-cytotoxicity assays (Fig. 5). The frequency of cytolytic cells correlated with the severity of the clonal GVH-like syndrome and weight loss in the marrow-transplanted AKR mice (i.e., IVB4 > IIID6 > none). Lytic activity in the spleens of mice injected i.p. with clone IVB4 was very low, but cytotoxic cells could be detected after brief expansion in IL-2 (data not shown). Mice given B10.BR marrow alone had minimal numbers of CTL in

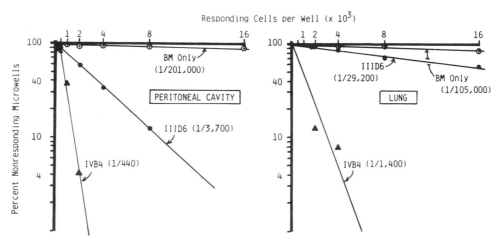

Figure 5   Recovery of cytolytic T-cell clones from B10.BR → AKR allogeneic bone marrow chimeras. Irradiated AKR hosts were given B10.BR bone marrow i.v. alone or followed by i.p. or i.v. injection of B10.BR-derived cytolytic T-cell clones (IVB4 and IIID6). Details on the injection schedule and doses can be found in Table 6. Thirteen days after marrow transplantation the peritoneal cavity of mice given cloned cells i.p. was lavaged, and the lungs of mice given cloned cells i.v. were collected and processed as described elsewhere (32). Recovered cells were used as responders in limiting dilution microcytotoxicity assays with irradiated AKR cells as stimulators; chromium-labeled AKR lymphoblasts were used as target cells. The values in parentheses are the frequencies of cytolytic cells recovered from the peritoneal cavity of i.p. injected mice (left panel) or the lungs of i.v. injected mice (right panel).

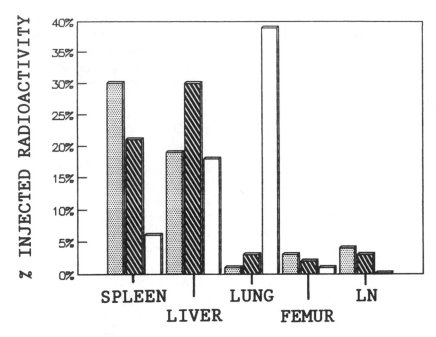

Figure 6 Distribution of cytolytic effector cell populations injected i.v. into irradiated allogeneic recipients. Irradiated (9 Gy) AKR mice were injected with chromium-labeled cells obtained from the spleens of unimmunized B10.BR mice (uncultured cells) (▨), with LAK cells generated by culture of C57BL/6 spleen cells in recombinant IL-2 for 72 hrs (▨), or with a B10.BR-derived T-cell clone (IC3) (▭). Data are presented as the mean percentage of total injected radioactivity (corrected for isotope decay) present in the indicated tissues at 24 hr after injection.

the tissues examined (less than one CTL per 100,000 cells) (Fig. 6). Thus, most (or all) of the lytic activity in mice given cloned cells was derived from the injected CTL clones.

Studies on the migration in vivo of parenterally (i.v.) injected T-cell clones showed that they did not localize in the spleen as well as "fresh" uncultured T cells (Fig. 6). This abnormal migration pattern appeared to increase in proportion to their length of time in culture and was independent of the tissue source of the T cells (i.e., spleen or lymph node) (33,34). The propensity of cultured or cloned T cells to localize in the lungs following i.v. injection may account for some of the immunopathologic effects seen (33). Abnormal migration also poses a significant technical problem in the design of experiments to evaluate antileukemic reactivity of CTL clones grown in vitro, because the effector cells must encounter the tumor cells in order to kill them by a direct cell mediated lytic mechanism. The paucity of cells in the spleen, femur, and lymph nodes are of particular concern.

In summary, the data described here (Table 6) and elsewhere (31) demonstrate that some CTL clones mediate a lethal GVH-like syndrome (e.g., miHA-specific IVB4 and Qa-1-specific IA3) while other clones with putatively similar target specificities did not (e.g., IIID6 and WRL-A3). To date, we have not identified a functional characteristic which distinguishes CTL clones that cause GVH-like disease from those that do not, although the clones with GVH reactivity tend to have slightly higher antigen-driven proliferation, suggesting that persistence and/or expansion in vivo may contribute to the degree of GVH-like damage. Further study with additional clones is needed to confirm this association and to identify lymphokines that might be produced by the GVL/GVH-reactive clones. The latter point is of particular importance since there is evidence that lymphokines, such as tumor necrosis factor, may act as mediators of GVH-associated immunopathology (other chapters in this volume). Cytolytic activity may not be the sole or most important functional property of cells contributing to GVHD.

B. GVL Reactivity of CTL Clones that Recognize Host Antigens

The data presented in the previous section show that the severity of antihost (GVH) reactivity can be manipulated on a clonal level by altering the dose and route of CTL clone injection and/or by selection of target antigen specificity and functional properties of the clones used. Thus, it seemed possible to "titrate" a clonal GVH reaction in an attempt to obtain a beneficial GVL effect. In this section, we describe the results of our attempts to do this using two CTL clones. WRL-A3 was an H-2-unrestricted CTL clone specific for Qa-1^b, a class I MHC-molecule encoded in the T1a/Qa region on mouse chromosome 17 (31). Qa-1^b is present on both normal and leukemic AKR lymphoblasts, but not all host tissues. IVB4 was an H-2D^k-restricted CTL clone that recognized an unidentified miHA present on both normal and leukemic T-cells of AKR mice (Fig. 5). Both of these clones were derived from B10.BR anti-CBA mice and were Thy 1$^+$ and Lyt-2$^+$.

A modification of the bioassay system described in Table 1 was used in the initial studies to assess the GVL reactivity of CTL clones in vivo without concern for engraftment or GVH-associated mortality (31). The antileukemic reaction was allowed to proceed for only 3-4 days, then to determine the level of leukemia remaining in the "primary" AKR hosts, the spleen and lung tissues from each animal were separately transferred i.p. into individual "secondary" AKR recipients. Lung tissues were examined in addition to the spleens because migration studies showed that significant numbers of cultured CTL accumulate within the lung but not the spleen (33,34, and Fig. 6). Antileukemic reactivity of CTL clones in vivo can be assessed more accurately in lung tissues than in the spleen; however, elimination of leukemia from the spleen is a better indicator of systemic "cure." The concentration of cultured CTL found in the spleen is influenced by the dose of cells injected i.v. (31) and by the length of time in culture (34).

Using the modified GVL bioassay, we found that both IVB4 and WRL-A3 cells significantly reduced, but did not eliminate, leukemia from the lungs and spleens of AKR hosts within 3-4 days (Table 7). Failure of CTL clones to completely eradicate leukemia from host tissues was attributed to their altered migration in vivo (Fig. 6) and the consequent paucity of effector cells in target tissues (e.g., the spleen) rather than loss of viability or functional capability (31). Despite such technical limitations, these results demonstrate on a clonal level that miHA and Qa-1 specific CTL can mediate an antileukemic reaction in vivo.

We next sought to determine whether a clonal GVH-like reaction could be manipulated in leukemia-bearing hosts to obtain a therapeutic GVL effect within the context of an allogeneic bone marrow transplant. Immunosuppressed leukemic AKR mice were given B10.BR bone marrow cells alone or followed by i.v. and i.p. injection of increasing doses of the miHA-specific CTL clone IVB4 (Table 8) (20). B10.BR marrow alone failed to prevent leukemia progression; all mice were dead within 15 days. Leukemic AKR hosts given the highest dose of IVB4 CTL (total = 18 × 10^6) developed an acute GVH-like

Table 7 Reactivity of miHA- and Qa-1-Specific CTL Clones Against AKR Leukemia as Measured In Vivo Using a Bioassay System[a]

CTL effector	Bioassay tissue	N mice cured/ N mice transplanted	MST (days) (range of deaths)
None	Lungs	0/12 (0%)	33 (18–48)
	Spleen	0/13 (0%)	34 (20-67)
IVB4[b] (anti-miHA)	Lungs	3/5 (60%)	>90* (36,38)
	Spleen	3/5 (60%)	> 90* (39,57)
WRL-A3[c] (anti-Qa-1)	Lungs	17/18 (94%)	>90* (72)
	Spleen	3/18 (17%)	58* (24-86)

[a]Lung and spleen cell suspensions were transferred from irradiated leukemic AKR hosts (see Table 1) to healthy AKR secondary recipients 3-4 days after injection of the CTL effector clones shown. The primary AKR hosts were considered "cured" of leukemia in the tissues examined if no leukemia developed in the secondary host within 90 days. * = Significant ($p < 0.05$) increase in median survival time (MST). Data adapted from (50).

[b]10×10^6 IVB4 cells were injected i.v. on days 0 and 2.

[c]5×10^6 WRL-A3 cells were injected i.v. on day 0.

wasting syndrome. All of these mice died within 9 days (MST = 5.5 days), having lost approximately one-third of their body weight. The mice were severely lymphopenic with no clinically evident leukemia. Stepwise reductions in the total dose of IVB4 cells resulted in decreased GVH reactivity as measured by loss of body weight after one week. Mice given the lowest dose of IVB4 cells (total = 3×10^6) showed virtually no body weight loss relative to the marrow controls; however, in the absence of a clinically evident clonal GVH reaction, these mice relapsed and died within the same time frame as control mice given B10.BR marrow only. Intermediate doses of IVB4 cells (6 to 12×10^6 total cells) caused mild to moderate GVH disease (23% body weight loss and only one death in the first 10 days). Mice in these two groups had a 117% increase in expected life span (in comparison to mice given marrow alone), although they ultimately succumbed to leukemia progression. Based on the results of in vivo bioassays (Table 7) and migration studies (Fig. 6) noted earlier, failure to completely eradicate leukemia in these mice was attributed to the inability to achieve an adequate concentration of effector cells in lymphoid tissues. Although not curative, the results in Table 8 demonstrated that it was possible to manipulate the GVH reaction at a clonal level in order to obtain a GVL effect. Conversely, they also showed that under certain experimental conditions a single miHA-specific CTL clone, which can eliminate leukemia cells in vivo, was capable of causing lethal GVH disease.

C. GVL Reactivity of Lymphokine-Activated Killer Cells

CTL that recognize virus-associated cell surface antigen on highly immunogenic tumors in an antigen-specific manner have been described in various tumor models (e.g., 35-38). It is unlikely that such cells were responsible for the alloimmunization-induced GVL reaction described here, since the GVL reaction occurred within a short time (6 days) using cells from donors that had not been immunized with retrovirus-associated antigens. It is more likely that the leukemia-"specific" effector cells detected in the spleens of trans-

Table 8 Titration of Clonal GVH Reactivity Against a Minor Histocompatibility Antigen in an Attempt to Obtain a Therapeutic GVL Effect[a]

Clone cell dose (route)	Day 3			Day 7			Median survival time (days)	% ILS[c]
	N alive/ N treated	Ave. body wt.[b]	% change	N alive/ N treated	Ave. body wt.[b]	% change		
6 × 10^6 (i.v.)	3/4	21.9	−12%	1/4	17.0	−31%	5.5	−54%
12 × 10^6 (i.p.) / 4 × 10^6 (i.v.)	8/8	20.6	−17%	7/8	18.9	−23%	26.0	+117%
8 × 10^6 (i.p.) / 2 × 10^6 (i.v.)	4/4	22.5	− 9%	4/4	22.4	− 9%	26.0	+117%
4 × 10^6 (i.p.) / 1 × 10^6 (i.v.)	3/3	24.3	− 2%	3/3	23.8	− 3%	11.5	− 2%
2 × 10^6 (i.p.)								
None (BM only)	6/6	24.8	−	6/6	24.6	−	12.0	−

[a] Lethally irradiated (9 Gy) AKR mice were given 1×10^5 leukemia cells obtained from the spleens of AKR mice with advanced, spontaneous T-cell leukemia/lymphoma. One day later, 10×10^6 bone marrow (BM) cells from B10.BR donor mice were given alone or together with B10.BR-derived miHA-specific CTL (clone IVB4) at the doses and routes indicated. Preliminary data reported in (20).

[b] Surviving mice were weighed at 3 and 7 days after transplantation. Average body weight in grams and percent change relative to leukemic mice given BM only are shown.

[c] % ILS = percent increase in (median) life span relative to leukemic mice given B10.BR BM only.

planted mice (Fig. 2) are MHC-unrestricted lymphokine-activated killer (LAK) cells induced in the host. LAK cells are distinct from antigen-specific CTL in that they recognize cell surface molecules present on most, if not all tumors, i.e., they exhibit broad tumor specificity (39). In the mouse, LAK cell activity is generally attributed to cells with the phenotype Thy 1^+, $CD8^-$ (Lyt-2), $CD4^-$ (L3T4), and asialo GM_1^+, but variations have been reported (39).

Recent studies in our laboratory revealed that asialo GM_1^+ cells were essential to the GVL reaction following transplantation of spleen cells from alloimmunized donors (unpublished data). While pretreatment of an alloimmune donor (CBA anti-B10.BR) with antibody to the asialo GM_1 glycolipid in vivo did not affect the GVL reaction, treatment of the AKR host with anti-asialo GM_1 antibody posttransplant completely abrogated the GVL effect. However, if asialo GM_1^+ LAK cells are involved in the GVL reaction, they are dependent on activation of antigen-specific donor T cells for their activity. This conclusion is based on our results showing (a) that $Lyt-1^+2^+$ donor T cells also were essential to the GVL reaction (30 and Table 4), (b) that immunization with non-H-2-encoded alloantigens was required (27,29), and (c) that some of the lytic effectors detected before and after transplantation were antigen-specific (30 and Figs. 2 and 3). Because asialo GM_1 is not expressed exclusively on LAK cells, but also on activated T cells (40,41), it is not possible to conclude from our present data whether the GVL-reactive asialo GM_1^+ cells represent LAK cells, T cells, or both.

To determine whether LAK cells could mediate a therapeutic GVL effect in vivo, we induced LAK activity by culturing spleen cells in recombinant IL-2 (rIL-2) and used the activated cells in a therapeutic model in combination with total body radiation (TBR) and allogeneic bone marrow transplantation (Fig. 7). The LAK cells were activ-

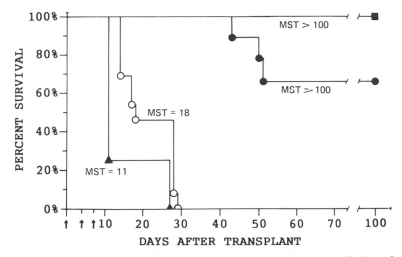

Figure 7 LAK cells activated in vitro mediated a therapeutically beneficial GVL reaction in vivo following allogeneic bone marrow transplantation. Leukemic AKR mice were given 9 Gy TBR followed 4 hr later by i.v. injection of H-2-compatible CBA/J bone marrow (1×10^7). Mice were given CBA marrow alone (○, $N = 13$) or followed by three injections i.v. of either CBA LAK cells (●, $N = 9$) (total of 1.1×10^8 cells) or spleen cells from alloimmunized CBA anti-B10.BR donors (■, $N = 10$) (total of 2.2×10^7 cells) on days 0, 4, and 7 (→). Control mice (▲, $N = 4$) were given leukemia only (no TBR, no transplant).

ated by culture of unprimed CBA spleen cells in rIL-2 (200 U/ml) for 72 hours. Lytic activity of the cells was measured at the time of transplant in standard CML assays using "NK-sensitive" YAC-1 tumor cells and "NK-resistant" AKR leukemia cells as targets (data not shown). Both of these targets are sensitive to LAK-mediated killing. All leukemia-bearing AKR mice that received CBA bone marrow alone died with progressive leukemia within 30 days (MST = 18 days) (Fig. 7). Repeated injection of LAK cells (without exogenous rIL-2) successfully eliminated leukemia in 67% of the host animals. Mice that died appeared to be clinically free of leukemia, but the actual cause of death was not determined. Shown for comparison as a "positive control" in Figure 7 is the survival curve for leukemic AKR mice that were given repeated injections of spleen cells from alloimmunized H-2-matched donors (CBA anti-B10.BR); all mice in this group survived leukemia-free to the end of the experiment. These results document that LAK cells activated in vitro exert an antileukemia effect in vivo. Under the experimental conditions used, this reaction was curative.

It should be noted that in vitro culture of murine splenocytes in rIL-2 for a short time (72 hr) did not significantly alter their in vivo migration patterns from that of uncultured spleen cells (Fig. 6). Thus, abnormal migration in vivo was not as much of a problem in experimental models of LAK effector cells (Fig. 7) as it was with CTL clones cultured for extended periods of time (e.g., clone IVB4 in Table 8). Nevertheless, our results using bioassay models demonstrate that a sufficient number of LAK cells must be present to eliminate leukemia from all host organs. In this experiment we achieved that goal by giving repeated injections of LAK cells without administering rIL-2. Current studies in our laboratory seek to determine the synergistic effect of rIL-2 and LAK cells given to leukemic hosts in the context of allogeneic or syngeneic bone marrow transplantation.

In our initial experiments (unpublished) we have not seen acute GVH mortality when allogeneic LAK cells or rIL-2 were given separately to irradiated hosts along with allogeneic H-2-matched bone marrow. These studies need to be repeated and extended before definitive conclusions about the use of LAK cells and/or rIL-2 for adoptive immunotherapy can be made. Other investigators have implicated NK/LAK cells in the pathologic manifestations of GVHD (42-44); however, activation of the NK/LAK cells may be dependent on the presence of alloreactive donor T cells and may not be causally related to GVHD. It is not yet clear whether lytic activity or lymphokine production is more important to the immunopathology of GVHD in such models.

IV. DISCUSSION AND CONCLUSIONS

In this chapter we have presented experimental evidence to indicate that GVL and GVH reactions in vivo can be mediated by distinct as well as identical cell populations. Figure 8 presents a conceptual diagram of the relationship between different lytic populations that contribute to the GVL reaction in vivo and T-cell population(s) that causes GVHD. Some GVL effector cells are antigen-specific CTL that recognize target antigens present on both normal host tissues and the leukemia (effectors A and B in Fig. 8). The target antigen(s) for these CTL may be expressed on all host tissues in addition to leukemia cells (effector A), or they may be present on all leukemia cells but restricted to only some normal tissues (for example, lymphoid/hematopoietic lineage cells as targets for effector B). Among the CTL clones described in this chapter, IVB4 and IIID6 could be considered typical of the former, while WRL-A3 and IA3 are representative of the latter. Other GVL effector cells may recognize target molecules that are unique to the leukemia cells

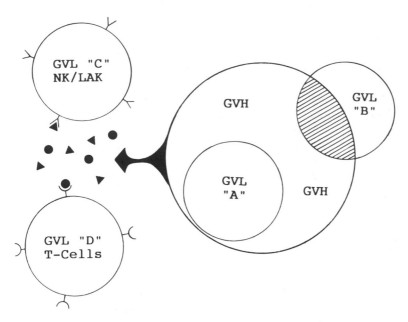

Figure 8 Conceptual diagram of the relationship between T cells that cause GVHD and effector subpopulations that mediate GVL reactivity ("A" thru "D") in vivo. GVH reactive cells may act directly (via lytic mechanisms) or indirectly (via secretion of various lymphokines, ●▲). GVL effector cells consist of subpopulations that are distinct from ("C" and "D") as well as included among ("A" and "B") cells that cause GVH disease. Some GVL/GVH effector cells have preferential GVL reactivity in vivo ("B"), even though they recognize a molecule present on normal host tissues.

through an MHC-unrestricted NK/LAK-type killing mechanism (effector C) or through an MHC-restricted antigen-specific T-cell mechanism (effector D).

We hypothesize that alloimmunization acts by selective activation of some or all of the GVL effector cells shown in Figure 8. Whether a therapeutic GVL reaction after alloimmunization occurs in the presence or absence of a lethal GVH reaction appears to depend on the number and nature of antihost (anti-AKR) reactive T-cell clones that are activated. Activation of a limited number of T-cell clones in experimental models by selective immunization with host alloantigens may be sufficient to induce a GVL reaction acting directly via CTL and/or indirectly via NK/LAK cells; however, if large numbers of T-cell clones specific or host tissues are activated, the GVL effect is associated with extensive organ damage. Although we have focused on lytic effector cells in this chapter, our hypothesis does not preclude a role for lymphokine secreting nonlytic (or lytic) T cells in either GVL or GVH reactivity.

On a clonal level we found great disparity in the ability of cytotoxic T-cell clones to cause or contribute to GVHD. For example, CTL clones IA3 (Fig. 4 and Table 6) and WRL-A3 (31) both recognized a class I molecule encoded in the Qa-region, yet they had markedly different patterns of GVH reactivity (severe vs. none, respectively) when given to susceptible hosts. Similarly, miHA-specific CTL clones IIID6 and IVB4 differed in their ability to cause GVHD in irradiated, marrow-transplanted AKR hosts, even though they had similar patterns of lytic and proliferative activity in vitro. The more severe reactivity of clone IVB4 may correspond to persistence and expansion of the clone in vivo as evidenced by higher CTL frequencies detected in LDA assays (Fig. 5). Tissue damage associated with the accumulation of cultured CTL in certain essential organs, especially the lungs and liver (Fig. 6), may account for some of the pathology observed. Involvement of naive T cells contained in the donor bone marrow or recruitment of other cell types also must be considered. Although our data show that some CTL clones specific for minor as well as class I (Qa-1) histocompatibility antigens can cause a lethal GVH-like syndrome, cytotoxicity alone is not sufficient. Our data does not allow any definitive conclusion regarding which functional property of a T-cell clone is requisite or sufficient to cause GVHD, although lymphokine production would seem to be the most likely candidate at present. Some cytotoxic T cells may alter their lytic activity in vivo under the influence of lymphokines. We have described class II antigen-specific T cells that up- and downregulate their lytic activity in the absence and presence of IL-2, respectively (53). These unique CTL were isolated from the spleens of H-2-incompatible allogeneic bone marrow chimeras (19). They suppressed GVH reactivity in vivo when in a nonlytic state (54); however, they reacted against host tissues and caused GVH-like disease when lytic (C. C.-Y. Shih, unpublished data).

suggest that lytic effector cells similar to those described here develop after allogeneic bone marrow transplantation in humans. Hercend and colleagues (45,46) have described activated NK cells that lyse autologous (patient's) leukemia in the peripheral blood following transplantation of T-cell-depleted allogeneic marrow. They suggest that activated NK (or LAK) cells might exert a direct antileukemia effect in vivo.

Van Rood et al. (47) have described CTL in the peripheral blood of allogeneic marrow recipients that are specific for class I molecules encoded telomeric to HLA-A on human choromosome 6. They suggest that these CTL play a role in chronic GVHD and might contribute to the decreased rate of leukemia relapse seen in marrow transplant patients who developed chronic GVHD. Another di-allelic locus, TCA, has been described by the same investigators (48). These genes code for differentiation markers expressed on leukemias and other malignancies and are examples of normal antigens that can mimic "leukemia-associated" antigens by virtue of their differential expression. CTL against these molecules may be similar to the murine Qa-1 specific clones described here (e.g., IA3 and WRL-A3). In the context of an allogeneic bone marrow transplant, these class I molecules may serve as preferential targets for GVL/GVH reactions in some, but not all donor-host combinations.

HLA-restricted CTL specific for miHA have been detected after allogeneic bone marrow transplantation in humans (49), but their precise role in the etiology of human GVHD has not been established. T-cell depletion of human bone marrow decreases the risk of developing GVHD (10-12). Although this could be attributed, in part, to the decreased generation of alloreactive cytotoxic T cells that recognize miHA, depletion of lymphokine-secreting T cells is likely to be of equal or greater importance. Exhaustive T-cell depletion of allogeneic marrow may remove T cells that are acting as direct effectors of a GVL reaction or acting indirectly through the activation and/or expansion of other cells (e.g., NK/LAK) or through facilitation of engraftment.

In conclusion, the complexity of the GVH syndrome that follows allogeneic bone marrow transplantation makes the task of successfully manipulating GVH-reactive cells to obtain a desired GVL effect extremely difficult. On an experimental level, we have demonstrated the existence of multiple GVL effector cells and examined strategies to take advantage of individual effector populations. With advances in T-cell-depletion procedures, availability of monoclonal antibodies and recombinant lymphokines, and increased understanding of various effector populations and mechanisms, successful clinical strategies also should be forthcoming. Even if we cannot predictably manipulate GVL/GVH reactive cells, we may still be able to use their effector molecules or lymphokines.

ACKNOWLEDGMENTS

This work was supported by grants no. CA-39854 and AI-22312 from the U.S. Public Health Service, by the Midwest Athletes Against Childhood Cancer Fund (Milwaukee), the American Cancer Society's Summer Student Oncology Clerkship, and the Cancer Center of the Medical College of Wisconsin. RLT was a recipient of Special Fellow and Scholar awards from the Leukemia Society of America, Inc. We are deeply indebeted to Mortimer M. Bortin for his help in starting and encouragement in pursuing these investigations.

REFERENCES

1. Bortin, MM, Rimm AA: Increasing utilization of bone marrow transplantation. Transplantation 1986;42:229-234.
2. Champlin RE, Gale RP: Role of bone marrow transplantation in the treatment of hematologic malignancies and solid tumors: Critical review of syngeneic autologous, and allogeneic transplants. Cancer Treat Repts 1984;69:145-161.
3. Gale RP, Champlin R: How does bone marrow transplantation cure leukaemia? Lancet 1984;2:28-30.
4. Odom LF, August CS, Githens JH, et al: Remission of relapsed leukaemia during a graft-versus-host reaction: A "graft-versus leukaemia reaction" in man? Lancet 1978;2:537-540.
5. Weiden PL, Fluornoy N, Thomas ED, et al.: Antileukemic effect of graft-versus-host disease in human recipients of allogeneic-marrow grafts. N Engl J Med 1979; 300:1068-1073.
6. Weiden PL, Sullivan KM, Fluornoy N, et al.: Antileukemic effect of chronic graft-versus-host disease: Contribution to improved survival after allogenic marrow transplantation. N Engl J Med 1981;304:1529-1533.
7. Weiden PL, Fluornoy N, Sanders JE, Sullivan KM, Thomas ED: Antileukemic effect of graft-versus-host disease contributes to improved survival after allogeneic marrow transplantation. Transplantation 1981;13:248-251.
8. Fefer A, Cheever MA, Thomas ED, et al.: Bone marrow transplantation for refractory acute leukemia in 34 patients with an identical twin. Blood 1981;57:421-430.
9. Barnes DWH, Corp MJ, Neal FE: Treatment of murine leukaemia with X rays and homologous bone marrow. British Med J 1956;2:626-627.
10. Prentice HG, Blacklock HA, Janossy G, et al.: Depletion of T-lymphocytes in donor marrow prevents significant graft-vs-host disease in matched allogeneic leukemic marrow transplant recipients. Lancet 1984;1:472-476.
11. Filipovich AH, Vallera DA, Youle RJ, et al.: Ex-vivo treatment of donor bone marrow with anti-T-cell immunotoxins for prevention of graft-versus-host disease. Lancet 1984;1:469-472.
12. Waldman H, Or R, Hale G, et al.: Elimination of graft-versus-host disease by in vitro depletion of alloreactive lymphocytes using a monoclonal rat anti-human lymphocyte antibody (Campath-1). Lancet 1984;2:483-486.

13. Mitsuyasu RT, Champlin RE, Gale RP, et al.: Treatment of donor bone marrow with monoclonal anti-T-cell antibody and complement for the prevention of graft-versus-host disease: A prospective, randomized, double-blind trial. Annals Int Med 1986;105:20-26.

14. Apperley JF, Jones L, Hale G, et al.: Bone marrow transplantation for patients with chronic myeloid leukaemia: T-cell depletion with Campath-1 reduces the incidence of graft-versus-host disease but may increase the risk of leukaemic relapse. Bone Marrow Transpl 1986;1:53-66.

15. Goldman JM, Gale RP, Horowitz MM, et al.: Bone marrow transplantation for chronic myelogenous leukemia in chronic phase: Increased risk for relapse associated with T-cell depletion. Annals Int Med 1988;108:806-814.

16. Truitt RL, Ash RC: Manipulation of T-cell content in transplanted human bone marrow: Effect on GVH and GVL reactions. In *Cellular Immunotherapy of Cancer*, edited by Truitt RL, Gale RP, Bortin MM. Alan R Liss, New York, 1987; pp. 409-421.

17. Horowitz MM, Gale RP, Sondel PM, et al.: Graft-versus-leukemia reactions following bone marrow transplantation in humans. Blood 1990;Feb., in press.

18. Butturini A, Bortin MM, Gale RP: Graft-versus-leukemia following bone marrow transplantation. Bone Marrow Transpl 1987;2:233-242.

19. Truitt RL, Shih C-Y, LeFever AV: Manipulation of graft-versus-host disease for a graft-versus-leukemia effect after allogeneic bone marrow transplantation in AKR mice with spontaneous leukemia/lymphoma. Transplantation 1986;41:301-310.

20. Truitt RL, LeFever AV, Shih C-Y: Graft-versus-leukemia reactions: Experimental models and clinical trials, In *Progress in Bone Marrow Transplantation*, edited by Gale RP, Champlin RE. Alan R Liss, New York, 1987;pp. 219-232.

21. Meredith RF, OKunewick JP: Possibility of graft-vs-leukemia determinants independent of the major histocompatibility complex in allogeneic marrow transplantation. Transplatation 1983;35:378-385.

22. Bortin MM, Truitt RL, Rimm AA: Nonspecific adoptive immunotherapy of T cell acute lymphoblastic leukemia in AKR Mice: A model for the treatment of T cell leukemia in man, In *The Handbook of Cancer Immunology*, Vol. 5,*Immunotherapy*, edited by Waters H. Garland STPM Press, New York, 1978; pp. 403-429.

23. Bortin MM: Graft versus leukemia, In *Clinical Immunobiology*, Vol. 2, edited by Bach FH, Good RA. Academic Press, New York, 1974; pp. 287-306.

24. Sullivan KM, Storb R, Buckner CD, et al.: Graft-versus-host disease as adoptive immunotherapy in patients with advanced hematologic neoplasms. N Eng J Med 1989;320:828-834.

25. Bortin MM, Truitt RL: AKR T cell acute lymphoblastic leukemia: A model for human T cell leukemia. Biomedicine 1977;26:309-311.

26. Bortin MM, Truitt RL, Rimm AA, Bach FH: Graft-versus-leukaemia reactivity induced by alloimmunisation without augmentation of graft-versus-host reactivity. Nature 1979;281:490-491.

27. Truitt RL, Shih C-Y, Rimm AA, et al.: Alloimmunization of H-2-compatible donors for adoptive immunotherapy of leukemia: Role of H-2, Mls, and non-H-2 antigens, In *The Potential Role of T Cells in Cancer Therapy*, edited by Fefer A, Goldstein A. Raven Press, New York, 1982;pp. 21-30.

28. Truitt RL, Shih C-Y, Kaehler DA, et al.: Graft-versus-leukemia and graft-versus-host reactivity following alloimmunization of MHC-compatible donor mice, In *Recent Advances in Bone Marrow Transplantation*, edited by Gale RP. Alan R. Liss, New York, 1983;pp. 243-253.

29. Bortin MM, Truitt RL, Shih C-Y, et al.: Alloimmunization for induction of graft-

versus-leukemia reactivity in H-2-compatibile donors: Critical role for incompatibility of donor and alloimmunizing strains at non-H-2 loci. Transpl Proc 1983; 15:2114-2117.

30. Truitt RL, Shih C-Y, LeFever AV, et al.: Characterization of alloimmunization-induced T lymphocytes reactive against AKR leukemia in vitro and correlation with graft-vs-leukemia activity in vivo. J Immunol 1983;131:2050-2058.

31. Glasebrook AL, Sarmiento M, Loken MR, et al.: Murine T lymphocyte clones with distinct immunological functions. Immunol Rev 1981;54:225-266.

32. LeFever AV, Truitt RL, Shih C-Y: Reactivity of in vitro expanded alloimmune cytotoxic T lymphocytes and Qa-1 specific cytotoxic T lymphocytes against AKR leukemia in vivo. Transplantation 1985;40:531-537.

33. LeFever AV, Truitt RL, Shih C-Y, et al.: Migration patterns and functional activity of cloned cytotoxic T lymphocytes in syngeneic and allogeneic mice. Transplantation 1984;37:410-417.

34. LeFever AV, Truitt RL: Migration of cytotoxic effector cells, In *Cellular Immunotherapy of Cancer*, edited by Truitt RL, Gale RP, Bortin MM. Alan R. Liss, New York, 1987; pp. 313-324.

35. Cheever MA, Greenberg PD, Fefer A: Specific adoptive therapy of established leukemia with syngeneic lymphocytes sequentially immunized in vivo and in vitro and nonspecifically expanded by culture with interleukin-2. J Immunol 1981;126: 1318-1322.

36. Dailey MO, Pillemer E, Weissman IL: Protection against syngeneic lymphoma by a long-lived cytotoxic T-cell clone. Proc Natl Acad Sci USA 1982;79:5384-5387.

37. Green WR: The in vitro generation of H-2-restricted cytotoxic T cells to AKR/ Gross leukemia virus-induced tumors. I. Requirement for stimulation with allogeneic leukemia cells in vivo. J Immunol 1982;128:1043-1049.

38. Weiss A, Brunner KT, MacDonald HR, Cerotini J-C: Antigenic specificity of the cytolytic T lymphocyte response to murine sarcoma virus-induced tumors. III. Characterization of cytolytic T lymphocyte clones specific for Moloney leukemia virus-associated cell surface antigens. J Exp Med 1980;152:1210-1225.

39. Herberman RB, Hiserodt J, Vujanovic N, et al.: Lymphokine-activated killer cell activity: characteristics of effector cells and their progenitors in blood and spleen. Immunol Today 1987;8:178-181.

40. Stout RD, Schwarting GA, Suttles J: Evidence that expression of asialo-GM_1 may be associated with cell activation: Correlation of asialo-GM_1 expression with increased total cellular RNA and protein content in normal thymocyte and spleen cell populations. J Immunol 1987;139:2123-2129.

41. Ting C-C, Hargrove ME, Wunderlich J, Loh N-N: Differential expression of asialo-GM_1 on alloreactive cytotoxic T lymphocytes and lymphokine-activated killer cells. Cell Immunol 1987;104:115-125.

42. Ghayur T, Seemayer TA, Lapp WS: Kinetics of natural killer cell cytotoxicity during the graft-versus-host reaction. Transplantation 1987;44:254-260.

43. Ghayur T, Seemayer TA, Kongshavn AL, Gartner JG, Lapp WS: Graft-versus-host reactions in the beige mouse: An investigation of the role of host and donor natural killer cells in the pathogenesis of graft-versus-host disease. Transplantation 1987;44:261-266.

44. Charley MR, Mikhael A, Bennett M, Gilliam JN, Sontheimer RD: Prevention of lethal, minor-determinate graft-vs-host disease in mice by in vivo administration of anti-asialo GM_1. J Immunol 1983;131:2101-2103.

45. Hercend T, Takvorian T, Nowill A, et al.: Characterization of natural killer cells with antileukemia activity following allogeneic bone marrow transplantation. Blood 1986;67:722-728.

46. Delmon L. Ythier P, Moingeon P, et al.: Characterization of antileukemia cells' cytotoxic effector function: Implications for monitoring natural killer responses following allogeneic bone marrow transplantation. Transplantation 1986;42:252–256.

47. van Rood JJ, Goulmy E, van Leeuwen A: The immunogenetics of chronic graft versus host disease and its relevance to the graft versus leukemia effect, In *Cellular Immunotherapy of Cancer*, edited by Truitt RL, Gale RP, Bortin MM. Alan R. Liss, New York, 1987;pp. 433–438.

48. van Leeuwen A, Schrier PI, Giphart MJ, et al.: TCA: A polymorphic genetic marker in leukemias and melanoma cell lines. Blood 1986;67:1139–1142.

49. Goulmy E, Blokland E, Pool J, et al.: Correlation between cytotoxic T-cell responses and graft-versus-host disease. Bone Marrow Transpl 1986;1(Sup. 1):138.

50. Truitt RL, LeFever AV, Shih C-Y: Analysis of effector cells in the graft-versus-leukemia reaction and their relation to graft-versus-host disease, In *T-cell Depletion in Allogeneic Bone Marrow Transplantation*, edited by Martelli MF, Grignani F, Reisner Y. Ares-Serono Symposia, Rome, 1988; pp. 73–85.

51. Shih C-Y, Truitt RL, Bortin MM: Genetic and cellular aspects of alloimmunization-induced graft-versus-leukemia reactivity, In *B and T Cell Tumors*, edited by Vitetta E, Fox CF. Academic Press, New York, 1982; pp. 493–497.

52. Jenkins RN, Aldrich CJ, Landolfi NF, Rich RR: Correlation of Qa-1 determinants defined by antisera and by cytotoxic T lymphocytes. Immunogenetics 1985;21:215–225.

53. Shih CC-Y, Truitt RL: Down-regulation of L3T4$^+$ cytotoxic T-lymphocytes by interleukin-2. Science 1987;238:344–347.

54. Shih CC-Y, Truitt RL: Prophylaxis of graft-vs-host disease by adoptive transfer of a class II antigen-specific murine T-cell clone. In *Cellular Immunotherapy of Cancer*, edited by Truitt RL, Gale RP, Bortin MM. Alan R. Liss, New York, 1987; pp. 439–447.

11

Intestinal Graft-vs.-Host Reaction

Allan McI. Mowat and Michelle V. Felstein*
Western Infirmary, University of Glasgow
Glasgow, Scotland

I. INTRODUCTION

Early studies of graft-vs.-host reaction (GVHR) quickly identified intestinal damage as an important component of host disease (1). Most animals with severe GVHR developed diarrhea, and this feature has remained one of the characteristic signs of Graft-vs.-Host Disease (GVHD), both in man and in experimental animals. Nevertheless, the exact mechanisms responsible for intestinal damage have not yet been fully elucidated. Indeed, it can be argued that the intestinal pathology itself has not been detailed adequately, and intestinal GVHR remains much more poorly understood than many of the other complications of GVHD. There are several possible reasons for this. First, many studies have not discriminated between intestinal alterations that represent true consequences of GVHR and those that are artefacts of the particular experimental system under study. As a result, there has been no generally acceptable set of indices that can be used as specific measures of the local disease. Second, the fact that the nature of the intestinal pathology is highly dependent on the model used has not been fully appreciated. Furthermore, the mucosal features vary markedly with time, even within a single experimental model, and it is unwise to extrapolate from the intestinal changes found in the dying (or even dead) animals studied by many authors. Finally, it should be remembered that the intestine is not only the largest lymphoid tissue in the body, but, as part of the mucosal immune system, it represents a distinct component of the host immune response. Therefore, measurements of systemic immune responsiveness in animals with GVHR may not reflect events within the intestine and the immuno-pathogenesis of intestinal GVHR can only be investigated accurately at the local level.

Present affiliation: Clinical Research Centre, Harrow, Middlesex, England

This chapter will review the intestinal pathology that characterizes GVHD in experimental animals in the light of the issues raised above. By detailing the sequence of pathological events, we will provide evidence that certain aspects of mucosal pathology are particularly characteristic of intestinal GVHR and can be used to measure the local immune response. This system will then provide the basis for our discussion of the mechanisms responsible for the intestinal damage in experimental GVHR.

II. THE INTESTINE AND ITS IMMUNE SYSTEM

A. Epithelial Pathophysiology

The gut-associated lymphoid tissues (GALT) are not only the largest immune compartment in the body, but also contain populations of lymphoid cells whose origin and function are distinct from cells in other tissues (for reviews see Refs. 2-4). Furthermore, this enormous population is in intimate contact with a specialized epithelial layer whose function is essential for the survival of the animal (Fig. 1). Both the epithelial and lymphoid cells in the gut are constantly changing, and it follows that local immune responses can produce rapid and profound changes in intestinal structure and function (Fig. 2). In this section, we will review aspects of intestinal immunology and physiology which are important for a clear understanding of enteropathy in GVHR. As virtually all studies of experimental GVHR have examined only the small intestine, we shall confine our attention to this part of the gut.

The principal function of the small intestine is the digestion and absorption of food material. These activities are performed by a wide range of enzymes found principally on the microvilli, which comprise the "brush border" on the luminal surface of columnar enterocytes. Any form of insult that compromises the production and function of these cells will inevitably have profound consequences for the well-being of the host. The functional unit of the small intestine is the villus (Figs. 1 and 2), which comprises a cylinder consisting of sheets of enterocytes. The profusion of these finger-like processes greatly increases the surface area of epithelial cells available for digestive functions. Atrophy or disruption of this villus architecture is an important cause of intestinal failure. As we shall describe, GVHR is one of the most potent means of producing this type of intestinal pathology.

The enterocytes that form the villus move upwards in continuous sheets from their origin in the crypts of Lieberkuhn, where a self-renewing population of stem cells normally balances loss of effete enterocytes from the villus tip (Figs. 1 and 2). In the steady state in normal animals, around 10 new cells are produced in each crypt per hour, and the migration of enterocytes from the crypt to the villus tip takes 2-3 days. However, when epithelial cell damage or increased cell loss occurs, both the production of new cells by the crypts and their subsequent migration can be rapidly and dramatically increased. In this way, secondary alterations in epithelial cell renewal form the principal means of repairing damage to mature enterocytes. In addition, certain stimuli can have direct effects on crypt cell turnover. These repair mechanisms probably evolved as a means of eliminating parasites that have attached to the epithelium, we shall see that similar effects also occur in GVHD.

Villus atrophy frequently occurs in association with these alterations in crypt cell kinetics, but increased production of new epithelial cells can itself interfere with intestinal function. When enterocytes leave the crypts, they are immature, with no microvilli

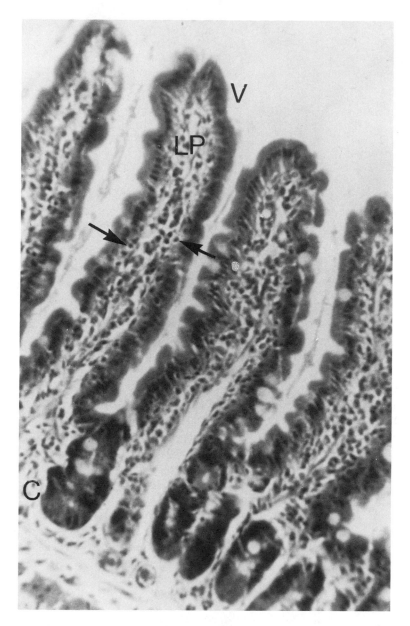

Figure 1 The appearance of the normal small intestine. The villus (V) is clothed by a layer of columnar epithelial cells which arise from dividing cells in the crypts (C). The lamina propria (LP) is separated from the epithelium by a basement membrane and contains a wide variety of lymphoid cells. Intraepitheial lymphocytes (arrows) are found between the epithelial cells (H and E ×500).

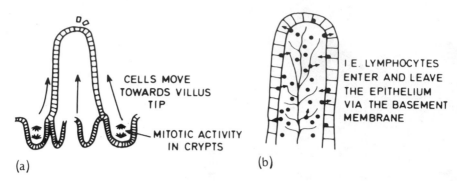

Figure 2 The villus/crypt unit as a dynamic structure showing cell movements in the intestinal epithelium: (a) epithelial cells and (b) lymphocytes. Enterocyte loss from the villus tip is normally balanced by continual upward movement of new cells produced in the crypts. Lymphocytes move constantly in and out of the epithelium.

and poorly developed enzymes. However, as the cells enter the villus compartment they differentiate rapidly and acquire the normal ability to digest and absorb foods. Conditions that enhance crypt cell turnover or enterocyte migration result in the appearance of a large number of recently derived, immature cells on the part of the villus normally covered by mature cells. As a result, there is an effective decrease in absorptive surface area.

The features discussed above illustrate how pathogenic insults can alter intestinal function either by direct damage to villus enterocytes or by interfering with the dynamic balance between epithelial cell renewal and differentiation. One further potential means of causing intestinal damage is to disrupt the tissues that underly the epithelium. The three-dimensional structure of the villus is highly dependent on the integrity of its basement membrane and associated ground substance. In addition, these mesenchymal structures play an important role in maintaining epithelial function. Thus, inflammatory insults which harm these elements are likely to have profound effects on epithelial behavior. Finally, the epithelium is invested closely by a complex network of blood vessels, as well as autonomic and peptidergic nerves, and the normal function of these elements is essential for intestinal integrity.

B. Mucosal Lymphoid Cells

The preceding section has highlighted the dynamic relationships between different epithelial and stromal components involved in maintaining the health of the intestine. To this must be added the effects of the large numbers of lymphoid cells found within the mucosa.

The most cursory microscopic examination reveals that the lamina propria which underlies the epithelium contains a wide variety of lymphoid and myeloid cells (Fig. 1). Many of these cell types are identical to those found in peripheral lymphoid tissues, with macrophages, eosinophils, and basophils particularly well represented in the mucosa. In addition, there are numerous B lymphocytes, T lymphocytes, plasma cells, and mast cells, but many of these appear to be distinct from their peripheral counterparts. The predominance of IgA-producing B cells in the intestine is well known, and up to 90% of plasma cells within the mucosa are committed to IgA synthesis (5). These cells are also derived from a distinct population of precursors within the GALT.

Mucosal T cells may also form a discrete population of lymphocytes and are found within two separate compartments. Those in the lamina propria have a $CD4^+:CD8^+$ ratio of 2:1 and are generally believed to contain a large number of functional helper T cells (3,4). Interestingly, lamina propria T cells congregate close to the crypts and are thus in an ideal position to modulate crypt cell behavior. The intestinal epithelium also contains a large population of T cells, which is particularly relevant to the present chapter. Fifteen to twenty percent of cells in the epithelium are lymphocytes. This is not only the single largest population of lymphocytes in the immune system, but intraepithelial lymphocytes (IEL) have many unusual characteristics which suggest they may be unique. Virtually all IEL are $CD3^+$, but up to 80% are $CD8^+$ and there are <10% $CD4^+$ T cells. Around 50% of $CD8^+$ IEL do not express pan T cell markers, such as CD5 in man or Thy 1 in mice, and approximately 2/3 contain cytoplasmic granules (6). There are no B cells, plasma cells, or macrophages within the epithelium, thus emphasizing how different this population is from the T cells found in the adjacent lamina propria. IEL lie between epithelial cells on the basement membrane and appear to move rapidly in and out of this compartment (Fig. 3). Their close proximity to the enterocytes suggests that IEL should play an important role in the pathogenesis of epithelial damage. Although this is supported by the increased number of IEL in immunologically based disorders such as celiac disease and GVHR (see below), their functions remain to be clarified. IEL can be persuaded to show cytotoxic T-lymphocyte (CTL) activity and secrete lymphokines in

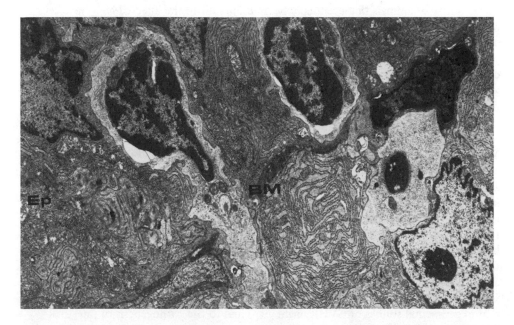

Figure 3 Electron-microscopic appearance of two intraepithelial lymphocytes, one of which is crossing into the epithelium through the basement membrane (BM) ($\times 16,000$) (E_p epithelial cell nucleus).

vitro, but these activities are weak (7-10), and IEL from most species do not respond to mitogens (11,12). The recent reports that IEL contain a large number of T cells confirms the unusual nature of this population but does not clarify their function (13).

Mucosal mast cells (MMC) are a further population of intestinal effector cells which differ from the equivalent cells in the periphery and which are important in GVHR. MMC occur predominantly in the lamina propria and differ from classical connective tissue mast cells in staining pattern, chemical content, and response to mast cell activators (14,15). They contain little or no histamine and secrete a serine protease (mast cell protease II) which is antigenically different from that found in peripheral mast cells (16). The differentiation and function of MMC are highly dependent on T lymphocytes, and MMC hyperplasia is a characteristic feature of cell mediated responses to intestinal parasite infections (14,17). Their exact role in other intestinal immune responses remains to be clarified.

In these sections, we have attempted to show how the intestinal mucosa may react to inflammatory stimuli and have highlighted the distinct populations of immune effector cells which are in close contact with the epithelial elements of the gut. The ways in which these interactions can produce intestinal pathology in GVHR will be an important focus of later sections.

III. INTESTINAL GVHR IN EXPERIMENTAL ANIMALS

A. Occurrence

The earliest descriptions of GVHR in animals come from the classical experiments on neonatal tolerance to allogeneic cells performed by Medawar and his colleagues (1,18). The majority of animals that eventually became tolerant to the injected allogeneic cells went through a characteristic runting syndrome, which was often fatal and was associated with skin disease, severe weight loss, and wasting. This runting disease was also accompanied by diarrhea, and it appeared that intestinal damage was an important cause of the clinical deterioration. Subsequent studies which began to define the basis of this "graft-vs.-host" disease also noted the presence of diarrhea (19), and since then this sign has provided one of the most important indicators of both clinical and experimental GVHD.

Intestinal disease has been described in all species in which GVHR has been examined, and there seems to be little evidence of interspecies differences in susceptibility. Most information on this condition pertains to mouse and man, and in this review we will concentrate on studies performed in rodent models, particularly those in mice. Where appropriate, we will highlight points which we consider of relevance to clinical GVHD in man, but it should be noted that the intestinal pathophysiology of rodents may not necessarily reproduce that of man. Humans are large, long-lived omnivores whose intestine has evolved different strategies from those employed by the essentially vegetarian laboratory rodent. As a result, there are important differences in intestinal flora and in the structure of both the intestinal epithelium and its associated lymphoid tissues. It is also difficult to reproduce exactly the characteristic syndromes of acute and chronic GVHD found in man. Nevertheless, with these reservations in mind, we hope to show that experimental studies of GVHR might give clues to the pathogenesis of intestinal GVHR under clinical conditions. Furthermore, we will attempt to illustrate how intestinal GVHR in experimenal animals provides a useful model of other enteropathies associated with local cell mediated immune (CMI) responses.

B. Clinical Features of Intestinal GVHR

Intestinal GVHR offers a potentially very useful means of examining mechanisms of intestinal dysfunction in immunologically mediated enteropathy. As noted above, diarrhea is the cardinal sign of intestinal GVHR and is seen in most animals with severe disease. Several mechanisms may account for this feature (Table 1). First, damage to enterocytes produces deficiency of several of the epithelial cell enzymes required for absorption of sugars (20,21). The resulting increased amounts of intact sugar left undigested in the lumen lead to osmotic water loss. Second, the damaged small intestine has a large number of immature or abnormal enterocytes (see below), and this may lead to decreased reabsorption of ions and water by the epithelium. This has not been examined directly in GVHR, but such cholera-like effects have been observed in IgE-mediated intestinal damage (22) and can be responsible for considerable water loss. Colonic damage in GVHR could also potentially interfere with normal water absorption mechanism but has not been studied in detail. Finally, the damaged epithelium may become hyperpermeable to serum and tissue proteins, with a concomitant loss of water. A protein-losing enteropathy of this type is evidenced by low serum proteins and increased intestinal loss of intravenously injected ^{51}Cr in mice with severe GVHR (23). There is also increased fecal loss of the serum protein α_1-antitrypsin in human GVHD (24), and irradiated mice with acute GVHR have increased loss of the tracer material ^{125}I-PVP from serum (25).

The profound metabolic consequences of the diarrheal loss of fluid, ions, and protein are complicated by the malabsorption of all essential nutrients. This is caused partly by the deficiencies in epithelial cell enzymes and by the loss of mature, absorptive surface area due to villus atrophy. A final harmful effect of GVHR on intestinal function is to increase the permeability of the epithelium to materials within the lumen. Increased uptake of large, orally administered molecules such as proteins and sugars is a nonspecific consequence of several forms of intestinal inflammation, including GVHR (26; Strobel, S., personal communication). Animals with GVHR also have evidence of increased serum levels of endotoxin, presumably derived from intestinal bacteria (27). Together, the diarrhea, malabsorption, and altered intestinal permeability are major causes of morbidity and mortality in GVHR.

C. Distribution of Intestinal Pathology

The studies reviewed elsewhere in this volume show that human GVHD can affect the entire gastrointestinal tract, sparing few sites from the mouth to the rectum and causing

---

Table 1 Possible Mechanisms for Diarrhea in Intestinal GVHR

Small intestine:

Disaccharidase deficiency in epithelium due to enterocyte damage → ↑ luminal sugars + ↑ osmotic water loss

Increased proportion of immature enterocytes → enzyme deficiency + abnormal water transport

Protein + water exudation through hyperpermeable epithelium

Large intestine:

Damage to colonic enterocytes → ↓ water reabsorption

---

lesions in several of the associated exocrine glands, including the pancreas and salivary glands. Unfortunately, there is little information of this kind from studies of experimental GVHR. The colon and ileum appear to be the worst affected areas of the bowel in acute GVHD in man (28), and one early study reported that the ileum was the most seriously damaged site in neonatal mice with acute GVHR (29). Although this was not confirmed by a subsequent report of GVHR in adult, unirradiated mice (23), increased susceptibility of the ileum and large bowel would be consistent with the greater bacterial load in these tissues and with the apparently deleterious effect of bacteria on the pathogenesis of GVHD (see below). Colonic disease has also been reported in severely affected mice (23), but its incidence in other models of GVHR is unclear. Similarly, the scleroderma-like lesions found in the esophagus and tongue in one study of rats undergoing a chronic form of GVHR across minor histocompatibility differences have not been examined subsequently (30). As there are no other reports of the distribution of intestinal GVHR in experimental animals, it remains uncertain if the pathology in these models is as widespread as that in human GVHD. Nevertheless, it seems reasonable to conclude that the apparent restriction of experimental GVHR to the small intestine reflects the interests of the relevant workers and the relative accessibility of the various parts of the gut in the different species, rather than true differences in pathogenesis. In this review, we shall concentrate on small intestinal damage, but as small bowel GVHR seems to provide a useful model for immune mediated damage to this organ, there is clearly a case for more detailed examination of intestinal GVHR in other sites.

IV. NATURE OF THE INTESTINAL PATHOLOGY

A. Epithelial Damage

Initial studies of homologous disease in mice noted severe intestinal inflammation, with macroscopic ulceration of the ileum and colon associated with focal degeneration of the crypts (18,31). Later, more detailed studies found intestinal dilatation and bloody exudates during acute GVHR in mice. These changes were accompanied by severe villus atrophy, crypt necrosis, and increased extrusion of necrotic cells from the villus tip (23, 29,32,33). Most research on human GVHD has also emphasized this destructive pattern of intestinal damage, and it is widely assumed that the pathology is simply due to a direct cytotoxic attack on mature, villus enterocytes. That this is not the case is demonstrated by studies which have examined the evolution of intestinal damage during GVHR models

---

Table 2 Pathological Features of Intestinal GVHR in Experimental Animals

Early:

      Increased crypt cell mitotic activity
      Crypt lengthening (± villus lengthening)
      Increased counts of intraepithelial lymphocytes, MMC

Late:

      Villus atrophy
      Continued crypt hyperplasia → ↑ crypt cell turnover
      Crypt cell necrosis (stem cell apoptosis)
      Loss of mucosal lymphoid cells

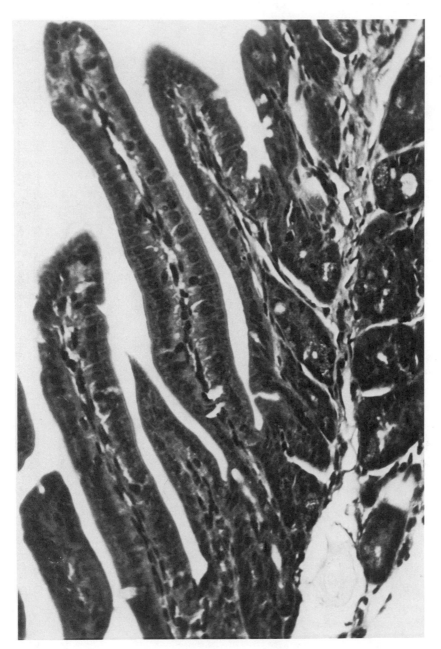

Figure 4 Proliferative enteropathy in murine graft-versus-host reaction. There is crypt lengthening and increased numbers of mucosal lymphoid cells, but no villus atrophy or enterocyte damage (HPE ×320).

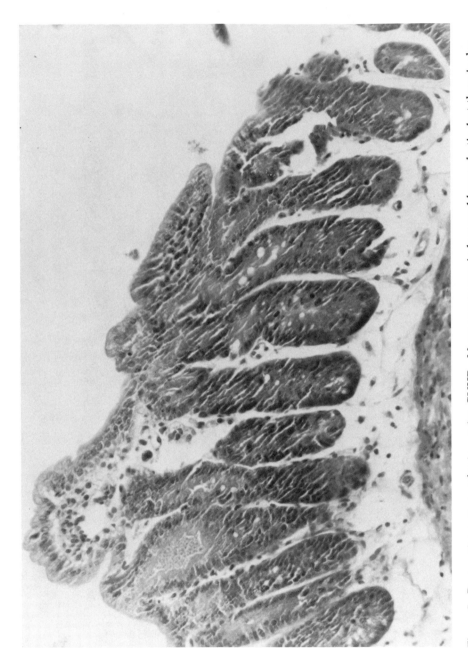

Figure 5   Destructive enteropathy in murine GVHR. Many crypts remain long and hyperplastic, but there is also necrosis of individual enterocytes and severe villus atrophy. The mucosa is devoid of lymphoid cells (HPE X320).

of varying intensity. We will attempt to show here that there are two distinct phases of enteropathy in experimental GVHR (Table 2): (1) A proliferative stage, which is characterized by increased epithelial cell turnover, crypt hypertrophy, and infiltration of the mucosa by lymphoid cells. This type of pathology is not accompanied by villus atrophy or damage to mature enterocytes (Fig. 4). This form of intestinal GVHR may be the only evidence of gut disease in mature, immunocompetent hosts and also comprises the early phase of damage in more severe models of GVHR. (2) In neonatal or immunocompromised hosts, a second phase of enteropathy ensues, in which the rapid development of villus damage may or may not be accompanied by continued crypt hyperplasia. The lymphoid cell infiltrates also disappear (Fig. 5).

1. Crypt Cell Pathology

Crypt cells are the principal target of small intestinal GVHR, irrespective of the type of enteropathy. As noted above, focal necrosis and degeneration of individual crypts has long been recognized in models of severe GVHR, and this is a highly characteristic feature of the terminal stages of intestinal damage. However, even in early studies, these destructive changes were often associated with histological evidence of crypt lengthening and increased mitotic activity (23,29). Wall et al. (32) then showed that the uptake of ^{3}H-TdR was greatly enhanced in crypts of both the jejunum and ileum of newborn mice with GVHR. As this hyperplasia was always accompanied by marked villus atrophy, it was concluded that the increased crypt cell mitotic activity was an attempt to repair the loss of mature enterocytes. Nevertheless, these studies examined intestinal pathology at only one time and in animals which were already acutely ill. It was not until 1977 that elegant studies by Elson et al. (34) demonstrated that crypt hyperplasia could occur in the absence of detectable villus atrophy and so suggested that stimulation of crypt cell production rate (CCPR) might be a direct consequence of GVHR. Although this work examined a single timepoint using relatively insensitive methods, the conclusions were supported by subsequent work using a sensitive stathmokinetic technique to measure epithelial cell turnover and villus/crypt architecture throughout the course of a GVHR in neonatal (CBA $\times$ BALB/c)F_1 mice. This approach showed that there was an increase in CCPR in the jejunum during the first 5-7 days of GVHR, and this preceded any evidence of villus atrophy (35). Nevertheless, significant villus damage did occur in this model, and so it remained possible that an earlier, undetected phase of villus atrophy had been the initial stimulus to crypt cell proliferation. This criticism was addressed in a subsequent timecourse study of intestinal GVHR in slightly older mice of the same strain (36). Under these conditions, there was a significant increase in CCPR within 2-3 days of inducing the GVHR. This progressed until the peak of the GVHR during the 2nd week and then resolved completely (Fig. 6). It is important to note that these animals never had villus atrophy and, in fact, conventional histology revealed no evidence of any damage to mature enterocytes whatsoever (Fig. 4). We have made similar observations of crypt hyperplasia in the absence of villus atrophy during many subsequent studies of intestinal GVHR in mature, unirradiated mice. Direct stimulation of crypt cell production rate (CCPR) is undoubtedly the principal consequence of GVHR under these circumstances.

Enhanced proliferation is not the only direct effect of GVHR on the biology of intestinal epithelial cells and their precursors (Table 3). Two separate studies have shown that enterocytes leaving the crypts of mice with GVHR do so at a much increased rate and so migrate more rapidly up the villus (21,32). This probably reflects a greater upward pressure arising from the enlarged crypt cell population, rather than increased cell

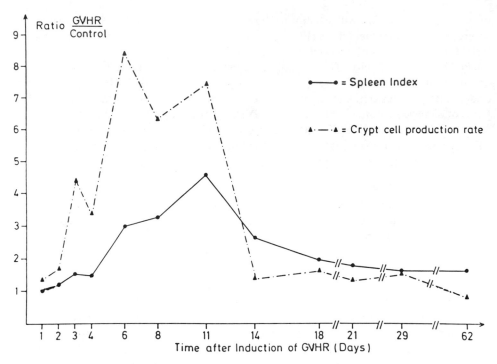

Figure 6 Progress of crypt hyperplasia in proliferative GVHR. Crypt cell production rate in jejunum of 6-7-day-old (CBA × BALB/c)F$_1$ mice with GVHR, expressed as a ratio to that in controls. The CCPR develops in parallel with the splenomegaly in these same animals.

loss. This idea is supported by our own observations that a GVHR is associated with crypt hyperplasia frequently produces villus lengthening, indicating an absolute increase in the number of villus enterocytes under these circumstances (unpublished observations). As we have discussed above, one consequence of the more rapida appearance of recently formed enterocytes on the villus is that the proportion of cells with mature enzyme function will be decreased. This has been confirmed in GVHR, where jejunal lactase and aminopeptidase activities do not develop until much higher up the villus than normal (21). Interestingly, however, the increased production of immature cells is balanced partly by a concomitant enhancement in the rate of differentiation of new enterocytes. Sucrase activity is enhanced in GVHR, and it has been noted that the architecture of the small intestine in neonatal mice with GVHR has a more "adult" appearance than

Table 3 Effects of GVHR on Behavior of Intestinal Crypt Cells

Increased proliferation rate

Enhanced migration onto villus

More rapid differentiation of enzymes

Induction of expression of class II MHC molecules

Ultimately, suppression of proliferation + necrosis

that of age-matched controls (30). In addition, Lund et al. (21) showed that enzyme differentiation in individual cells actually occurred more rapidly in GVHR than in normal mice. Thus, the immunological insult of the GVHR not only alters the mitotic activity of enterocytes but also modifies the subsequent differentiation of these cells.

Enhanced expression of class II MHC molecules by the epithelium is a further effect of GVHR on enterocyte differentiation. Class II MHC molecules are expressed both in the cytoplasm and on the surface of small bowel villus enterocytes in most species (2,37). In normal animals, this is usually at a low level and is restricted to mature epithelial cells. There is no expression of Ia molecules by normal crypt cells. However, the pattern of Ia expression is altered dramatically in the intestine of rats and humans with acute GVHR. Villus enterocytes not only produce many more Ia molecules, but this phenomenon now involves the entire epithelium, including the crypts (38). This effect is of course similar to that found in other tissues during GVHR, and an identical pattern is observed in the intestine during parasite infections, as well as in human enteropathies such as celiac disease (38,39). The basis of this effect on enterocytes has not been elucidated, but it is interesting to note that the conditions which enhance Ia expression are all associated with marked increases in crypt cell mitotic activity. Therefore, the increased production of class II MHC molecules in GVHR may reflect an effect on enterocyte differentiation similar to that noted above for epithelial cell enzymes. It seems likely that these effects are mediated at the level of the appropriate genes, and it would be rewarding to perform parallel studies of gene expression and epithelial cell turnover and differentiation during GVHR.

2. Evolution of Villus Damage

Together, these finding indicate the profound noncytolytic effects which GVHR can have on cell function in the intestine and emphasize that the primary effects of a GVHR on the intestine are to modify the behavior of crypt cells. Nevertheless, the ability of GVHR to produce more severe changes should not be underestimated. Villus atrophy is a highly characteristic feature of intestinal GVHR and, in many cases, there can be complete loss of the normal villus architecture (Fig. 5). As we have noted earlier, many workers have made the implicit assumption that villus damage represents the primary lesion of intestinal GVHR. Other pathological features are then considered as secondary events, or as epiphenomena. We would argue that the evidence for this hypothesis is lacking and suggest that it is villus atrophy which is the secondary consequence of GVHR (Table 2). As we have noted earlier, villus atrophy occurs only in severe forms of GVHR, such as those found in neonatal or irradiated hosts or in certain unirradiated adults. Its appearance seems to correlate well with the development of the more severe features of systemic GVHR, such as weight loss and runting (40,41,104). In virtually all models of intestinal GVHR which ultimately cause villus atrophy, this is associated with a particularly intense period of crypt hyperplasia, which reaches its peak shortly before villus atrophy can be demonstrated. These findings suggest that villus atrophy represents a more severe and progressive form of the same process which initially causes crypt hyperplasia. One possible explanation for this dould be that a period of very intense crypt hyperplasia creates a hyperdynamic, unstable mucosa, which cannot maintain the column of mature enterocytes necessary for intact villus architecture. An alternative possibility is suggested by a recent study of GVHR in irradiated (CBA $\times$ BALB/c)F_1 mice, which indicated that a distinct phase of crypt cell injury signals a sudden transition from a proliferative to a destructive form of enteropathy (40). In these experiments, mice developed significant

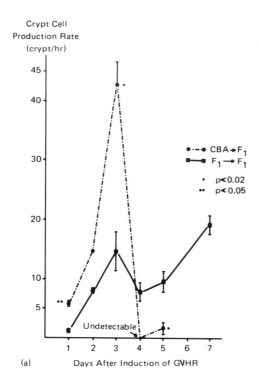

(a)

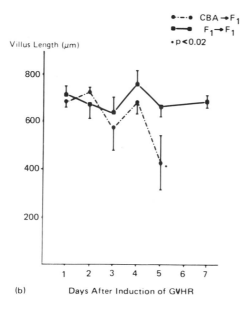

(b)

Figure 7   Development of crypt hyperplasia (a) and villus atrophy (b) during a destructive GVHR in irradiated mice. A large increase in crypt cell production rate occurs very quickly and before villus damage is seen.

crypt hyperplasia within 1-2 days of inducing the GVHR, and this rose to a very high level by 3-4 days (Fig. 7). Villus atrophy appeared only on day 5 and was accompanied by a sudden cessation in crypt cell mitotic activity, rather than the further rise in CCPR which would be anticipated if crypt cell turnover was merely responding to epithelial cell damage. Thereafater, progressive mucosal destruction occurred, with marked evidence of the crypt necrosis and ulceration. However, the villus enterocytes remained remarkably intact until the mucosa was almost entirely necrotic. We have subsequently observed a similar association between inhibition of CCPR and the appearance of villus atrophy in other models of acute GVHR in mice.

Many earlier studies also emphasized the presence of crypt lesions in advanced intestinal GVHR (23,29,33), and others have suggested that crypt stem cells, rather than villus enterocytes, are the principal target of this form of GVHR (42,43). Proof of this idea requires detailed ultrastructural analysis of the epithelial lesions of acute GVHR. Unfortunately, there are few such studies and the findings are often conflicting. Examination by light microscopy shows necrosis of individual crypt cells which has been characterized as apoptosis of the basal cells (43). However, whether the damaged cells are the crypt stem cells has not been proven. It is also unclear whether mature villus enterocytes are damaged at all during GVHR, as some workers have found these cells to be vacuolated (23,29,44), while others have found intact microvillus borders and little evidence of enterocyte damage (32). Clearly, more detailed EM analysis of enterocytes in intestinal GVHR is needed.

In summary, the intestinal epithelium provides an important target for the pathogenic effects of GVHR and most evidence seems to favor the idea that crypt cells are the principal focus of this attack. Initially, the immune stimulus produces a proliferative enteropathy characterized by increased crypt cell proliferation, migration, and differentiation, but with few effects on mature enterocytes (Table 2). In severe cases, this early phase intensifies rapidly and progresses to a destructuve disorder associated with cessation of crypt cell mitotic activity and crypt necrosis. Only at this stage does villus atrophy and damage to mature enterocytes appear, and we propose that these events are secondary to the alterations in crypt cell turnover and function.

B. Pathology of Nonepithelial Structures in Intestinal GVHR

Direct damage to the functioning, epithelial tissues of the gut has obvious and important consequences for the host, but many components of the extracellular matrix and underlying tissues are also involved in maintaining the integrity of the intestine. Although there have been no direct studies of the effects of GVHR on intestinal basement membrane (BM) or local microvasculature, damage to these tissues can be seen readily in animals with acute GVHR. Thickening of the basement membrane occurs early in GVHR, but later, the BM appears to disintegrate as villus atrophy develops (unpublished observations). It is not clear whether the BM damage contributes to or is merely secondary to the evolving mucosal destruction. Damage to local blood vessels may also be important in intestinal GVHR. Swelling of the intestinal vascular endothelium has been noted in irradiated mice with severe GVHR (43) and hemorrhagic exudates are present during the terminal stages of intestinal GVHR (29,44). We have recently found that mice dying of GVHR have evidence of segmental ischaemia (unpublished observations). It therefore seems possible that immune-mediated destruction or occlusion of the local blood supply contributes to the failure of intestinal function in GVHR.

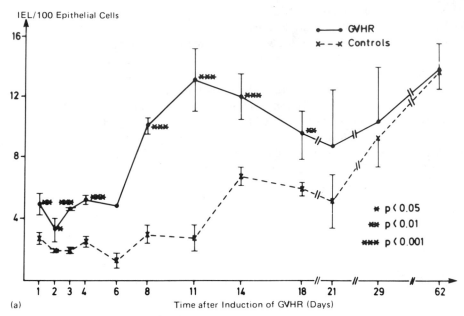

(a)

Figure 8 Behavior of intraepithelial lymphocyte populations in different forms of intestinal GVHR. IEL counts increase rapidly in both proliferative (a) and destructive (b) enteropathy. However, the IEL counts remain increased for some time in the proliferative GVHR in unirradiated (CBA X BALB/c)F_1 mice, while IEL disappear rapidly as GVHR progresses in irradiated F_1 hosts given CBA donor cells (b).

C.   Effects of GVHR on Intestinal Lymphoid Cells

1.   General

One of the most characteristic features of GVHR is its ability to disrupt the structure and function of the immune system. It would be surprising therefore if such a large lymphoid organ as the gut were to escape this damage. In parallel with their assessment of epithelial pathology, initial studies on intestinal GVHR emphasized atrophy of Peyer's patches and depletion of mucosal lymphoid cells (18,19,29,45). Loss of lymphoid elements undoubtedly occurs in the terminal phase of intestinal GVHR (Fig. 5) and is found frequently on examination of humans with acute GVHD (28,47). Nevertheless, these findings are again biased by studying late stages of severe disease using nonquantitative methods. Some microscopic studies did report that early, acute GVHR in mice was associated with infiltration of the mucosa by lymphoblasts (23,44), but the nature and origin of these cells was not determined. More recent work has shown there is marked infiltration of the lamina propria by T lymphocytes during several different models of murine GVHR and this correlates with the severity of mucosal damage. Interestingly, the majority of infiltrating T cells are found near the crypts, the major targets of the GVHR. Both donor and host T cells can be found in this infiltrate, with the relative proportions depending on the type of model under investigation (42,46). Infiltration of the gut by donor T cells and the epithelial damage can be prevented by local irradiation of the PP, suggesting that these cells are derived from intestinal, rather than peripheral lymphoid tissues (46). These results are consistent with the hypothesis that intestinal GVHR reflects local activation of donor T lymphoblasts within the intestinal lymphoid tissues.

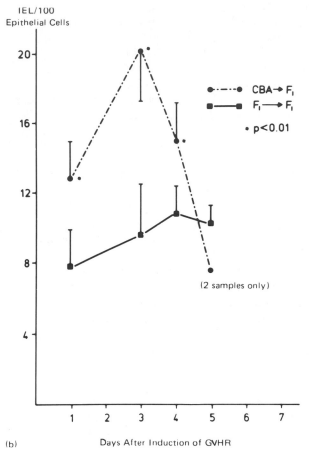

IEL/100
Epithelial Cells

CBA→F$_1$

F$_1$⟶F$_1$

• p<0.01

(2 samples only)

(b)   Days After Induction of GVHR

Figure 8 (continued)

2. Intraepithelial Lymphocytes

An important component of the lymphocytic infiltration of the gut in GVHR is an increased proportion of intraepithelial lymphocytes. Indeed, counts of IEL have proved to be an important quantitative means of assessing intestinal GVHR. An increased IEL count is one of the earliest detectable signs of intestinal GVHR, occurring within 24 hours of inducing GVHR in neonatal or irradiated mice and continuing to rise in parallel with the other proliferative features of GVHR, such as crypt hyperplasia and splenomegaly (36,40). Subsequent changes in IEL count then depend on the type of intestinal GVHR (Fig. 8). Whereas the IEL count falls to normal after the peak of the GVHR in mice undergoing an entirely proliferative enteropathy, a GVHR which causes villus atrophy and mucosal destruction is associated with almost complete loss of IEL (Fig. 8) (36,40,48). The origin of the increased number of IEL in GVHR has not been determined precisely, but the majority seem to be of host origin (42; Mowat and Micklem. unpublished). As in normal animals, the majority of IEL in GVHR are CD8$^+$ and many of these are Thy 1$^-$ (42; Mowat and Micklem, unpublished). These findings suggest that the initial increase in IEL count in GVHR reflects recruitment of a host-derived population which is analogous to that found in normal animals. These cells may then be eliminated subsequently by antihost cytolytic mechanisms. Nevertheless, the possibility that donor lymphocytes also gain access to the epithelium cannot be excluded. The donor T lymphoblasts which infiltrate the lamina propria in GVHR have a very similar phenotype ot IEL and have been noted close to the crypt epithelium (42). Furthermore, the thoracic duct of mice with GVHR contains donor-derived CD8[+] T lymphoblasts, which migrate to the epithelium (42,46,49). The relative contribution of host and donor cells to the increased number of IEL remains to be clarified, as does the role of these cells in intestinal GVHR.

3. Other Lymphoid Cells

The altered populations of IEL and lamina propria T lymphoblasts are accompanied by changes in other mucosal lymphoid cells. Although it is difficult to count many of these cell types, the general finding is that severe GVHR ultimately leads to depletion of many of the lymphoid cells found in the normal intestine. Of particular interest, the loss of lamina propria plasma cells (50) could account for the IgA deficiency that has been noted in clinical GVHD (51) and, by compromising local defense mechanisms, may contribute to intestinal damage. The reported depletion of Ia[+] macrophages and dendritic cells (42) is a further possible factor in producing dysfunction of the intestinal immune system. Although the timing of these events has not been detailed in earlier work, recent studies of acute GVHR in mice have shown that the atrophic pattern of mucosal damage is preceded by an early phase of enhanced IgA production and increased number of IgA plasma cells (Watret and Ferguson, unpublished). Once again, there is evidence that intestinal GVHR occurs in a biphasic manner.

Hyperplasia of mucosal mast cells is a further indicator of the proliferative consequences of intestinal GVHR. Several studies have reported an increase in MMC in rodent GVHR, and this may reflect recruitment and differentiation of precursors within the mucosa (36,42,46,52). In parallel, there is an increase in serum levels of interleukin 3 (IL-3) (53), while the intestine and serum show increased levels of the mucosal mast cell specific protease II (Fig. 9). The exact timecourse of the MMC hyperplasia remains to be confirmed, but there is some evidence that the increased number of MMC parallels other proliferative changes of GVHR (see below). Whether there is subsequent depletion of host-derived MMC, as found with IEL and IgA plasma cells, is not known.

4. Organized Lymphoid Tissues

The organized tissues of the GALT are also involved in the intestinal phase of GVHR and show a similar biphasic pattern of damage. As we have noted, depletion and atrophy of Peyer's patches is a characteristic feature of late, acute GVHR and, of course, this may contribute to depletion of mucosal lymphocytes. However, we have also found that the presence of a GVHR accelerates the development of PP in isografts of fetal small intestine implanted under the kidney capsule of mice (47). Thus, the depletion of PP may be preceded by initial lymphoid hyperplasia. Interestingly, the crypts supplying the dome epithelium of PP also share the biphasic pattern of crypt hyperplasia and atrophy found elsewhere during intestinal GVHR (54).

In conclusion, the pattern of damage to intestinal lymphoid tissues parallels that found in the associated epithelium. As in other, peripheral lymphoid organs, there is an early period of infiltration by donor T lymphoblasts and an associated proliferation of many host-derived immune cells. In mild forms of GVHR, this proliferation may be the

SERUM   JEJUNUM

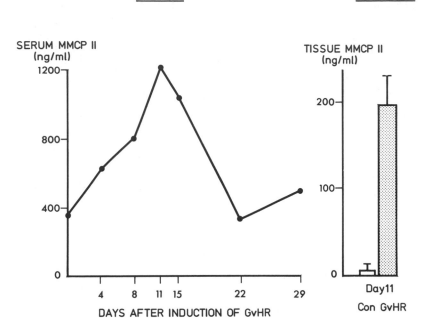

Figure 9 Increased mouse mucosal mast cell-specific protease II levels in the serum and small intestinal mucosa of adult (CBA × BALB/c)F_1 mice with proliferative GVHR.

only abnormality, but in acute, destructive models of GVHR there is progression to the lymphoid depletion often thought to be the principal feature of GVHR.

V. MECHANISMS OF INTESTINAL GVHR

The immunologic basis of systemic GVHR is covered extensively elsewhere in this volume, and we shall restrict the present discussion to mechanisms relating specifically to intestinal GVHR. In many instances, there are close similarities between the systemic and intestinal forms of the disease, but there are differences in several, important areas. In this review, we will first address the cellular and genetic factors which determine the induction of intestinal GVHR, before discussing local and systemic effector mechanisms.

A. Cellular and Genetic Basis of Intestinal GVHR

1. Donor Cell Requirements

Studies of the T-lymphocyte subsets and genetic incompatibilities responsible for inducing intestinal GVHR have lagged behind those in systemic GVHR. Initial work on a fully allogeneic GVHR in neonatal (CBA × BALB/c)F_1 mice showed that Lyt-1^+2^- T cells were alone responsible for inducing the increased IEL count in GVHR. Although both Lyt-1^+2^+ and Lyt-1^+2^- T cells were needed to induce full crypt hyperplasia, Lyt-1^+2^- cells themselves caused a significant degree of crypt hyperplasia. An important and consistent finding was that Lyt-1^-2^+ T cells had no ability to induce intestinal GVHR alone

(12). These results were interpreted as evidence that Lyt-1⁻ DTH effector T cells were essential for inducing intestinal pathology in GVHR, but that in interaction with Lyt-1^+2^+ (? precursors) cells was required to produce the full syndrome. As Lyt-1 is probably present on all mouse T cells and cannot be used as a reliable marker of helper/inducer T cells (55), subsequent studies therefore used Lyt-2 (CD8) and L3T4 (CD4) as nonoverlapping markers of class I and II major histocompatibility complex (MHC) restricted T lymphocytes. Employing this approach, Guy-Grand et al. (42) studied acute GVHR in three models of acute GVHR in (C3H × DBA/2)F_1 hosts. Their results showed that both $CD4^+$ and $CD8^+$ donor T cells could induce some degree of intestinal GVHR in all models, although individual differences were noted. While $CD4^+$ cells were much more efficient at inducing crypt hyperplasia, as well as Ia expression by crypts and infiltration by donor T lymphoblasts in irradiated hosts, only $CD8^+$ cells induced significant alterations in unirradiated adults and were more efficient than $CD4^+$ cells in newborn hosts. Interestingly, however, $CD8^+$ cells seemed to infiltrate the mucosa more efficiently, suggesting that $CD4^+$ cells were more pathogenic on a cell-for-cell basis. In addition, only $CD4^+$ cells induced marked increases in IEL count or hyperplasia of MMC. Unfortunately, these studies did not detail the evolution of the individual features of GVHR, but they are consistent with the idea that both $CD4^+$ and $CD8^+$ can mediate intestinal GVHR in fully allogeneic models. This is supported by our own recent experiments, which suggest that both $CD4^+$ and $CD8^+$ cells are neeed for intestinal GVHR in (CBA × BALB/c)F_1 neonates (Fig. 10). However, preliminary findings show that the relative contribution of the two subsets varies both with the strain used and the type of pathology examined. Together with the results of Guy-Grand, our findings suggest that each population of donor T cells may act via different effector mechanisms.

2. Genetic Basis

Studies of the phenotype of donor T cells responsible for inducing intestinal GVHR have been complemented by examination of its genetic basis. Experiments in irradiated B10 congenic mice showed that villus atrophy, crypt hyperplasia, and increased intestinal permeability only occurred in a GVHR induced across a class II MHC incompatibility at either I-E or I-A (25). No intestinal pathology was induced by class I incompatibilities. However, these studies did observe some systemic disease in class I restricted GVHR and so it was possible that some intestinal damage had been overlooked by the histological analysis used. That this was not the case was shown by our own experiments in B10 congenic mice using sensitive morphometric techniques (12). This work demonstrated that crypt hyperplasia and increased IEL counts during GVHR in unirradiated adult mice were entirely I-A-restricted and that class I MHC disparities induced no intestinal GVHR. We and others have subsequently confirmed that crypt hyperplasia, increased IEL counts, crypt cell Ia expression, and MMC hyperplasia are entirely class II-restricted in the more severe GVHR occurring in newborn F_1 mice (42,56). These findings are clear evidence that class II MHC alloantigens are essential to induce intestinal GVHR. Nevertheless, it should be recalled that both $CD4^+$ and $CD8^+$ cells could cause intestinal GVHR in fully allogeneic mice and there is also some evidence that some intestinal GVHR can be induced by a class I MHC disparity, provided enough donor T cells are injected into irradiated recipients (42).

The relative ability of class I and II MHC alloantigens to induce intestinal GVHR has been examined more closely using the strong alloantigenic stimuli presented by mutant MHC molecules (105). In these studies, highly purified $CD8^+$ or $CD4^+$ T cells from

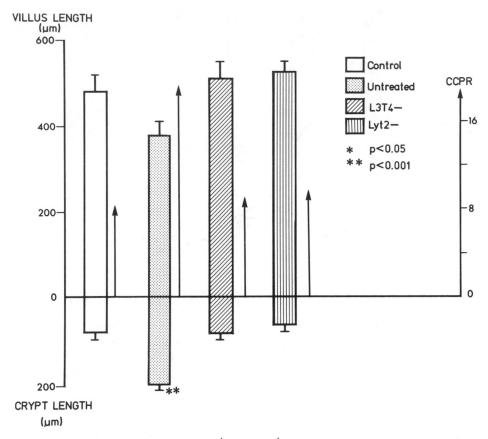

Figure 10 Requirement for both CD8$^+$ and CD4$^+$ donor T cells in the induction of intestinal GVHR in (CBA × BALB/c)F$_1$ mice. Villus and crypt lengths and CCPR in jejunum of mice given unseparated, CD4- or CD8-depleted donor cells.

C57Bl/6 (B6) mice caused intestinal GVHR in (B6 × bm1)F$_1$ or (B6 × bm12)F$_1$ mice carrying mutant H-2K and I-A molecules, respectively. Although both T-cell subsets caused crypt hyperplasia and villus atrophy during a destructive GVHR in irradiated hosts, as well as an entirely proliferative enteropathy in neonatal mice, CD4$^+$ T cells were consistently more efficient at inducing intestinal GVHR (Fig. 11). Furthermore, only CD4$^+$ T cells caused early mortality and induced an increased IEL count in GVHR. As has been shown for systemic GVHR and allograft rejection (57,58), the ability of CD4$^+$ and CD8$^+$ T cells to induce intestinal GVHR was entirely restricted by the appropriate MHC incompatibility. Together, these results indicate that, under appropriate conditions, both class I and II MHC alloantigens can stimulate intestinal GVHR, but that class II MHC restricted CD4$^+$ T cells appear to be the more potent inducers of intestinal GVHR.

3. Relative Effects of MHC Restriction

These studies also provided several pieces of evidence that class I and II MHC-restricted T cells cause different forms of intestinal pathology. First, an increase in IEL counts only

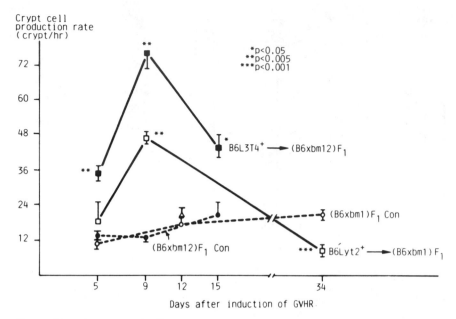

Figure 11 Class II MHC alloantigens are more potent inducers of intestinal GVHR than class I MHC alloantigens. Progress of crypt hyperplasia in irradiated (B6 × bm1)F$_1$ mice carrying an H-2K^b class I MHC mutation and in (B6 × bm12)F$_1$ mice with an I-A^b class II MHC mutation after transfer of highly purified B6 CD8$^+$ or CD4$^+$ T cells, respectively.

occurred in a class II MHC-restricted GVHR. Secondly, mice with a class I-restricted GVHR did not develop the acute disease that killed class II-restricted GVHR mice within 2–3 weeks but suddenly developed a lethal, wasting disorder after 5–6 weeks. This late GVHR was accompanied by intestinal villus atrophy, but the crypt hyperplasia normally found when villus atrophy complicates GVHR was absent. Indeed, mice with this late disorder had crypt atrophy and suppressed crypt cell mitotic activity (Fig. 11). Again, these studies suggest that CD4$^+$ and CD8$^+$ cells may play distinct roles at different stages of intestinal GVHR.

Recent experiments in (C57Bl × DBA/2)F$_1$ (BDF$_1$) mice suggest that these different effects of CD4$^+$ and CD8$^+$ T cells may both be required for intestinal GVHR across fully allogeneic differences (104). When BDF$_1$ mice are given B10 parental cells, an acute GVHR develops, which causes anemia, weight loss, and frequently death. In contrast, the same number of DBA/2 parental cells produces a GVHR which is associated with prolonged lymphoid hyperplasia and autoantibody production, but there is no weight loss or death (59). Recent work has shown that these different forms of disease occur because DBA/2 animals have fewer and less efficient CD8$^+$ cells than B10 mice (60). Thus, it is of some interest that BDF$_1$ mice given B10 cells develop severe intestinal GVHR with villus atrophy and crypt hyperplasia as well as a biphasic increase and loss of IEL. In contrast, induction of a GVHR with DBA/2 cells produces no lesions of intestinal GVHR. Thus, the presence of both CD4$^+$ and CD8$^+$ T cells seems to be required to induce intestinal damage in this GVHR.

4. Minor Histocompatibility Differences

The majority of studies of the genetic basis of intestinal GVHR have concentrated on MHC incompatibilities, and there are no detailed experiments on GVHR across minor histocompatibility differences. Mild crypt hyperplasia and villus edema has been reported in irradiated, minor antigen incompatible (DBA/2 × B10.D2)F_1 mice with GVHR (44), and there are anecdotal reports of diarrhea in some other models of GVHR directed at minor histocompatibility differences. However, there are marked differences in the outcome of systemic GVHR across different minor histoincompatibility antigens (61) and it is probably impossible to predict how frequently intestinal GVHR will occur in different strain combinations. Clearly, more detailed work is required on intestinal pathology under these circumstances.

B. Local Mechanisms in Intestinal GVHR

1. Nature of the Local Cell-Mediated Immune Response

In common with other alloreactive responses, the principal question in intestinal GVHR has been whether cytotoxic T-cell activity or delayed-type hypersensitivity is the mechanism responsible for the gut pathology. Much of the data discussed in the preceding section emphasized the importance of class II MHC-restricted T cells in the induction of intestinal GVHR. Classically, CTL responses are predominantly class I MHC-restricted, and so these findings could implicate DTH as the principal pathogenic mechanism. Nevertheless, we have also discussed evidence that class I MHC-restricted CD8$^+$ T cells are also required to induce intestinal GVHR. Furthermore, it is now clear that there is no absolute correlation between the phenotype and function of individual T-cell subsets (62), and this kind of phenotypic approach may not help elucidate the exact mechanisms involved in T-cell-mediated immunopathology.

Understanding the functional basis of intestinal CMI responses is complicated further by the knowledge that the rules governing systemic and intestinal immunity may be different. Thus, measurements of systemic effector mechanisms will probably not reflect intestinal responses. Unfortunately, it is also difficult to characterize mucosal effector T cells directly. As we have noted, the majority of the donor T lymphoblasts found in the lamina propria of the gut of mice with acute GVHR directed at full MHC differences are CD8$^+$ (42). In addition, T cells with CTL activity have been isolated from the mucosa of mice with acute GVHR (42). Together these findings could indicate that while CD4$^+$ T cells are necessary for the *induction* of intestinal GVHR, their role may merely be to recruit CD8$^+$ CTL which act as the local effector cells. Nevertheless, it should be noted that in an acute GVHR induced by class II MHC-restricted T cells, the lamina propria T lymphoblasts are predominantly CD4$^+$ (42); yet these mice still sustain significant intestinal pathology. Thus, phenotypic investigations of mucosal T cell infiltrates clearly do not give a clear answer as to which functional mechanisms are responsible for intestinal GVHR.

The resolution of these issues at the cellular level may ultimately require cellular markers which correlate absolutely with function, such as lymphokine production, presence of CTL-specific esterases (63), or sensitivity to lysosomotropic agents which eliminate cytotoxic lymphocytes (64). Nevertheless, certain experimental approaches have provided some evidence which may point to the pathogenic mechanisms involved. Our own work on the intestinal damage which occurs in most strains of adult, unirradiated F_1 mice has given strong indirect support for the role of DTH. In these studies, crypt hyperplasia and increased IEL counts occurred in the absence of antihost CTL in the gut or other lymphoid tissues (65). Furthermore, the evolution of the intestinal alterations paralleled exactly the evolution of splenomegaly, a feature which probably reflects the nonspecific, proliferative consequences of GVHR (36). An important finding was that identical intestinal changes occurred in parental strain mice made chimeric for F_1 bone marrow cells, despite the fact that the intestinal epithelium of these animals remains syngeneic to the parental donor T cells. In contrast, F_1 mice made chimeric for donor BM had no evidence of intestinal GVHR after injection of donor T cells (66). Further experiments showed that class II MHC-disparate BM cells of F_1 origin could induce intestinal GVHR in parental animals. These findings indicated that the crypt hyperplasia and increased IEL counts could not be due to a direct attack by donor CTL in the intestinal tissue itself, but rather it was secondaary to recognition of recirculating, Ia^+ "passenger leukocytes" of BM origin. Although an earlier study did not find intestinal GVHR in $F_1 \rightarrow$ parent BM chimeras (67), this report was poorly documented, and the "bystander effect" of GVHR on the gut has been confirmed by an alternative type of experiment. In these studies, pieces of fetal small intestine of parental type were implanted under the kidney capsule of adult F_1 hybrid mice. After some weeks, grafts of this kind develop relatively normal intestinal architecture of donor type (68) but are infiltrated by recirculating BM-derived cells of host origin. When a GVHR was induced in the F_1 hosts by injection of parental lymphocytes, the donor-type grafts showed increased in IEL count, CCPR, and crypt length which were similar to those found in the host jejunum (34,48). These experiments show that the gut itself does not need to present an allogeneic stimulus to the alloreactive donor cells and suggest that the alterations such as crypt hyperplasia are due to nonspecific soluble mediators released during a DTH response directed at BM-derived cells.

The experiments described above dealt entirely with a form of GVHR in which crypt hyperplasia was the only epithelial lesion. Thus, it could be argued that the more severe type of damage typified by villus atrophy might be due to distinct pathogenic mechanism, such as direct attack on enterocytes by CTL. This idea would appear to be consistent with the fact that several models of acute GVHR produce villus atrophy and are associated with high levels of specific antihost CTL activity, both in the gut and other lymphoid tissues (40,41). Nevertheless, this correlation is not absolute. Five- to six-day old noenates also develop villus atrophy in GVHR, but have no CTL activity (41), while treatment of mice with $2'$-deoxyguanosine prevents villus atrophy but has no effect on CTL activity in GVHR (see below). Further evidence against a role for CTL in causing villus atrophy comes from the finding that the ability of different class I MHC mutations to induce acute, intestinal GVHR in irradiated mice correlates with their ability to induce $CD8^+$ helper T cells, rather than their recognition by CTL (Mowat and Sprent, submitted). Finally, we and others have shown that T-cell infiltration, villus atrophy, crypt hyperplasia, and crypt cell necrosis can all occur as bystander phenomena in fetal intestine of donor type implanted in mice with acute GVHR (Fig. 12) (33,40,46). Therefore, the bulk of available evidence argues against an essential role for CTL in any of the intestinal lesions of GVHR.

2. Role of Soluble Mediators

The findings that intestinal GVHR can occur even when specific CTL cannot attack the gut epithelium are indirect evidence that soluble mediators released during the DTH response are responsible for the pathology. Recent work has provided more direct support

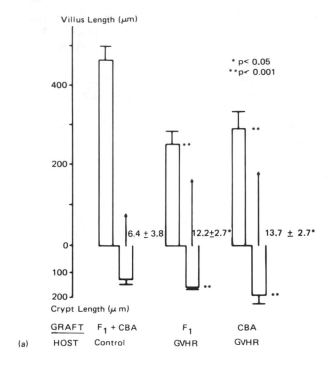

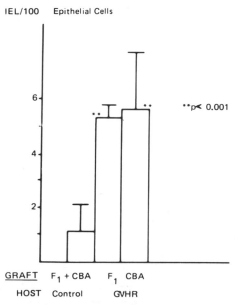

Figure 12 Intestinal GVHR occurs as a "bystander phenomenon." Mucosal architecture (a) and IEL counts (b) in grafts of fetal (CBA × BALB/c)F_1 or CBA small intestine implanted in irradiated (CBA × BALB/c)F_1 mice given CBA donor cells. Villus atrophy, as well as increases in CCPR, crypt length, and IEL count occur, irrespective of whether the gut grafts are syngeneic to the donor.

for this hypothesis. First, Guy-Grand et al. have found that mucosal lymphocytes isolated from mice with acute GVHR produce lymphokines, including interleukin 2 (IL-2), Il-3, and γ-interferon (γ IFN). In addition, it has been shown that an acute GVHR in mice is associated with increased levels of TNF in serum (69), while both crypt hyperplasia and villus atrophy in GVHR can be prevented by treating mice with antibodies against tumor necrosis factor (TNF) (43) or γIFN (Fig. 13). Anti-IFN also prevents the increased IEL count in GVHR. Finally, we have shown recently that treatment of mice with the α/β-interferon-inducer, polyinosinic-polycytydylic acid, exacerbates the intestinal consequences of murine GVHR (Fig. 14) but has no effect on CTL activity (56).

The exact ways in which cytokines could damage the gut remain highly speculative. As there is ample evidence that meditors such as TNF, α/βIFN, and γIFN can modify the proliferation and differentiation of other, nonlymphoid cells (70-73), these agents could account directly for the altered proliferation and differentiation of crypt cells seen in GVHR. Their undoubted cytostatic functions may also be responsible for the inhibition of crypt cell proliferation and ultimate crypt cell necrosis characteristic of severe GVHR. Furthermore, IFN is an obvious candidate to explain the enhanced expression of class

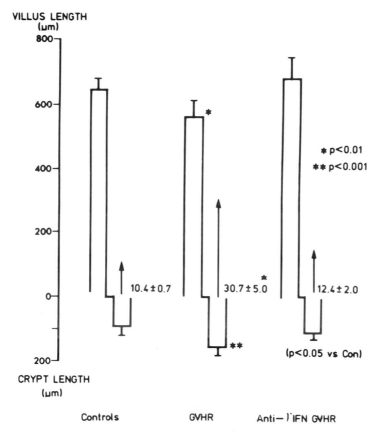

Figure 13 Prevention of intestinal GVHR by antibodies to γ-interferon. BDF$_1$ mice given B6 donor cells develop villus atrophy, crypt lengthening, and increased CCPR compared with controls. Anti-γIFN-treated hosts have virtually no mucosal pathology.

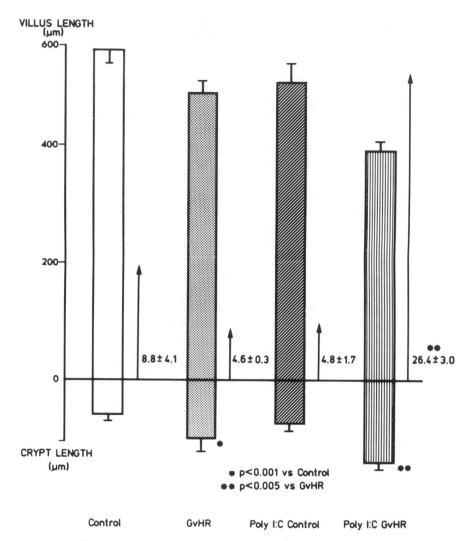

Figure 14 Exacerbation of intestinal GVHR by enhancing production of α/β-interferon with polyinosinic:polycytydylic acid. Neonatal (CBA × BALB/c)F_1 mice with GVHR only have an increased crypt length compared with controls, but poly I:C treated GVHR mice also have villus atrophy and a large increase in CCPR.

II MHC molecules by enterocytes in GVHR. Finally, TNF and IFN are known to have profound effects on endothelial cells and fibroblasts (71,74,75) and we have already discussed the potentially harmful effects of interfering with the normal functions of these cells. Clearly, there is a need to examine directly the effects of these, and other cytokines on intestinal epithelial cell function.

3. Role of Nonspecific Effector Cells

Recruitment and activation of nonspecific effector cells is an alternative way in which inflammatory cytokines could produce gut damage in GVHR. The potential importance of this pathway is suggested by the large number of macrophages, eosinophils, and other inflammatory cells in the intestinal mucosa, but only two of these cell types have been studied directly in GVHR.

As we have discussed, hyperplasia of mucosal mast cells is a feature of many experimental models of GVHR and probably reflects recruitment by IL-3. Although the hyperplasia of MMC was initially detected using histological techniques, more recent work has shown increased amounts of the MMC-specific protease II in the serum and intestinal mucosa of both rats and mice with GVHR (Fig. 9) (52). This protease release occurs in association with either destructive or proliferative enteropathy and in unirradiated mice, protease levels correlated precisely with the development of splenomegaly (Newlands, GFJ, Mowat, A McI, Miller, RP, submitted). Their function of MMC in intestinal GVHR is unclear. However, it is significant that the natural substrate of MMC-specific protease II appears to be the type IV collagen found in the intestinal basement membrane (76). Therefore, MMC-derived enzymes may contribute to the enteropathy of GVHR by interfering with the normal function of the BM which helps maintain the integrity of the epithelium. Other mediators released from MMC may also help explain the altered intestinal permeability found in GVHR.

The other nonspecific effector cells that have received attention in GVHR are NK cells. Enhanced NK cell activity by peripheral lymphocytes has been described in many studies of experimental GVHR (65,77,78) and this is accompanied by activation of NK cells within isolated populations of IEL (65). The enhanced NK activity by IEL parallels other features of proliferative enteropathy in unirradiated adult mice with GVHR and is preceded by a systemic antihost DTH response (79). That mucosal NK cells are an important nonspecific effector mechanism in intestinal GVHR is supported by the fact that treatment of unirradiated adult mice with anti-asialo G_{M1} (AsG_{M1}) antibody prevents the crypt hyperplasia normally found in GVHR (80). Although the interpretation of these results is potentially confused by the expression of AsG_{M1} on CTL as well as NK cells (81), it should be noted that the effects of anti-AsG_{M1} on intestinal pathology were examined in a model of GVHR in which CTL cannot be detected. For these reasons, selective depletion of NK cells probably is the explanation for the ability of anti-AsG_{M1} to inhibit intestinal GVHR. An interesting, additional finding from this study was that control mice treated with the antibody had slightly lower IEL counts than normal mice (80), suggesting that AsG_{M1}^{+} IEL may be involved directly in the pathogenesis of intestinal GVHR.

It is important to note that the effects of anti-AsG_{M1} on intestinal GVHR were examined in a model which produced hyperplasia in the absence of villus atrophy. Rapid and marked activation of NK cells does occur in models of GVHR which cause villus atrophy, but this is usually a transient feature which accompanies the other early, proliferative changes of GVHR, including crypt hyperplasia. Indeed, the onset of villus atrophy is consistently associated with complete loss of NK cell activity (40). Although these findings suggest that NK cells may be involved only in the proliferative consequences of GVHR in the gut, depletion of NK cells is extremely effective in preventing systemic disease in severe, destructive forms of GVHR (82,83). Therefore, it remains possible that activation of NK cells is a necessary, early component of severe GVHR-induced enteropathy.

The ways in which NK cells could influence intestinal pathology are unknown, but could reflect their known ability to produce inflammatory cytokines (84,85). Alternatively, a direct interaction between NK cells and crypt stem cells could involve the cytolytic machinery of NK cells.

4. Other Immune Mecahnisms

In addition to different effector T-cell mechanisms, there is some evidence that suppressor T-cell (T_s) activity may be involved in certain features of GVHR. Gleichmann and colleagues have argued that allospecific T_s are responsible for the anemia, weight loss, and lymphoid atrophy found in unirradiated BDF_1 mice given C57Bl donor cells (59). As we have discussed, these mice also develop a severe enteropathy with intense crypt hyperplasia and villus atrophy, and we have found recently that the intestinal changes can be inhibited by treating host mice with $2'$-deoxyguanosine (dGuo) (Felstein and Mowat, submitted). This agent is believed to have selective effects on T_s (86), a finding confirmed by our own studies. In addition, dGuo had no effect on the generation of other immune effector mechanisms in GVHR, including CTL. Thus, T_s may be responsible for the later, atrophic stages of intstinal GVHR, perhaps by switching off turnover of BM and crypt stem cells.

This hypothesis is supported by findings that a GVHR induced by an incompatibility at the I-J locus in mice occasionally causes villus atrophy in association with inhibition of crypt cell turnover and decreased IEL counts (12,56). The I-J locus has been associated with T_s function in many experimental systems and an I-J-restricted GVHR has been shown previously to activate immunosuppressive phenomena (12,87-89). Therefore, our results could support a possible role for T_s in producing mucosal atrophy in GVHR. Howeever, current problems in establishing T_s as a separate population of T cells and in identifying the genetic basis of the I-J locus (90) mean that experiments on effector functions of I-J-restricted T_s must be interpreted with care. An apparent role for "T_s" in intestinal GVHR could merely reflect release of inhibitory mediators by conventional effector T cells at a particular stage of differentiation.

Throughout this review, we have concentrated entirely on the role of T lymphocytes and T-dependent effector mechanisms in intestinal GVHR. There are no studies of the role of antibodies in the pathogenesis of intestinal GVHR, but the production of allo-antibodies does not correlate with the analogous enteropathy found in rejecting allo-grafts of gut (91). There is also evidence from other experiments that antibody-dependent mechanisms cannot produce the type of intestinal pathology found in GVHR (92).

C. Host Factors in Intestinal GVHR

The outcome of GVHR is clearly dependent on the host animal under study. Although much of this influence reflects the ability of different host alloantigens to activate donor T cells, several other host factors appear to influence the development of intestinal GVHR in experimental animals.

1. Intestinal Microflora

The beneficial effect of bowel decontamination on survival after clinical BMT has been well documented but the role of the intestinal flora on organ-specific consequences of experimental GVHR are less clear. Several workers have reported that germ-free mice or mice with a gut flora consisting entirely of anaerobes have markedly less mortality due to acute GVHR than conventional animals. In parallel, removal of aerobic gut flora prevents much of the liver and gut damage normally associated with severe GVHR (93,94). If these animals are subsequently returned to conventional conditions or associated with gram-negative aerobes, mortality and tissue damage due to GVHR reappear. Recent studies have also shown that administration of LPS or *E. coli* exacerbates systemic GVHR in irradiated mice, while passive immunization with antibody to *E. coli* has a mild, beneficial effect (95,96). Together, these findings suggest that gram-negative aerobes in the gut flora are critical for the pathogenesis of GVHR. Nevertheless, it should be noted that the beneficial effect of the germ-free state only applies to the early stages of acute GVHR. Eventually, these animals show mortality rates and pathology which are similar to, if not higher than those in conventional hosts (93,94,27). Furthermore, the effects of exogenous LPS or passive immunization with anti-*E. coli* antibody were generally small and were mainly restricted to GVHR across minor histocompatibility antigen differences (95,96).

The role of infection in intestinal GVHR is of particular importance in view of the close proximity of the intestinal flora to the epithelial structures. Early studies suggested that the characteristic necrotic lesions of established GVHR were due to local abcesses which had formed due to mucosal penetration of organisms (94). However, as we have discussed, crypt hperplasia, villus atrophy and lymphocytic infiltration occur in sterile, antigen-free grafts of small intestine implanted under the kidney capsule of mice with GVHR (Fig. 12) (34,48). Thus, although it may undoubtedly occur, local infection is clearly not necessary for the development of GVHR-specific lesions within the intestine. One explanation for the apparently paradoxical evidence on the role of intestinal flora may come from work showing that crypt degeneration only occurs in sterile explants of gut if these are placed in hosts with a conventional microflora (33). Although originally interpreted as evidence that an immune response against cross-reacting antigens on epithelia and intestinal organisms caused intestinal damage in GVHR, there is no evidence to support this theory. Rather, it seems more likely that bacterial products influence the level of systemic antihost immune responsiveness. Enterobacteria produce several agents with adjuvant activity, and it has long been known that animals with GVHR have increased levels of circulating endotoxin (27). Thus, initial damage to the gut caused by GVHR may allow increased absorption of bacterial products which then exacerbate the tissue lesions by virtue of their ability to enhance ongoing immune responses. An additional, but not necessarily exclusive possibility is that the increased levels of bacterial endotoxin cause release of TNF (71,97), whose enteropathic properties in GVHR have been discussed above. In conclusion we consider that there is insufficient evidence to support a direct role for local infection in intestinal GVHR, but we suggest that release of intestinal bacterial products may play an important secondary role in the pathogenesis of severe GVHR.

There are no studies on the role of local viruses in intestinal GVHR in experimental animals. However, Coxsackie virus A1 has been shown to cause intestinal damage after human BMT (98), while the studies of Grundy et al. (99) have highlighted the synergistic ability of CMV to cause severe lung disease in experimental GVHR. These potential complicating effects of both bacterial and viral infections are particularly serious considerations in view of the local and systemic immune deficiencies which can occur in GVHR.

2. Endogenous Host Factors

The role of endogenous, host-derived factors in the outcome of intestinal GVHR is illustrated by the different outcomes of a GVHR in different types of host using the same donor-host strain combination. Studies of this nature have shown that intestinal pathology is much more severe when the hosts used are irradiated, athymic, or very immature. Under each of these circumstances, (CBA × BALB/c)F_1 mice not only develop much more intense crypt hyperplasia than that found in intact, adult hosts, but develop villus atrophy which is not usually a feature of this model of GVHR (40,41,100). There seem to be two possible explanations for this phenomenon. First, the hosts that develop severe intestinal damage all lack a normal T-lymphocyte system and so may be defective in the mechanism by which host T cells are thought to resist the proliferation of alloreactive donor T cells (101). This idea is supported strongly by the enhanced GVHR found in athymic mice. In addition, the susceptibility of neonatal mice to the development of villus atrophy in GVHR alters rapidly during the period of the first week of life (41) when mature host T cells are seeding the intestinal and peripheral lymphoid tissues (102). An alternative possibility is that the intestine of compromised hosts is unusually susceptible to the effects of GVHR. Irradiation has particularly profound effects on the function and renewal of the intestinal epithelium, while rapid alterations in mucosal architecture occur during the early neonatal period. In common with GVHR, the major maturational changes affect crypt cell function and a synergistic effect on intestinal damage can readily be imagined. Thus, the more severe intestinal GVHR in compromised hosts may be due to factors both within the immune system and the gut. Irrespective of the mechanisms involved, the interaction between the host and an ongoing GVHR has important implications for the conditioning regimes used in human BMT.

VI. CONCLUSIONS

The data discussed in this review have highlighted the profound effects which experimental GVHR can have on the small intestine. In addition, we have shown that the pattern of intestinal damage is sufficiently reproducible that certain aspects of the mucosal pathology can be used as sensitive indices to measure this form of GVHR. Together with the ability of a GVHR to generate a wide range of different immune effector functions, these features mean that studies of intestinal GVHR can provide a useful means of assessing the immunopathological potential of different subsets of T-lymphocyte and other lymphoid effector cells. In addition, the pattern of intestinal pathology in GVHR reproduces that found in naturally occurring enteropathies which cause villus atrophy, crypt hyperplasia, and increased numbers of MMC and IEL and which are associated with local CMI reactions (92). These include gluten-sensitive enteropathy, cow's milk protein intolerance, several parasite infections, Crohn's disease, and of course, acute intestinal GVHR after allogeneic BMT in man. As the mechanisms underlying the intestinal damage in many of these diseases are unknown, intestinal GVHR in animals offers a flexible model to study the pathogenesis of T-lymphocyte-mediated enteropathy under experimental conditions.

A hypothetical pathogenesis of intestinal GVHR is illustrated in Fig. 15. This is based primarily on the evidence that the self-renewing crypt stem cell is the principal target of intestinal GVHR. As we have discussed, the intestinal epithelium does not itself seem to induce this process, and we have proposed that the intestinal pathology occurs as a bystander effect of soluble cytokines released by DTH effector cells that are activated by class II MHC alloantigens on bone marrow-derived stimulator cells (Fig. 15). Together, the short biological half-life of most cytokines and the close association between intestinal pathology and the presence of infiltrating T lymphoblasts suggests that the enteropathic mediators are produced locally. However, the site of induction of donor T cells is unclear. Ia[+] dendritic cells and macrophages are abundant within the mucosa (103), but there is also evidence that the donor T lymphoblasts found in the mucosa during GVHR are derived from precursors activated within the PP (46). Alternatively, the possibility remains that intestinal GVHR is a local effect of highly active cytokines released during the systemic immune response.

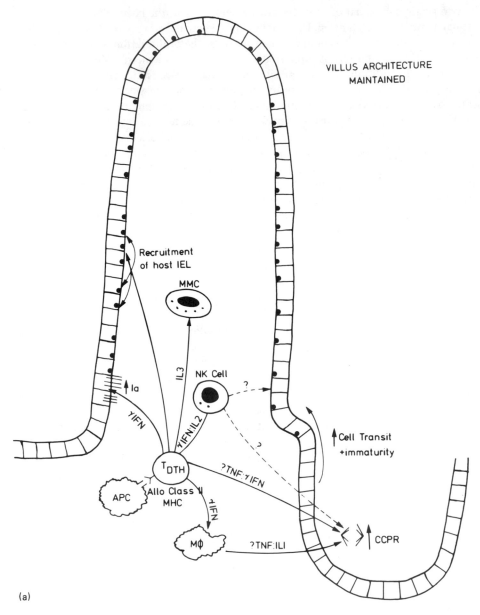

Figure 15 Mechanisms of enteropathy in GVHR: See text for details. (a) Phase 1-proliferative and (b) phase 2-destructive.

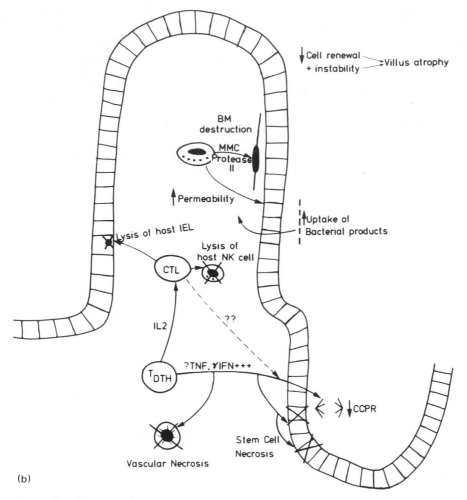

(b)

Figure 15 (continued)

    We suggest there are several ways in which these factor may produce the characteristic pathology and compromise intestinal function (Fig. 15). First, there could be direct effects on crypt cell behavior, with an initial stimulation of proliferation and differentiation. This will be manifested initially by microscopic evidence of crypt lengthening and hyperplasia, but prolonged increases in cell turnover may ultimately lead to accelerated villus cell loss due to an increase in upward pressure from newly formed crypt cells. As a result, the mucosa may become hyperdynamic and unstable, normal villus architecture will not be maintained, and there will be a loss of effective absorptive surface area. Malabsorption and nutritional defects will also be favored by the presence of a higher proportion of immature cells being pushed onto the villus surface by the enhanced CCPR. Villus atrophy may also be produced in the later stages of the DTH response, because alterations in the amount or type of cytokines may lead to suppressed crypt cell proliferation and hence a failure to compensate for enterocyte loss. Intestinal fibroblasts and endothelial cells may provide further targets for the direct effects of enteropathic cytokines. The intestinal architecture is highly dependent on the normal function of these cells and modulation of their activity by the interferons or TNFs and could have profound effects on epithelial cell function. The final way in which inflammatory mediators may damage the intestine is by recruitment of nonspecific effector cells, and we have presented evidence that MMC and NK cells may be two components of this phenomenon. Other inflammatory cells are surely also involved, but their roles remain to be elucidated.

The pathways we have outlined are speculative and are undoubtedly oversimplified. Nevertheless, we hope that our discussion may not only provide a framework for further studies of the complex interactions involved in intestinal GVHR, but will also suggest potential areas of future research in others forms of immunopathology.

ACKNOWLEDGMENTS

The work quoted in this chapter was supported by the Medical Research Council (U.K.), The Coeliac Trust, and ConaCyt (Mexico).

REFERENCES

1.   Billingham RE, Brent L, Medawar PB: Acquired tolerance of skin homografts. Ann NY Acad Sci 1955;59:409-498;
2.   Mayrhofer G: Physiology of the intestinal immune system, In *Local Immune Responses of the Gut*, edited by Newby TJ, Stokes CR. CRC Press, Boca Raton, FL, 1984; pp. 1-96.
3.   Parrott DMV: The structure and organisation of lymphoid tissue in the gut, In *Food Allergy and Intolerance*, edited by Brostoff J, Challacombe SJ. Bailliere Tindall, London, 1987; pp. 3-26.
4.   Mowat A McI: The cellular basis of gastrointestinal immunity, In *Immunopathology of the Small Intestine*, edited by Marsh NN. John Wiley & Sons, 1987; pp. 41-72.
5.   Lamm ME: Cellular aspects of immunoglobulin A. Adv Immunol 1976;22:223-290.
6.   Mowat A McI, MacKenzie S, Baca ME, Felstein MV, Parrott DMV: Functional characteristics of intraepithelial lymphocytes from mouse small intestine. II. In vivo and in vitro responses of intraepithelial lymphocytes to mitogenic and allogeneic stimuli. Immunology 1900;58:627-634.
7.   Davies MDJ, Parrott DMV: Cytotoxic T cells in small intestinal epithelial, lamina propria and lung lymphocytes. Immunology 1981;44:367-371.
8.   Ernst PB, Befus AD, Bienenstock J: Leukocytes in the intestinal epithelium: an unusual immunological compartment. Immunol Today 1985;6:50-55.
9.   Ernst PB, Clark DA, Rosenthal KL, Befus AD, Bienenstock J: Detection and characterization of cytotoxic T lymphocyte precursors in the murine intestinal intraepithelial leukocyte population. J Immunol 1986;136:2121-2126.
10. Dillon SB, MacDonald TT: Functional characterisation of Con A responsive Lyt 2 positive mouse small intestinal intraepithelial lymphocytes. Immunology 1986; 59:389-396.
11. Dobbins WO: Human intestinal intraepithelial lymphocytes. Gut 1986;27:972-985.
12. Mowat A McI, Borland A, Parrott DMV: Hypersensitivity reactions in the small intestine. 7. The intestinal phase of murine graft-versus-host reaction is induced by Lyt 2⁻ T cells activated by I-A alloantigens. Transplantation 1986;4:192-198.

13. Goodman T, Lefrancois L: Expression of the $\gamma\delta$ T-cell receptor on intestinal CD8$^+$ intraepithelial lymphocytes. Nature 1988;333:855-858.

14. Jarrett EEE, Haig DM: Mucosal mast cells in vivo and in vitro. Immunology Today 1984;5:115-119.

15. Befus AD, Pearce F, Bienenstock J: Intestinal mast cells in pathology and host resistance, In *Food Allergy and Intolerance*, edited by Brostoff J, Challacombe SJ. Bailliere Tindall, London, 1987; pp. 88-102.

16. Woodbury RG, Gruzenski GM, Lagunoff D: Immunofluorescent localization of a serine protease in rat small intestine. Proc Natl Acad Sci USA 1978;75:2785-2789.

17. Miller HRP: The protective mucosal response against gastrointestinal nematodes in ruminants and laboratory animals. Vet Immunol Immunopathol 1984;6:176-259.

18. Billingham RE: The biology of graft-versus-host reactions. Harvey Lectures 1967; 62:21-79.

19. Simonsen M. Graft versus host reactions. Their natural history and applicability as tools of research. Progr Allergy 1962;6:349-467.

20. Hedberg CA, Reiser S, Reilly RW: Intestinal phase of the runting syndrome in mice. II. Observations on nutrient absorption and certain disaccharidase abnormalities. Transplantation 1968;6:104-110.

21. Lund, EK, Bruce MG, Smith MW, Ferguson A: Selective effects of graft-versus-host reaction on disaccharidase expression by mouse jejunal enterocytes. Clinical Science 1986;71:189-198.

22. Perdue MH, Chung M, Gall DG: Effect of intestinal anaphylaxis on gut function in the rat. Gastroenterol 1984;86:391-397.

23. Cornelius EA: Protein-losing enteropathy in the graft-versus-host reaction. Transplant 1970;9:247-252.

24. Weisdorf SA, Salati LM, Longsdorf JA, Ramsay NKC, Sharp HL: Graft-versus-host disease of the intestine: a protein losing enteropathy characterized by fecal α_1-anti-trypsin. Gastroenterol 1983;85:1076-1081.

25. Pequet P-F: GVHR elicited by products of class I or class II loci of the MHC: analysis of the response of mouse T lymphocytes to products of class I and class II loci of the MHC in correlation with GVHR-induced mortality, medullary aplasia and enteropathy. J Immunol 1985;135:1637-1643.

26. Turner MW, Boulton P, Shields JG, Strobel S, Gibson S, Miller HRP, Levinsky RJ: Intestinal hypersensitivity reactions in the rat. I. Uptake of intact protein, permeability to sugars and their correlation with mucosal mast cell activation. Immunology 1988;63:119-124.

27. Walker RI: The contributionof intestinal endotoxin to mortality in hosts with compromised resistance: A review. Exp Haematol 1978;6:172-184.

28. Slavin RE, Woodruff JM: The pathology of bone-marrow transplantation, In Pathology Annual, edited by Sommers SC. Appleton-Century-Crofts Pub., 1974; pp. 291-344.

29. Reilly RW, Kirsner JB: Runt intestinal disease. Lab Intest 1965;14:102-107.

30. Beschorner WE, Tutschka PJ, Santos GW: Chronic graft-versus-host disease in the rat radiation chimera. I. Clinical features, haematology, histology and immuno pathology in long-term chimeras. Transplantation 1982;33:393-399.

31. Gorer PA, Boyse EA: Pathological changes in F_1 hybrid mice following transplantation of spleen cells from donors of the parental strains. Immunol 1959;2: 182-193.

32. Wall AJ, Rosenberg JL, Reilly RW: Small intestinal injury in the immunologically runted mouse. Morphologic and autoradiographic studies. J Lab Clin Med 1971; 78:833-834A.

33. van Bekkum DW, Knaan S: Role of bacterial microflora in development of intestinal lesions from GVHR. J Natl Canc Inst 1977;58:787-790.

34. Elson CO, Reilly RW, Rosenberg IH: Small intestinal injury in the GVHR: an innocent bystander phenomenon. Gastroenterol 1977;72:886-889.

35. MacDonald TT, Ferguson A: Hypersensitivity reactions in the small intestine. III. The effects of allograft rejection and of GVHD on epithelial cell kinetics. Cell Tiss Kinet 1977;10:301-312.

36. Mowat A McI, Ferguson A: Intraepithelial lymphocyte count and crypt hyperplasia measure the mucosal component of the graft-versus-host reaction in mouse small intestine. Gastroenterology 1982;83:417-423.

37. Bland PW: MHC class II expression by the gut epithelium. Immunology Today 1988;9:174-178.

38. Barclay AN, Mason DW: Induction of Ia antigen in rat epidermal cells and gut epithelium by immunological stimuli. J Exp Med 1982;156:1665-1676.

39. Arnaud-Battandier F, Cerf-Bensussan N, Amsellem R, Schmitz J: Increased HLA-DR expression by enterocytes in children with coeliac disease. Gastroenterology 1986;19:1206-1212.

40. Mowat A McI, Felstein MV, Borland A, Parrott DMV: Experimental studies of immunologically mediated enteropathy. Delayed type hypersensitivity is responsible for the proliferative and destructive enteropathy in irradiated mice with graft-versus-host reaction. Gut 1988;29:949-956.

41. Felstein MV, Mowat A McI: Experimental studies of immunologically mediated enteropathy. IV. Correlation between immune effector mechanisms and type of enteropathy during a graft-versus-host reaction in neonatal mice of different ages. Clin Exp Immunol 1988;72:108.

42. Guy-Grand D, Vassalli P: Gut injury in mouse graft-versus-host reaction. Study of its occurrence and mechanisms. J Clin Invest 1986;77:1584-1595.

43. Piguet P-F, Grau GE, Allet B, Vassalli P: Tumor necrosis factor/cachectin is an effector of skin and gut lesions of the acute phase of graft-vs-host disease. J Exp Med 1987;166:1280-1289.

44. Rappaport H, Khalil A, Halle-Pannenko O, Pritchard L, Dantchev D, Mathe G: Histopathologic sequence of events in adult mice undergoing lethal graft-versus-host reaction developed across H-1 and/or non-H-2 histocompatibility barriers. Am J Pathol 1979;96:121-142.

45. Nowell PC, Cole LJ: Lymphoid pathology in homologous disease of mice. Transplant Bull 1959;6:435.

46. Guy-Grand D, Griscelli C, Vassalli P: The mouse gut T-lymphocyte, a novel type of T-cell: Nature, origin and traffic in mice in normal and graft-versus-host conditions. J Exp Med 1978;148:1661-1677.

47. Slavin RE, Santos GW: The graft-versus-host reaction in man after bone marrow transplantation: Pathology, pathogenesis, clinical features and implications. Clin Immunol Immunopathol 1973;1:472-498.

48. Mowat A McI, Ferguson A: Hypersensitivity reactions in the small intestine. 6. Pathogenesis of the graft-versus-host reaction in the small intestinal mucosa of the mouse. Transplantation 1981;32:238-243.

49. Sprent J: Fate of H-2 activated T-lymphocytes in Syngeneic Hosts. I. Fate in lymphoid tissues and intestines traced with ^{3}H-thymidine, ^{125}I-deoxy-uridine and [51]chromium. Cell Immunol 1976;21:278-302.

50. Gold JA, Kosek J, Wanek N, Bauer S: Duodenal immunoglobulin deficiency in graft-versus-host disease (GVHD) mice. J Immunol 1976;117:471-476.

51. Cunningham-Rundles C, Brandeis WE, Safai B, O'Reilly R, Day NK, Good RA: Selective IgA deficiency and circulating immune complexes containing bovine proteins in a child with chronic graft-versus-host disease. Am J Med 1979;67:883-890.

52. Ferguson A, Cummins AG, Munro GH, Gibson S, Miller HRP: Intestinal mucosal

mast cells in rats with graft-versus-host reaction. Adv Exp Med Biol 1988;216A: 625-634.

53. Crapper RM, Schrader JW: Evidence for the in vivo production and release into the serum of a T cell lymphokine, persisting-cell stimulating factor (PSF), during graft-versus-host reactions. Immunology 1986;57:553-558.

54. Klein RM, Clancy J, Sheridan K: Acute lethal graft-versus-host disease stimulates cellular proliferation in Peyer's patches and follicle associated ileal epithelium of adult rats. Virch Arch (B) 1984;47:303-311.

55. Ledbetter JA, Rouse RV, Micklem HS, Herzenberg LA: T-cell subsets defined by expression of Lyt 123 and Thy 1 antigens. Two parameter immunofluorescence and cytotoxicity analysis with monoclonal antibodies modifies current views. J Exp Med 1980;152:280-295.

56. Felstein MV: Ph.D. Thesis, University of Glasgow, 1988.

57. Sprent J, Schaefer M, Lo D, Korngold R: Properties of purified T cell subsets. II. In vivo responses to class I vs class II H-2 differences. J Exp Med 1986;163:998-1011.

58. Rosenberg AS, Mizuochi T, Sharrow SO, Singer A: Phenotype, specificity and function of T cell subsets and T cell interactions involved in skin allograft rejection. J Exp Med 1987;165:1296-1315.

59. Gleichmann E, Pals ST, Rolink AG, Radaszkiewicz T, Gleichmann H: Graft-versus-host reactions: clues to the etiopathology of a spectrum of immunological diseases. Immunol Today 1984;5:324-332.

60. Via CS, Sharrow SO, Shearer GM: Role of cytotoxic T lymphocytes in the prevention of lupus-like disease occurring in a murine model of graft-versus-host disease. J Immunol 1987;139:1840-1849.

61. Korngold R, Sprent J: Variable capacity of L3T4$^+$ T cells to cause lethal graft-versus-host disease across minor histocompatibility barriers in mice. J Exp Med 1987;165:1552-1564.

62. Sprent J, Webb SR: Function and specificity of T cell subsets in the mouse. Adv Immunol, in press.

63. Henkart PA, Berrebi GA, Takayama H, Munger WE, Sitkovsky MV: Biochemical and functional properties of serine esterases in acidic cytoplasmic granules of cytotoxic T lymphocytes. J Immunol 1987;139:2398-2405.

64. Thiele DL, Charley MR, Calomeni JA, Lipsky PE: Lethal graft-vs-host disease across major histocompatibility barriers: requirement for leucyl-leucine methyl ester sensitive cytotoxic T cells. J Immunol 1987;138:51-57.

65. Borland A, Mowat A McI, Parrott DMV: Augmentation of intestinal and peripheral natural killer cell activity during the graft-versus-host reaction in mice. Transplantation 1983;36:513-519.

66. Mowat A McI: Ia$^+$ bone marrow derived cells are the stimulus for the intestinal phase of murine graft-versus-host reaction. Transplantation 1986;42:141-144.

67. Cornelius EA, Martinez C, Yunis EJ, Good RA: Haematological and pathological changes induced in tolerant mice by the injection of syngeneic lymphoid cells. Transplant 1968;6:33-44.

68. Ferguson A, Parrott DMV: Growth and development of antigen-free grafts of fetal mouse intestine. J Path 1972;106:95-101.

69. Bayston K, Faulkner L, Cohen J: Serum amyloid P in experimental GVHD. Abstract presented at meeting on Cellular mechanisms in infection immunity. Elsinore, Denmark, 1988.

70. Trinchieri G, Perussia B: Immune interferon: a pleiotropic lymphokine with multiple effects. Immunol Today 1986;6;131-136.

71. Le J, Vilcek J: Tumor necrosis factor and interleukin 1: cytokines with multiple overlapping biolocial activities. Lab Invest 1987;56:234-248.

72. Paul NL, Ruddle NH: Lymphotoxin. Ann Rev Immunol 1988;6:407–438.
73. Weetman AP, Rees AJ: Synergistic effects of recombinant tumour necrosis factor and interferon-gamma on rat thyroid cell growth and Ia antigen expression. Immunology 1988;63:285-289.
74. Pober JS, Collins T, Gimbrone MA, Libby P, Reiss CS: Inducible expression of class II major histocompatibility antigens and the immunogenicity of vascular endothelium—Overview. Transplantation 1986;41:141-146.
75. Freundlich B, Bomalaski JS, Neilson E, Jimenez SA: Regulation of fibroblast proliferation and collagen synthesis by cytokines. Immunol Today 1986;7:303-307.
76. Woodbury RG, Neurath H: Purification of an atypical mast cell protease and its levels in developing rats. Biochemistry 1978;17:4298-4304.
77. Roy C, Ghayur T, Kongshavn PAL, Lapp WS: Natural killer activity by spleen lymph node and thymus cells during the graft-versus-host reaction. Transplantation 1982;34:144-146.
78. Kubota E, Ishikawa H, Saito K: Modulation of F_1 cytotoxic potentials by GVHR. Host and donor-derived cytotoxic lymphocytes arise in the unirradiated F_1 host spleens under the condition of GVHR-associated immunosuppression. J Immunol 1983;131:1142-1148.
79. Mowat A McI, Borland A, Parrott DMV: Augmentation of natural killer cell activity by anti-host delayed-type hypersensitivity during the graft-versus-host reaction in mice. Scand J Immunol 1985;22:389-399.
80. Mowat A McI, Felstein MV: Experimental studies of immunologically mediated enteropathy. II. Role of natural killer cells in the intestinal phase of murine graft-versus-host reaction. Immunology 1987;68:179-183.
81. Suttles J, Schwarting GA, Stout RD: Flow cytometric analysis reveals the presence of asialo G_{M1} on the surface membrane of alloimmune cytotixic T lymphocytes. J Immunol 1986;136:1586-1591.
82. Charley MR, Mikhael A, Bennett M, Gilliam JN, Sontheimer RD: Prevention of lethal, minor-determinate graft-host disease in mice by the in vivo administration of anti-asialo GM_1. J Immunol 1983;131:2101-2103.
83. Varkila K: Depletion of asialo-GM1$^+$ cells from the F_1 recipient mice prior to irradiation and transfusion of parental spleen cells prevents mortality to acute graft-versus-host disease and induction of anti-host specific cytotoxic T cells. Clin Exp Immunol 1987;69:652-659.
84. Handa K, Suzuki R, Matsui H, Shimizu Y, Kumagi K: Natural killer (NK) cells as a responder to interleukin 2 (IL2). II. IL2-induced interferon production. J Immunol 1983;130:988-992.
85. Kasahara T, Djeu JY, Dougherty SF, Oppenheim JJ: Capacity of human large granular lymphocytes to produce multiple lymphokines: interleukin 2, interferon and colony stimulating factor. J Immunol 1983;131:2379-2385.
86. Bril H, Van Den Akker Th.W, Molendijk-Lok BD, Bianchi ATJ, Benner R: Influence of 2'-deoxyguanosine upon the development of DTH effector T cells and suppressor T cells in vivo. J Immunol 1984;132:599-604.
87. Zinkernagel RM: Activation or suppression of bactericidal activity of macrophages during a graft-versus-host reaction against I-A and I-J region differences, respectively. Immunogenetics 1980;10:373-382.
88. Liew FY: Regulation of delayed-type hypersensitivity. VII. The role of I-J subregion gene products of delayed-type hypersensitivity to major histocompatibility antigens by specific suppressor T cells. Eur J Immunol 1981;11:883-888.
89. Mowat A McI, Lamont AG, Strobel S, MacKenzie S: The role of antigen processing and suppressor T cells in immune responses to dietary proteins in mice. Adv Exp Med Biol 1987;216A:709-719.

90. Murphy DB: The I-J puzzle. Ann Rev Immunol 1987;5:405-428.

91. Elves MW, Ferguson A: The humoral immune response to allografts of foetal small intestine in mice. Br J Exp Path 1975;56:454-458.

92. Mowat A McI: The immunopathogenesis of food sensitive enteropathies, In *Local Immune Responses of the Gut*, edited by Newby TJ, Stokes CR. CRC Press, FL, 1984; pp. 199-225.

93. Jones JM, Wilson R, Bealmear PM: Mortality and gross pathology of secondary disease in germfree mouse radiation chimeras. Rad Res 1971;45:577-588.

94. van Bekkum DW, Roodenburg J, Heidt PJ, van der Waalt D: Mitigation of secondary disease of allogeneic mouse radiation chimeras by modification of the intestinal microflora. J Nat Canc Inst 1974;52:401.

95. Moore RH, Lampert IA, Chia Y, Aber VR, Cohen J: Influence of endotoxin on graft-versus-host disease after bone marrow transplantation across major histocompatibility barriers in mice. Transplantation 1987;43:731-736.

96. Moore RH, Lampert IA, Chia Y, Aber VR, Cohen J: Effect of immunisation with *Escherichia coli* J5 on graft-versus-host disease induced by minor histocompatibility antigens in mice. Transplantation 1987;44:249-253.

97. Kawakami M, Cerami A: Studies of endotoxin-induced decrease in lipoprotein lipase activity. J Exp Med 1981;154:631.

98. Buckner CD, Clift RA, Sanders JE, Meyers JD, Counts GW, Farewell VT, Thomas ED: Protective environment for marrow transplant recipients. A prospective study. Ann Intern Med 1978;89:893-901.

99. Grundy JE, Shanley JD, Shearer GM: Augmentation of graft-versus-host reaction by cytomegalovirus infections resulting in interstitial pneumonitis. Transplantation 1985;39:548-553.

100. Mowat A McI, Felstein MV, Baca ME: Experimental studies of immunologically mediated enteropathy. III. Severe and progressive enteropathy during a graft-versus-host reaction in athymic mice. Immunology 1987;61:185-188.

101. Bellgrau D, Wilson DB: Immunological studies of T-cell receptors. I. Specifically induced resistance to graft-versus-host disease in rats mediated by host T-cell immunity to alloreactive parental T cells. J Exp Med 1978;148:103-114.

102. Chanana AD, Schaedeli J, Hess MW, Cottier H: Predominance of theta-positive lymphocytes in gut-associated and peripheral lymphoid tissues of newborn mice. J Immunol 1973;110:283-285.

103. Mayrhofer G, Pugh CW, Barclay AN: The distribution, ontogeny and origin in the rat of Ia positive cells with dendritic morphology and of Ia antigen in epithelia, with special reference to the intestine. Eur J Immunol 1983;13:112-122.

104. Mowat A McI, Felstein M: Experimental studies of immunologically mediated enteropathy. V. Destructive enteropathy during an acute graft-versus-host reaction in adult BDF_1 mice. Clin Exp Immunol 1989; in press.

105. Mowat A McI, Sprent J: Induction of intestinal graft-versus-host reactions across mutant major histocompatibility antigens by T lymphocyte subsets in mice. Transplant 1989;47:857-863.

12

Cutaneous Graft-vs.-Host Disease

Beatrix Volc-Platzer and Georg Stingl
University of Vienna Medical School
Vienna, Austria

I. INTRODUCTION

Graft-versus-host disease (GVHD) occurs mainly after allogeneic bone marrow transplantation (BMT), which within the past years has evolved from a last-resort experimental therapy to a first-line treatment for various hematologic and nonhematologic disorders. Despite matching for major histocompatibility (HLA) antigens and prophylactic regimens with immunosuppressive drugs, e.g., methotrexate (MTX) and cyclosporine A (CsA), GVHD occurs in one third to one half of BM recipients. GVHD is a clinical syndrome affecting three major target organs: the gut, the liver, and the skin. Clinicopathologic events within the skin are termed cutaneous GVHD (cGVHD) and the underlying pathogenetic event occurring within target tissues is the "graft-vs.-host reaction" (GVHR). Originally, a GVHR was defined as the interaction of immunocompetent cells of a donor with MHC (major histocompatibility complex)-incompatible cells or tissues of a severely immunosuppressed host (1). This strict definition, i.e., the obligatory requirement of histoincompatibility between donor and host, is no longer tenable since reports exist of acute GVHD arising in recipients of not only allogeneic BM but also syngeneic BM from identical twins (2,3). Experimental models for "syngeneic GVHD" (4)indeed suggest that pathogenic mechanisms other than MHC-restricted cytotoxicity are responsible for tissue necrosis in GVHD. Within this chapter we will describe the clinicopathological features of cGVHD based on animal models and immunopathologic studies of human cGVHD and construct a model for pathogenetic events occurring in this disease.

II. CLINICAL, HISTOPATHOLOGIC, AND IMMUNOPATHOLOGIC ASPECTS OF ACUTE AND CHRONIC CUTANEOUS GVHD

Cutaneous GVHD occurs in both an acute and a chronic form; criteria have been established which allow a classification of cGVHD according to both the type of clinical

Table 1 Acute cGVHR-Clinical Staging

Grade I:	Macularpapular rash involving <25% of the body surface
Grade II:	Macularpapular rash involving >25% of the body surface
Grade III:	Erythroderma
Grade IV:	Toxic epidermal necrolysis-(TEN) like appearance

manifestation as well as the severity of the disease (Tables 1,2) (5-8). Acute cGVHD occurs within the first 3 months after BMT, usually within the first 4 weeks but occasionally as early as 5 days after BMT. Furthermore, acute cGVHD may persist until day 100 after BMT and even longer. Prodromal signs include itching, pain upon pressure, and retroauricular as well as palmoplantar erythema. The predominant feature of early and less severe acute cGVHD is a macular papular rash predominantly involving the central portion of the face ("malar" area), lateral aspects of the trunk, outer surfaces of the extremities, hands and feet, and, occasionally, the axillary and inguinal regions. In certain patients the rash may progress to involve the entire integument, and in most severe, but fortunately rare, instances may lead to the clinical picture of toxic epidermal necrolysis (TEN) (9). Even the experienced dermatologist may encounter difficulties in distinguishing early signs of acute cGVHD from certain drug-induced or viral rashes. In most but not all instances the histopathological evaluation of a skin biopsy may establish the diagnosis of acute cGVHD (see below).

The clinicopathological appearance of chronic cGVHD is quite different from that of acute cGVHD. Chronic cGVHD is frequently, but not regularly, preceded by the acute form of the disease. It usually develops later than day 100 after BMT and may follow the acute form either immediately or after a disease-free interval. The mucocutaneous manifestations of chronic GVHD clinically resemble a wide variety of skin diseases (7) including lichen planus (10,11), lichen sclerosus and atrophicus (Volc-Platzer et al., manuscript in preparation), sicca syndrome (12), and subacute cutaneous lupus erythematosus (Volc-Platzer et al., unpublished observation). In the more advanced stage of the disease, features of systemic scleroderma (7) localized (13), disseminated (12) or predominate, may occasionally involve the underlying fascia, and may thus mimic "eosinophilic fasciitis" (12).

Cytopathic changes of keratinocytes (KC) are the most striking histopathologic feature of acute cGVHD; they range from focal basal cell vacuolization and dyskeratosis or eosinophilic degeneration of scattered epidermal cells to frank necrosis of the entire malpighian layer (Table 3). These epithelial changes, which are not confined to the epidermis but are also found within hair follicle and sebaceous gland epithelium in synchrony with the epidermal lesions, are usually accompanied by a slight-to-moderate

Table 2 Acute cGVHR-Histologic Staging

Grade I:	Basal cell vacuolization
Grade II:	Basal cell vacuolization, single necrotic KC (mummified cells with satellite lymphocytes)
Grade III:	Subepidermal clefts, numerous necrotic KC
Grade IV:	Necrosis of the entire epidermis and complete separation from the dermis

Table 3 Symptoms and Complications of Chronic GVHD

Symptoms	Frequency (%)
skin involvement (dyspigmentation, erythema, lichenoid rashes, scleroderma-like appearance)	90-100
Sicca syndrome including stomatitis and ocular involvement	80
Sicca syndrome with ocular involvement alone	75-80
esophagitis	35-40
serositis	20
myositis	10
bacterial infections	70
weight loss	50
contractures	40

mononuclear cell infiltrate of the papillary dermis. Characteristically, these infiltrating lymphocytes are often clustered around dyskeratotic/necrotic KC ("satellite necrosis"). However, there is usually a striking discrepancy between the pronounced epidermal changes and the rather poor cellular infiltration within the papillary dermis.

Again, if should be remembered that histopathological changes similar to those seen in grade I/grade II acute cGVHD may also be observed after administration of cytotoxic drugs, total body irradiation (14,15), and in the course of viral infections.

Histopathologically, chronic cGVHD is characterized by both cytopathic changes of basal KC and by a pronounced epidermal thickening (i.e., acanthosis), probably resulting from increased KC proliferation, and thus resembles lichen planus. However, the mononuclear cell infiltrate within the papillary and upper reticular dermis is less severe than in "idiopathic" lichen planus and pronounced around dermal blood vessels, hair follicles, and sweat glands. As the disease progresses, the density of the mononuclear cell infiltrate decreases, whereas fibrotic/sclerotic changes within the dermis as well as atrophic changes within the epidermis become increasingly prominent (7,16).

The original assumption that the GVHR is immunologic in nature led several investigators to search for pathologic immune phenomena in the organs affected by this reaction. In both acute and chronic cGVHD IgM and complement components are reportedly deposited along the dermoepidermal junction (17). In addition, recipients of HLA-identical BM have been reported with circulating IgM antibodies cytotoxic for epithelial, but not for lymphoid cells (18). The pathogenetic significance of either event is presently unknown.

In the more recent past, the immunophenotype of resident and passenger cells of GVHD skin biopsies has been extensively studied by using appropriate mAbs in various immunolabeling procedures (19-24).

In acute cGVHD, epidermal Langerhans cells (LC)* as assessed by their surface antigens CD45, CD1a, CD4, HLA-DR, DQ & DP are greatly reduced in number. The few remaining LC are morphologically altered as evidenced by a rounded shape and blunt den-

---

*LC are bone-marrow–derived, dendritic leukocytes with potent antigen-presenting capacity (25).

drites. In the mouse system, there exists evidence that in acute cGVHD LC are numerically reduced and impaired in their antigen-presenting function (26,27). This defect appears to be a consequence of the acute GVHD and cannot be solely explained by the conditioning regimens (e.g., total body irradiation, cyclophosphamide) which by themselves also exert an injurious effect on the LC population.

A most prominent immunohistologic feature of lesional skin biopsies from patients with acute cGVHD is the aberrant expression of class II alloantigens by the KC (19,21, 22). While we find HLA-DR antigens—in addition to the cytoplasmic invariant chain (22) within the KC cytoplasm—and, to a lesser extent, HLA-DP antigens to be expressed rather regularly, we never detected HLA-DQ antigens on KC surfaces (22). Although the significance of HLA-DR/DP-bearing KC for the pathogenesis of acute cGVHD is not yet clear, this pathologic immune phenomenon is of great diagnostic importance as HLA-DR expression by KC precedes the first histopathologic changes in 50% of patients with acute cGVHD (22). In certain cases, there was a striking difference between the paucity of histopathologic changes (Fig. 1) and the prominent band-like expression of HLA-DR antigens by KC (Fig. 2).

Most recently, it has been reported that in certain skin diseases exhibiting HLA-DR-reactive KC (e.g., lichen planus) KC express the intercellular adhesion molecule 1 (ICAM-1) (28,29). In lesional skin biopsies of a few patients with acute cGVHD, we have most recently observed the occurrence of anti-ICAM-1 reactivity of KC, similar in distribution to that seen with anti-HLA-DR reagents.

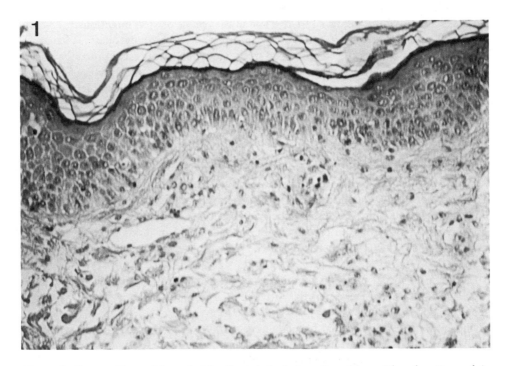

Figure 1 Intraepidermal lymphoid cells and single keratinocytes with pyknotic nuclei within a biopsy from a macularpapular rash occurring 14 days after BMT. (H and E staining, ×150)

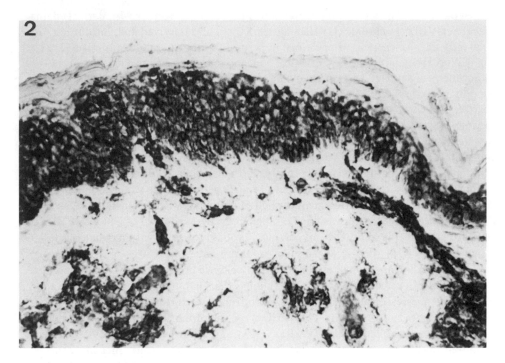

Figure 2 Anti-HLA-DR: striking band-like reactivity of keratinocytes within a serial skin section from the same biopsy. (3-step immunoperoxidase, ×150)

As opposed to these consistent observations on phenotypic alterations of KC in acute cGVHD, the exact phenotype of infiltrating mononuclear cells is not yet well defined. Several authors including ourselves have found that the majority of infiltrating lymphocytes have the CD3$^+$/CD8$^+$ phenotype (19-22). This, however, does not mean that these CD3$^+$/CD8$^+$ cells are the actual effector cells of acute cGVHD, as we and others (19-22) found that the lymphocytes surrounding necrotic KC are not only of the CD3$^+$/CD8$^+$/CD4$^-$, but also frequently of the CD3$^+$/CD4$^-$/CD8$^-$ ("double-negative") phenotype. The immunophenotype of the skin cells in chronic cGVHD shows both similarities and dissimilarities to that seen in acute cGVHD. Within chronic cGVHD lesions, KC almost uniformly express abundant quantities of HLA-DR antigens and ICAM-1 moieties (22; Volc-Platzer et al., manuscript in preparation) and infiltrating T lymphocytes are predominantly CD3$^+$/CD8$^+$ (22). In contrast to acute cGVHD, however, the density of CD1a$^+$ epidermal LC is within normal limits in most patients (22).

III. PATHOGENETIC EVENTS

What is (are) the mechanism(s) leading to the predominating histopathologic feature of cGVHD, i.e., the "dying" keratinocyte? This phenomenon includes vacuolization of basal KC, scattered single cell necrosis (dyskeratosis, "mummified" cells), clefts between epidermis and dermis due to confluent necrosis of basal KC, and frank necrosis of the entire epidermis. These changes are predominantly found—together with dermal edema—in acute cGVHD. In chronic cGVHD, injured KC are also observed and, in addition, one frequently encounters signs of epidermal hyperproliferation and dermal fibrosis (7).

In order to construct a hypothetical concept about the events occurring in the pathogenesis of acute cGVHD, it should be remembered that the epidermal injury may not only occur in the presence, but also in the virtual absence of a significant mononuclear cell infiltrate. Although it is conceivable that cell-to-cell contact is needed for a possible cytotoxic effect of lymphocytes against KC (satellite necrosis), the occurrence of widespread KC necrosis cannot be explained by such a mechanism. It rather appears that soluble mediators released by activated "immunocytes" in the skin or, even, at distant organs, are primarily responsible for the epithelial damage. The fact that the development of an acute GVHD—induced in a semiallogeneic mouse strain combination—can be prevented by in vivo treatment of the BM recipients with an antiserum against TNF-α (30) suggests that this cytokine can be one of the mediators of acute cGVHD. The pathogenetic role of other cytokines most probably present within cutaneous lesions of acute GVHD (IL-1, IFN-γ) remains unclear at present.

The question as to whether donor or host cells are predominantly responsible for KC damage still awaits clarification. The findings that, in both human and murine allogeneic BMT, pretreatment of donor BM with anti-pan T cell reagents results in a decreased incidence and/or severity of cGVHD show that donor cells are required to elicit the final effector mechanisms of cGVHD (31,32). This, however, does not necessarily mean that the allogeneic or even syngeneic (4) donor cells are directly mediating the tissue injury seen in acute cGVHD. In fact, there exist arguments for the contribution of host cells in the development of acute cGVHD in that pretreatment of recipient animals with antiserum against asialo-GM1 reduces the severity of acute cGVHD considerably (33). Following this reasoning, host lymphocytes residing in the target tissues (i.e., the skin) could become activated by donor cells and/or their products and would finally cause epithelial injury. In fact, there is recent evidence that the skin, particularly the epidermis, harbors a population of CD3$^+$ T lymphocytes. From studies on hematopoietic cells in normal skin we know that the majority of these CD3$^+$ T lymphocytes are CD8$^+$, are situated between the basal KC, their highest numbers being observed in volar skin (Foster et al., 33a), which are the sites first involved when GVHD develops. Possibly as a consequence of immunodysregulation induced by transient loss of circulating CD8$^+$ cells (34) (or transient increase and relative predominance of CD4$^+$ cells), these skin T cells would be activated and as so-called autocytotoxic cells (35) mediate KC damage. Enhancement of this phenomenon by LFA-1/ICAM-1 interaction (29,36) appears likely since ICAM-1 expression is observed on either foci of KC or in a band-like distribution within the epidermis of cGVHD lesions.

Our own immunocytochemical studies provide some evidence for the contribution of host cells in the developing cGVHD: in allogeneic murine bone marrow chimeras it has been shown that the resident epidermal LC population is replaced by donor cells (37). In agreement with these findings we detected the male Y-body in epidermal LC of a woman who had received for the treatment of severe aplastic anemia BM from her HLA-matched brother (38). To our surprise, however, we failed to detect the Y-body in lymphocytes infiltrating the skin in this particular patient, which supports the concept that host cells are important effector cells of cGVHD.

The pathogenetic events operative in the development of chronic cGVHD appear different from those leading to acute cGVHD. On the basis of the above data, acute cGVHD is primarily the result of immunodysregulation and not necessarily dependent upon histoincompatibility between donor and host. In contrast, histoincompatibility— at least for minor histocompatibility (miHA) antigens—appears to play a major role in the development of chronic cGVHD in that this syndrome has never been reported following syngeneic or autologous BMT (neither in the animal nor in the human situation). Evidence exists that T cells generated from skin GVH lesions occurring 1-2 months after allogeneic BMT responded to pretransplant recipient cells in a fashion typical for sensitized T cells (39). This indicates that T-cell sensitization against "altered-self" or allogeneic determinants occurs already in the early posttransplant period.

Since chronic cGVHD is in most instances a long-lasting disease, the question arises: "What keeps this process going?" IFN-gamma known to be released by activated T cells (40) either circulating or present within the inflammatory infiltrate, has been shown not only to enhance but also to induce the expression of the adhesion-molecule ICAM-1 (29) as well as of class II alloantigens, by cells which under normal conditions do not express these molecules (41,42). The aberrant expression of ICAM-1 by KC in addition to enhanced expression of this adhesion molecule by endothelial cells may well be responsible for the recruitment of lymphocytes into the skin, thereby increasing the numbers of cells participating in the inflammatory process. The perpetuation of cGVHD activity may further be supported by the usually large number of class II antigen-expressing KC, which by in vitro experiments have been shown to stimulate T-cell blasts (43), thereby substantially augmenting cell mediated immune mechanisms. These activated T cells and/or their products may well induce increased cytokine production by skin cells (predominantly KC), e.g., IL-1, IL-6, GM-CSF, TNF-α, TGF-α. TGF-S (25). It seems reasonable to speculate that such an altered cytokine secretion pattern contributes to the main pathologic features of chronic cGVHD, i.e., epidermal acanthosis as well as fibrosis.

IV. SUMMARY

Acute and chronic skin GVHD appear to be different diseases from clinical, histopathologic, and probably pathogenetic viewpoints. Acute cGVHD is not necessarily the consequence of an antigen-triggered immune response and rather a sequela of immune dysregulation caused by differences in maturation between the various donor cell subpopulations. The direct mechanisms responsible for tissue injury are not entirely clear but probably involve cytokines such as TNF-α. Chronic cGVHD, on the other hand, is much more likely to be due to specific immune response primarily due to miHA differences, and bears many features of autoimmune diseases involving the skin as well.

REFERENCES

1. Billingham RE: The biology of graft-versus-host reactions. Harvey Lect 1966;62: 21-72.
2. Rappaport J, Reinherz E, Mihm M, Lopansri S, Parkman R: Acute graft-versus-host disease in recipients of bone marrow transplants from identical twin donors. Lancet 1979;II:717-720.
3. Gluckman E, Devergie A, Solier J, Saurat JH: Graft-versus-host disease in recipients of syngeneic bone marrow. Lancet 1980;I:253-254.
4. Glazier A, Tutschka PJ, Farmer EA, Santos GW: Graft-versus-host disease in cyclosporin A-treated rats after syngeneic reconstitution. J Exp Med 1983;158:1–8.

5. Glucksberg H, Storb R, Fefer A, Buckner CD, Neiman PE, Clift RA, Lerner KG, Thomas ED: Clinical manifestations of graft-versus-host-disease in human recipients of marrow from HLA-matched sibling donors. Transplantation 1974;18: 295-304.

6. Lerner KG, Kao GF, Storb R, Buckner CD, Clift RA, Thomas ED: Histopathology of graft-versus-host-reaction (GVHR) in human recipients of marrow from HLA-matched sibling donors. Transplant Proc 1974;6:367-371.

7. Shulman HM, Sale GE, Lerner KG, Barker EA, Weiden PL, Sullivan K, Gallucci B, Thomas ED, Storb R: Chronic cutaneous graft-versus-host disease. Am J Pathol 1980;91:545-570.

8. Sullivan KM, Parkman R: The pathophysiology and treatment of graft-versus-host disease. Clinics in Hematol 1983;12:775-789.

9. Peck GL, Herzig GP, Elias PM: Toxic epidermal necrolysis in a patient with graft-vs-host reaction. Arch Dermatol 1972;105:561-569.

10. Touraine R, Revuz J, Dreyfus B, Rochant H, Mannoni P: Graft versus host reaction and lichen planus. Br J Dermatol 1975;92:589.

11. Saurat JH, Didierjean L, Gluckman E, Bussel A: Graft versus host reaction and lichen planus-like eruption in man. Br J Dermatol 1975;92:591-592.

12. Lawley TJ, Peck GL, Montsopoulos HM, Gratwohl AA, Deisseroth AB: Scleroderma, Sjögren-like syndrome, and chronic graft-versus-host disease. Ann Int Med 1977;87:707-709.

13. Van Vloten WA, Scheffer E, Dooren LJ: Localized scleroderma-like lesions after bone marrow transplantation in man: a chronic graft-versus-host reaction. Br J Dermatol 1977;96:337-341.

14. Sale GE, Lerner KG, Barker EA, Shulman HM, Thomas ED: The skin biopsy in the diagnosis of acute graft-versus-host disease in man. Am J Pathol 1977;89: 621-636.

15. Hymes SA, Simonton SC, Farmer EA, Beschorner WB, Tutschka PJ, Santos GW: Cutaneous busulfan effects in patients receiving bone marrow transplantation. J Cut Pathol 1985;12:125-129.

16. Janin-Mercier A, Saurat JH, Bourges M, Sohier J, Didierjean L, Gluckman E: The lichen planus-like and sclerotic phases of the graft versus host disease in man: an ultrastructural study of six cases. Acta Dermatovener 1981;61:187-193.

17. Tsoi M, Storb R, Jones E, Weiden PL, Shulman H, Witherspoon R, Atkinson K, Thomas ED: Deposition of IgM and complement at the dermo-epidermal junction in acute and chronic graft-versus-host disease in man. J Immunol 1982;120: 1485-1492.

18. Merrit CB, Mann DL, Rogentine GN: Cytotoxic antibody for epithelial cells in human graft-versus-host disease. Nature 1971;232:638-639.

19. Lampert IA, Janossy G, Suitters AJ, Bofill M, Palmer S, Gordon Smith E, Prentice H, Thomas JA: Immunologic analysis of the skin in graft-versus-host disease. Clin Exp Immunol 1982;50:123-131.

20. Sloane JP, Thomas JA, Imrie SF, Easton DF, Powles RL: Morphological and immunohistochemical changes in the skin in allogeneic bone marrow recipients. J Clin Pathol 1984;37:919-930.

21. Lever R, Turbitt M, MacKie R, et al.: A prospective study of the histological changes in the skin in patients receiving bone marrow transplants. Br J Dermatol 1986;114:161-170.

22. Volc-Platzer B, Rappersberger K, Mosberger I, Hinterberger W, Emminger-Schmidmeier W, Radaszkiewicz T, Wolff K: Sequential immunohistologic analysis of the skin following allogeneic bone marrow transplantation. J Invest Dermatol 1988; 91:162-168.

23. Perreault D, Pelletier M, Landry D, Gyger M: Study of Langerhans cells after allogeneic bone marrow transplantation. Blood 1984;63:807-811.
24. Murphy GF, Merot Y, Tong AKF, Smith B, Mihm MC Jr: Depletion and repopulation of epidermal dendritic cells after allogeneic bone marrow transplantation in humans. J Invest Dermatol 1985;84:210-214.
25. Stingl G, Hauser C, Tschachler E, Groh V, Wolff K: Immune functions of epidermal cells. In *Immune Mechanisms in Cutaneous Disease*, edited by Norris DA. Marcel Dekker, New York; 1989.
26. Breathnach SM, Shimadas, Kovac Z, Katz SI: Immunological aspects of acute cutaneous graft-versus-host disease: decreased density and antigen-presenting function of Ia$^+$ Langerhans cells and absent antigen-presenting function of Ia$^+$ keratinocytes. J Invest Dermatol 1986;86:226-234.
27. Breathnach SM, Katz SI: Efect of X-irradiation on epidermal immune function: decreased density and alloantigen presenting capacity of Ia$^+$ Langerhans cells and impaired production of epidermal cell derived thymocyte activating factor (ETAF). J Invest Dermatol 1985;85:538-553.
28. Dustin ML, Rothlein R, Bhan AK, Dinarello CA, Springer TA: Induction by IL-1 and interferon γ, tissue distribution, biochemistry, and function of a natural adherence molecule (ICAM-1). J Immunol 1986;137:245-254.
29. Dustin ML, Singer KH, Tuck DT, Springer TA: Adhesion of T lymphoblasts to epidermal keratinocytes is regulated by interferon-γ and is mediated by intercellular adhesion molecule 1 (ICAM-1). J Exp Med 1988;167:1323-1340.
30. Piguet P-F, Grau GE, Allet B, Vassalli P: Tumor necrosis factor/cachectin is an effector of skin and gut lesions of the acute phase of graft-vs.-host disease. J Exp Med 1987;166:1280-1289.
31. Korngold R, Sprent J: Lethal graft-versus-host disease after bone marrow transplantation across minor histocompatibility barriers in mice. Prevention by removing mature T cells from marrow. J Exp Med 1978,148:1687-1698.
32. Neudorf S, Filipovich A, Ramsay N, Kersey J: Prevention and treatment of acute graft-versus-host disease. Semin Haematol 1984;21:91-100.
33. Charley MR, Mikhael A, Bennet M, Gilliam JN, Sontheimer RD: Prevention of lethal, minor-determinate graft-host disease in mice by the in vivo administration of anti-asialo-GM$_1$. J Immunol 1983;131:2101-2105.
33a. Foster CA, Yokofeki H, Rappersberger K, Koning I, Volc-Platzer B, Rieger A, Coligan JE, Wolff K, Stiugl G: Human epidermal T cells predominately belong to the lineage expressing α/S T cell receptor. J Exp Med 1900;in press.
34. Reinherz EL, Parkman R, Rappaport J, Rosen FS, Schlossmann SF: Aberrations of suppressor T cells in human graft-versus-host disease. N Engl J Med 1979;300:1061-1068.
35. Parkman R, Rappaport J, Rosen FS: Human graft-versus-host disease. J Invest Dermatol 1980;74:276-279.
36. Krensky AM, Robbins E, Springer TA, Burakoff SJ: LFA-1, LFA-2 and LFA-3 antigens are involved in CTL-target-conjugation. J Immunol 1984;132:2180-2182.
37. Katz SI, Tamaki K, Sachs DH: Epidermal Langerhans cells are derived from cells originating in the bone marrow. Nature 1979;282:324-326.
38. Volc-Platzer B, Stingl G, Wolff K, Hinterberger W, Schnedl W: Cytogenetic identification of allogeneic epidermal Langerhans cells in a bone-marrow-graft-recipient. N Engl J Med 1984;310:1123-1124.
39. Reinsmoen NL, Kersey JH, Bach FH: Detection of HLA restricted anti-minor histocompatibility antigen(s) reactive cells from skin GVHD lesions. Human Immunol 1984;II:249-257.

40. Kelso A, Glasebrook AL: Secretion of interleukin 2, macrophage activating factor, interferons, and colony-stimulating factor by alloreactive T lymphocyte clones. J Immunol 1984;132:2924-2931.
41. Volc-Platzer B, Stingl G: HLA-DR synthesis and expression by human keratinocytes, In *Exp Çlin Photoimmunol.*, edited by Daynes RA, Krueger G. CRC Press, Boca Raton, FL, 1986; pp. 119-126.
42. Auböck J, Romani N, Grubauer G, Fritsch P: HLA-DR expression on keratinocytes is a common feature of diseased skin. Br J Dermatol 1986;114:465-472.
43. Niederwieser D, Auböck J, Troppmair J, Herold M, Schuler G, Boeck G, Lotz J, Fritsch P, Huber C: IFN-γ mediated induction of MHC antigen expression on human keratinocytes and its influence on in vitro alloimmune responses. J Immunol 1988;140:2556-2564.

13

Tumor Necrosis Factor and Graft-vs.-Host Disease

Pierre-Francois Piguet
Centre Medical Universitaire
Geneva, Switzerland

I. THE ELUSIVE PATHOGENESIS OF GVHD

Graft-vs-Host Disease (GVHD) is a complex disease resulting from the introduction of foreign T lymphocytes into an immunocompromised host. It principally consists of runting (or cachexia), atrophy of the lymphohematopoietic organs (leading to infection and hemorrhage), and damage to the epithelia, with necrosis of epithelial cells. The pathogenesis of these alteration is obscure; although they are undoubtedly triggered by the foreign T lymphocytes (1), the relationship between the donor T lymphocyte and the damaged organ is far from clear. Indeed, GVHD lesions are extremely difficult to explain on the basis of accepted patterns of T-cell function, such as cell mediated lymphosis (CML) or the delayed-type hypersensitivity reaction (DTH) (2). Thus, the recent identification of tumor necrosis factor (TNF), a cytokine whose production is increased by the activation of T lymphocytes and which can induce cachexia and cell necrosis, has improved our understanding of the pathogenesis of these lesions.

II. TNF: A CYTOKINE WITH CYTOPATHIC PROPERTIES

Initially, TNF was investigated as a factor capable of inducing tumor necrosis. However, since the purification of the protein (3) and the cloning and expression of the gene in *E. coli* (4,5), interest in TNF has increased far beyond its ability to damage tumors. TNF-alpha is a 17.5 kD protein, encoded by a gene that is closely associated with the major histocompatibility complex (MHC). Macrophages are the major source of this cytokine in physiological circumstances, but several other cell types, including T lymphocytes (6), NK cells (7) and mast cells (8), have been reported to produce TNF. Recent articles have reviewed the cellular and molecular biology of TNF (9-12). This chapter will highlight primarily the properties of TNF observed in rodents in vivo.

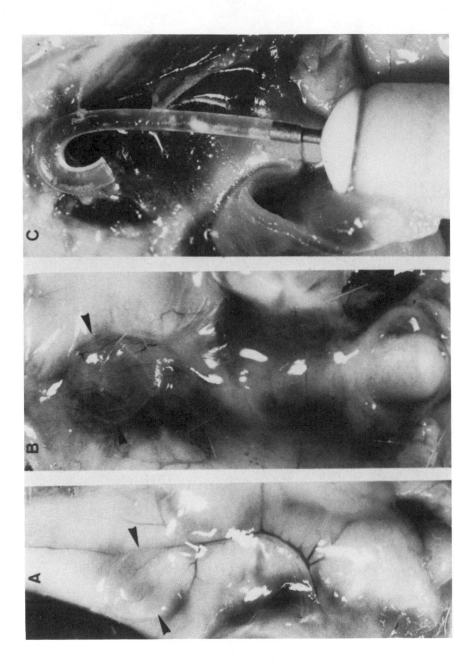

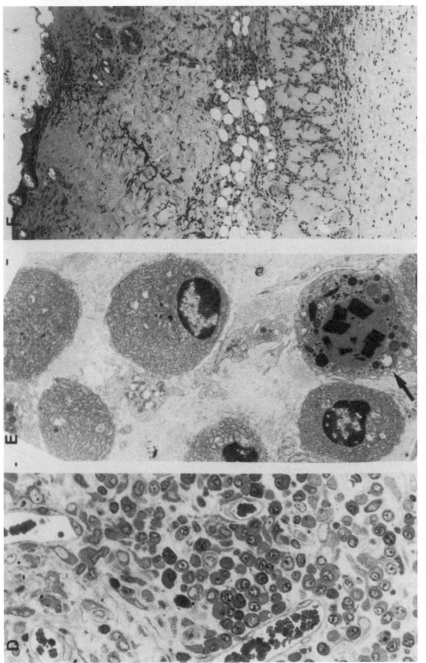

Figure 1 Infusion of mouse rTNF in continuous hypodermic perfusion during 7 days using an osmotic pump connected to a cannula. (A,B,C) Macroscopic aspect: (A), solvent only; (B), mouse rTNF at 0.8 μg/day. The area of infusion has induced the formation of a tissue mass (arrows); (C), mouse rTNF at 4 μg/day. There is complete necrosis of the surrounding tissue. (D and E) Light electron microscopy of the mass shown in B, with blood vessels and fibroblasts having an abundant RE. One cell is undergoing apoptotic degeneration (arrow). (F) Light microscopy of the border of the necrotic area shown in panel C.

Injection of human rTNF in rodents leads to fever, shock, intravascular coagulation, and disseminated necrosis. These effects resemble those produced by endotoxemia (13-17). Susceptibility to TNF can be increased by galactosamine (18) or adrenalectomy (19); it can be decreased by cyclooxygenase inhibitors (14,16). Human rTNF strongly synergizes with LPS and IL-1 to induce hemorrhagic necrosis in mice (20). Repeated injections induce cachexia and the breakdown of the fatty tissue (21). Thus, the administration of TNF in vivo affects many organs: hemopoietic tissues (myeloid reaction), the intestinal tract (hemorrhagic necrosis), the liver (midzonal necrosis), and the lung (alveolar damage).

In our studies, mouse rTNF (22) has been administered to mice in continuous perfusion through an osmotic pump (Fig. 1). When infused at a rate of 4 μg/day, mouse rTNF induces necrosis of the surrounding tissue. The lesion appears as a coagulation necrosis which affects the dermis, epidermis, striated muscle, and bone; in short, the whole thoracic wall is involved (Fig. 1 C and F). Mouse rTNF is much more necrotizing than human rTNF when administered to mice and is toxic alone; no synergism with LPS or Il-1 appears to be required (20, and our own experiments). Different strains of mice vary in their susceptibility of necrosis; B10 are highly susceptible while CBA are relatively resistant. The necrosis is resistant to various treatments including indomethacine, irradiation or anti LPS IgG, anticoagulant therapy, passive immunization with anti-LPS antibodies, or the removal of leukocytes and platelets from the circulation. However, local necrosis can be completely prevented by injection of anti-TNF IgG. TNF therefore appears to be a cytokine with extraordinary and possibly unique necrotizing properties when given in vivo.

When the dose of TNF is decreased (e.g., to 0.8 μg/day), continuous infusion of TNF induces the formation of a tissue mass made of fibroblasts and blood vessels (Fig. 1 B and D). TNF can therefore also act as a growth factor for fibroblast and endothelial cells, as previously reported (23,24). However, even when TNF administration induces cellular proliferation, it also increases the number of cells undergoing apoptotic degernation: these alterations are evident among fibroblasts (Fig. 1E) and within lymphohematopoietic organs. Apoptosis is a normal process evident within tissues with a high turnover rate, such as the epithelium of the digestive tract and the thymus (25,26). It can be recognized on electron microscopy (EM) by a condensation of the nuclear and cytoplasmic organelles, followed by fragmentation of the nucleus despite the presence of an intact cell membrane. These alterations have been interpreted as an active self-destructive process that may subserve some homeostatic function (26).

Evidence for an important role for TNF in various pathological processes is suggested by the results of the passive immunization with anti-TNF antibodies. This treatment prevents the lethal effects of LPS injections, and thus TNF appears to be the principal endogenous effector of the endotoxin toxicity (27). It also prevents the hemorrhagic necrosis of brain venulae that occurs during cerebral malaria (28). This complication is elicited by the response of CD4[+] T lymphocytes to the parasite (29). TNF may therefore also be an important component of T-cell-mediated immunopathologic reactions.

III. GVHD INCREASES THE PRODUCTION OF TNF

GVHD does not lead to a detectable increase of serum TNF activity (30) as is the case with endotoxemia or a malarial infection. However, many cells, particularly endothelial cells, are capable of binding TNF (31) and therefore a lack of serum activity does not ex-

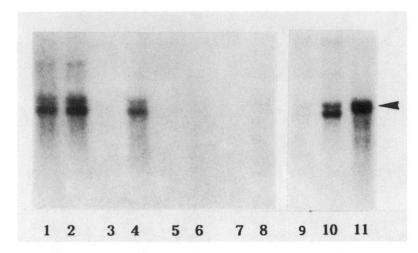

Figure 2 Northern blot analysis of the TNF-alpha mRNA. Lanes 1–10 were loaded with
4 μg of the RNA extracted from the organs of F_1 B10 X CBA mice, 15 days after irradiation and injection of B10 T-depleted BMC (i.e., controls, odd-numbered lanes) or BMC
and T lymphocytes (i.e., GVHR, even-numbered lanes). 1 and 2, spleen; 3 and 4, lung; 5
and 6, skin; 7 and 8, gut; 9 and 10, lungs from another experiment; 11, lung from a normal mice, injected i.v. with 100 μg of LPS 60' before sacrifice. Arrow, the position of the
18S.

clude an increase of the production of the cytokine in GVHD. A possible role for TNF
is suggested by Northern blot analysis, which indicates that GVHD markedly increases
TNF mRNA levels (Fig. 2). In this experiment, mice were lethally irradiated and reconstituted either with T-depleted bone marrow cell (BMC) alone or with BMC plus T lymphocytes, which led to lethal GVHD in 20-30 days (30,32,33). RNA was extracted from
various organs 15 days after bone marrow transplantation and probed for TNF mRNA.
An increase in the TNF mRNA level in mice with GVHD was easily detectable within the
spleen and the lung (Fig. 2, tracks 2, 4, 10) and much less so in the skin and gut (Fig. 2,

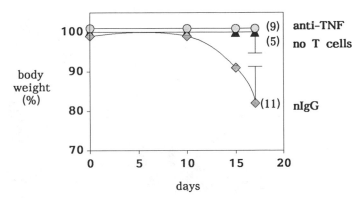

Figure 3 Body weight, in % of the controls, of mice injected with T-depleted BMC; 0–0
or BMC and T lymphocyte (i.e., GVHR) treated with nonimmune IgG or anti-TNF IgG.

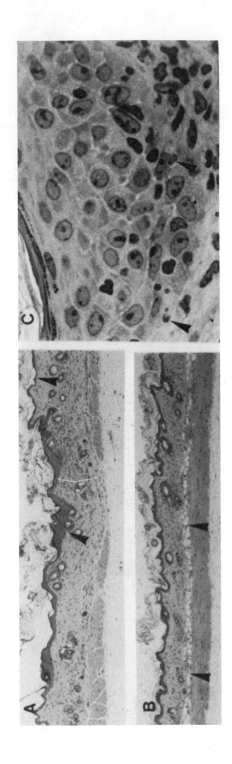

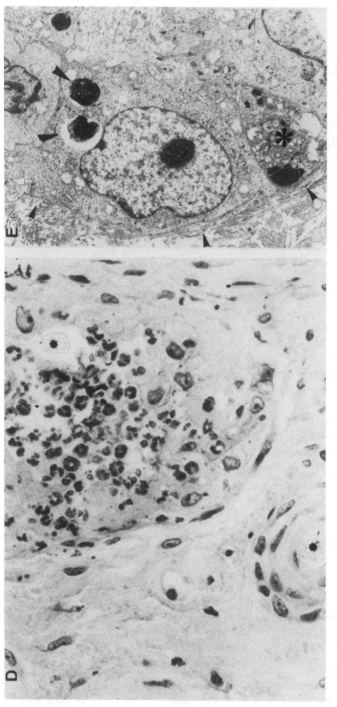

Figure 4 Skin from mice with GVHD (day 15), treated with nonimmune (A) or anti-TNF (B) IgG. (A) Foci of epidermal atrophy and regeneration (arrows) and the absence of hypodermic fat are evident. (B) The hypodermic fat is present (arrow), and the epidermis has a regular thickness. (C) Detail of a lichenoid regeneration, with isolated cell necrosis (arrows). (D) Two hair follicles (star) from a GVHR mouse; one is necrotic with numerous epithelial cells in fragmentation resembling polymorphonuclear leukocytes. (E) EM aspect of a keratinocyte located above the basement membrane (arrows) with two large apoptotic bodies (wide arrows). Nearby, the remnant of a disintegrated cell (star).

tracks 6 and 8). A lethal dose of LPS (100 μg, injected i.v.) induces an increase in TNF mRNA comparable to GVHD (Fig. 2, tracks 10 and 11). There are two notable differences, however, between the induction of TNF message by LPS and by GVHD: (1) the increase of TNF transcription is short-lived after LPS injection (detectable only for 2-3 hr after injection), whereas the mRNA induced by GVHD can still be detected up to 25 days after bone marrow transplantation (BMT); (2) the TNF mRNA induced by T lymphocytes is of a smaller size than that induced by LPS (Fig. 2, tracks 10 and 11).

IV. INFLUENCE OF THE PASSIVE IMMUNIZATION WITH ANTI-TNF IgG ON GVHD

The following experiments have been described elsewhere (30,34) and will only be briefly reviewed here. Results are based on the administration of approximately 2 mg/week of deaggregated polyclonal rabbit anti-TNF-alpha IgG to mice with GVHD after BMT. These antibodies have no detectable cross-reaction towards TNF-beta. As previously mentioned, such injections prevent the necrosis and morbility elicited by the continuous mouse rTNF (4 μg/day). The aspects of GVHD that are affected by anti-TNF antibody injections are enumerated below.

1. *Mortality*. The antibody treatment delays the GVHD-induced mortality. This delay has been observed in various donor-host strain combinations, involving major histocompatibility differences, minor loci only, or differences limited to MHC class I or II products.

2. *Cachexia (or runting)*. GVHD is associated with a loss of 20-30% of the body weight together with the disappearance of hypodermic fat. Passive immunization with anti-TNF antibodies prevents the weight loss and preserves hypodermic fat stores (Figs. 3 and 4, A and B).

3. *Hemopoietic failure*. GVHD turns off the hemopoietic reconstitution after BMT (33). The presence of anti-TNF IgG increases the rate of hemopoietic reconstitution by increasing both the total splenic cellularity and the frequency of stem cells (CFU-S) in the spleen (unpublished observations).

4. *Epidermal GVHD*. The epidermal lesions of GVHD appear on low-power microscopy as regions of epidermal atrophy and regeneration (lichenoid reaction (Fig. 4A))

Table 1 Epithelial Lesion of GVHD: Effect of α-TNF

BMT	Treatment	Epidermis		Gut		Lung mitosis
		necrosis	mitosis	necrosis	mitosis	
BMC	—	11(8)	2.5(1)	0.2(0.1)	0.7(0.2)	0.02(0.02)
BMC + T	nIg	64(37)	4.2(3)	0.8(0.4)	1.6(0.3)	4.00(2.34)
BMC + T	α-TNF	23(17)	2.6(2)	0.4(0.3)	0.6(0.4)	2.50(0.80)

CBA × B10 F_1 mice were injected with B10 T-depleted BMC (control) or with BMC and T lymphocytes (GVHD). They were injected on day 7 with 2 mg of rabbit IgG and killed on day 15. Epidermis and gut: number of necrotic cell or of mitotic figures/microscopic field × 10^{-2}. Lung: number of alveolar mitosis/microscopic field × 10^{-2}. Results are the mean (±SD) of the value of 5 or more individual mice examined on day 15 after BMT (B10 vs CBA × B10F_1 strain combination).

and at the cellular level as the chnges in keratinocyte (5) (Fig. 4C,D,E). By electron microscopy (EM), damaged keratinocytes show features of apoptotic degneration (Fig. 4E). These alterations are significantly prevented by anti-TNF IgG (Fig. 4A and B and Table 1).

5. *Intestinal GVHD.* By light microscopy, the alterations induced by GVHD are characterized by hypertrophy (i.e., enlargement of the small bowel (30)) and by architectural changes in the mucosa (elevation of the crypts and atrophy of the villae (Fig. 5A and B)). At the cellular level, there is an increase in both the number of necrotic enterocytes and in mitotic regeneration (Fig. 5C and D and Table 1). The necrosis within the crypts shows features of apoptosis (Fig. 5E and F). Injections of anti-TNF markedly prevents these alterations (Table 1 and Fig. 5A and B).

6. *GVHD-induced alveolar damage.* Alveolae are not a recognized target of the acute phase of GVHD (35,36). However, in some strain combinations, GVHD induces a severe alveolitis, characterized by alveolar hemorrhage (Fig. 6A), damage of both endothelial and epithelial cells, and an increase of the alveolar mitotic index (34) (Fig. 6B,D,E). These alterations, which are not distinguishable from those produced by a 3-day infusion of mouse rTNF at a rage of 4 μg/day (22), are partially prevented by anti-TNF antibodies (Fig. 6C and Table 1).

7. *Anti-TNF IgG does not effect T lymphocyte activation.* The presence of anti-TNF IgG does not prevent the activation of the parental T lymphocytes injected in an irradiated F_1 recipient (30). This indicates that the blockade of the GVHD-induced tissue damage does not occur at the level of the T-cell response but rather "downstream" at the level of TNF-mediated damage.

8. *Anti-TNF IgG does not affect the chronic phase of GVHD.* We have explored the influence of anti-TNF antibodies upon hepatitis, which develops 25 days after BMT in our GVHD models. Antibodies had no detectable influence upon chronic hepatocellular damage.

9. *Anti-TNF does not affect hybrid resistance (HR).* In some strain combinations, hemopoietic reconstitution is delayed by the "resistance" of the irradiated host to the bone marrow graft (37). HR affects both parental bone marrow cells (BMC) and T lymphocytes injected into irradiated F_1 recipients (38). The radioresistant host cell(s) responsible for HR are not yet clearly identified and might comprise cells of the monocytic and LGL or NK lineages. Presence of anti-TNF does not markedly diminish HR to parental hemopoietic grafts (unpublished observations).

V. CELLULAR ORIGIN AND STIMULI OF TNF SECRETION

A. T Lymphocytes

TNF can be produced by T-cell lines in vitro (6), but it is rather unlikely that donor T lymphocytes are the major source of the cytokine during the GVHD; they are low producers when compared to macrophages, and their number is too low within GVHD-affected organs. Indeed, when GVHD lesions are severe and the transcription of TNF mRNA is markedly increased (e.g., 15 days after BMT), the presence of donor T cells with significant antihost activity is extremely difficult to detect. In fact, the disease cannot be transferred by lymphoid cells isolated from the organ of diseased animals as has been observed by initial investigations of GVHD (39) and by ourselves (unpub-

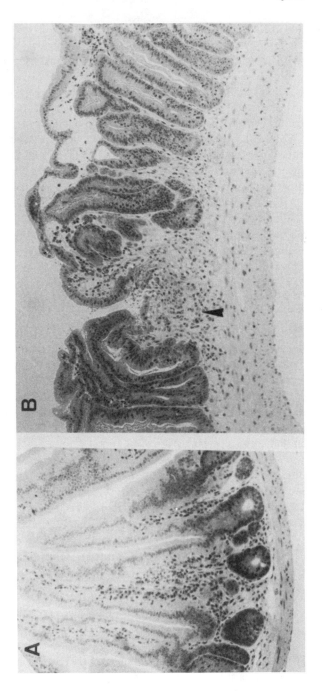

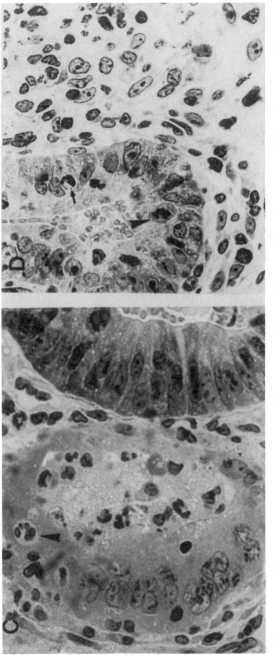

Figure 5 Duodenal mucosa of GVHD mice treated with anti-TNF (A), or control IgG (B-E). Elevation of the crypts, flattening of the villae, and a disintegrated crypt (arrow) are evident in B. (C) Two adjacent crypts, one showing disintegrative changes with numerous fragmented cells. (D) A severely damaged crypt (left) has isolated necrosis and mitotic cells (arrows); the remnant of an already disintegrated crypt is seen on the right. (E) EM of an enterocyte in mitosis and apoptotic enterocytes (arrows). (F) Bottom of a crypt with two apoptotic enterocytes (arrows) in absence of lymphoid infiltration. (G) Low magnification of the upper crypt showing two dead enterocytes (arrows) in coagulation necrosis.

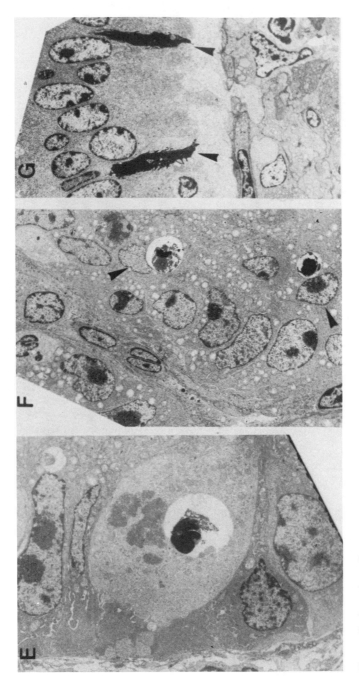

Figure 5 (continued)

lished observations). Furthermore, the frequency of antihost T lymphocytes detectable by limiting dilution analysis (LDA) is always below 10^{-4} (32).

B. Cells of Other Lineages Activated by T-Cell-Derived Lymphokines

Macrophages, which appear to be the most significant source of TNF, can be increased in number and/or activated to secrete TNF by a variety of cytokines such as GM-CSF, interleukin-3, and interferon-gamma. Infusion of mice with rGM-CSF increases the TNF mRNA level in various organs (unpublished observations). Antibodies to GM-CSF (in association with anti-IL-3) prevent the elevation of the serum TNF level associated with cerebral malaria (40).

Anti-GM-CSF IgG also attenuates the epidermal lesions of the acute phase of GVHD (unpublished observation). IFN gamma has been shown to increase the production of TNF by macrophages in vitro, but antibody to IFN gamma, which prevents cerebral malaria, does not attenuate the acute phase of GVHD and, in fact, exerbates it (unpublished observation). Infusion of recombinant human interleukin-2 (IL-2) to mice increases the number of large granular lymphocytes (LGL) in various organs, including epithelia (42). The number of LGL also increases in epithelia and mucosa during GVHD, where they are suspected of playing a pathogenic role (34,43,44). A role for IL-2 during GVHD is also supported by the protective influence of the passive immunization with anti-IL-2 receptor antibody (45).

C. Endogenous LPS

LPS is a potent inducer of the secretion of TNF by macrophages (11), and one might therefore suspect that GVHD favors the entry of LPS into the circulation from the gut, thereby increasing the production of TNF. Administration of LPS to mice has been reported to influence the course of GVHD (46). It is difficult, however, to explain the increase of the production of TNF via endogeneous LPS because LPS injections do not induce an the same TNF mRNA as GVHD (Fig. 2) and because injection of LPS induces mainly vascular lesions, whereas GVHD produces epithelial lesions with only moderate vascular participation.

VI. FEATURES OF CELL NECROSIS INDUCED BY GVHD

As GVHD and the perfusion of TNF share the capacity to induce disseminated cell necrosis, this aspect of GVHD will be discussed in more detail.

A. Difficulties of Quantification

The evaluation of the incidence of epithelial cell necrosis is rather imprecise because the lethally damaged cells are relatively "short-lived," i.e., the period of time between the recognizable damage and the complete cellular disintegration is relatively short. In addition, the evaluation of the number of isolated necrotic cells per microscopic field does not take into account the more massive necrosis, which is frequently observed (see

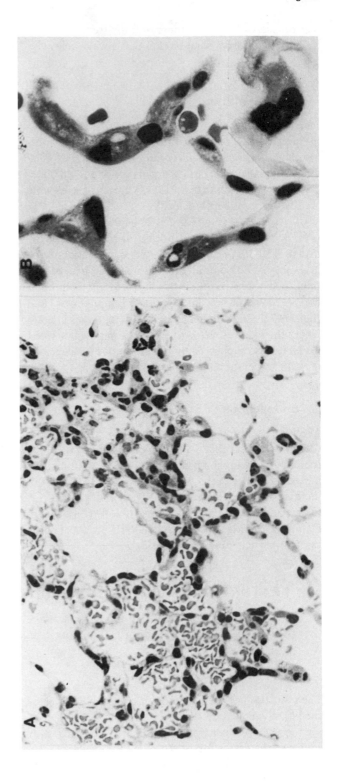

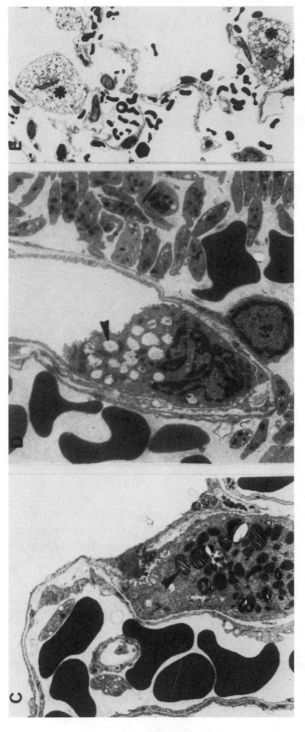

Figure 6   (A) Alveolar hemorrhage. (B) Necrosis of the alveolar septa from mouse with GVHD treated with anti-TNF IgG; a type 2 epithelial cell contains lamellated bodies (arrows). (C) EM of an alveolar septa and mitotic figure (insert). (D) Alveolar GVHD, showing platelet aggregation (right) and a damaged type 2 epithelial cell with a fragmented nucleus and emptied lamallated bodies (arrow). (E) Alveolar GVHD, showing the detachment of dying alveolar cells (star).

B. Epithelial Cell Necrosis in Different BMT Conditions

Table 2 summarizes our past studies on the conditions leading to lethal GVHD and to an increase in cell necrosis after BMT. GVHD to both MHC or non-MHC produces cellular necrosis. It can be induced by either $CD4^+$ or the $CD8^+$ T lymphocytes (47). In addition an HVGR can also lead to detectable necrosis in some strain combinations; thus, the transfer of T-cell-depleted BMC from an F_1 donor to an irradiated parental recipient can induce lesions that are basically similar to those of GVHD (Table 2). This observation suggests that the response of the irradiated host against the graft can be self-damaging.

C. Apoptotic Degeneration

EM studies have described the cellular necrosis of GVHD as apoptotic degeneration (48), but the distinction between apoptosis and the other forms of necrosis has frequently been omitted. As apoptotic degeneration is a normal process that is evident in tissue with a rapid turnover rate (see Section II), GVHD (and the administration of TNF) may induce the acceleration of a normal physiologic process.

D. Cell Necrosis Affects Either Isolate Cells or Whole Structures

Cells undergoing apoptotic degeneration are frequently found in isolation (Figs. 4E, 5E,F, 6D). In addition, the necrosis may take the form of crypt or follicilar "pseudo-abscesses" (so-called follicular GVHD) (49). These lesions correspond to a synchronized necrosis of large numbers of cells, resulting in the fragmentation of epithelial surfaces which resembles polymorphonuclear infiltration (see Fig. 4D and 5B,C,D). GVHD-induced alveolitis can also evolve toward the necrosis of the whole alveolar septa (Fig. 6B).

E. Epithelial Necrosis Preferentially Affects Germinal Cells

This notion has been suggested by studies of the epidermal cell necrosis of human GVHD, which are predominantly located within the rete ridge (50). In the intestinal mucosa, apoptotic degeneration is evident among enterocytes from the crypts (Fig. 5E and F), which also contains germinal cells (51). Apoptosis of a mitotic figure can be observed (Fig. 5E). Enterocytes in coagulation necrosis (i.e., "aged" dead cells, Fig. 5G) are observed along the villae. In light of the migration of enterocytes from the crypt up to the villae (51), these findings suggest that the initial enterocyte damage occurred within the crypt.

F. Cell Necrosis Associated with an Increase of Cellular Regeneration

Cell necrosis and regeneration appear closely associated, but each organ has its peculiarities (see Table 1). In the alveolar epithelium, which has a very low turnover rate, GVHD causes a striking increase in the mitotic rate. The necrosis is extremely difficult to score in this organ because the damaged cells detach from the basement membrane and disintegrate as floating cells. In the intestinal mucosae, where the turnover rate is normally rapid, the effect induced by GVHD is modest (Table 1). An increase of the mitotic rate could be considered to be a compensation for the reduction of the life expectance of the differentiated cells (52) and thus could represent an indirect evaluation of cell death.

Table 2 Epithelial Lesions Induced by Various Histocompatibility Loci and by CD-4 or CD-8T Lymphocytes

| Donor | | Host | | | | | Epidermal |
BMC	T	(rx)	Donor/host	Treatment	MST	Enteropathy	necrosis
B10	0	B10	–	–	>80	1.0(0.1)	1.0
(CBA × B10)F1	0	B10	H-2 + lm	–	>80	3.1(1.1)	2.1(0.3)
CBA	0	CBA	–	–	>80	1.0(0.1)	1.0(0.6)
(CBA × B10)F1	0	CBA	H-2 + lm	–	>80	1.1(0.2)	1.2(0.4)
B10	0	(CBA × B10)F1	H-2 + lm	–	>80	1.0(0.1)	1.0
B10	B10, 10^6	(CBA × B10)F1	H-2 + lm	–	19	1.5 (0.3)	3.0(2.0)
B10	B10, 10^6	(CBA × B10)F1	H-2 + lm	αCD-8	27	1.8(0.5)	3.0(2.0)
B10	B10, 10^6	(CBA × B10)F1	H-2 + lm	αCD-4	34	3.8(1.0)	4.0(3.0)
B6H-2k	0	CBA	lm	–	>80	1.0(0.2)	1.0
B6H-2k	B6H-2k, 10^6	CBA	lm	–	25	1.4(0.8)	14.8(6.4)
B6H-2k	B6H-2k, 10^6	CBA	lm	αCD-8	35	0.9(0.4)	9.5(3.2)
B6H-2k	B6H-2k, 10^6	CBA	lm	αCD-4	40	0.9(0.4)	4.4(3)
B10.A(6R)	0	B10.AQR	MHC class II	–	>80	1.0(0.3)	1.0
B10.A(6R)	B10.A(6R), 10^5	B10.AQR	MHC class II	–	16	1.4(0.2)	6.3(3.9)
B10.A(6R)	B10.A(6R), 10^5	B10.AQR	MHC class II	αCD-8	12	0.9(0.1)	30.5(3.0)
B10.A(6R)	B10.A(6R), 10^5	B10.AQR	MHC class II	αCD-4	18	1.4(0.4)	7.0(3.0)
B10.A	0	B10.A(2R)	MHC class I	–	80	1.0(0.1)	1.0
B10.A	B10.A(2R), 5×10^6	B10.A(2R)	MHC class I	–	19	1.0(0.1)	3.7(2.1)
B10.A	B10.A(2R), 5×10^6	B10.A(2R)	MHC class I	αCD-8	25	1.2(0.2)	9.2(4.2)
B10.A	B10.A(2R), 5×10^6	B10.A(2R)	MHC class I	αCD-4	30	2.5(1.2)	3.6(1.7)

MST = mean survival time. lm = minor Poci.
Enteropathy has been scored as the ratio of the increase of the length of the crypts compared to the BMC controls. Epidermal necrosis, number of isolated necrotic cells/microscopic field $\times 10^{-2}$. Treatment with the anti-CD monoclonal antibodies has been performed both in vitro and in vivo (47). Results are the mean of 5 or more mice examined on day 15.

VII. T-CELL-INDUCED AND TNF-MEDIATED TISSUE DAMAGE (T-TNF)

Our studies of the role of TNF in GVHD and in cerebral malaria have led us to hypothesize the existence of a T-cell-induced, TNF-mediated type of tissue damage (T-TNF). In contrast to the classical concepts of CML and DTH, which require the presence of the T lymphocyte inside the lesion and the specific recognition of the affected cell, the T-TNF type of damage requires neither; the activation of T lymphocytes can lead, by the diffusion of TNF, to the damage of distant organs without immunologic recognition in situ. This concept helps to explain phenomena which are not easily explained by the classical notion of T-cell-mediated immunity:

A. Epithelial Cell Necrosis Without Lymphocyte Contact or the Problem of "Isolated Cell Necrosis"

Lymphocyte-target cell contact might not always be required for epithelial cell necrosis. Contacts between leukocyte (i.e., a lymphocyte or a large granular leukocyte) and necrotic keratinocytes have been observed (44,53), but the significance of this contact is difficult to determine. In my own study of the necrosis of the crypts on electron micrographs, the cells in apoptotic degeneration were not more frequently in contact with an intraepithelial lymphocyte than those unaffected (see Fig. 5F). Furthermore, the more massive necrosis such as intestinal crypt disintegration, epidermal follicular GVHD, and diffuse alveolar damage occur without significant lymphocytic infiltration (Fig. 4B, 5C and D, 6B). It therefore seems reasonable to envision that diffusion of TNF across the basement membrane might play a role. TNF might be produced either by cells from the chorion or submucosa, or even from cells farther away, such as spleen or the lung cells, as these organs appear to be the major TNF producers (Fig. 2).

B. Runting or Cachexia

The rapid breakdown of the hypodermic fat in absence of a local inflammtory reaction fits with the concept of a T-TNF type of systemic disease.

C. Specificity of Tissue Damage Induced by GVHD and HVGR

GVHD enteropathy has previously been described as the damage of an "innocent bystander"; donor T cells can damage intestinal grafts of the donor as well as the host genotype (43,54). This absence of specificity at the effector level is best explained by the diffusion of a nonspecific cytopathic mediator. Similarly, lesion of the HVGR described above might be explained by a "backward" induction of TNF in the BM—derived F_1 donor by radioresistant host T cells. In our experiments, the lesions are more severe in the F1B10 than in the F1CBA strain combination, a difference which might be due to the greater susceptibility of the B10 to TNF-induced necrosis (see Section II).

D. Role of MHC Class I or II Loci and T Lymphocyte Subclasses

If there are indeed quantitative differences in the number of T lymphocytes required to induce lethal GVHD to different MHC class I or II antigens (33,55), the lesions, such as cell necrosis and cachexia, are surprisingly similar whatever the locus involved (47). Both $CD4^+$ and $CD8^+$ T lymphocytes are capable of increasing cell necrosis in GVHD (in fact,

the CD4$^+$ "helpers" are more efficient inducers of cell necrosis than the CD8$^+$ "killers")
and the resultant tissue alterations are disappointingly similar (47). We suspect both T
lymphocyte subsets (and response elicited by either class I or II MHC loci) are capable of
increasing the production of TNF by the secretion of cytokines such as GM-CSF and may
therefore produce similar lesions.

VIII. CONCLUSIONS

I have presented evidence indicating that TNF plays a key role as an effector of the lesions of the acute phase of GVHD. There are: (1) infusion of TNF can mimic many of
the manifestations of the acute phase of GVHD, notably cell necrosis and cachexia, (2)
GVHD increases the production of TNF; and (3) passive immunization with anti-TNF
antibodies prevents GVHD lesions. This interpretation simplifies the understanding of a
complex disease, whose different manifestations might be related to the effect of a diffus-
ible mediator with cytopopathic properties.

ACKNOWLEDGMENTS

I express my gratitude to G. Grau, P. Vassalli, and J. H. Saurat for a critical reading of the
manuscript, to V. DuBose for its preparation, and to A. F. Rochat, M. C. Peclet, G. Ley-
vraz, and C. Vesin for their technical collaboration. This work is supported by grant no.
3.650.87 from the Swiss National Science Foundation.

REFERENCES

1. Korngold R, Sprent J: Lethal graft-versus-host disease after bone marrow trans-
    plantation across minor histocompatibility barriers in mice. Prevention by re-
    moving mature T cells from the marrow. J Ex Med 1978;148:1687-1698.
2. Gale RP: Graft-versus-host disease. Immunol Rev 1985;88:193-214.
3. Aggarwal BB, Kohr WJ, Hass PE, Moffat B, Spender SA, Henzel WJ, Bringman
    TS, Nedwin GE, Goddel DV, Harkins RN: Human tumor necrosis factor. Pro-
    duction, purification and characterization. J Biol Chem 1985;260:2345-2354.
4. Carswell EA, Old LJ, Cassel RI, Green S, Fiore N, Williamson B: An endotoxin-
    induced serum factor that causes necrosis of tumors. Proc Natl Acad Sci USA
    1975;72:3666-3670.
5. Pennica DG, Nedwin E, Hayflick JS, Seeburg PH, Derynck R, Palladino MA, Kohr
    WJ, Aggarwal BB, Goeddel DV: Human tumor necrosis factor: precursor struc-
    ture, expression and homology to lymphotoxin. Nature (London) 1984;312:724-
    729.
6. Cuturi MC, Murphy M, Costa-Giomi MP, Weinman R, Perussia B, Trinchieri G:
    Independent regulation of tumor necrosis factor and lymphotoxin production by
    human peripheral blood lymphocytes. J Exp Med 1987;165:1581-1594.
7. Degliantoni G, Murphy M, Kobayashi M, Francis MK, Perussia B, Trinchierei G:
    Natural killer (NK) cell-derived hematopoietic colony-inhibiting activity and
    NK cytotixic factor. Relationship with tumor necrosis factor and synergism with
    immune interferon. J Exp Med 1985;162:1512-1530.
8. Young JDE, Liu CC, Butler G, Cohn ZA, Galli SC: Identification, purification and
    characterisation of a mast cell-associated cytolytic factor related to tumor necrosis
    factor. Proc Natl Acad Sci USA 1987;84:9175-9179.

9. Beutler B, Cerami A: Cachectin: more than a tumor necrosis factor. N Engl J Med
    1987;316:379-385.
10. Le J, Vilcek J: Biology of disease. Tumor necrosis factor and interleukin 1: cyto-
    kines with multiple overlapping activities. Lab Invest 1987;56:234-248.
11. Beutler B, Cerami A: Tumor necrosis, cachexia, shock, and inflammation: A com-
    mone mediator. Ann Rev Biochem 1988;57:505-519.
12. Old LJ: Tumor necrosis factor. Scientific American 1988;258.5:41-49.
13. Tracey K, Beutler B, Lowry SF, Merryweather J, Wolpe S, Milsark IW, Hariri RJ,
    Fahey TJ, Zentella A, Albert G, Shires TG, Cerami A: Shock and tissue injury in-
    duced by recombinant human cachectin. Science 1986;234:470-474.
14. Talmadge JE, Bowersox O, Tribble H, Lee SH, Shepard M, Liggit D: Toxicity of
    tumor necrosis factor is synergistic with gamma-interferon and can be reduced with
    cyclooxygenase inhibitors. Am J Path 1987;128:410-425.
15. Remick DG, Kunkel RG, Larrick JW, Kunkel SL: Acute in vivo effects of human re-
    combinant tumor necrosis factor. Lab Invest 1987;56:583-590.
16. Kettelhut IC, Fiers W, Goldberg AL: The toxic effects of tumor necrosis factor in
    vivo and their prevention by cyclooxygenase inhibitors. Proc Natl Acad Sci USA
    1987;84;4273-4277.
17. Dinarello CD, Cannon JG, Wolf SM, Bernheim HA, Beutler B, Cerami A, Figari IS,
    Palladino MA, O'Connor JV: Tumor necrosis factor (cachectin) is an endogenous
    pyrogen and induces production of interleukin 1. J Exp Med 1986;163:1433-1450.
18. Lehman V, Freudenberg MA, Galanos C: Lethal toxicity of lipolysaccharide and
    tumor necrosis factor in normal and D-galactosamine-treated mice. J Exp Med 1987;
    165:657-663.
19. Bertini R, Bianchi M, Ghezzi P: Adrenalectomy sensitizes mice to the lethal effects
    of interleukin 1 and tumor necrosis factor. J Exp Med 1988;167:1708-1712.
20. Rothstein JL, Schreiber H: Synergy between necrosis factor and bacterial products
    causes hemorrhagic necrosis and lethal shock in normal mice. Proc Natl Acad Sci
    USA 1988;85:607-611.
21. Tracey KJ, Wei H, Manogue KR, Fong Y, Hesse DG, Hguyen HT, Kuo GC, Beutler B,
    Cotran RS, Cerami A, Lowry SF: Cachectin/tumor necrosis factor induces cachexia,
    anemia and inflammation. J Exp Med 1988;167:1211-1227.
22. Piguet PF, Grau GE, Allet B, Kapanci Y, Vassalli P: Diffuse alveolar damage elicited
    by perfusion with tumor necrosis factor (TNF). Int Arch Allerg Immunol (abstract)
    1986;83:18.
23. Frater-Schroder M, Risau W, Hallmann R, Gautschi P, Bohlen P: Tumor necrosis
    factor type alpha, a potent inhibitor of endothelial cell growth in vitro, is angiogenic
    in vivo. Proc Natl Acad Sci USA 1987;84:5277-5281.
24. Leibovich SJ, Polverini PJ, Shepard HM, Wiseman DM, Shively V, Nuseir N: Macro-
    phage-induced angiogenesis is mediated by tumor necrosis factor-alpha. Nature
    1987;329:630-632.
25. Duvall E, Wyllie AH: Death and the cell. Immunology Today 1986;7:115-119.
26. Kerr JFR, Bishop CJ, Searle J, Harmon BV, Bishop CVV: Apoptosis. In *Perspective
    in Mammalian Cell Death*, edited by Potten CS. Oxford Science Publication, 1987;
    pp. 93-128.
27. Beutler BI, Milsark W, Cerami A: Passive immunisation against cachectin/tumor
    necrosis factor (TNF) protects mice from the lethal effect of endotoxin. Science
    (Wash, D.C.) 1985;229:869-871.
28. Grau GE, Fajardo L, Piguet PF, Allet B, Lambert PH, Vassalli P: Tumor necrosis
    factor (cachectin) as an essential meditor in murine cerebral malaria. Science 1987;
    237:1210-1212.
29. Grau GE, Piguet PF, Engers HD, Louis JA, Vassalli P, Lambert PH: L3T4[+] T lym-

phocyte play a major role in the pathogenesis of murine cerebral malaria. J Immunol 1986;137:2348-2354.

30. Piguet PF, Grau GE, Allet B, Vassalli P: Tumor necrosis factor/cachectin is an effector of skin and gut lesions of the acute phase of the graft-vs-host disease. J Exp Med 1987;166:1280-1289.

31. Nawroth PP, Stern DM: Modulation of endothelial cell hemostatic properties by tumor necrosis factor. J Exp Med 1986;163:740-745.

32. Piguet PF: Clonal analysis of the T lymphocytes involved in parent versus F1 graft-versus-host reaction. Immunogenetic 1984;20:71-81.

33. Piguet PF: GVHR elicited by products of class I or class II loci of the MHC: analysis of the response of mouse T lymphocytes to products of class I and class II loci of the MHC in correlation with the GVHR-induced mortality, medullary aplasia and enteropathy. J Immunol 1985;135:1637-1643.

34. Piguet PF, Grau GE, Collart MA, Vassalli P, Kapanci Y: Pneumopathies of the graft-versus-host-reaction: Alveolitis associated with an increased level of TNF mRNA and chronic interstitial pneumonitis. Lab Invest 1989;61:37-45.

35. Rappaport H, Khall H, Halle-Pannenko O, Pritchard L, Dantchev D, Mathe G: Histopathologic sequence of events in adult mice undergoing lethal graft-versus-host-reaction developed across H-2 and/or non H-2 histocompatibility barriers. Am J Path 1979;96:121-142.

36. Hackman RC: The pathology of bone marrow transplantation, in *Masson monographs in diagnostic pathology*, edited by Sale GE, Shulman HM, no 9. 1984; pp. 156-162.

37. Cudkowicz G, Nakamura I: Genetics of the murine hemopoietic-histocompatibility system: an overview. Trans Proc XV 1983;2058-2063.

38. Elkins WL, Quant MM: Regulatory effect of H-2 region in the graft vs host response: F1 hybrid resistance to alloreactive T cells. J Immunol 1981;127:1459-1462.

39. Grebe SC, Streilein JW: Graft-versus-host-reactions. Adv Immunol 1976;22:185-186.

40. Grau GE, Kindler V, Piguet PF, Lambert PH, Vassalli P: IL3 and GM-CSF are intermediates in increased TNF production during experimental cerebral malaria. J Exp Med 1988;168:1499-1504.

41. Collart MA, Bellin D, Vassalli JD, de Kossodo S, Vassalli P: Gamma interferon enhances macrophage transcription of the tumor necrosis factor/cachectin, interleukin 1, and urokinase genes, which are controlled by a short-lived repressor. J Exp Med 1986;164:2113-2118.

42. Piguet PF, Grau GE, Irle C, Vassalli P: Administration of interleukin-2 to mice enhances production of hemopoietic and natural killer cells. Eur J Immunol 1986;16: 1257-1261.

43. Guy-Grand D, Vassalli P: Gut injury in mouse graft versus host reaction: its occurrence and mechanisms. J Clin Invest 1986;77:1584-1595.

44. Guillen FJ, Ferrara J, Hancock WW, Messadi D, Fonferko E, Burakoff SJ, Murphy GF: Acute cutaneous graft-versus-host-disease to minor histocompatibility antigens in a murine model Evidence that large granular lymphocytes are effector cells in the immune response. Lab Invest 1986;55:35-42.

45. Ferrara JL, Marion A, McIntyre JF, Murphy GF, Burakoff SJ: Amelioration of acute graft versus host disease due to minor histocompatibility antigens by in vivo administration of anti interleukin-2 receptor antibody. J Immunol 1986;137:1874-1877.

46. Skopinska E: The effect of the *Escherichia coli* lipopolysaccharide (endotoxin) on the graft-versus-host reaction in mice. Ann Med Sect Pol Acad Sci 1986;21:185-192.

47. Piguet PF, Janin-Mercier A, Vassalli P, Saurat JH: Epidermal lesions of the GVHR:

evaluation of the role of different MHC and non MHC loci and of the Ly-2$^+$ and L3T4$^+$ T lymphocytes. J Immunol 1987;139:406-410.

48. Slavin RE, Woodruff JM: The pathology of bone marrow transplantation. Pathology Annual 1974;9:291-296.

49. Friedman KJ, LeBoit PE, Farmer ER: Acute follicular graft-vs-host reaction. A distinct clinicopathologic presentation. Arch Dermatol 1988;124:688-691.

50. Sale GE, Shulman HM, Galucci BB, Thomas ED: Young rete ridge keratinocytes are preferred targets in cutaneous graft-versus-host disease. Am J Pathol 1985;118:278-287.

51. Ijiri K, Potten CS: Cell death in cell hierarchies in adult mammalian tissues. In *Perspectives on Mammalian Cell Death*, edited by Potten CS. 1987; pp. 326-356.

52. Bowden DH: Alveolar response to injury. Thorax 1981;36:801-804.

53. Sale GE, Galucci BB, Schubert MM, Sullivan KM, Thomas ED: Direct ultrastructural evidence of target-directed polarization by cytotoxic lymphocytes in lesions of human graft-versus-host disease. Arch Pathol Lab Med 1987;111:333-336.

54. Mowat AM, Ferguson A: Hypersensitivity reactions in the small intestine. Transplantation 1981;32:238-243.

55. Sprent J, Schaefer M, Lo D, Korngold R: Properties of purified T cell subsets. II. In vivo responses to class I vs. class II H-2 differences. J Exp Med 1986;163:998-1011.

14

Monoclonal Antibody Therapy for the Prevention of Graft-vs.-Host Disease

Herman Waldmann, Geoffrey Hale, Stephen R. Cobbold, Mike Clark, Shixin Qin, Richard Benjamin, and Martin J. S. Dyer
University of Cambridge
Cambridge, England

I. INTRODUCTION

Graft-vs.-Host Disease (GVHD) is a major complication of allogeneic bone marrow transplantation (BMT), which has limited the therapeutic use of BMT to relatively well-matched donor-recipient combinations. Even in this setting GVHD accounts for significant morbidity and mortality despite prophylactic therapy with immunosuppressive drugs. As the disease is mediated by T cells contained within the donor marrow inoculum it should be a simple matter to remove these T cells and thus eliminate the problem. The practical realities are that GVH reactions are part of a more complex series of processes that are finely balanced. These other processes include host reactivity to the marrow graft itself (HVG) as well as the so-called graft-vs.-leukemia (GVL) effect. It is important for the future of clinical BMT and its potential applications in producing transplantation tolerance and ameliorating autoimmunity that we fully understand the cellular and molecular basis of these phenomena. However this does not mean that we should avoid finding independent strategies to prevent GVHD, to prevent marrow graft rejection, and to treat leukemia. Ultimately a combination of therapeutic maneuvers directed towards both the donor marrow as well as to the recipient could be used to prevent GVHD without risk of rejection or leukemia relapse. This chapter will address the possibility of using monoclonal antibodies (MAbs) as agents to control these three interacting elements in BMT.

Monoclonal antibody technology has made it possible to produce reagents which can react with desired populations of lymphocytes while sparing stem cells. The clinical application of MAbs requires an understanding of how best to use them to kill cells or block their function. MAbs alone cannot kill but act to focus natural effector systems, in particular complement and Fc-receptor-bearing accessory cells, to the target. We have sought to exploit this knowledge to ablate cell populations both in vivo and in vitro. This has led us to study the role of T lymphocytes and their subsets in GVHD and in marrow rejection in animal models and to apply this knowledge to the clinical setting.

This chapter will begin by considering the features of MAbs that make them most effective as lytic agents. We will progress to a discussion of how MAbs to defined T cell subsets have been used to ablate populations in the mouse and to summarize the information this has provided on the T cells participating in GVHD and HVG reactions. We then review the clinical experience of the CAMPATH* (Cambridge Pathology) users group in using the human complement fixing MAb CAMPATH-1 for purging allogeneic marrow prior to grafting; and finally we discuss the development of lympholytic MAbs for possible in vivo conditioning in humans.

II. MONOCLONAL ANTIBODIES AS AGENTS TO CONTROL LYMPHOCYTE FUNCTIONS

MAbs may be used to control lymphocytes by ablating relevant cells or by perturbing the functions of critical receptors, adhesion molecules, or their ligands.

A. Monoclonal Antibodies as Ablative Agents

1. Harnessing the Complement System

The complement cascade is initiated by the binding of C1q to the antigen-antibody complex. Consequent to this, cells may be killed by clearance through binding to C3b receptors on cells of the macrophage/granulocyte series or through the assembly of directly lytic "terminal" components in their membrane. The important variables that influence the success or otherwise of homologous complement activation are antibody isotype, the target antigen itself, and various "restriction factors" that act to limit lysis of cells by homologous complement. In certain instances appropriate combinations of MAbs may demonstrate synergy in lysis (1,2); and for certain target antigens the use of univalent MAbs may permit lysis where bivalent reagents fail (3,4).

Isotype

The use of class-switch variants of chimeric recombinant antibodies coupled with abundant data from myeloma proteins and MAbs suggest that for the three species available (mouse, rat, human) there is a definite subclass hierarchy for lysis which is related but not identical to the hierarchy for C1q binding (5-7). IgM antibodies are high in the hierarchy in all species. If we consider IgG antibodies, then the approximate order is mIgG2a $\geqslant$ IgG2b $>$ IgG3 $>$ IgG1 for both C1q binding and lysis (5). For rat IgGs it is rIgG2b $>$ IgG2c $>$ IgG1 $>$ IgG2a for C1q binding and rIgG2b $>$ IgG1 $>$ IgG2c = IgG2a for lysis (7) (although we have an example of a class-switch variant where IgG2a was more lytic than IgG1 (8)). For human IgGs the hierarchy is huIgG1 $>$ IgG3 $>$ IgG2 $>$ IgG4 for lysis and huIgG3 $>$ IgG1 $>$ IgG2 $>$ IgG4 for C1q binding (6).

Target Antigen

The density of the target antigen has long been known to be an important factor in complement lysis (9). However, there are clearly other aspects of the target antigen that dictate whether or not lysis can occur (10). The feature of "good or permissive" antigens is that they allow very efficient activation of C1 compared to "poor" antigens of comparable site density. The proportion of human lymphocyte surface molecules that are "permissive" as targets for complement lysis is small. A particularly effective specificity is that defined by the CAMPATH 1 series of rat MAbs, which are able to lyse human lymphocytes with human complement (11-13). The special convenience of being able to use donor complement as a complement source has meant the evolution of a remarkably simple and rapid way of purging lymphocytes from human marrow allografts (14) (Sec. IV).

It should, however, be stressed that good C1 activation *per se* may not always be sufficient to guarantee lysis. This is the case for the rIgG2b MAb CAMPATH3 reactive with human CD3 (4). Lysis was only effective with the univalent but not with the bivalent form. The rate-limiting step appeared to be in the terminal stages of the lytic pathway (after C3 deposition). It seems as though here the interaction of the target antigen with the bivalent form of antibody has resulted in the cell somehow being protected from lysis.

2. Lysis by Cells Expressing Fc Receptors

Knowledge of the diversity and function of Fc receptors is accumulating rapidly (15). However, it is still unclear which Fc receptors are relevant to destruction of antibody coated cells in vivo. Again the use of monoclonal antibodies—MAb class-switch variants and recombinant antibodies—has demonstrated a hierarchy of Ig binding to these as follows: for the high affinity huFcRI receptor on monocytes and macrophages, that hierarchy is known for human antibodies as huIgG1 $\geq$ IgG3 > IgG4 $\gg$ IgG2 (16). For both the widely expressed HuFcγRII receptor and also for the huFcγRIII, the rank Ig binding is huIgG1 = IgG3 $\gg$ IgG2 and IgG4 (17,18).

There is uncertainty as to what in vitro test may best identify an antibody with a chance of being lytic in vivo. Several groups have used ADCC with human K-cells for this purpose. There is now data for all three species of MAb. For mouse Igs the rank order is IgG3 > IgG2a > IgG2b $\gg$ IgG1 (19). For rat this is rIgG2b = IgG1 $\gg$ IgG2a > IgG2c (7,8), and for human it seems to be IgG1 > IgG3 > IgG4 > IgG2 (6,20).

The point of this short review of effector systems is to emphasize that selection of antibodies for lysis need not be a purely empirical process. As we better know the rules for harnessing these effector mechanisms, then so can we design or select better MAbs for use in this field.

3. Lymphocyte Depletion with Monoclonal Antibodies Administered In Vivo

Animal Models

Our laboratory has for many years been investigating ways of killing lymphocytes in vivo. We have largely focused on rat monoclonal antibodies and have attempted to determine which isotypes are the most effective. This work is largely reviewed elsewhere (21,22), and suffice it to say that rIgG2b and possibly rIgG1 seem far more effective than the other subclasses. The impressive ability of rat IgG2b MAbs to mouse CD4 and CD8 to deplete these subsets from peripheral lymphoid tissues has made it possible to create mice depleted of appropriate subsets for experimental use (23). In adoptive transfer studies where lymphocytes are transferred from one mouse to another it has been possible simply to coat the inocula with rIgG2b MAbs to Thy-1, CD4, or CD8 to guarantee elimination of those cells through recipient effector mechanisms (22,24,25). It will be apparent to the reader that such simple manipulations make it possible to establish which T cells participate in GVHD and in marrow rejection. Information derived from such studies will be presented in Sec. III.

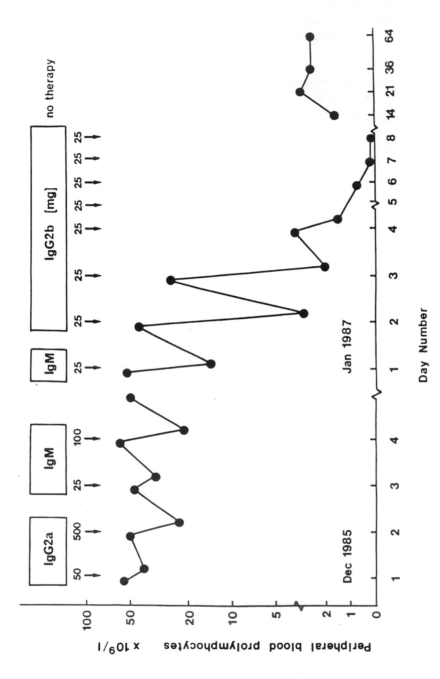

Figure 1 The effects of MAbs of different rat isotypes against the CAMPATH-1 antigen. A patient with BCLL had been treated unsuccessfully in 1985 with intravenous infusions of rIgG2a and rIgM antibodies to the CAMPATH 1 antigen. By 1987 the disease had progressed to a prolymphocytic transformation, and further therapy was instituted with the rIgM again and subsequently with the rIgG2b class-switch variant (doses in mg are shown in the figure). The rIgG2b produced substantial clearance of blood lymphocytes. (Further information can be obtained from Dyer et al. (26).)

Humans

There is surprisingly little clinical data available to demonstrate effective depletion of lymphocytes by MAbs. Perhaps the most lytic of the rodent anti-human lymphocyte antibodies described so far is the pan-lymphocyte rat MAb CAMPATH 1G (8). This is one of a series of CAMPATH-1 MAbs of various isotypes, all of which have the capacity to activate human complement to bring about lymphocyte lysis in vitro. However, the rIgG2b form is far more effective than the rIgM or rIgG2a forms at lysis of lymphocytes in vivo (26). This is shown in Figure 1. Here a patient with prolymphocytic leukemia was treated sequentially with the IgM, IgG2a, and then the rIgG2b MAb. The rIgG2b has exactly the same variable region gene as the rIgG2a as it was actually derived as a class-switch·variant from the IgG2a form. The rIgG2b variant (CAMPATH 1G) produced a profound depletion of lymphocytes from blood, spleen, and bone marrow. Recently a "reshaped" human IgG1 form of this antibody has been created by the recombinant DNA approach (20) and this too has exquisite lympholytic properties in vivo (27) (Fig. 2). It has the theoretical advantage of being less likely to evoke an antiglobulin response and

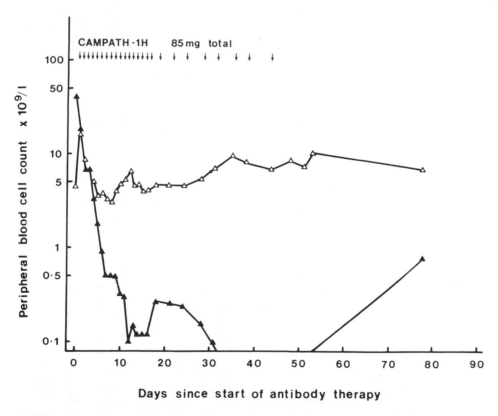

Figure 2 The effect of CAMPATH-1H in clearing blood lymphocytes from a patient with non-Hodgkin's lymphoma. Antibody was infused over 2-4 hours on the days shown and levels of lymphocytes (closed triangles) and neutrophils (open triangles) measured. The lymphocytes which reappeared in day 78 were normal. The patient remains in remission some 4 months following the termination of MAb therapy. (From Hale et al. (27).)

is therefore a potentially invaluable drug for the control of human immune funtion as well as for the serotherapy of leukemia and lymphoma. The application of the CAMPATH-1 series of monoclonal antibodies to the area of marrow allografting will be developed in Sec. IV.

B. Monoclonal Antibodies to Block Lymphocyte Functions

T cells function by interacting with other cells. These interactions require the participation of a large range of membrane receptors for recognition of antigen, adhesion, and perception of growth factors. Interference with these receptor activities may alter the way T cells respond to antigens and this may have therapeutic benefit. Superficially one might imagine that receptor blockade would be a transient phenomena that might disappear with removal of antibody. However, in practice animal models have told us that there may be real scope for the use of blocking MAbs to prevent immune responses while permitting tolerance to take place. We have shown that administration of CD4 MAbs to mice will allow tolerance to be induced to both the therapeutic MAb itself as well as to foreign proteins such as human gamma globulin (HGG) given at the same time (28-31). Depletion of CD4 cells was not necessary as F(ab)$_2$ fragments (30) and nonlytic or rIgG2a CD4 MAbs would also do it (Qin et al, unpublished data). Similar data have been obtained for LFA-1 MAbs in producing tolerance to HGG (30) and for CD8 MAbs in producing tolerance to class I-restricted minor transplantation antigens (32) (see Sec. III.C). Clearly it does seem possible to influence the decision ON or OFF that T cells make when they confront antigen. Such a selective approach to control of GVHD and marrow rejection may have a major therapeutic benefit without incurring the penalty of gross T-cell depletion in already heavily immunocompromised recipients. The feasibility of using nondepleting CD4 and CD8 MAbs to allow permanent acceptance of marrow grafts is considered further in Sec. III.C.

III. MONOCLONAL ANTIBODIES TO PREVENT ALLO-RE-ACTIVITY IN BONE-MARROW TRANSPLANTATION

A. Subsets Involved in GVHD

The classical animal model of GVHD has been the transfer of spleen and marrow cells from P1-type donors into lethally irradiated (P1 X P2)F$_1$ recipients. In this setting removal of T cells from the donor inoculum prevents GVHD and allows normal hemopoietic reconstitution. This model has permitted identification of the T-cell subsets responsible for GVHD. Using alloantisera, Korngold and Sprent showed that GVHD over certain minor-mismatched combinations was mediated by CD8 cells (33). Mason (34) reported that CD4 cells and to a lesser extent CD8 cells were able to cause GVHD across major barriers in the rat. Vallera et al. (35) and Korngold and Sprent (36) suggested that lethal GVHD across complete MHC barriers involved predominantly Lyt-1 cells and not CD8 cells. Cobbold et al. (25), using coating MAbs or inocula from MAb-depleted donors, were able to show that CD8 cells could be the dominant effectors of GVHD in certain MHC-mismatched combinations. GVHD could be induced in the absence of any help from CD4 cells. This, together with the previous alloantisera data, suggested that both CD4 and CD8 subsets could mediate GVHD independently. Sprent and Korngold subsequently showed that purified populations of CD4 and CD8 cells would mediate GVHD with CD4 cells biased to recognition of class II-restricted determinants and CD8 cells to class I (37).

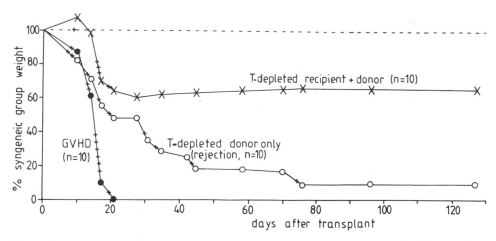

Figure 3 Depletion of both recipient and donor T cells improves survival of P1-into-P2 MHC-mismatched marrow transplants. Adult thymectomized BALB/c mice were used as the donors of bone marrow and spleen cells (10^7 of each). These were not depleted in the GVHD control group (●), but in other groups they were given MAbs to deplete CD4 and CD8 cells. Donor cells were then infused i.v. to lethally irradiated CBA euthymic recipients (4 hr after 850 rads), themselves either undepleted (○) or depleted of CD4 and CD8 cells 5 days before transplantation (X). Data are expressed as % of the group weight of syngeneic controls. Mice that died were counted as having zero weight. (From Cobbold et al. (25).)

B. Marrow Rejection in Mice

T-cell purging of the marrow/spleen inocula in the P1-into-P2 situation turned out to be more complex. Thierfelder et al. (24) observed that coating doses of rIgG2b anti-Thy1 could prevent death in the P1-into-(P1 × P2)F_1 combination but were not effective for fully allogeneic combinations. However, very high doses of anti-Thy1 MAb given together with the spleen/marrow inoculum not only prevented GVHD but allowed complete donor chimerism and long-term survival. We speculated that excess antibody had continued to work in the recipient and must have depleted recipient T cells that had been spared by irradiation. To confirm this we pretreated both donors and recipients with rIgG2b CD4 and CD8 MAbs some days before transplantation and were able to show similar long-term survival of P1-into-P2 (Fig. 3) or (P1 × P2)F_1-into-(P1 × P3)F_1 recipients (25). This was conclusive evidence that irradiated recipients still had functional T cells with the capacity to reject. We subsequently demonstrated that the in vivo administration of CD4 and CD8 MAbs would even allow engraftment in MHC-mismatched combinations where recipients had received only 600 rads of irradiation (Fig. 4). Animals that received the CD4 and CD8 MAbs together showed virutally complete donor-type reconstitution. Controls that had received the foreign marrow without any MAb conditioning all survived but exhibited viruially complete autologous recovery (38). Recipient pretreatment with neither CD4 nor CD8 MAb alone was sufficient to permit donor engraftment and hemopoiesis. Again recipients survived with recovery of their own hemopoietic system. This means that both CD4 and CD8 cells can reject marrow grafts independently. The role each plays will of course depend on the genetic differences between host and donor. Another valid conclusion was that the balance of

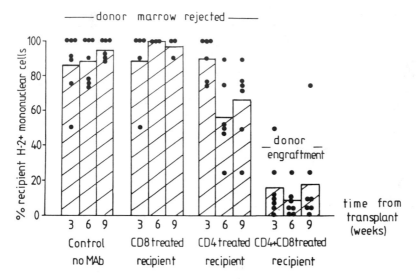

Figure 4 Chimerism in CD4- and CD8-depleted recipients of allogeneic marrow. Groups of CBA/Ca mice (14-18 weeks old) were depleted with CD4 and CD8 MAbs alone or in combination, and then irradiated with 600 rads of irradiation. They were infused with T-cell-depleted marrow and spleen cells as in Fig. 3. The levels of recipient-type chimerism were measured 3, 6, and 9 weeks after transplantation. Individual mice are shown as closed circles, while open circles depict a low white cell count. The % mean of recipient type cells is indicated by the blocks. (Data from Ref. 38.)

donor vs. recipient type haemopoiesis is related to the balance of donor vs recipient allo-reactivity. GVH would seem to favor donor, and HVG would favor recipient-type (i.e., autologous) recovery. These findings may have some relevance to interpretation of the finding that the risk of leukemia relapse is increased following T-cell purging of human marrow.

C. Bone Marrow Grafts to Produce Transplantation Tolerance in the Adult

In the previous examples of successful P1-into-P2 marrow grafts, we observed (38) that the recipients were tolerant to subsequent grafts of donor-type skin. This really was not surprising as virtually all T cells in these animals were of donor type. However, recognizing the power of in vivo T-cell depletion with MAbs, we sought to establish whether it was possible to achieve long-term partial chimerism and tolerance with minimal or no irradiation. We argued that if we could control GVH and HVG reactions with mono-clonal antibodies, then this should be feasible in the adult mouse. We have examined a series of minor-mismatch combinations and have found that indeed this is possible. For example, B10.BR marrow can be used to tolerize CBA mice such that these animals can later accept B10.BR skin (32) (Fig. 5). As before, it was necessary to condition recipients with a combination of CD4 and CD8 MAbs in order for chimerism to be established. So effective was this protocol that all components (MAbs; marrow and skin) could be administered simultaneously. Indeed, we were able to achieve transplantation tolerance across the B10.A-into-CBA/Ca combination (single class I plus multiple minor differences) (32), a genetic combination similar to that used successfully by Med-

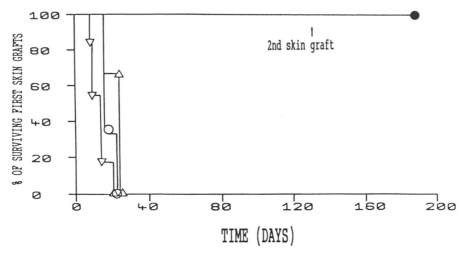

TIME (DAYS)

Figure 5 Tolerance to multiple minor transplantation antigens induced by the combination of CD4 and CD8 MAb therapy and marrow transplantation. CBA/Ca mice ($n = 6$) received either CD4 ($\triangle$); CD8 ($\bigcirc$); both CD4 and CD8 MAbs on days 0, 3, and 5 plus 1 X 10^7 marrow and 1 X 10^7 spleen T-cepleted cells 2 hr after the first MAb injection. Control mice ($\triangledown$) received no MAb. B10.BR skin was grafted 3 weeks later. The MST of the groups were: CD4 depleted, 16 days; CD8 depleted, 16 days. In the group which had been pretreated with both CD4 and CD8 MAbs ($\bullet$), a second B10.BR skin graft was transplanted 130 days after the first. Both the first and second grafts have remained healthy for a further 200 days. (From Ref. 32.)

awar and his colleagues for the neonate. We were able to show that animals tolerized in this way exhibitied long-term low-level chimerism. In this case however, the T cells that reemerged were predominantly recipient type. Therefore these T cells were truly tolerant of donor antigens. We could achieve tolerance of each of the T-cell subsets without necessarily depleting it. The inclusion of a lytic rIgG2b with a nonlytic rIgG2a was sufficient to produce tolerance, irrespective of which was directed to CD4 and which to CD8 (Table

Table 1 Depletion of Neither CD4 nor CD8 T-cells is Necessary for Tolerance to Be Induced Within Any One of the Respective Subsets

Monoclonal antibody treatment	PBL Lymphocytes			Graft survival (MST)
	%CD4	%CD8	%Thy-1[+]	
IgG2a CD4 IgG2b CD8	31.5	1.3	52.5	>100
IgG2a CD4 IgG2a CD8	26.4	12.5	56.7	12
IgG2b CD4 IgG2a CD8	1.7	15.3	19.8	>100
IgG2b CD4 IgG2b CD8	4.3	6.5	3.5	>100
PBS	39.8	12.5	47.0	9.8

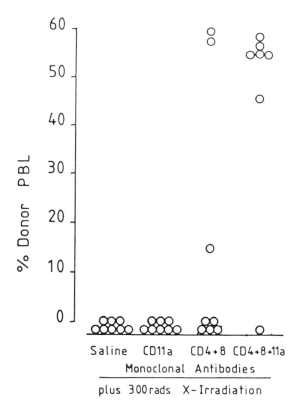

Figure 6 Chimerism can be established across whole MHC and minor mismatch combinations using only 300 rads of X-irradiation in conditioning recipients, if this is combined with MAb therapy with CD4, CD8, and CD1a MAbs. CBA/Ca mice received 300 rads X-irradiation followed by 2×10^7 T-depleted BALB/c marrow cells. Mice then received MAb therapy as shown. CD4+8 was 1 mg of an equal mixture of MAb YTS 169.4; YTS 156.7 (both CD8); YTS 191.1, and YTA 3.1 (both CD4) given on days 0 (i.v.), 1, and 3. CD11a was 250 μg of the nondepleting FD441.8 MAb given on days 0 (i.v.), 3, 5, 7, and 9. All mice were bled on day 80, and their percentage PBL staining for donor H-2 type ($H-2^d$) was determined by cytofluorograph Y. (From Benjamin, Qin, Cobbold, and Waldmann, unpublished.)

1). Clearly each of the T-cell subsets can be tolerized to minor transplantation antigens if blockaded through these two adhesion molecules.

If blockade could be used to tolerize alloreactive cells in bone marrow transplants, then there would be no need to "purge" as presently practiced. This may again have repercussions on leukemia control as there would be sufficient T cells available to devise ways to achieving "bystander" GVL effects.

We are currently analyzing to what extent the immunosuppressive effects of irradiation can be replaced by MAbs for complete (MHC plus minor) mismatches. We have for the BALB/c-into-CBA/Ca combination been able to reduce the requirement for irradiation to 300 rads by using a combination of CD4, CD8, and CD11a MAbs (Benjamin, Qin, Cobbold, and Waldmann, unpublished). As shown in Figure 6, we were able to with MAb therapy with CD4, CD8, and CD11a MAbs. CBA/Ca mice received 300 rads

achieve long-term chimerism in this difficult combination without the need for any other myelotoxic agents. These data suggest that similar antibody strategies applied in the conventionally conditioned patient may also control the alloreactive phenomena which currently prejudice successful transplantation.

Norman CBA/ca mice (n = 6) were given 15 days of treatment with equal amounts of each MAb (0.5 mg/day in total per mouse) as well as 1×10^7 B10.BR marrow cells at the beginning of treatment. Five days after the last MAb injection, mice from each group were bled and their blood lymphocytes (PBL) analyzed by flow cytometry. Numbers given are the percentage of positive cells. Three weeks later all mice were grafted with B10.BR tail skin to determine if they were tolerant. Mean graft survival time (MST) is shown. Data are from Qin et al. (32).

IV. CLINICAL DATA

A. The Use of CAMPATH-1M for the Prevention of GVHD

GVHD affects the majority of recipients of HLA-matched bone marrow transplants (39) despite the prophylactic use of immunosuppressants. This makes mismatched transplantation virtually impossible. Animal models have shown that GVHD can be abolished by purging of T cells from donor bone marrow. We have developed a simple procedure for removing lymphocytes (including T cells) from human marrow (11,14) using the rIgM MAb CAMPATH-1M. This antibody is extremely lytic with human complement and was developed to explore the value of complete purging (rather than selective purging as previously discussed). In theory the MAb should be easy to use since it could simply be added to the marrow suspension and transfused into a sea of recipient complement. In practice we wished to assess the degree of T-cell depletion and to attempt to correlate this with outcome. We therefore opted to add donor serum as a complement source to accomplish lysis in vitro. A pilot study was conducted in collaboration with Shimon Slavin (14). This showed that GVHD could be eliminated without any need for prophylactic drug immunosuppression. However we observed that late graft failure occured in 2 out of the 10 patients transplanted and postulated that this was a result of residual host resistance uncompromised by GVH reactions. Subsequently several other centers reported graft failure using other T-cell purging techniques. Following this pilot study many centers in the UK and Europe participated in a larger study. This CAMPATH users group comprising 20 centers has recently reported on a total of 441 matched sibling transplants followed for a minimum of 100 days (40,41). These data will be briefly reviewed here again. The median age of this series was 29 years and the distribution by disease was: ALL 98, AML 128, CGL 188, and others 27. All marrow samples were treated with a single round of CAMPATH-1M and 25% donor serum as complement. This purging protocol can certainly be improved on (42), but as conducted the overall depletion was still good with the final inoculum containing a mean of 0.7% of E-rosetting cells. Failure to deplete T cells was seen in a few instances where insufficient free Ca^{++} had been left in the diluent to permit complement activity. The median number of nucleated cells infused was 2.3×10^8/kg. Engraftment was obtained in 393 patients with a median time to 0.5×10^9 neutrophils of 19 days. Table 2 shows the outcome for acute and chronic GVHD in this group.

The incidence of acute GVHD was 18% grade 1, 8% grade 2, and 8% grade 3/4. The percentages were based on the 335 patients who survived to day 100 with durable engraftment or suffered GVHD but died before day 100. Prophylactic CyA did not im-

Table 2 The Effect of CAMPATH-1 M Marrow Purging on the Incidence of GVHD and Graft Failure

GVHD prophylaxis	No. of patients	Acute GVHD				Chronic GVHD			Graft failure	
		0	1	2	3/4	0	M	S	Complete	Partial
180 CyA, 3 Mtx	181	93	35	13	9	98	28	3	20	3
none	260	127	26	14	18	128	13	4	44	4
Total	441	220	61	27	27	226	41	7	64	7

Patients were scored 0 for GVHD only if they survived 100 days (acute) or 120 days (chronic) without GVHD but with durable engraftment. Data from Hale and Waldmann for CAMPATH users (41). 0 = none, M = moderate, S = severe.

prove the incidence of GVHD. An infusion of residual T cells of more than 4×10^6/kg did correlate with GVHD. The incidence of chronic GVHD was very low (15% mild/ moderate and 3% severe). These figures are based on the percentage of 274 patients who survived 120 days with durable grafts. Chronic GVHD did seem to correlate positively with the use of prophylactic CyA. It is possible that this reflects impairment of mechanisms concerned with generation of immunologic tolerance (43).

The incidence of graft failure was far higher than would be expected for unpurged transplants, 15% of all grafts. A further 3% were deemed partial failure because graft function was restored following immunosuppressive treatment. Of the 108 patients who received prophylactic TLI as an additional component of the conditioning (44), there were 12 (11%) graft failures, while in the 333 who did not there were 59 cases of failure (18%). There can be little doubt that these graft failures were due to residual host resistance (rejection) because only 1 out of 49 patients whose autologous marrow had been purged in the same way have failed to engraft (40).

Previous studies have shown that GVHD is negatively correlated with relapse and that relapse may be more common after transplants from identical twins (45,46). International Registry data now also suggest significant risk of relapse followng T-cell purging in leukemia (47). Detailed analysis of our data in acute leukemia would still be premature based on our small sample. Actuarial probabilities of survival and remaining in remission at 2 years are shown in Table 3 together with the results of CGL (41). The results in the latter show a clear increase in the relapse risk following CAMPATH-1 purging.

Multivariate analysis of the CGL data revealed three risk factors for relapse. These were higher dose-rate irradiation ($p = 0.02$), slow engraftment ($p = 0.02$), and lack of any form of GVHD ($p = 0.01$). The reliability of the irradiation data is uncertain and could be confounded by other intercenter variations. There are at least two nonexclusive hypotheses for the antileukemic effect of donor T cells. They may exert a cytotoxic effect against leukemic cells (conventional wisdom) or, as we have previously proposed (48), alloreactivity may determine the balance between host and donor hemopoiesis (see Sec. III.B). As CGL is a stem cell disease, events that favor host hemopoiesis (autologous recovery) would also favor relapse. Removal of donor T-cell would shift the balance of reactivity to HVG, thus biasing recipient-type hemopoiesis.

Table 3 Actuarial Probabilities of Survival and of Remaining in Remission at 2 Years

	No. of patients	Survival (%)	Chance of remaining in remission (%)
ALL 1st remission	36	60 ± 10	80 ± 10
AML 1st remission	90	42 ± 8	74 ± 10
CGL 1st chronic phase	142	69 ± 6	71 ± 7
with any GVHD	44	77 ± 8	86 ± 8
without GVHD	83	73 ± 7	63 ± 9
engraft < 26 days	98	74 ± 6	78 ± 7
engraft > 25 days	29	75 ± 13	52 ± 18

Probabilities were calculated by the log-rank method. Data from Hale and Waldmann for CAMPATH users (41).

V. PROSPECTS

Undoubtedly the rIgM, rIgG2b, and huIgG1 forms of CAMPATH 1 are all agents that can be used in BMT to prevent GVHD and rejection. The two IgG versions are powerful lympholytic agents in vivo and for this reason may have a role in BMT for lymphoid leukemias where residual resistance and leukemia could be reduced in the conditioning period. We are hopeful that in the other forms of leukemia marrow rejection may also be controlled so that any elements of "hemopoietic competition" dictated by residual alloreactivity would be removed. Present regimes of drug prophylaxis for GVHD are still inadequate and do not allow progress to the mismatch situation which would make BMT available to a wider population. In our view there is a need to maintain the momentum gained by the knowledge that alloreactivity is preventable and to urgently establish novel antileukemic strategies. There is a unique opportunity within the BMT arena to evolve new MAb-based therapies that will target residual leukemic cells without concern for normal host stem cells that would anyway have been ablated by irradiation.

Improved control of alloreactivity in BMT also has tremendous potential in a range of nonmalignant conditions from rescue in aplastic anemia to the establishment of chimerism in organ transplantation. We can be optimistic that the more we come to know about the rules for best use of MAbs to direct immune responses and kill tumor targets, the closer we will be to realizing this potential.

ACKNOWLEDGMENTS

The work described here was carried out with support of the Medical Research Council, the Leukaemia Research Fund, and Wellcome Biotech. Ltd. CAMPATH-1* is a trademark of Wellcome Biotech.

REFERENCES

1. Hughes-Jones NC, Gorick BD, Howard JC: The mechanism of synergistic complement-mediated lysis of rat red cells by monoclonal IgG antibodies. Eur J Immunol 1983;13:635-640.
2. Bindon CI, Hale G, Clark MR, Waldmann H: Therapeutic potential of monoclonal antibodies to the leukocyte common antigen: Synergy and interference in complement-mediated lysis. Transplantation 1985;40:538-544.

3. Cobbold SP, Waldmann H: Therapeutic potential of monovalent monoclonal antibodies. Nature 1984;308:460-462.

4. Clark M, Bindon C, Dyer M, Friend P, Hale G, Cobbold S, Calne R, Waldmann H: The improved lytic function and in-vivo efficacy of monovalent monoclonal CD3 antibodies. Eur J Immunol 1989;19:381-388.

5. Oi VT, Vuong TM, Hardy R, Reidler J, Dangl J, Herzenberg LA, Stryer L: Correlation between segmental flexibility and effector function of antibodies. Nature 1984; 307:136-140.

6. Bruggemann M, Williams GT, Bindon CI, Clark MR, Walker MR, Jefferis, R, Waldmann H, Neuberger MS: Comparison of the effector functions of human immunoglobulins using a matched set of chimeric antibodies. J Exp Med 1987;166:1351-1361.

7. Bruggemann M, Teale C, Bindon C, Clark M, Waldmann H: A matched set of rat/mouse chimeric antibodies. J Immunol 1989;142:3145-3150.

8. Hale G, Cobbold SP, Waldmann H, Easter G, Matejtschuk P, Coombs RRA: Isolation of low-frequency class-switch variants from rat hybrid myelomas. J Immunol Meth 1987;103:59-67.

9. Circolo A, Borsos T: Lysis of hapten-labeled cells by anti-hapten IgG and complement: effect of cell surface hapten density. J Immunol 1982;128:1118-1121.

10. Bindon CI, Hale G, Waldmann H: Importance of antigen specificity for complement mediated lysis by monoclonal antibodies. Eur J Immunol 1988;18:1507-1514.

11. Hale G, Bright S, Chumbley G, Hoang T, Metcalf D, Munro AJ, Waldmann H: Removal of T cells from bone marrow for transplantation: a monoclonal antilymphocyte antibody that fixes human complement. Blood 1983;62:873-882.

12. Hale G, Hoang T, Prospero T, Watt SM, Waldmann H: Removal of T cells from bone marrow for transplantation: comparison of rat monoclonal anti-lymphocyte antibodies of different isotypes. Mol Biol Med 1983;1:305-319.

13. Hale G, Swirsky DM, Hayhoe FGJ, Waldmann H: Effects of monoclonal anti-lymphocyte antibodies in vivo in monkeys and humans. Mol Biol Med 1983;1:321-334.

14. Waldmann H, Or R, Hale G, Weiss L, Cividalli G, Samuel S, Manor D, Brautbar C, Polliack A, Rachmilewitz EA, Slavin S: Elimination of graft versus host disease by in vitro depletion of alloreactive lymphocytes using a monoclonal rat anti-human lymphocyte antibody (CAMPATH-1). Lancet 1984;2:483-486.

15. Unkeless JC, Scigliano E, Freedman VH; Structure and function of human and murine receptors for IgG. Annu Rev Immunol 1988;6:251-281.

16. Huber H, Douglas SD, Nusbacher J, Kochwa S, Rosenfield RE. IgG subclass specificity of human monocyte receptor sites. Nature 1971;229:419-420.

17. Simmons D, Seed B: The Fc gamma receptor of natural killer cells is a phospholipid-linked membrane protein. Nature 1988;333:568-570.

18. Stengelin S, Stamenkovic I, Seed B: Isolation of cDNAs for two distinct human Fc receptors by ligand affinity cloning. EMBO J 1988;7:1053-1059.

19. Kipps IJ, Parham P, Punt J, Herzenberg LA: The importance of immunoglobulin isotype in human antibody dependent cell-mediated cytotoxicity (ADCC) directed by murine monoclonal antibodies. J Exp Med 1985;161:1-17.

20. Riechmann L, Clark MR, Waldmann H, Winter G: Reshaping human antibodies for therapy. Nature 1988;332:323-327.

21. Waldmann H: Manipulation of the immune system with monoclonal antibodies. Annu Rev Immunol 1989;7:407-444.

22. Cobbold SP, Barel D, Waldmann H: Manipulating the immune system with monoclonal antibodies, in *T Cell Activation and Disease*, edited by Feldmann M, Lamb J. Wiley, New York, 1989;147-175.

23. Cobbold SP, Jayasuriya A, Nash A, Prospero TD, Waldmann H: Therapy with monoclonal antibodies by elimination of T-cell subsets in vivo. Nature 1984;312: 548-551.
24. Thierfelder S, Cobbold S, Kummer U, Waldmann H, Schuh R: Antilymphocytic antibodies and marrow transplantation. VII. Two of nine monoclonal anti-Thy-1 antibodies used for pretreatment of donor marrow suppressed graft-versus-host reactions without added complement. Exp Hematol 1985;13:948-955.
25. Cobbold S, Martin G, Waldmann H: Monoclonal antibodies for the prevention of graft-versus-host disease and marrow graft rejection: The depletion of T-cell subsets in vitro and in vivo. Transplantion 1986;42:239-247.
26. Dyer MJS, Hale G, Hayhoe FGJ, Waldmann H: Effects of CAMPATH-1 antibodies in vivo in patients with lymphoid maligancies; influence of antibody isotype. Blood 1989;73:1431-1439.
27. Hale G, Dyer MJS, Clark MR, Phillips JM, Marcus R, Riechmann L, Winter G, Waldmann H: Remission induction in non-Hodgkin lymphoma with rehsaped human monoclonal antibody CAMPATH-1H. Lancet 1988;ii:1394-1399.
28. Benjamin R, Waldmann H: Induction of tolerance by monoclonal antibody therapy. Nature 1986;320:449-451.
29. Benjamin RJ, Cobbold SP, Clark MR, Waldmann H: Tolerance to rat monoclonal antibodies: implications for serotherapy. J Exp Med 1986;163:1539-1552.
30. Benjamin RJ, Qin S, Wise MP, Cobbold SP, Waldmann H: Monoclonal antibodies for tolerance induction: a possible role for the CD4 (L3T4) and CD11a (LFA-1) molecules in self-non-self discrimination. Eur J Immunol 1988;18;1079-1088.
31. Qin S, Cobbold S, Tighe H, et al.: CD4 monoclonal antibody pairs for immunosuppression and tolerance induction. Eur J Immunol 1987;17:1159-1165.
32. Qin S, Cobbold S, Benjamin R, Waldmann H: Induction of classical transplantation tolerance in the adult. J Exp Med 1989;169:779-794.
33. Korngold R, Sprent J: Lethal GVHD across minor histocompatibility barriers: mature of the effector cells and role of the H2 complex. Immunol Rev 1983;71: 5-30.
34. Mason DW: Subsets of T cells in the rat mediating lethal graft-versus-host disease. Transplantation 1981;32:222.
35. Vallera DA, Soderling CC, Kersey JH: Bone marrow transplantation across major histocompatibility barriers in mice. III. Treatment of donor grafts with monoclonal antibodies directed against Lyt determinants. J Immunol 1982;128:871-875.
36. Korngold R, Sprent J: Surface markers of T cells causing lethal graft-versus-host disease to class I versus class II H-2 differences. J Immunol 1985;135:3004.
37. Korngold R, Sprent J: T cell subsets and graft-versus-host disease. Transplantation 1987;44:335-339.
38. Cobbold SP, Martin G, Qin S, Waldmann H: Monoclonal antibodies to promote marrow engraftment and tissue graft tolerance. Nature 1986;323:164-166.
39. Storb R, Thomas ED: Graft-versus-host disease in dog and man: the Seattle experience. Immunol Rev. 1985;88:215-238.
40. Hale G, Cobbold S, Waldmann H: T cell depletion with CAMPATH-1 in allogeneic bone marrow transplantation. Transplantation 1988;45:753-759.
41. Hale G, Waldmann H: CAMPATH-1 for prevention of graft-versus-host disease and graft rejection. Summary of results from a multi-centre study. Bone Marrow Transplantation 1988;3(Suppl 1):11-14.
42. Frame JN, Sheehy D, Cartegena T, Cirrincione C, O'Reilly R, Kernan NA: Optimal conditions for in vitro T cell depletion of human marrow by CAMPATH-1 plus complement as demonstrated by limiting dilution analysis. Bone Marrow Transplantation 1989;4:55-61.

43. Cheney RT, Sprent J: Capacity of cyclosporine to induce auto-graft-versus-host disease and impair intrathymic T cell differentiation. Transplant Proc 1985;17: 528-530.

44. Slavin S, Or R, Naparstek E, Cividalli G, Weshler Z, Weiss L, Mumcuoglu M, Engel-hard D, Aker M, Pollack A, Ben-Yehuda A, Brautbar C, Hale G, Waldmann H: New approaches for the prevention of rejection and graft-vs-host disease in clinical bone marrow transplantation. Israel J Med Sci 1986;22:264-267.

45. Weiden PL, Flournoy N, Thomas ED, et al.: Antileukemic effect of graft-versus-host disease in human recipients of allogeneic marrow grafts. New Engl J Med 1979;300: 1068-1073.

46. Weiden PL, Sullivan KM, Fluornoy N, et al.: Antileukemic effect of chronic graft-versus-host disease: contribution to improved survival after allogeneic marrow trans-plantation. New Engl J Med 1981;304:1529-1533.

47. Ringden O: for the Advisory Committee of the IBMTR. Graft-versus-leukaemia reac-tions in early leukaemia. Bone Marrow Transplantation 1988;3(Suppl 1):216.

48. Waldmann H, Hale G, Cobbold S: The immunobiology of bone marrow transplanta-tion, in *Leucocyte Typing III: white cell differentiation antigens.* edited by McMi-chael AJ, et al. Oxford University Press, Oxford, 1987; pp. 932-937.

15

Thalidomide Treatment for Graft-vs.-Host Disease

Georgia B. Vogelsang
The Johns Hopkins Univeristy School of Medicine
Baltimore, Maryland

I. INTRODUCTION

Thalidomide (N-phthalimidoglutarimide) is best known as an unsuspected teratogenic agent. Thalidomide also has immunosuppressive properties, which were first recognized about the time of withdrawal of thalidomide from clinical use. Although small clinical trials in a variety of autoimmunity diseases continued to take place, this finding was not aggressively pursued. We have found that thalidomide is a very effective agent for treating and preventing GVHD in animal models. We have begun human trials with thalidomide.

Thalidomide was introduced as a sedative in 1956 (1). Because of the lack of toxicity in rodent studies and the lack of overdose-suicide potential, thalidomide rapidly became a frequently prescribed drug. It was sold under several trade names and was added to many other drugs for its sedative effects. In 1961 the drug was withdrawn after it was associated with fetal anomalies. The unusual nature of these birth defects (phocomelia—small or absent limbs with or without other abnormalities) enabled investigators to associate the introduction of thalidomide with the sudden increase in this rare constellation of anomalies. Further work with thalidomide showed that the teratogenic effects are species-specific (i.e., not seen in rodents, but found in rabbits). Thalidomide was the drug that demonstrated the need for extensive preclinical screening and has been credited with launching the Food and Drug Administration into meaningful drug regulation.

About the time of thalidomide removal, reports of neuropathies appeared in the literature (2). It is still difficult to ascertain the prevalence of the problem, since the majority of patients receiving the drug have Hansen's disease (see below). The neuropathy is usually described as having a stocking-glove distribution with sensory changes predominating (3). There have been no direct relationships with dose and exposure; however, the majority of patients have received the drug for many months to years. Older patients seem more frequently affected. The neuropathy has not always reversed on discontinuing the drug (2).

II. IMMUNOLOGIC EFFECTS OF THALIDOMIDE

Sheskin made the first reports of the immunologic activity of thalidomide (4). He noted that patients with reactional lepromatous leprosy (a syndrome characterized by erythematous nodules and systemic symptoms such as fever, malaise, weight loss, iritis, neuritis, adenopathy, acute epididymo-orchitis, and proteinura) receiving thalidomide as a sedative had rapid relief of their systemic symptoms. Because of the impressive responses, the World Health Organization sponsored a controlled trial showing the effectiveness of thalidomide in lepromatous leprosy (5). How thalidomide exerts these effects in Hansen's disease is not known. As recently reviewed by Hastings, animal models suggest that thalidomide inhibits IgM synthesis, inhibits neutrophil chemotaxis, and decreases phagocytosis (6). These may be important in blocking the systemic effects of lepromatous leprosy.

Multiple other conditions of possible immunologic origin have responded to thalidomide (7). Diseases with reported responses include actinic prurigo, discoid lupus erythematous, aphthous stomatitis, Behcet's syndrome, pyroderma gangrenosum, ulcerative colitis, and prurigo nodularis. The difficulty obtaining thalidomide has prevented most investigation into its use in autoimmune disorders. Most reports of its use have been in patients who have failed conventional therapy.

The possible immunologic effects of thalidomide were postulated to be related to the teratogenic effects. It was suggested that thalidomide may not be toxic to the fetus but rather an immunosuppressive agent that prevented the "rejection" of abnormal fetuses. Although this idea did not account for the specificity of the anomalies, the species specificity, or why deformed fetuses were immunogenic, it did spawn some early work on the immunologic properties of thalidomide. Hellman et al. (8) reported that thalidomide prolonged graft survival. Since then about equal numbers of investigators have found a beneficial effect as have found no effect on graft survival (9-13). Field et al. (14) first suggested that thalidomide may be useful in GVHD. They measured spleen weight as an index of GVHD in a parent into F_1 hybrid model and found equivocal improvements in animals receiving thalidomide. In most of the studies quoted above, significant experimental design problems existed, resulting in contradictory results. Thalidomide is rapidly hydrolyzed. Thus, in experiments giving the drug in drinking water, little or no drug was actually administered. In other experiments, the drug was given i.p. in methylcellulose. Given this way, the majority of the drug actually remains unabsorbed in the peritoneal cavity. Moreover, in all of these experiments, the drug was given only for several days. Experiments in our laboratory with skin grafts have shown a doubling of graft survival time when thalidomide was given twice a day by gavage in vegetable oil (15). Preliminary studies with a cardiac allograft model have shown prolonged graft survival also. Thus, there is some evidence that these early investigators were correct that thalidomide does have some ability to prolong graft survival, but experimental flaws prevented definitive demonstration.

III.   EFFECTS ON EXPERIMENTAL GVHD

Because of the suggestions of immunologic activity and the relative lack of side effects, we have conducted experiments using thalidomide in a major mismatch rat model of GVHD to ascertain its immunosuppressive effects (15-19). This model is a well-established one and was used with the initial work with CsA (20). Lewis rats after marrow lethal total body irradiation (TBI) received TR1-incompatible ACI marrow and within 2 weeks developed acute GVHD. Untreated, most animals succumb to GVHD. In the first series of experiments, animals were treated with thalidomide once GVHD was documented by clinical appearance (erythematous skin, weight loss, bilirubinuria) and at least grade 2 GVHD histologically on skin biopsy. The results of these experiments are shown in Table 1. As can be seen, the majority of animals responded to therapy. Once therapy was discontinued after 40 days, the animals remained stable chimeras with no flare of disease occurring. These results look promising when compared to similar work done with CsA. In this same model, we were unable to rescue animals with CsA once GVHD was apparent. Initial work by Borel et al. (21) suggested that animals developing GVHD after completion of an initial course of CsA responded to a second course. Tutschka et al. (20) could not confirm these results. Moreover, in both the rat and dog, if therapy was delayed 3 to 5 days posttransplant, CsA was unsuccessful in preventing or treating GVHD (20,22).

In the next series of experiments, thalidomide was administered at 50 mg/kg/day or 100 mg/kg/day starting the day of major mismatched transplant (ACI marrow into lethally irradiated Lewis recipients). Prophylaxis was successful in the majority of animals (Table 2). The animals developing GVHD had mild cutaneous GVHD, which responded to continued thalidomide therapy. Again, this work looks promising when compared to CsA. CsA given at a dose of 12.5 mg/kg prevents GVHD in this model. However, when the CsA is discontinued almost all animals develop GVHD. All of the thalidomide-treated animals remained stable chimeras after cessation of therapy at day 40 and accepted ACI skin grafts while rejecting the third-party BN skin grafts. Control animals receiving 12.5 mg/kg/day of subcutaneous CsA developed acute GVHD once CsA was stopped. All of these animals were subsequently rescued with thalidomide (50 mg/kg/day). Dose titration studies have shown that 50 mg/kg/day dose to be the most successful (Table 3). Animals receiving 1 mg/kg, 5 mg/kg, 10 mg/kg, and 25 mg/kg all developed GVHD. All animals responded to continued therapy, however, the higher the dose of thalidomide,

Table 1   Treatment of Acute GVHD

Evaluable animals	Thalidomide therapy	Animals without GVHD		
		Day 14	Day 40	Day 100
28	none	0	–	–
48	50 mg/kg × 40 days	0	46[a]	46
17	100 mg/kg × 40 days	0	16[a]	16

GVHD = acute Graft-vs.-Host Disease; MHC = major histocompatibility complex.

[a]Animals died of acute GVHD and infection.

Table 2 Prophylaxis of Acute GVHD

Evaluable animals	CsA prophylaxis	Thalidomide prophylaxis	Animals without GVHD		
			Day 14	Day 40	Day 100
12	None	None	0	—	—
24	12.5 mg/kg	None	24	24	4
64	None	50 mg/kg	54[a]	64	64

[a]Animals developed mild GVHD which responsed to continued therapy.

the more rapid the response and, overall, the less severe the disease. These results suggest that there is a dose response to thalidomide. When CsA is given in a similar fashion, there is a sharp breakpoint around 10 mg/kg dose. Doses less than this are equally ineffective. At 10 mg/kg about half of the animals develop GVHD. At 12.5 mg/kg, none of the animals develop GVHD.

Pharmacokinetic studies using an HPLC assay have been preformed in conjunction with the above studies (18). Dose levels, plasma levels, and efficacy were correlated. These studies show that at the lowest effective dose of 50 mg/kg/day, a level about 8 µg/ml was obtained in the animals.

Subtherapuetic doses of CsA and thalidomide were given to determine if there was any interaction between CsA and thalidomide (18). Animals receiving low doses of thalidomide or low doses of CsA developed acute GVHD, as shown in Table 4. Animals receiving the low dose combinations had a lower incidence of GVHD. Measurement of blood levels of CsA and thalidomide in these animals failed to show that metabolism of the drugs had been altered in such a way as to increase effective blood levels. These studies combined with the studies showing that thalidomide could be used after CsA show that there is no apparent antagonism between the two drugs.

Chimerism in all of the above models was shown by the permanent (>100 days) acceptance of ACI skin grafts with rejection of third-party BN skin grafts. The chimeric animals failed to respond to donor ACI or recipient Lewis lymphocytes but did respond to BN lymphocytes in mixed lymphocyte cultures. Adoptive transfer experiments were

Table 3 Thalidomide Dose Response

Evaluable animals	Thalidomide Dose mg/kg	Animals without GVHD				
		Day 14	Day 21	Day 28	Day 35	Day 42
6	0	0	0	—	—	—
8	1	0	0	2	5	8
6	5	0	5	6	6	6
6	10	0	5[a]	5	5	5
3	25	0	3	3	3	3
6	50	6	6	6	6	6

[a]One animal died of viral infection after recovery from mild GVHD.

Table 4 Combination Low-Dose Thalidomide plus CsA Prophylaxis of GVHD

Evaluable animals	CsA prophylaxis	Thalidomide prophylaxis	Animals without GVHD		
			Day 14	Day 40	Day 100
8	2.5 mg/kg	None	0	—	—
12	2.5 mg/kg	1 mg/kg	6[a]	12	12
12	2.5 mg/kg	5 mg/kg	9[a]	12	12
13	2.5 mg/kg	10 mg/kg	12[a]	13	13
8	5 mg/kg	None	0	—	—
10	5 mg/kg	1 mg/kg	7[a]	10	10
14	5 mg/kg	2.5 mg/kg	12[a]	14	14
19	5 mg/kg	5 mg/kg	18[a]	19	19

[a]Animals developed mild GVHD which responded to continued therapy.

also performed. Lethally irradiated Lewis rats and WF rats received fresh ACI marrow plus splenocytes from thalidomide-treated chimeras (Lewis rats with ACI marrow). The Lewis rats did not develop GVHD but did accept an ACI skin graft while rejecting a third-party BN skin graft. WF animals died of acute GVHD. These data suggest that thalidomide permitted the development of specific suppressor cells, an observation similar to that seen with CsA.

The animal model was also used to explore the use of thalidomide in chronic GVHD (19). The histopathology and immunology of chronic GVHD in this MHC-mismatched rat model has been well characterized (23). This model has never been used as a therapeutic model in the past. Animals with chronic GVHD were treated with 1.5 mg/kg azathioprine and 1 mg/kg prednisone every other day (standard therapy), thalidomide 50 mg/kg/day, or CsA 7.5 mg/kg/day (9). Therapy was administered for 6 weeks. Of 7 animals receiving standard therapy, 3 died or had progressive disease, 2 had a 50% improvement, and 2 had 100% improvement. Of 11 animals treated with thalidomide, 1 died and the remaining had complete responses. Of the animals treated with CsA, 8 died and the remaining 3 were complete responders. Once therapy was discontinued, 2 animals in both the prednisone/azathioprine group and CsA relapsed with chronic GVHD. Preliminary experiments with low dose combination thalidomide and CsA show the same synergy as was seen in acute GVHD. Combinations of thalidomide with prednisone and azathioprine failed to show additional benefit. Although a larger number of animals need to be treated, these results suggest that thalidomide may also have utility in treating chronic GVHD.

IV. CLINICAL TRIALS

Because of the encouraging results in animals models, a phase I/II trial of thalidomide for patients failing first line therapy with acute or chronic GVHD has been started (24). With the initial patients entered on the study it became evident that the thalidomide levels were lower than anticipated, especially in patients with acute GVHD. Dosing had been based on pharmacologic data from the time of introduction of the drug which employed a colorometric assay. Because of the low levels obtained, we performed normal volunteer pharmacokinetic studies using HPLC methodology to measure the thalidomide.

These studies showed that both the rate of absorption and maximal absorption is quite variable after a single oral dose. The degree of sleepiness did not correlate with peak absorption. Thus, although it may limit the dosage given as the patient becomes more tolerant to the effects of the drug, sleepiness is not a good biologic indicator of absorption. Because of these findings in normal volunteers, we are currently trying to determine a better dosing schedule. Specifically, we are seeing if a less frequent dosing schedule or a "weighted" schedule with most pills taken at night will provide as good or better drug therapy.

Because of the difficulties of absorption in patients with damaged guts with acute GVHD and the need to rapidly treat these very ill patients, an intravenous formulation of the drug is being actively pursued.

Despite these difficulties with the pharmacokinetics, the trial, particularly in chronic GVHD, has continued. Although still early, responses in patients who have failed multiple agents have been seen. Responses have been seen in patients with lichenoid, sclerodermatous, oral, ocular, and hepatic involvement with GVHD. One patient with myasthenia gravis and chronic GVHD also appears to have benefitted. These patients are unique in that they have survived for an average of 2 years with this disease. Other investigators are also reporting responses in patients treated with thalidomide. Thalidomide levels have been used to assure adequate dosing. Further follow-up will be necessary to determine the extent and durability of these responses. If these trials continue to be successful, a trial comparing thalidomide standard therapy is planned.

V. MECHANISTIC STUDIES

The mechanism of the immunologic effects of thalidomide has not been fully explored. As mentioned earlier, there have been several lines of investigation including the effects of thalidomide on antibody synthesis, neutrophil chemotaxis, and graft rejection. Little is known about the cellular or molecular mechanism of action of thalidomide in particular as it relates to cellular immunity. One pertinent finding is the absolute decrease of $CD4^+$ and increase in $CD8^+$ cells in normal volunteers receiving thalidomide (25). These findings are similar to those seen in our laboratory in normal animals receiving CsA.

Exploring the mechanism of action of thalidomide in vitro has been difficult. Thalidomide is a small, nonpolar molecule. This has caused two major problems. First, thalidomide is very insoluble. Thus, it is difficult to directly determine the immunologic effects of thalidomide on cells. Second, thalidomide, once in solution, hydrolizes rapidly. These two problems have made it difficult to determine if native thalidomide or a metabolite are the active compound. Extensive work has been done with analogues which suggest that the phthalimide ring structure must be intact for the drug to retain activity. Work in this animal model of GVHD has shown that phthalimide is capable of preventing but not treating GVHD (7). Aminoglutethamide (a glutamide derivative) is incapable of either preventing or treating GVHD. To date, a satisfactory thalidomide derivative has not been found, although the search for a nonteratogenic (and hopefully more soluble) compound continues.

As another method of exploring the immunologic properties, we have synthesized a fluorescent thalidomide derivative (17). The binding of this thalidomide derivative to normal peripheral blood lymphocytes is strikingly similar to the binding of fluorescent, dansylated cyclosporine. With both drugs, there is a small intensely binding group of cells (brights) and a large, less intensely binding group of cells (dims). The lymphocytes

Table 5 Characterization of Cells Based on Staining Characteristics

	Danylated CsA		Fluorescent thalidomide	
	Bright	Dims	Bright	Dims
Helper T cells	−	+	−	+
Cytotoxic T cells	−	+	−	+
Suppressor T cells	+	−	+	−
IL-2 stimulation	−	+	−	+
Mitogenic stimulation	−	+	−	+
Alloantigen	−	+	−	+

identified by each drug are the same (i.e., the cells which stain brightly with cyclosporine also stain intensely with thalidomide). The two groups have been functionally and phenotypically characterized (Table 5). The brights for both drugs appear to be antigen-specific suppressor cells. The dims for each drug contain precursor cytotoxic lymphocytes.

Current work is directed at identification of intracellular binding proteins for each drug. At least two binding proteins have been identified for CsA—calmodulin and cyclophilin. While the relative amount of calmodulin within a cell is relatively constant, the concentration of cyclophilin varies greatly and is inversely proportional to the CsA sensitivity. Thus, cyclophilin appears to be a negative regulator. Early work suggests that these proteins may also be important in how thalidomide affects cells.

There are many similarities between thalidomide and CsA. The last similarity which will be recounted here is the ability to use both drugs to induce syngeneic GVHD. Basically, when either drug is given after a syngeneic transplant, a syndrome clinically and histologically indistinguishable from allogeneic GVHD occurs. We are using this model to better understand how self-recognition occurs.

Thus, although thalidomide and CsA are strikingly different compounds chemically, the similarities between the two are remarkable. The ability to use two different compounds to probe alloreactivity and transplantation tolerance (allogeneic GVHD and its resolution) as well as auto-recognition (syngeneic/autologous GVHD) should result in significant advances in our understanding of immunologic regulation.

ACKNOWLEDGMENT

Supported in part by grants CA 44783 and CA 15346 from the National Cancer Institute. Dr. Vogelsang is a Special Fellow of the Leukemia Society of America.

REFERENCES

1. Kunz W, Keller H, Muckter H. N-Phthalyl-glutaminsaure-inid: Experimentelle Untersuchungen an einem neuen synthetischen Product mit sedtiven Eigenschaften. Arzneimittelforsch 1956;6:426-430.
2. Fullerton PM, O'Sullivan OJ. Thalidomide neuropathy: A clinical electrophysiological and histological followup. N Neurol, Neurosurg, and Psychiat 1968;31:543-551.
3. Mellin GW, Katzenstein M. The saga of thalidomide. New Engl J med 1962;267:1184-1193, 1238-1244.

4. Sheskin J. Thalidomide in treatment of lepra reactions. Clin Pharmacol Ther 1965;6: 303-306.
5. Iyer CGS, Languillon J, Ramunujam K, Tarabini-Castellani G, Terencia de las Aguas J, Bechelli L, et al. WHO coordinated short term double blind trial with thalidomide in the treatment of acute lepra reaction in male lepromatous patients. Bull WHO 1971;45:719-732.
6. Hasting RC. Kellersberger memorial lecture 1979: Immunosuppressive/anti-inflammatory thalidomide analogues. Ethiop Med J 1980;18:65-71.
7. Barnhill RL, McDougall AC. Thalidomide: Use and possible mode of action in reactional lepromatous leprosy and various other conditions. J Am Acad Dermatol 1982;7:317-323.
8. Hellman K. Effect of thalidomide on the immunological response in local lymph nodes after a skin homograft. Lancet 1966;1:1134-1136.
9. Playfair JHC, Leuchare E, Davres AJS. Effect of thalidomide on skin graft survival. Lancet 1963;1:1003-1004.
10. Bore PJ, Scothorne RJ. Effect of thalidomide on survival of skin homografts in rabbits. Lancet 1966;1:1240-1242.
11. Florsheim GL. Another chance for thalidomide. Lancet 1966;1:207.
12. Dukor P, Dietrich FM. Immunosuppression by thalidomide. Lancet 1967; 1:569-570.
13. Mouzas GL, Gershon RK. The effect of thalidomide on skin allografts in mice: survival of the grafts. Transplantation 1968;6:476-478.
14. Field EO, Gibbs JE, Tucker DF, Hellmann K. Effect of thalidomide on the graft versus host reaction. Nature 1966;211:1308-1310.
15. Vogelsang GB, Hess AD, Gordon G, Santos GW. Treatment and prevention of acute graft-versus-host disease with thalidomide in a rat model. Transplantation 1986;41:644-647.
16. Vogelsang GB, Taylor S, Gordon G, Hess AD. Thalidomide, a potent agent for the treatment of graft-versus-host disease. Transplant Proc 1986;18:904-907.
17. Vogelsang, GB, Hess AD, Gordon G, Brundrett RB, Santos GW. Thalidomide—induction of transplantation tolerance. Transplant Proc 1987;19:2658-2661.
18. Vogelsang GB, Wells MC, Santos GV, and Hess AD. Combination low dose thalidomide and cyclosporine prophylaxis for acute graft-versus-host disease. Transplant Proc 1988;20:226-228.
19. Vogelsang GB, Hess AD, Friedman K, Santos GW. Therapy of chronic graft-versus-host disease in a rat model. Blood 1986;68(Suppl. 1):1020.
20. Tutschka PJ, Beshorner WE, Hess AD. Use of cyclosporine a (CsA) in a rat model of allogeneic marrow transplantion. Blut 1980;25(Suppl):241-253.
21. Borel JF, Feyer, C, Gubler HU, Statelin H. Biological effects of cyclosporin A: a new anti-lymphocytic agent. Agents Actions 1976;6:468-475.
22. Deeg HJ, Storb R. Experimental marrow transplantation, in *Cyclosporin A*, edited by White DJG. Elsevier Biomedical, Amsterdam, 1982;pp. 121-134.
23. Beschorner WE, Tutschka PJ, Santos GW. Chronic graft-versus-host disease in the rat radiation chimera. I. Clinical presentation, hematology, histology, and immunopathology in long term chimeras. Transplantation 1982;33:393-397.
24. Vogelsang GB, Hess AD, Ling T, Brundrett RB, Colvin OM, Wingard JR, et al. Thalidomide therapy of chronic graft-versus-host disease. Blood 1987;70(Suppl. 1):1116.
25. Gad SM, Shannon EJ, Krotoski WA, Hastings RC. Thalidomide induces imbalances in T-lymphocyte sub-populations in the circulating blood of healthy males. Lepr Rev 1985;56:35-39.

PART II
Clinical Graft-vs.-Host Disease

Introduction

H. Joachim Deeg
University of British Columbia and
Vancouver General Hospital
Vancouver, British Columbia, Canada

Kerry Atkinson
St. Vincent's Hospital
Sydney, New South Wales, Australia

As shown in Part I, extensive studies in animal models have investigated the principles of bone marrow transplantation and have established a foundation upon which to build clinical transplant protocols. Animal and in vitro human models have allowed us to recognize, with increasing sophistication, mechanisms of cell-cell interaction, cell activation, modulation, and regulation, and a network of cytokines. These tools should enable us to solve, eventually, the remaining hurdles of transplantation. The following chapters show not only where marrow transplantation has succeeded, but also where old problems remain or new ones have developed.

The first clinical bone marrow transplants carried out in the mid-1950s by E. D. Thomas showed that many observations made in murine models could be extrapolated to the clinical situation; for example, patients given marrow infusions from donors other than monozygotic twins were likely to develop "secondary disease" now called Graft-vs.-Host Disease (GVHD). These manifestations were similar to those observed in mice, involving mostly skin, intestinal tract, and liver.

Initially the use of marrow transplantation was restricted to patients with far advanced leukemia. However, it is of interest to recall that at this time G. Mathe also attempted marrow transplantation in victims of a radiation accident at Vinka, Yugoslavia. On a smaller scale, this situation was similar to that 30 years later at Chernobyl. However, the Vinka accident preceded the introduction of histocompatibility typing; it was not until the mid-1950s that Jean Dausset described antibodies in the sera of pregnant women that showed preferential reactivity with leukocytes from the fetus's father. Antigens recognized by those antibodies were subsequently termed human leukocyte antigens (HLA); they are encoded for by a series of genes, termed the major histocompatibility complex (MHC), on the short arm of chromosome 6.

In the 1960s several observations relevant to the genetics and the mechanism of GVHD were reported. Pediatricians observed neonates with manifestations of severe

immunodeficiency that were apparently not genetically determined. Findings resembled
those in mice which were neonatally injected with allogeneic cells and developed runt
disease. Babies with hydrops fetalis given intrauterine or postnatal exchange transfusions could develop florid GVHD. It was recognized that the relative immunoincompetence of fetuses and neonates allowed for engraftment of maternal cells via materno-
fetal transfusion in utero or of third-party donor cells administered via exchange transfusions. These conditions, therefore, fulfilled the requirements for the development of
GVHD as formulated by R. Billingham: (1) administration of immunocompetent donor
cells; (2) histoincompatibility between donor and recipient; and (3) inability of the recipient to destroy or inactivate the transfused or transplanted cells.

In 1968 Epstein and colleagues in Seattle were the first to show the importance
of histocompatibility typing for the outcome of bone marrow transplantation in randomly bred dogs. At about the same time the first successful allogeneic transplant was
carried out by Good and colleagues in a boy with Wiskott-Aldrich syndrome. Rodent
models developed by Santos et al. and van Bekkum et al. and a canine model developed
by Thomas et al. and Storb et al. paved the way for the development of clinical protocols
not only for the conditioning of patients, but also for the postgrafting prevention of
GVHD by agents such as cyclophosphamide or methotrexate (MTX).

The next two decades saw the rapid development of clinical transplantation, growing from an initial few centers to several hundred transplant units worldwide, with more
than 4000 allogeneic transplants being performed annually. Postgrafting GVHD prophylaxis at the beginning of this modern era of bone marrow transplantation utilized either
intermittent cyclophosphamide or MTX. With these regimens, 50-70% of patients still
developed acute GVHD. In 1974 Glucksberg et al. described a grading system for the
disease, taking into consideration involvement of skin, intestinal tract, and liver (as well
as overall performance of the patient), based on pathological and clinical parameters.

The following 24 chapters of this book deal with clinical GVHD as we know it
today. Chapters 16 through 30 focus on the acute form of the disease. Deeg and Cottler-
Fox (Chapter 16) introduce the topic by describing the clinical spectrum and the pathophysiology of acute GVHD. There is evidence that the introduction of cyclosporine
(CSP) has modified the clinical appearance of GVHD; if CSP is combined with other
agents such as MTX or glucocorticoids, the overall incidence of acute GVHD after transplantation of marrow from an HLA-identical sibling is reduced to about 20% and severe
or lethal manifestations are rare. The incidence of chronic GVHD is less affected. With
HLA-nonidentical transplants the incidence of acute GVHD remains high despite combination regimens, although mortality appears to have decreased. The mechanisms of
tolerance and acute GVHD in clinical marrow transplantation are still incompletely
understood. Evidence for nonspecific suppressor cells (suppressor mechanisms) in GVHD
and a specific suppressor mechanism in the development of tolerance has been presented,
although attempts at cloning suppressor cells have been unsuccessful. The role of natural
suppressor cells is still unclear. Conceivably clonal anergy as described in murine models
is also operational in man. In addition to cellular considerations, a rapidly evolving cytokine network may contribute to our understanding: for example, there is evidence that
tumor necrosis factor is involved in acute GVHD, and blocking its action may interfere
with the manifestations of GVHD. Thus, the use of monoclonal antibodies directed at
soluble mediators may be helpful for prevention and treatment of GVHD.

Snover (Chapter 17) gives a detailed review of histological criteria used to establish
the diagnosis of acute GVHD. In the skin it is difficult, early after diagnosis, to differen-

tiate GVHD from chemoradiotherapy-induced changes and occasionally drug, or virus-related alterations. He emphasizes that the lesions may vary in different areas and different layers of the skin. Similarly, the intestinal tract may show manifestations related to causes other than GVHD. A particular variant of necrosis is the so-called "exploding crypt cell," most readily recognized in the rectum. Otherwise, biopsies of the small intestine are more reliable. The broadest differential diagnosis has to be considered in the liver. One finding Snover emphasizes as almost diagnostic is that of "endothelialitis," an infiltration of endothelium by lymphocytes quite similar to that seen in organ graft rejection. The most important finding with acute GVHD in any organ, however, is that of epithelial necrosis; lymphocytic infiltration may be absent. The involvement of other organs such as lungs, heart, and kidney remains controversial.

The next four chapters deal with the prevention of GVHD. Jacobs (Chapter 18) gives an overview of some experimental and clinical data and the rationale for donor pretreatment with CSP in an attempt to prevent GVHD in the recipient. This approach is intriguing. There are animal data suggesting that pretreatment of the donor with CSP or monoclonal antibodies directed, for example, at NK cells may reduce the probability of GVHD in the recipient. Such an approach would avoid manipulation of marrow in vitro and immunosuppressive treatment of patients in vivo. Ethically this would be acceptable only if the treatment was without risk to the donor.

Martin and Kernan (Chapter 19) give a comprehensive discussion of the concept of T-cell depletion with an assessment of the present advantages and disadvantages. Three to four log depletions of T cells from donor marrow can be achieved. It is important to assess remaining T lymphocytes by methods such as limiting dilution analysis. It appears that approximately 10^5 T cells/kg are generally tolerated without inducing GVHD. However, since different methods are being used and since it is not clear in man which lymphocyte subset triggers GVHD, the numbers of relevant T cells transplanted in different studies may vary widely. Of concern are the observations of an increased incidence of graft failure and leukemic recurrence with T-cell-depleted marrow. The mechanisms involved (donor T-cell antihost reactivity, altered lymphokine secretion, etc.) require further study. The rate of immunoreconstitution is usually not affected, although there can be delayed generation of cytotoxic T cells during the first 6 months. It has also been suggested that the incidence of EBV-related lymphoproliferative disorders may be increased in these patients. Additional studies on lymphocyte subpopulations (in donor bone marrow and in the patient following engraftment) and on cytokines are necessary.

Gluckman (Chapter 20) reviews chemotherapeutic regimens utilized for the prevention of GVHD. Emphasis is on CSP and combinations of CSP with other drugs such as MTX or glucocorticoids, combinations that have reduced the incidence of acute GVHD to around 20% after genotypically HLA-identical transplants. There are data to suggest that this figure may be even lower with the addition of I.V. immunoglobulin. The incidence of chronic GVHD has been less affected and remains at approximately 25-50%.

Finally, Vossen and Heidt (Chapter 21) present data on gnotobiotic measures used for the prevention of GVHD. Although this approach has been highly effective in murine models (as discussed in Part I of this book), it is not without problems in the clinical setting. The authors suggest that complete decontamination is more effective than selective decontamination and, in children, can reduce the incidence of acute GVHD after transplantation of unmanipulated marrow to 5%. Additional, prospectively randomized studies are desirable.

The next four chapters deal with the impact of immunogenetics and antiviral immune responses on the development of GVHD. Beatty and Herve (Chapter 22) present an overview of the role of histocompatibility antigens in the development of GVHD. The difference in GVHD with syngeneic (0%) and genotypically HLA-identical allogeneic transplants (20-50%) illustrates the impact of non-MHC antigens, which are very poorly defined. There is a clear increase in the incidence of GVHD with increasing degrees of HLA disparity between donor and recipient. While the administration of CSP and MTX had a beneficial effect with class I differences, it did not with class II differences. Microvariants of traditional HLA-A and B alleles are currently being studied, and their impact on GVHD remains to be determined. The same is true for newly described class I antigens (HLA-E) and HLA-B-associated transcripts or tumor necrosis factor.

This analysis is expanded in the next chapter by Herve, Cahn, and Beatty (Chapter 23), discussing the clinical impact of histoincompatibility on the development of GVHD. Clearly, GVHD is more frequent with HLA-nonidentical transplants (96% with a one haplotype disparent donor) than with HLA-identical transplants. Therefore, aggressive efforts at GVHD prevention via T-cell depletion were made. This, however, resulted in failure of sustained engraftment—in some studies in more than 50% of patients. Intensification of conditioning regimens can overcome this hurdle only partially, and at the expense of increased toxicity. It will be necessary to determine more precisely which donor T cells are beneficial to engraftment (hopefully without triggering GVHD) and which host cells oppose engraftment. This should facilitate the development of new regimens of monoclonal antibodies directed at donor or host cells (or both). The authors also suggest that selective B-cell depletion may reduce the risk of lymphoproliferative disorders with EBV-positive donors.

Rappeport (Chapter 24) then reviews syngeneic and autologous GVHD and the current concepts regarding its mechanism. Syngeneic GVHD was first reported 10 years ago and was thought to be due to T-cell dysregulation posttransplant and possibly virus-induced recipient cell modifications. Subsequently, extensive animal studies have revealed that CSP treatment and radiation-induced thymic damage interfere with the normal intrathymic maturation pathway and elimination of autoreactive cells. Although autologous and syngeneic transplant recipients generally do not receive CSP, many do receive irradiation. No cases of syngeneic GVHD have been observed in patients with aplastic anemia (conditioned with cyclophosphamide or given marrow without preceding conditioning).

There are solid data supporting a correlation of GVHD and infections, and there are studies showing a beneficial effect of gnotobiosis on GVHD prevention. Ringden summarizes data (Chapter 25) suggesting a correlation between donor (and patient) anti-herpesvirus immune status and the development of acute and chronic GVHD. It is hypothesized that, for example, in virus-positive recipients, immune donor cells might kill virus-infected cells, whereas nonimmune donor cells would undergo clonal expansion, thus increasing the risk of GVHD. Furthermore, activated cells might secrete cytokines, such as interferon, leading to the increased expression of histocompatibility antigens as targets for GVHD on patient cells. In addition, cross-reactive antigens (for example class I-like structures on CMV) may lead to an expansion of alloreactive cells. Although controversial, these data may explain some aspects of syngeneic or autologous GVHD that are otherwise difficult to understand.

In Chapter 26 Henslee describes modalities of treatment for acute GVHD. Classically, in patients given GVHD prophylaxis with MTX or cyclophosphamide, glucocorticoids were used for the treatment of established acute GVHD, with response rates of about 30%. Similar results were obtained with antithymocyte globulin (ATG), whereas combinations of ATG and CSP were beneficial in 60% of patients. Since most patients currently receive CSP prophylaxis, this approach is no longer an option. It appears, nevertheless, that those patients have a high response rate with either ATG or glucocorticoids. Anti-T-lymphocyte monoclonal antibodies have also been tested extensively. However, given alone they usually result in only transient responses. There is encouraging data with immunotoxin-conjugated monoclonal antibodies, both in patients given T-cell-depleted and T-cell-replete marrow grafts. Other agents, such as thalidomide, appear to have little effect on acute GVHD.

Yee (Chapter 27) supplements the preceding chapters by providing an overview of the pharmacological monitoring of immunosuppressive drugs in transplant patients. Although there has never been a randomized study comparing the efficacy of immunosuppression with a control group of patients not given immunosuppression, almost all patients given T-cell-replete marrow grafts do receive some immunosuppressive drug. It is of interest that MTX, historically the most widely used agent, is being monitored in regards to potentially toxic serum levels; however, dose and time-dependent therapeutic target ranges have never been clearly determined. Currently the most widely used drug is CSP. MTX has been compared to CSP in randomized studies but results have been ambiguous. There are wide patient-to-patient variations of CSP blood/plasma levels, and it has been difficult to establish clearly toxic and therapeutic ranges. Nevertheless, available data suggest that serum trough levels above 200 ng/ml reduce the risk of acute GVHD. If CSP is determined on whole blood, levels should be about twice as high. Toxicity is substantial, affecting kidneys, liver, the central nervous system, the skin, the cardiovascular system, and other organs. Other agents such as glucocorticoids given alone or ATG have played only a limited role in GVHD prophylaxis.

Bowden (Chapter 28) reviews infectious problems in patients undergoing bone marrow transplantation. While during the period of neutropenia immediately following transplantation all patients are highly susceptible to infections, patients with GVHD are at risk during their entire course. This is due to impaired immunoreconstitution, the immunosuppressive effect of GVHD itself, and immunosuppressive treatment, as well as breakdown of mechanical barriers (oral and intestinal mucosa). In earlier studies gramnegative organisms were responsible for most infections. Currently gram-positive bacteria, in particular staphylococci, are cultured frequently not only in patients with chronic but also with acute GVHD. Various fungal species and viruses, in particular herpesviruses, contribute to morbidity. The empiric use of broad spectrum antibiotics at the onset of fever, the addition of amphotericin B, and the prophylactic use of agents such as acyclovir have markedly reduced the incidence of fatal infections. This has been further helped by isolation of patients in laminar air flow rooms and by intravenous immunoglobulin administration. Prolonged treatment with cotrimoxazole has prevented not only *P. carinii* pneumonia but also other late infections. Better GVHD prevention may further reduce the incidence of infection.

Spitzer (Chapter 29) reviews the experience with transfusion-induced GVHD, not only in patients immunosuppressed by cytotoxic antitumor chemotherapy but also in neonates, patients after surgery, and certain nonmalignant diseases. A feature more striking in transfusion-induced GVHD as compared to posttransplant GVHD is that of marrow suppression, often contributing to the patient's death. The onset is often abrupt (median day 8). Leukocytes from patients with CML appear to be more potent in inducing GVHD than cells from normal donors, although it is not clear how many lymphocytes are necessary to trigger GVHD. Therapy, with glucocorticoids, has generally been unsuccessful, and more than 80% of reported patients have died. Transfusion-induced GVHD can be prevented by gamma-irradiation of the transfusion products.

In Chapter 30 Kernan analyzes the problem of graft failure after T-cell-depleted bone marrow transplantation. With HLA-nonidentical transplants, host cell reactivity is directed to disparate HLA antigens on donor cells; with HLA-identical transplants, the target antigens are entirely unknown. It is also not clear whether an increased recurrence of leukemia, reported in some series, is due to the same mechanism (reemergence of host cells in general) or is a separate phenomenon as suggested by murine experiments. Conceivably, the addition of growth factors after transplantation might be beneficial, although at least one study in mice suggests the opposite. This area clearly requires further investigation.

Chapters 31 to 39 deal predominantly with chronic GVHD. Atkinson (Chapter 31) reviews the clinical spectrum of chronic GVHD. The recognized manifestations of this symdrome have expanded over the past decade to include not only skin, mucous membranes, gastrointestinal tract, and liver but also serous membranes, muscle, lungs, kidneys, and even the nervous system. There are also ample data showing involvement of the hemopoietic system, often in the form of thrombocytopenia. Lymphoid hypoplasia, autoantibody production, and autoimmune disorders illustrate involvement of the immune system. The incidence of chronic GVHD has been reported to be 25-50%, and in older age groups even 70%. Chronic GVHD can be of the limited form (skin with or without liver involvement; good prognosis) or extensive (poorer prognosis) or can occur as a progression from acute GVHD after a quiescent interval or even de novo, which carries the best prognosis.

Shulman (Chapter 32) reviews the pathology and histology of chronic GVHD. He emphasizes the dynamic nature of chronic GVHD, both in regard to its time course and patterns of presentation. Lymphocytic infiltrates, often rich in $CD8^+$ cells, are frequently seen early in the course but may be missing completely at a more advanced stage. The picture in the skin, for example, can be that of hyperproliferation and acanthosis or hypoproliferation and atrophy. Stimulation of host fibroblasts by donor cells may lead to proliferation, and the release of cytokines, for example Il-4, may contribute to increased collagen production, and interferon release may result in increased expression of histocompatibility antigens on host cells. The impact of other cytokines is currently being investigated.

In Chapters 33 and 34, Atkinson describes risk factors and pathogenesis of chronic GVHD. Chronic GVHD appears to involve both alloreactivity and autoimmunity. For example, donor T cells can become sensitized to host tissue, as shown by in vitro reactivity (despite HLA identity), a finding further substantiated by the characterization of non-HLA antigens which can serve as targets. Activated donor cells can interact directly with host targets and destroy them. A thymus damaged by conditioning or GVHD may not be able to eliminate autoreactive cells, thus allowing for the development of autoimmune disorders. Chronic GVHD is more frequent in patients who previously had acute GVHD. Additional risk factors, even in patients without preceding acute GVHD, were increasing patient age, donor buffy coat infusion or a T-cell-replete marrow graft, and, in male patients, transplantation from an alloimmunized female donor. Thrombocytopenia at the time of diagnosis of chronic GVHD heralds a poor prognosis.

The natural history of untreated extensive chronic GVHD is unfavorable, with only 20% of patients surviving with Karnofsky scores ≥70%. It is important, therefore, to recognize the disease early. This is discussed by Loughran and Sullivan (Chapter 35). It is, indeed, possible to identify among asymptomatic patients without physical findings those who are likely to develop clinical GVHD. These patients with subclinical GVHD, at day 100 posttransplant, show abnormal light microscopic findings in skin and oral mucosa along with deposits of C3 and IgM, as well as a decrease in IgA plasma cells in lip biopsies. These patients tend to be older, have serum bilirubin values in excess of 1 mg/dl, and had previous acute GVHD or received prednisone after day 50 posttransplant. Disappointingly, early institution of treatment did not prevent the development of overt disease. Nevertheless, it appears useful to identify these patients for closer follow-up examinations. Recent data suggest that it may also be important to obtain a preliminary function test to diagnose early obliterative bronchiolitis; the disease may respond to immunosuppression but not to treatment directed at obstructive lung disease.

In Chapter 36 Lum reviews the impact of GVHD on immune recovery after transplantation. All patients undergoing bone marrow transplantation require at least 3-6 months for their immune system to show signs of maturation and up to 2 years for complete reconstitution. Frequently T lymphocytes fail to provide helper function and show excess suppression. In addition, B cells do not respond to neoantigens even in the presence of normal helper cells. There is also impaired chemotaxis of neutrophils. Immunoreconstitution may be further delayed in patients given T-cell-depleted grafts. In patients with chronic GVHD, immunoreconsitution is even further delayed, and abnormal suppressor function and low CD4/CD8 ratios may persist for years. There are impaired primary and secondary immune responses to specific antigens, and there is no switch from IgM to IgG antibody, although IgG levels may actually be high. B-cell defects may be further aggravated in HLA-incompatible transplants. Chronic GVHD also interferes with transferred immunity, as well as the response to vaccines.

Sanders (Chapter 37) reviews the effects of chronic GVHD on growth and fertility. Currently available data indicate that most endocrinological and developmental problems are related to total body irradiation, used as part of the conditioning regimen since only very minor problems are generally observed in patients prepared with chemotherapy alone. It appears, however, that GVHD, and possibly its treatment with glucocorticoids, adds further to growth inhibition. However, often no catch-up growth is observed even after discontinuation of treatment. GVHD also does not appear to affect fertility, although GVHD-related complications such as vaginitis can develop.

Treatment of chronic GVHD may not be necessary in patients with limited disease but is mandatory in patients with extensive disease since only 20% of those untreated are expected to survive (Chapter 38). Historical evidence suggested that cytotoxic therapy (e.g., azathioprine, procarbazine) is superior to glucocorticoids. However, a recent randomized study failed to show an advantage of a combination of prednisone plus azathioprine versus prednisone alone. In fact, there were more infectious complications with the combination, and survival was inferior. Thus, prednisone remains the mainstay of treatment for standard risk chronic GVHD and should be given for at least 9 months. Patients who fail to respond or those with thrombocytopenia may benefit from combinations of prednisone and CSP. All patients should receive infection prophylaxis, usually with cortimoxazole (or penicillin). Refractory patients may respond to the addition of azathioprine, to thalidomide, or to modalities such as ultraviolet A irradiation after sensitization with methoxypsoralen. A benefit of immunoglobulin administration has, so far, not been proven.

Finally Weiden and Horowitz (Chapter 39) review evidence in favor of the one potentially beneficial effect of GVHD in patients with malignant diseases—the graft-vs.-leukemia effect. Such an effect was demonstrated 30 years ago in murine models. Weiden and colleagues first showed in 1979 that patients transplanted for leukemia had a lower probability of disease recurrence if they developed GVHD (acute or chronic or both). This observation appeared to be supported by the fact that patients given transplants from monozygotic twin donors had a higher probability of relapse than patients transplanted from HLA-identical allogeneic donors. Subsequent investigations revealed that a graft-vs.-leukemia effect was quite prominent with some diagnoses (e.g., ALL) but less so with others (e.g., AML). Furthermore for any diagnosis the effect was strong for patients at high risk for relapse (acute leukemia transplanted in relapse, CML in blast transformation) but not significant in good risk patients. In high-risk patients the graft-vs.-leukemia effect was reflected in improved survival. It was of note that only clinically overt (but not subclinical) GVHD conveyed an antileukemia effect. Despite these observations, however, a randomized study in which GVHD was allowed to develop by design failed to show a net benefit of GVHD on probability of disease-free survival. Currently ongoing studies are expected to yield additional information on the role of T cells and allogenicity. However, so far it has not been possible to separate GVHD from a graft-vs.-leukemia effect.

In summary, these chapters show that despite controversies and uncertainties regarding the pathogenesis and prevention of GVHD, a great deal has been learned. In addition, they describe ongoing research that may further advance the field in the near future.

16

Clinical Spectrum and Pathophysiology of Acute Graft-vs.-Host Disease

H. Joachim Deeg
University of British Columbia and
Vancouver General Hospital
Vancouver, British Columbia, Canada

Michele Cottler-Fox
National Institutes of Health
Bethesda, Maryland

I. INTRODUCTION

Bone marrow transplantation consists of an infusion of viable lymphohemopoietic cells from one individual into another (1). Although attempts have been made at enriching for pluripotent stem cells capable of repopulating the recipient with cells of all lineages, the general approach is still to infuse a mixture of cells which, among others, contains lymphohemopoietic stem cells. This mixture also contains immunocompetent cells that are removed from their self environment and transferred into a nonself (foreign) milieu. It was noted already in early investigations that transplantation of lymphohemopoietic cells was relatively nonproblematic if the donor was syngeneic to the recipient (2). However, if the donor was histoincompatible, recipients, although achieving hemopoietic reconstitution, would usually develop skin changes, diarrhea, and weight loss (3), and die with a syndrome termed "secondary disease." Similar observations were made by Billingham and Brent (4) in mice neonatally transplanted with allogeneic spleen cells; these animals developed diarrhea, skin lesions, growth retardation, hypoplasia of the lymphatic organs, and hepatocyte necrosis and died from "runt disease." The larger the number of lymphocytes transfused, the more severe the disease or the earlier it developed (5). These observations have been summarized classically by Billingham in the three requirements necessary for the development of GVHD (6): (a) infusion of immunocompetent cells; (b) histocompatibility differences between donor and recipient; and (c) inability of the recipient to destroy donor cells.

The early work of Gowans (7) in a rat model suggested that GVHD was triggered by small lymphocytes contained in thoracic duct lymph. Subsequent work by others (8,9) confirmed this impression, and the work by McGregor (10) indicated that "marrow" cells, although incapable of inducing GVHD by themselves, gave rise to the cells (lymphocytes) which eventually triggered GVHD.

It is of note, nevertheless, that allogeneic marrow transplants can be carried out successfully between individuals other than identical twins. For example, among dogs given a transplant from a DLA-identical littermate, approximately 45% survive without GVHD without even having received postgrafting immunosuppression (11). Recent clinical trials indicate that even some human patients may be able to receive an allogeneic HLA-identical transplant without postgrafting immunosuppression and do not develop clinically significant GVHD (12). Thus, there may be donor-host combinations where, for reasons yet to be determined, tolerance develops without patients ever showing evidence of GVHD. Class et al. (13) recently observed that renal transplant recipients frequently failed to become sensitized and develop antibodies against the noninherited maternal HLA haplotype, a finding resembling that of neonatal tolerance in mice. It is tempting to speculate that marrow transplantation from a donor whose mother shares HLA antigens with the transplant recipient might result in a low incidence of GVHD. Such a situation would exist, for example, if two siblings had inherited the same paternal haplotype but different maternal haplotypes, respectively. Nevertheless, the likelihood of developing GVHD increases with the degree of histoincompatibility between donor and recipient (14), conceivably more so for class II than for class I major histocompatibility complex (MHC) antigen differences (15). The incidence of GVHD is reduced in both MHC identical and nonidentical transplant recipients who receive T-lymphocyte-depleted marrow (16) or are given immunosuppressive treatment after grafting (17).

II. CLINICAL SPECTRUM

A. Causes of GVHD

It is readily apparent that the conditions for the development of GVHD exist in settings other than allogeneic marrow transplantation. During pregnancy, paternal histocompatibility antigens expressed in the fetus reside for prolonged periods of time in the HLA haploidentical mother (18,19). Although the fetus enjoys a particularly privileged immunological status, there are instances where a materno-fetal transfusion can lead to a GVHD-like reaction in the fetus. It has been postulated, for example, that certain syndromes of immunodeficiency, clearly a feature of GVHD, are due to such intrauterine reactions (20). In addition, iatrogenic GVHD has been described following exchange transfusions in fetuses with hydrops fetalis (21). Similarly, any random donor transfusions given to a patient receiving immunosuppressive therapy, for example, for the treatment of Hodgkin's disease, carry the risk of GVHD due to the recipient's inability to reject transfused cells (22). Recent reports show that the requirements for GVHD are also fulfilled in some instances of organ transplantation, in particular after intestinal transplants where lymphoid cells presumably from the Peyer's patches are capable of attacking the immunosuppressed transplant recipient (23). Individual cases of GVHD have been associated with liver (24) or heart-lung transplants (25), presumably induced by lymphocytes from lymphatic tissue transplanted along with the organ. Most frequently, however, GVHD occurs in the setting of allogeneic marrow transplantation, and most investigations into GVHD have dealt with marrow transplant recipients.

B. Kinetics of GVHD

As in animal models, GVHD in man can develop early or late after transplantation (1). Accordingly, the disease has been separated into acute and chronic forms. Such a division is somewhat artificial. GVHD with features of the acute disease can develop with considerable delay, for example, after withdrawal of cyclosporine, not only after syngeneic but also after allogeneic transplantation (26,27). Conversely, GVHD with all characteristics of the chronic form can develop rather early after transplantation (1,28). It appears, therefore, that clinical (and occasionally laboratory) features characterize the disease form better than the time of onset (29).

Patients may develop only acute or chronic GVHD or may experience both forms of the disease (1,28), as shown schematically in Figure 1. The present chapter deals only with acute GVHD. (Chronic GVHD is discussed in Chapter 32.)

Human acute GVHD usually develops within 2-8 weeks of marrow transplantation in patients given genotypically HLA identical marrow grafts, and some form of GVHD prophylaxis (1,17). In patients receiving no GVHD prophylaxis (12,30) or transplanted from an HLA nonidentical donor (31,40) GVHD may develop hyperacutely within a few days of transplantation. Generally, the appearance of GVHD is preceded by evidence of donor marrow engraftment. However, occasionally signs of GVHD may develop in the absence of clear signs of engraftment (empty marrow, no rise in peripheral blood cell counts) or in the presence of "lymphoid engraftment" only. Thus, although one may be inclined to take the development of GVHD as an indicator of engraftment, it does not constitute proof of functional hemopoietic reconstitution. Perhaps this should not be surprising since GVHD by itself may inhibit hemopoiesis.

C. Target Organs of Acute GVHD

The classically recognized target organs of acute GVHD in man are skin, gastrointestinal tract, liver, and lymphatic organs (31-37). Although other tissues such as mucous membranes, conjunctivae, exocrine glands, and bronchial tree may also be involved, generally only involvement of skin, intestinal tract, and liver is used for clinical grading of acute GVHD (37-39) (Fig. 2).

The onset of acute GVHD is usually marked by a maculopapular rash often involving palms, soles, and ears, although it can begin in other areas of the body, such as back, shoulders, or face. The rash may then spread and involve the entire body surface. The lesions can remain distinct or become confluent, with the appearance of diffuse total body erythema. Usually the rash is pruritic, and patients may experience pruritus before a rash is visible. There may be an associated rise in body temperature. In more severe cases bullae can form, and via dermo-epidermal separation, large surface areas can desquamate, leading to denudation reminiscent of burn injuries. This is associated with significant protein loss and risk of superinfection. Occasionally the major complaint of patients

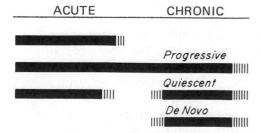

Figure 1 Presentation of chronic GVHD relative to acute GVHD.

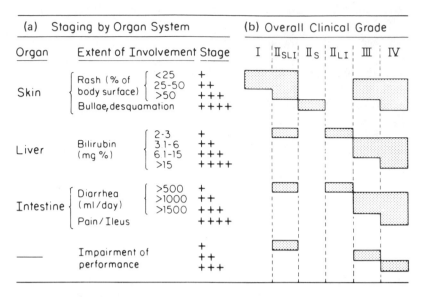

Figure 2 Clinical grading of acute GVHD: (a) summarizes the staging by organ system; (b) shows the overall clinical grade. With grade I, only the skin can be involved. With more extensive involvement of the skin or involvement of liver and intestinal tract and impairment of the clinical performance status, either alone or in any combination, the overall grade advances from II to IV. Some investigators consider it worthwhile to subdivide the overall grade II into one category including patients with skin involvement only (II_S), or liver and intestinal without skin involvement (II_{LI}). Patients with grade II_S may have a better prognosis than patients with other grade II diseases. Liver dysfunction also includes transaminase and alkaline phosphatase elevations. However, it appears difficult to correlate the extent of enzyme abnormality with the prognosis of GVHD. Some investigators prefer to grade intestinal involvement according to body weight: + = 10-15, ++ = 16-20, +++ = 21-25, and ++++ ≥ 26 ml/kg/day of diarrhea. (Modified from Deeg and Storb (38) and Vogelsang et al., personal communication.)

is burning in palms and soles, aggravated by weight bearing. These symptoms may worsen or may be triggered by the administration of cyclosporine, particularly when it is given intravenously (40).

With the fully developed picture of GVHD, the diagnosis should be unequivocal. However, if only a maculo-papular skin rash is present, the diagnosis may be in doubt. As discussed in Chapter 17, even a skin biopsy may not be diagnostic during the first 2-3 weeks after transplantation since histologic changes due to chemoradiotherapy can be indistinguishable from those seen with GVHD (41). Similarly, infections, especially of viral etiology and drug reactions, for example, to semi-synthetic penicillins and cotrimoxazole, must be excluded.

Hepatic and intestinal involvement may become manifest concurrently with or following skin involvement. Isolated liver or intestinal involvement is uncommon. Similarly, it is uncommon to see liver or gut involvement before skin disease is apparent (35-37). Nevertheless, it is in most instances the severity of liver and especially intestinal tract involvement that determines the prognosis (42).

Liver dysfunction may develop within days but more commonly within 2-4 weeks of transplantation. Generally there is a gradual rise of both direct and indirect bilirubin, which may peak at any level (see Fig. 2) and in extreme cases may reach values of $\geqslant 40$ mg/dl (684 μmol/L). In parallel there is usually a rise in alkaline phosphatase and transaminases (SGOT [AST], SGPT [ALT]) to as little as twice or as much as 10–20 times normal values. The gamma-glutamyl transpeptidase may be elevated even if other enzymes remain in the normal range. The liver may be enlarged, but patients rarely complain of pain.

The differential diagnosis of liver dysfunction is broader than with skin involvement. Mild to moderate liver function abnormalities, especially in the immediate posttransplant period, may be related to chemoradiotherapy used for conditioning, and mild elevations of bilirubin (mostly indirect) and lactate dehydrogenase may be seen even in patients conditioned with cyclophosphamide alone. Those abnormalities tend to regress spontaneously within days. Of greater concern is the development of veno-occlusive disease of the liver (43). This vascular complication usually occurs within 1-2 (rarely 3) weeks of transplantation, and typically presents with weight gain, right upper quadrant pain, abdominal distension, icterus and alkaline phosphatase elevation out of proportion of transaminase abnormalities. Other causes of hepatic dysfunction which may coexist with GVHD include infection (e.g., bacterial septicemia, cytomegalovirus), drug toxicity (e.g., cyclosporine), or parenteral nutrition (44).

Causes of intestinal disease after marrow transplantation are legion. GVHD frequently presents with diarrhea and nausea, sometimes abdominal pain, or even paralytic ileus (45). The bowel wall is edematous (46), the lumen may be fluid-filled, and the transit time can be extremely short. The stool is usually watery, green-brown; it can be overtly bloody or only show a guaiac positive reaction. In severe cases the picture may resemble cholera.

Many patients, particularly those conditioned with irradiation, will have diarrhea during the immediate posttransplant period. If this course is protracted, an infectious cause (e.g., *Clostridium difficile*) must be excluded, and the development of intestinal GVHD, presenting with the same symptoms and findings, must be considered.

Gross and histologic pathological findings of acute GVHD are reviewed in detail elsewhere (see Chapter 17). Briefly, the skin shows basal cell vacuolar degeneration and necrosis, dyskeratosis, spongiosis, eosinophilic body formation of epidermal cells, focal epidermo-dermal separation, occasionally progressing to complete epidermal loss. Typical hepatic lesions include eosinophilic necrosis of hepatocytes and necrosis of small bile duct epithelium. Grading of the lesions is generally based on bile duct findings since parenchymal lesions vary widely. Lesions in the gastrointestinal tract range from necrosis of single mucosal epithelial cells to crypt abscesses and diffuse mucosal denudation (47).

D. Prognosis

Acute GVHD profoundly affects the overal prognosis after marrow transplantation. For example, among patients grafted for severe aplastic anemia, approximately 90% of those with no or only minimal (grade I) acute GVHD survive compared to 60% of those with grades II-III, and none of those with grade IV disease (48). Mortality is usually related to infectious complications as a result of the profound immunodeficiency associated with GVHD and its immunosuppressive therapy. Occasionally a patient may die from hepatic failure or an abdominal catastrophe such as bowel performation or intestinal hemorrhage.

III. RISK FACTORS

GVHD does not develop uniformly in all allogeneic transplant recipients, and severity varies in those who do show manifestations of the disease. What is the basis for such differences? Will it be possible eventually to prevent GVHD in all transplant recipients? Several risk factors associated with the development of GVHD in both animal models and human marrow transplantation have been recognized (49-54); others may still await identification.

A. Histoincompatibility

Allogeneic marrow transplants can be carried out successfully between individuals other than identical (syngeneic) twins. Several recent clinical trials indicate that some patients may be able to receive allogeneic, HLA-identical marrow grafts without postgrafting immunosuppression and not develop clinically significant GVHD (12). Nevertheless, it is clear that the likelihood of developing GVHD increases with the degree of histoincompatibility between donor and recipient (14).

The Seattle group has recently updated its experience in patients given unmanipulated bone marrow grafts from HLA genotypically nonidentical donors (55). While with *phenotypic* HLA identity the incidence of acute GVHD was not different from that seen with genotypically HLA identical transplants (about 35%), the probability of developing GVHD increased from one (60%) to two (75%) to three antigen (90%) mismatched transplants. Survival, however, was not adversely affected with one HLA antigen difference, and mortality was increased only when donor and patient differed for two or three antigens (14). Similar results were reported by Powles et al. (56). Differences for HLA-DR (class II), and especially for DR plus B (class I and II) carried the highest risk. These observations raise the possibility that class III antigens, located on human chromosome 6 in between HLA-B and DR, may also play a significant role in the development of GVHD (57). Although investigations in regards to complement factors are currently lacking, there are data from murine models suggesting that tumor necrosis factor (TNF), also encoded in the region between HLA-B and D, may be involved in the development of GVHD (58). The HLA-DR region has also been implicated as important in the development of GVHD after transplantation from unrelated volunteer donors (15).

B. Infusion of Lymphocytes

A clear relationship between the number of spleen cells (containing a large proportion of lymphocytes) but not marrow cells (containing only few lymphocytes) transplanted, and the incidence and severity of GVHD in mice was demonstrated in early experiments by van Bekkum and colleagues (2). Storb and colleagues showed that cross-circulation between DLA incompatible dogs (one of whom was lethally irradiated) not only resulted in rapid engraftment (proving the presence of hemopoietic stem cells in peripheral blood) but also in the hyperacute development of severe GVHD compatible with a role of lymphocytes in the development of GVHD (59). In fact, the infusion of thoracic duct lymphocytes alone (not containing hemopoietic stem cells) results in GVHD in lethally irradiated histoincompatible recipient dogs (H. J. Deeg, unpublished observations). The detrimental effect of donor lymphocytes on GVHD has long been recognized (60). However, there is also evidence that the addition of viable donor lymphocytes to the bone marrow inoculum facilitates engraftment (61-63), an observation that resulted in the hypothesis that a certain degree of GVHD may be necessary for engraftment to occur (see below). Based on data from their canine model, Storb and colleagues added donor lymphocytes to the transplant regimen of patients with severe aplastic anemia, thereby reducing the incidence of graft rejection from about 35% to 15% (64), and improving survival from 40-45% to about 70%. Concurrently, however, there was a significant increase in the incidence of chronic GVHD (from 33% to 66%), most notably the de novo form (65). The incidence of acute GVHD was only insignificantly increased. The bone marrow cell dose, although positively correlated with the probability of engraftment, did not contribute significantly to the development of GVHD (66).

In retrospect, these observations should not be surprising in view of the now recognized pivotal role of T lymphocytes in the development of GVHD. Consequently, efforts in recent years have been directed at inactivating or removing T lymphocytes rather than adding them to the transplant inoculum (67-76). Clearly, these approaches reduce the incidence of GVHD. However, T-cell depletion has also resulted in an increased probability of graft failure (67,71,73,75,77). Furthermore, there is now evidence that the extent of T-cell depletion or, alternatively, the *number* of donor T lymphocytes given to the recipient, correlates with the probability of developing GVHD (73,77,78). These data taken together have led to currently ongoing studies in which a certain number of lymphocytes, preferably a defined phenotype, is given to the transplant recipient with the hope of achieving both engraftment and prevention of GVHD (79,80).

C. Patient and Donor Age

Specific tolerance can be induced consistently in mice during fetal development and neonatally; tolerance is more difficult to induce in adult animals. This has been attributed to the recipient's immune status, more specifically thymic function.

Although clinical studies have been less systematic, available data show a correlation of age at transplantation and incidence of acute GVHD (Table 1). The reasons for this are not clear. However, it is possible that, as the thymus regresses with age, it may become less capable of "reeducating" donor-derived T lymphocytes to accept the host environment as self. There is also evidence that the thymus-derived hormone thymopoie-

Table 1 Incidence of Acute GVHD by Patient Age

Seattle[a]		IBMTR[b]	
Patient age (years)	Incidence (%)	Patient age (years)	Incidence (%)
≤10	6-26	<10	34 ± 4
11-20	26-40	10-19	37 ± 3
21-30	26-42	20-29	41 ± 3
31-40	42-57	30-39	45 ± 3
≥41	50-80	≥40	50 ± 7

[a]Storb and Thomas (96).

[b]Includes 4636 patients who had engraftment and survived at least 21 days posttransplant. The GVHD incidence overall differs significantly (p < 0.002). The data presented here were obtained from the Statistical Center of the International Bone Marrow Transplant Registry. The analysis has not been reviewed or approved by the Advisory Committee of the IBMTR.

tin is decreased in patients after marrow transplantation, and that this may correlate with the development of GVHD (81). However, the administration of thymosin fraction 5 after transplantation does not prevent GVHD nor accelerate immunoreconstitution (82). Additional evidence for the central role of a functional thymus in the establishment of tolerance derives from recent studies on syngeneic and autologous GVHD (27,83-87). This notion is further supported by the observation that the elimination of T cells with autoreactive T-cell receptors occurs in the thymus (88), and that cyclosporine interferes with this process (89). On the other hand, implantation of precultured thymic monolayers or epithelial cells, albeit generally not completely HLA identical with the marrow transplant recipient, has not reduced the incidence of GVHD after allogeneic marrow transplantation (90).

As described in detail elsewhere, colonization of the transplant recipient by bacterial or viral organisms may contribute to GVHD by way of cross-reactivity of host target cells and contaminating organisms (see Chapter 21) , recognized by donor T lymphocytes (91-93). Conceivably, therefore, older age may predispose to GVHD by means of offering a broader target range of colonizing organisms.

Since repair processes show some decline with age, it is also possible that tissue damage in older patients undergoes repair more slowly. Consequently, lesions produced in a bystander reaction might represent targets for a graft-vs.-host reaction longer than would be expected in a younger individual.

Donor age also has been invoked as a risk factor for GVHD in some (94,95) but not in other studies (96). Although there is a high correlation between donor and patient age in sibling transplants, the donor age is thought to be an independent factor by many investigators. The linkage to the development of GVHD is poorly understood. Possibly it is related to donor antiviral immunity leading to an anamnestic response of donor T lymphocytes against infected host cells (see Chapter 28).

D. Host Environment (Gnotobiosis)

Studies in murine models show that lethally irradiated, germ-free or decontaminated mice given marrow cells from germ-free donors develop no GVHD as compared to 100% GVHD fatality in control mice maintained in a conventional environment (91-93). It has been suggested that enterobacteria invading immunologically produced GVHD lesions of the intestinal mucosa (and possibly elsewhere) share antigenic determinants with host epithelial cells, enabling reactivation or amplification of alloreactive donor T-lymphocyte clones, initially primed against host lymphohemopoietic or epithelial cells. Consequently, a clinically inapparent graft-vs.-host reaction in the presence of these bacteria would progress and develop into more severe lesions manifested clinically as GVHD, for example, of the intestinal tract. Alternatively, damage to intestinal mucosa as a result of the chemoradiotherapy regimen used to prepare patients for transplantation may allow endotoxin from the gut microflora to enter the circulation and stimulate cytokine production by macrophages and lymphocytes either regionally or systemically. In a minor (non-H2) antigen mismatched mouse model, passive immunization with antiendotoxin for the first 21 days after transplantation protected against GVHD (92).

Clinical results in adult and pediatric patients with aplastic anemia suggest that skin and gut decontamination with antibiotics and placement in a protective environment such as laminar air flow isolation reduce the incidence of GVHD (98,99). In a nonrandomized, retrospective study from Seattle, isolation and decontamination reduced the cumulative incidence of acute GVHD from approximately 40% to 25% with a respective increase in survival from 70% to 85% (99). Similar studies have been undertaken in patients with lymphohemopoietic malignancies, but, although some advantages (such as fewer septicemias) were seen, no significant reduction in GVHD or improvement in survival was observed. The reasons are not clear. However, compared to patients with aplastic anemia, generally conditioned with cyclophosphamide alone, these patients usually received more intensive chemotherapy and total body irradiation. This, in turn, results in decreased compliance with the regimen of oral antibiotics and less successful decontamination. It is also possible that the more severe tissue damage induced by irradiation itself negates the potentially beneficial effects of isolation and decontamination.

E. Antiviral Immunity

Recent reports, mostly from Scandinavian countries, suggest that antiviral, especially anticytomegalovirus immunity of donor and host may also influence the development of GVHD (100) (see Chapter 25). It is certainly of note in this context that other recent clinical trials suggest that the incidence of cytomegalovirus infections is reduced by the prophylactic use of cytomegalovirus hyperimmune globulin or high dose intravenous immunoglobulin (101,102) and that this is associated with a reduced incidence of GVHD (103-105).

IV. IMMUNOLOGY

A. Cellular Immune Mechanisms

Immunologic events associated with GVHD or the development of tolerance have been studied in many models. It was thought initially that GVHD was prevented and tolerance established if host-reactive clones of donor origin were eliminated, a mechanism termed "clonal deletion" or, in a modified form, "clonal abortion." Additional data suggest that suppressor cells may play a role as well, possibly by mediating clonal abortion.

T lymphocytes mature in the thymus, where they acquire antigen receptors and differentiate into subpopulations with different functions including helper ($CD4^+$), suppressor ($CD8^+$) and cytotoxic T cells ($CD4^+$ or $CD8^+$). It has recently been shown that cells bearing T-cell receptors (TCRs) reactive to self are physically eliminated in the thymus, and possibly in the periphery as well (88). In irradiated mice transplanted with syngeneic marrow, the deletion occurs at a $CD4^+8^+$ precursor stage. Donor T lymphocytes, known to be responsible for triggering GVHD, obviously have not undergone negative selection for recipient (patient) self. Hence, they are expected to proliferate towards nonself (patient) antigens. These activated donor derived helper T ($CD4^+$) cells release cytokines, such as IL-2, and recruit additional cell types.

Although it is not clear which recipient cells provide the primary stimulus or target for donor T lymphocytes, there is evidence that macrophages (106) and natural killer cells (107) may be involved. The reaction between donor and recipient cells may be subclinical and result in tolerance, or it may progress to a clinical picture of GVHD. Since helper T cells recognize antigen in association with MHC class II molecules, it has been speculated that the presence of numerous antigen-presenting (dendritic) cells in the liver, intestinal tract, and skin may explain why these organs are the major targets in acute GVHD (108).

B. Helper T Cells

Peripheral blood T-cell profiles after marrow transplantation have been extensively investigated, initially with heteroantisera (109-111) and more recently with monoclonal antibodies (MAb) (112-115). The relative number of T lymphocytes was found to be normal
by 2 months following transplant; there was no correlation between T-cell levels and
GVHD. DeBruin and colleagues found unusually high numbers of immature T cells early
after transplant (112). The T helper ($CD4^+$) to suppressor ($CD8^+$) cell ratio (normally
2:1) was reversed in peripheral blood regardless of the presence of GVHD, and in fact
was also observed after syngeneic and autologous transplants. Reports differ in regards
to the normalization of the T-cell phenotypes. Friedrich and colleagues reported that the
$CD4^+$ and $CD8^+$ cell ratio quickly returned to normal in patients with an uncomplicated
course or those who resolved acute GVHD (113). Atkinson and collaborators found that
$CD4^+$ cells were depleted and remained so for over 2 years; $CD8^+$ cells began to recover
within 3 months after transplantation, and subsequently remained at normal or elevated
levels for years (114). Others observed that the course could vary (115). Although these
studies depict the imbalance of T-cell subset recovery postgrafting, they fail to shed light
on the immunopathologic development of GVHD.

C. Cytotoxic T Cells

Cytotoxic T cells ($CD4^+$ or $CD8^+$) are able to recognize and destroy allogeneic and virally
infected target cells through interaction with MHC molecules (usually class I) and nomi-
nal antigens on their surface.

　　　Parkman and colleagues investigated the in vitro capacity of chimera (donor-derived) lymphocytes during acute GVHD to lyse donor, host, or control fibroblasts labeled
with ^{14}C amino acids (116). Unfractionated donor lymphocytes did not lyse any of
those target cells, whereas unfractionated cells from chimeras with acute GVHD triggered
significant lysis of all targets, suggesting that target antigens were expressed on all cells
tested. Lysis was mediated by null cells bearing $C'3$ receptors. These cells were present
in blood of normal individuals and were reactive only when separated from suppressor
cells. Reinherz and colleagues showed that patients with acute GVHD lacked cells with
a suppressor (TH2) phenotype but cessation of acute GVHD coincided with the appearance of suppressor cells (111). On this basis it was postulated that acute GVHD was produced by donor autocytotoxic null lymphocytes when the level of suppressor cells was
low (116). It was further argued that acute GVHD could also develop in other clinical
settings, for instance during chemotherapy-induced neutropenia or in autologous or
syngeneic bone marrow transplantation, when manipulation of the immune system
produced a deficiency in suppressor cells such that regulation of autocytotoxic effector
cells was no longer possible. In that setting, conceivably, circulating T cells with suppressor phenotype are nonfunctional.

　　　Tsoi and colleagues investigated cytotoxicity to host fibroblasts by chimera cells
and the role of serum blocking factors early after grafting (117, 118). During the first
2 months postgrafting, mononuclear leukocytes from about one-half of the patients were
cytotoxic to host fibroblasts, and serum did or did not contain blocking activity. The
percentage of patients without cytotoxicity increased significantly with time posttransplant while the fraction of patients with cytotoxicity decreased. After one year, 89%
of patients showed neither cytotoxicity nor blocking by chimera serum compared to 11%
with both activities. Early postgrafting, there was evidence of a correlation between in

vitro cytotoxicity (of chimera cells against host fibroblasts) and the development of acute GVHD. Cells from 14 of 20 patients with acute GVHD were cytotoxic to host fibroblasts compared to 7 of 18 patients without acute GVHD. There was no correlation between the presence of blocking factors early postgrafting and acute GVHD.

D. Suppressor T Cells

"Suppressor" T cells (CD8$^+$) are thought to regulate the action of other T cells, B cells, and possibly other cell types. Their reactivity is usually, but not always, MHC class I restricted. They may be either specific or nonspecific. However, it has been difficult or impossible to clone T lymphocytes with the phenotype and function attributed to suppressor cells. In addition, recent evidence suggests that the "suppression" of antigen-specific B-cell function may be effected via killing of B cells by class II-restricted CD8$^+$ cytotoxic T cells (119,120). Analogous observations in human transplant recipients are still lacking. We will use the term suppression for the observed *effects* of cellular functions, while realizing that they may be mediated by cytotoxic cells or other mechanisms such as clonal anergy.

In human patients receiving methotrexate alone as GVHD prophylaxis, CD8$^+$ cell reconstitution has been noted to occur faster in those who develop acute GVHD (grades II-IV) than in those who do not (121). Indeed, a CD4$^+$/CD8$^+$ ratio of <2.0 on day 19 posttransplant has been described as being significantly correlated with acute GVHD (grades II-IV). Y-chromosome studies have shown these T cells to be of mixed donor and recipient origin (121). As in animal models, analyses are complicated by the fact that different postgrafting immunosuppressive regimens have been and continue to be used in various studies.

Extensive studies have been carried out in patients given HLA-identical marrow grafts and postgrafting immunosuppression with methotrexate (122,123). Before grafting, lymphocytes from the marrow donors did not respond to host cells. After grafting, lymphocytes (of donor origin) from one-third of marrow recipients with chronic GVHD showed proliferation in mixed leukocyte culture against host cells, which indicated that GVHD may be mediated by lymphocytes "sensitized" to minor histocompatibility antigens. In patients without GVHD, lymphocytes remained unresponsive to host cells. Nonspecific suppressor cells (i.e., lymphocytes that suppressed the proliferation of donor cells against cells from unrelated controls) were usually absent shortly after transplantation in patients with and without GVHD and in long-term survivors without GVHD, but present in approximately half the patients with chronic GVHD. Lymphocytes from long-term healthy recipients, but not from patients with chronic GVHD, suppressed specifically the response of donor lymphocytes to trinitrophenol-modified host leukocytes. These results strongly suggest that stable chimerism after HLA-identical allogeneic marrow grafting involves a specific suppressor mechanism.

Although many questions remain, it appears that in both histoincompatible animal models and HLA-identical human marrow transplant recipients, nonspecific suppressor cells are associated with the presence of GVHD, and specific suppressor cells result in the establishment of tolerance, possibly, as suggested by results in dogs, via clonal abortion.

In contrast to the failure to clone classic T suppressor cells, investigators have succeeded in cloning cells of a different phenotype, termed natural suppressor cells (124). In an animal model these cells were able to prevent GVHD (124). Similar (or identical) cells have been identified in other models and evidence has been presented suggesting that these cells mediate their function via interferon gamma (125). It is currently not clear whether analogous cells play a role in marrow transplantation in man.

E. NK Cells (Large Granular Lymphocytes)

NK cells are capable of killing virally infected, transformed, or other target cells to which they have not been previously sensitized. They are not restricted. Lopez and colleagues investigated NK activity against herpes simplex virus type 1-infected fibroblasts, NK (HSV-1), in patients before transplant (126). Patients with normal NK activity were more likely to develop GVHD postgrafting than those with low NK activity suggesting that pretransplant NK response might be predictive of a patient's risk of developing GVHD, and that the assay reflected host-dependent GVHD stimulator cell function. Livnat and colleagues, measuring NK activity against a K562 myeloblastoid cell line, NK (K562), found that about one-third to one-half of patients were deficient in NK activity before transplantation (127). After transplantation NK activity returned to normal between days 30 and 100 in most patients but was deficient in about 20% of patients beyond one year. There was no association between NK activity and acute or chronic GVHD. When these data were pooled no correlation between pretransplant level of NK (K562) and GVHD was found, but a significant correlation between NK (HSV-1) and the subsequent development of GVHD was observed (128) suggesting the existence of different effector cell populations mediating NK activity. Dokhelar and collaborators, using K562 targets, found a strong correlation between NK activity and acute GVHD, and suggested that NK cells were involved in the pathogenesis of acute GVHD (129).

In murine models there is evidence that donor NK cells are involved in the mechanism of GVHD, although this view is currently not undisputed (107). One might also speculate that poor graft function, occasionally associated with GVHD (130), is mediated by suppressor or NK cells.

F. Humoral Immune Mechanisms

Merritt and colleagues described the appearance, concurrently with the onset of GVHD, of a complement (C')-dependent cytotoxic IgM antibody active against epithelial but not lymphoid cells in the sera of three recipients of HLA-identical marrow (131). Several investigators found deposits of IgG, IgA, IgM, and C'3 at the dermo-epidermal junction and in blood vessel walls in patients with acute or chronic GVHD (132,133). Tsoi and colleagues reported that deposits of IgM and C'3 were significantly associated with GVHD: 39% of 88 patients with acute GVHD showed light deposits and 86% of patients with chronic GVHD showed heavy deposits of IgM (134).

Individual reports desribe the presence of a cold IgG lymphocytotoxin lysing lymphocytes from unrelated individuals but not donor or recipient lymphocytes during acute GVHD; others describe cold auto- and allolymphocytotoxins directed at non-HLA antigens on B and T lymphocytes in 50% of posttransplant sera (135,136). However, there was no consistent correlation of the present of lymphocytotoxins and GVHD. Opelz and colleagues detected lymphocytotoxins in about 50% of a small number of marrow-grafted patients (137). These IgM antibodies, reactive at 4°, 20°, and 37°C, developed posttransplant against non-HLA antigens on donor and chimera lymphocytes and, possibly, host lymphocytes. There was no significant correlation of the presence of antibodies and GVHD, although a relationship between patient survival and development of antibodies against chimera lymphocytes was suggested. In contrast to these findings,

Warren and colleagues found no lymphocytotoxic antibodies against donor lymphocytes in patients with sustained engraftment, except in two cases with mixed donor-host chimerism (138).

G. Syngeneic Acute GVHD

The classic tenet formulated by Billingham states that histocompatibility differences between donor and recipient must exist for GVHD to develop (6). However, as first reported by Rappeport and colleagues in 1979 (86), a GVHD-like syndrome can develop after syngeneic or autologous transplantation. Studies on cyclosporine treated marrow-transplanted rats and mice, which develop GVHD upon cyclosporine withdrawal, have shed durther light on this phenomenon (23,84,139). Significant thymic damage with medullary atrophy and loss of Ia$^+$ nurse cells play a central role in the development of syngeneic GVHD (139). Associated findings include a decrease in the number of T cells, especially helper cells, and the appearance of CD4/CD8 double positive or double negative cells as well as immature cells (with phenotypic markers otherwise only found on thymocytes) in peripheral blood (140,141). Recent studies indicate that cyclosporine interferes with deletion of cells expressing self-reactive T-cell receptor specificities (142). Although patients given syngeneic or autologous marrow grafts usually do not receive cyclosporine, these observations point toward mechanisms that may result in inappropriate self-reactivity and GVHD. An alternative suggestion is based on observations made in patients treated with LAK cells (143). After transplantation, activated T cells release IL-2, which may trigger nonspecific, potentially autoreactive effector cells (e.g., NK cells) capable of attacking and lysing autologous targets. One might argue against this that, if anything, IL-2 production and responsiveness by chimera cells have been found to be decreased (144).

V. PATHOPHYSIOLOGY

There is now convincing documentation that T cells contained in the donor marrow or subsequently derived from stem cells initiate the graft-vs.-host reaction and, directly or indirectly, lead to the manifestations of GVHD. The immunopathogenesis involves three steps (145): (a) recognition (afferent loop); (b) recruitment; and (c) effector phase (efferent loop).

In order for donor cells to be activated, they need to recognize antigens to which they can react. Classically, this includes MHC class I and II antigens expressed on host cells, most importantly of lymphohemopoietic lineage since only such cells can express immunogenicity. It is clear, however, that non-MHC antigens, viral antigens, and tissue-specific antigens such as epithelial cell (skin)-associated antigens can also be recognized. Conceivably, the latter may serve as targets in skin explant models such as those used by Vogelsang and collaborators (146) and Bagot and colleagues (147) to predict GVHD in HLA-identical transplant recipients. Furthermore, nonlymphohemopoietic cells, induced by cytokines (in particular gamma-interferon) to express Ia-like antigens, may also serve as recognition signals for donor T lymphocytes. Once activated, donor cells, by developing into effector cells or recruiting other cells as effectors, can then initiate the attack that leads to target organ damage and clinically apparent GVHD. Thus, the pathophysiology of acute GVHD may be understood by examining, first, how the different immunologically active cells interact or communicate and, second, how clinical maneuvers used to prevent or treat GVHD may inhibit these interactions or communications.

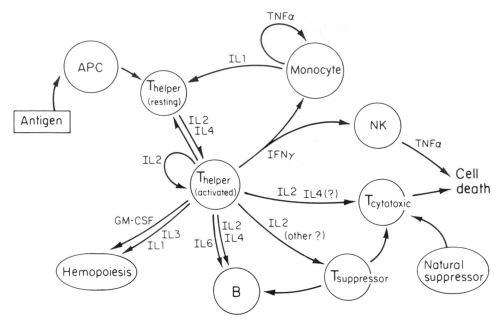

Figure 3 Cytokine network of acute GVHD. As discussed in the text, this scheme is largely based on data obtained in experimental models, and in some respects remains hypothetical. It appears, however, that donor T lymphocytes recognize host (allo)antigen, presumably under involvement of antigen presenting cells (APC). This results in an activation of T lymphocytes and other cell populations, mediated by cytokines. (I1 = interleukin; IFN = interferon; TNF = tumor necrosis factor; GM-CSF = colony stimulating factor granulocytes/macrophages; B = B lymphocytes; NK = natural killer cells.

Cells of the immune system interact directly or communicate via a cytokine network. Cytokines are polypeptides most of which were originally isolated from activated mononuclear cells. However, they are also produced by, and act on, cells of other lineages, and may act locally or have systemic effects (Fig. 3). As a result, additional cells are recruited, and various effector functions are triggered. One cytokine released by epithelial cells, epidermal-cell-derived thymocyte activating factor (ETAF), has properties similar to IL-1, including the stimulation of IL-2 secretion by $CD4^+$ T cells (148) resulting not only in clonal expansion of T cells but also in the stimulation of NK cells and B cells. Furthermore, as stated above, activated T cells produce interferon gamma (IFN), which enhances MHC class II (DR, Ia-like) antigen expression on macrophages and epithelial cells (skin, intestinal tract, bile ducts), further stimulating T-cell and NK-cell responses. Cells with (increased) MHC class II expression also serve as potent accessory (antigen-presenting) cells and bind to and direct the traffic of antigen specific T cells. In addition to IL-2, activated T cells produce IL-4 and IL-6, which stimulate B cells, and IL-3 and GM-CSF, which both stimulate marrow hemopoietic cells. Macrophages and IL-2-stimulated NK cells also produce tumor necrosis factor (TNF) alpha.

TNF, encoded by genes located within the MHC, functions in conjunction with IFN gamma to augment recognition of histocompatibility differences by inducing class II antigen expression on some cells, and upregulating constitutively expressed class I and class II antigens. While TNF from NK cells is generated in response to IL-2 released below) but whose quantification is even more difficult. It is therefore likely that the incidence of cell necrosis is underestimated.

by activated T cells, it is also secreted in response to IL-1 stimulation by virus particles, C5a, and bacterial endotoxin such as lipopolysaccharide. TNF acts to increase the adhesion of leukocytes to endothelial cells, leading to skin and gut infiltration by inflammatory cells. TNF may also cause apoptosis of isolated, less differentiated epithelial cells in gut and skin as well as increased cell division leading to hyperplasia. These data imply that TNF may be an important part of the final common pathway in the pathophysiology of acute GVHD. Direct evidence for a role of TNF in GVHD was recently presented by Piguet and colleagues (58). In a mouse model these workers showed that by using an antibody to recombinant mouse TNF, they were able to ameliorate or prevent the gut and skin lesions of acute GVHD.

The key event in the cytokine network with respect to GVHD, then, would appear to be activation of resting T cells. Any strategy aimed at limiting or preventing this activation might, thus, be expected to eliminate or lessen the severity of acute GVHD. A number of therapeutic maneuvers which work in this way have been used clinically with success: these include T-cell depletion of the donor marrow inoculum; selective gut decontamination and administration of prophylactic immunoglobulins; and immunosuppressive chemotherapy for the host pre- and posttransplant. Techniques which limit the ability of antigen presenting cells to function in this capacity, such as UV irradiation or heat inactivation (149), might also be predicted to have a role in preventing GVHD.

Cytokine production increases following T-cell activation. Thus, inhibition of cytokine production at the transcriptional or translational level, a block at the level of a second messenger from cell membrane to nucleus, block of cytokine receptors, or production of cytokine inhibitors are all strategies that might be expected to decrease GVHD. In fact, cyclosporine, one of the most useful prophylactic immunosuppressive drugs currently employed, blocks production of Il-2, IL-3, IL-4, IFN gamma, and possibly IL-1 mRNA at the nuclear level (150). UV irradiation, which interferes with intracellular calcium regulation, thus potentially blocking second messenger transmission between cell membrane and the nucleus, may also work at this level (151).

Methotrexate and prednisone, two drugs known to be useful in preventing or treating GVHD, may work at the next step in the cytokine network, i.e., cell proliferation in response to stimuli. Methotrexate is used early posttransplant, at a time when $CD4^+$ T cells are generally in excess of $CD8^+$ T cells, and may help to maintain a more favorable anti-GVHD balance of T helper:T suppressor cells. Prednisone, which is often given for a longer period of time or at the onset of GVHD, is known to have a lympholytic effect.

As of yet, little is known about blockade of cytokine receptors or inhibitory cytokines, and few efforts have been made at therapy with this aim (152,153). However, preliminary results in animal models indicate that there may be a role for monoclonal antibodies to T-cell receptors, IL-2 receptors, or pan-T-cell (CD5) receptors (154,155,156).

The last step in the cytokine network as we know it today is TNF production by macrophages and NK cells. Here, blockade of receptors for IFN gamma, by monoclonal or polyclonal antibodies, might be expected to have some degree of efficacy in preventing, reversing, or altering acute GVHD. Finally, a recent report on the use of rabbit antimouse recombinant TNF shows this to be the case (58). What signals might affect the function of natural suppressor cells (124-125) is currently under investigation.

VI. CONCLUSIONS

GVHD continues to be a frequent complication of HLA-compatible and -incompatible bone marrow transplantation; GVHD is seen infrequently in other clinical settings. Although classically described with allogeneic transplantation, a syndrome clinically, and often histologically, indistinguishable from acute GVHD can also be seen after syngeneic and even autologous marrow infusion. T lymphocytes play a pivotal role in triggering GVHD, however, the mechanism is still incompletely understood. Common to all settings is an imbalance of lymphocyte subsets, associated with allo- or autoreactivity. At least in part this appears to be related to thymic dysfunction and ineffective elimination of self-reactive T lymphocytes. In addition, there is evidence for abnormal production of or responsiveness to cytokines which may result in a nonspecific activation of NK cells. The role of natural suppressor cells requires further characterization. The developing understanding of the cytokine network of graft-host interactions may allow for refined manipulation via antibodies directed at cytokines or their respective receptors.

ACKNOWLEDGMENT

Supported in part by grants CA14626 and HL33859 awarded by the National Institutes of Health, Bethesda, MD.

REFERENCES

1. Deeg HJ, Klingemann H-G, Phillips GL: *A Guide to Bone Marrow Transplantation*. Springer-Verlag, Berlin, Heidelberg, New York, 1988.
2. van Bekkum DW, deVries JJ: *Radiation Chimaeras*. Logos, London, 1967.
3. Barnes DWH, Loutit JF: Spleen protection: the cellular hypothesis. In *Radiobiology Symposium*, edited by Bacq ZM. Butterworth, London, 1955; pp. 134–135.
4. Billingham RE, Brent L: A simple method for inducing tolerance of skin homografts in mice. Transplantation Bulletin 1957;4:67-71.
5. Santos GE, Cole LJ: Effect of donor and host lymphoid and myeloid tissue injections in lethally x-irradiated mice treated with rat bone marrow. J Natl Cancer Inst 1958;21:279-293.
6. Billingham RE: The biology of graft-versus-host reactions. Harvey Lectures, 1966-1967;62:21-78.
7. Gowans JL: The fate of parental strain small lymphocytes in F1 hybrid rats. Ann NY Acad Sci 1962;99:432-455.
8. Medawar PB: Introduction: definition of the immunologically competent cell. Ciba Foundation Study Group 1963;16:1-5.
9. Owens AH Jr, Santos GW: The induction of graft-versus-host disease in mice treated with cyclophosphamide. J Exp Med 1968;128:277-291.
10. McGregor DD: Bone marrow origin of immunologically competent lymphocytes in the rat. J Exp Med 1968;127:953-966.
11. Storb R, Rudolph RH, Kolb HJ, Graham TC, Mickelson E, Erickson V, Lerner KG, Kolb H, Thomas ED: Marrow grafts between DL-A-matched canine littermates. Transplantation 1973;15:92-100.
12. Lazarus HM, Coccia PF, Herzig RH, Graham-Pole J, Gross S, Strandjord S, Gordon E, Cheung N-KV, Warkentin PI, Spitzer TR, Warm SE: Incidence of acute graft-versus-host disease with and without methotrexate prophylaxis in allogeneic bone marrow transplant patients. Blood 1984;64:215-220.

13. Claas FHJ, Gijbels Y, van der Velden-De Munck J, van Rood JJ: Induction of B cell unresponsiveness to noninherited maternal HLA antigens during fetal life. Science 1988;241:1815-1817.

14. Beatty PG, Clift RA, Mickelson EM, Nisperos BB, Flournoy N, Martin PJ, Sanders JE, Stewart P, Buckner CD, Storb R, Thomas ED, Hansen JA: Marrow transplantation from related donors other than HLA-identical siblings. N Engl J Med 1985;313: 765-771.

15. Gingrich RD, Howe CWS, Goeken NE, Ginder GD, Kubler JW, Tewfik HH, Klassen LW, Armitage JO, Fyfe MA: The use of partially matched, unrelated donors in clinical bone marrow transplantation. Transplantation 1985;39:526-532.

16. Filipovich AH, Vallera DA, Youle R, Haake R, Blazar BR, Arthur D, Neville DM, Ramsay NKC, McGlave P, Kersey JH: Graft-versus-host disease prevention in allogeneic bone marrow transplantation from histocompatible siblings. Transplantation 1987;44:62-69.

17. Deeg HJ: Chemoprevention of graft-vs-host disease: effects on donor marrow and host environment. In *Bone Marrow Transplantation: Current Controversies*, UCLA Symposia on Molecular and Cellular Biology, New Series. Vol. 91. edited by Gale RP and Champlin R. Alan R. Liss, Inc., New York, 1989, pp. 441-453.

18. Hathaway WE, Fulginiti VA, Pierce CW, et al. Graft-vs-host reaction following a single blood transfusion. JAMA 1967;201:1015-1020.

19. Kadowaki JI, Zuelzer WW, Brought AJ, et al.: Lymphoid chimaerism in congenital immunological deficiency syndrome with thymic alymphoplasia. Lancet 1965; ii: 1152-1156.

20. Bastien J, Williams R, Ornelas W, Tani P, Thompson L: Maternal isoimmunization resulting in combined immunodeficiency and fatal graft versus host disease in an infant. Lancet 1984; i:1435-1437.

21. Naiman JL, Punnett HH, Lischner HW et al.: Possible graft-vs-host reaction after intrauterine transfusion for Rh erythroblastosis fetalis. N Engl J Med 1969;281: 697-701.

22. Pflieger H: Graft-versus-host disease following blood transfusions. Blut 1983;46:61-66.

23. Cohen Z, Silverman R, Levy G, Wassef R, Langer B: Clinical small intestinal transplantation using cyclosproine A and methylprednisolone. Transplant Proc 1987;19: 2588-2590.

24. Burdick JF, Vogelsang GB, Smith WJ, Farmer ER, Bias WB, Kaufmann SH, Horn J, Colombani PM, Pitt HA, Perler BA, Merritt WT, Williams GM, Boitnott JK, Herlong HK: Severe graft-versus-host disease in a liver-transplant recipient. N Engl J Med 1988;318:689-691.

25. Herman JG, Beschorner WE, Baughman KL, Boitnott JK, Vogelsang GB, Baumgartner WA: Pseudo-graft-versus-host disease in heart and heart-lung recipients. Transplantation 1988;46:93-98.

26. Powles RL, Clink HM, Spence D, Morgenstern G, Watson JG, Selby PJ, Woods M, Barrett A, Jameson B, Sloane J, Lawler SD, Kay HEM, Lawson D, McElwain TJ, Alexander P: Cyclosporin A to prevent graft-versus-host disease in man after allogeneic bone-marrow transplantation. Lancet 1980; 1:327-329.

27. Glazier A, Tutschka PJ, Farmer ER, Santos GW: Graft-versus-host disease in cyclosporin A-treated rats after syngeneic bone marrow transplantation. J Exp Med 1983; 158:1-8.

28. Sullivan KM, Parkman R: The pathophysiology and treatment of graft-versus-host disease. Clinics Haematol 1983;12:775-789.

29. Shulman HM, Sale GE: Pathology of acute and chronic cutaneous GVHD. In *The Pathology of Bone Marrow Transplantation*, edited by Sale GE, Shulman HM. Masson Publishing USA, Inc., New York, 1984; pp. 40-76.

30. Sullivan KM, Deeg HJ, Sanders J, Klosterman A, Amos D, Shulman H, Sale G, Martin P, Witherspoon R, Appelbaum F, Doney K, Stewart P, Meyers J, McDonald GB, Weiden P, Fefer A, Buckner CD, Storb R, Thomas ED: Hyperacute graft-v-host disease in patients not given immunosuppression after allogeneic marrow transplantation. Blood 1986;67;1172-1175.

31. Beschorner WE, Tutschka PJ, Farmer ER, Santos GW: Two histopathologic patterns of acute graft-versus-host disease in humans. Exp Hematol 1979;7:99.

32. Neudorf S, Filipovich A, Ramsay N, Kersey J: Prevention and treatment of acute graft-versus-host disease. Sem Hematol 1984;21:91-100.

33. Chomette G, Mathe G, Auriol M, Brocherion C, Pinaudeau Y: Le syndrome secondaire chez l'homme: etude anatomique de six cas de leucémies traités par greffe allogénique de moelle osseuse après irradiation totale. Virchows Archiv Abteilung B (Cell Pathology) 1970;349:98-114.

34. Kersey JH, Meuwissen HJ, Good RA: Graft versus host reactions following transplantation of allogeneic hematopoietic cells. Human Pathology 1971;2:389-402.

35. Glucksberg H, Storb R, Fefer A, Buckner CD, Neimann PE, Clift RA, Lerner KG, Thomas ED: Clinical manifestations of graft-versus-host disease in human recipients of marrow from HL-A matched sibling donors. Transplantation 1974;18:295-304.

36. Slavin RE, Santos GW: The graft versus host reaction in man after bone marrow transplantation: Pathology, pathogenesis, clinical features, and implication. Clin Immunol Immunopathol 1973;1:472-498.

37. Thomas ED, Storb R, Clift RA, Fefer A, Johnson FL, Neimann PE, Lerner KC: Bone marrow transplantation. N Engl J Med 1975;292:832-843, 895-902.

38. Deeg HJ, Storb R: Graft-versus-host disease: Pathophysiological and clinical aspects. Ann Rev Med 1984;35:11-24.

39. Vogelsang GB, Hess AD, Santos GW: Acute graft-versus-host disease: Clinical characteristics in the cyclosporine era. Medicine 1988;67:163-174.

40. Kennedy MS, Yee GC, Deeg HJ, Storb R, Thomas ED: Pharmacokinetics and toxicity of cyclosporine in marrow transplant patients. Transplant Proc 1983;15:2416-2418.

41. Sale GE, Lerner KG, Barker EA, Shulman HM, Thomas ED: The skin biopsy in the diagnosis of acute graft-versus-host disease in man. Am J Pathol 1977;89:621-635.

42. Deeg HJ, Loughran TP, Storb R, Kennedy MS, Sullivan KM, Doney K, Appelbaum FR, Thomas ED: Treatment of human acute graft-versus-host disease with antithymocyte globulin and cyclosporine with or without methylprednisolone. Transplantation 1985;40:162-166.

43. McDonald GB, Sharma P, Matthews DE: Venocclusive disease of the liver after bone marrow transplantation: diagnosis, incidence, and predisposing factors. Hepatology 1984;4:116-122.

44. McDonald GB, Shulman HM, Sullivan KM, Spencer GD: Intestinal and hepatic complications of human bone marrow transplantation, Parts I and II. Gastroenterology 1986;90:460-477, 770-784.

45. Sale GE, Shulman HM, McDonald GB, Thomas ED: Gastrointestinal graft-versus-host disease in man. A clinicopathological study of the rectal biopsy. Am J Surg Pathol 1979;3:291-299.

46. Fisk JD, Shulman HM, Greening RR, Mcdonald GB, Sale GE, Thomas ED: Gastrointestinal radiographic features of human graft-versus-host disease. Am J Roantgenol 1981;136:329-336.

47. McDonald GB, Sale GE: The human gastrointestinal tract after allogeneic marrow transplantation, In *The Pathology of Bone Marrow Transplantation*, edited by Sale GE, Shulman HM. Masson Publishing USA, Inc., New York, 1984; pp. 77-103.

48. Storb R, Pentice RL, Buckner CD, Clift RA, Appelbaum F, Deeg HJ, Doney K, Hansen JA, Mason M, Sanders JE, Singer J, Sullivan KM, Witherspoon RP, Thomas ED: Graft-versus-host disease and survival in patients with aplastic anemia treated by marrow grafts from HLA-identical siblings. Beneficial effect of a protective environment. N Engl J Med 1983;308:302-306.
49. Atkinson K, Farrell H, Cooley M, O'Flaherty E, Downs K, Biggs J: Human marrow T cell dose correlates with severity of subsequent acute graft-versus-host disease. Bone Marrow Transplantation 1987;2:51-57.
50. Bross DS, Tutschka PJ, Farmer ER, Beschorner WE, Graine HG, Mellits ED, Bias WB, Santos GW: Predictive factors for acute graft-versus-host disease in patients transplanted with HLA-identical bone marrow. Blood 1984;63:1265-1270.
51. Gale RP, Bortin MM, van Bekkum DW, Biggs JC, Dicke KA, Gluckman E, Good RA, Hoffman RG, Kay HEM, Kersey JH, Marmont A, Masaoka T, Rimm AA, van Rood JJ, Zwaan FE: Risk factors for acute graft-versus-host disease. Br J Haematol 1987; 67:397-406.
52. Ringden O, Nilsson B: Death by graft-versus-host disease associated with HLA mismatch, high recipient age, low marrow cell dose, and splenectomy. Transplantation 1985;40:39-44.
53. Bortin MM: Factors influencing the risk of acute graft-vs-host disease in man. In *Progress in Bone Marrow Transplantation*, edited by Gale RP, Champlin R. Alan R. Liss, Inc., New York, 1987; pp. 243-264.
54. Santos GW, Hess AD, Vogelsang GB: Graft-versus-host reactions and disease. Immunol Rev 1985;88:169-192.
55. Anasetti C, Beatty PG, Sanders J, Storb R, Thomas ED, Hansen JA: Graft versus host reaction, relapse and survival after HLA-nonidentical marrow transplants for malignancy. Exp Hematol 1988;16:495.
56. Powles RL, Morgenstern GR, Kay HEM, McElwain RJ, Clink HM, Barrett MH, Sloane J, Lumley H, Lawler SD, Dady PJ, Jameson B, Watson JG, Leight M, Hedley D, Filshie J: Mismatched family donors for bone-marrow transplantation as treatment for acute leukaemia. Lancet 1983; i:612-615.
57. Gingrich RD, Ginder GD, Goeken NE, Howe CWS, Wen B-C, Jussey DH, Fyfe MA: Allogeneic marrow grafting with partially mismatched, unrelated marrow donors. Blood 1988;71:1375-1381.
58. Piguet PF, Grau GE, Allet B, Vassalli P: Tumor necrosis factor/cachectin is an effector of skin and gut lesions of the acute phase of graft-vs-host disease. J Exp Med 1987;166:1280-1289.
59. Storb R, Epstein RB, Ragde H, Bryant J, Thomas ED: Marrow engraftment by allogeneic leukocytes in lethally irradiated dogs. Blood 1967;30:805-810.
60. Grebe SC, Streilein JW: Graft-versus-host reactions. A review. Adv Immunol 1976; 22:119-221.
61. Storb R, Epstein RB, Bryant J, Ragde H, Thomas ED: Marrow grafts by combined marrow and leukocyte infusions in unrelated dogs selected by histocompatibility typing. Transplantation 1968;6:587-592.
62. Deeg HJ, Storb R, Weiden PL, Shulman HM, Graham TC, Torok-Storb BJ, Thomas ED: Abrogation of resistance to and enhancement of DLA-nonidentical unrelated marrow grafts in lethally irradiated dogs by thoracic duct lymphocytes. Blood 1979;53:552-557.
63. Storb R: The role of T cells in engraftment: Experimental models, clinical trials. In *Progress in Bone Marrow Transplantation*, edited by Gale RP, Champlin R. Alan R. Liss, INc., New York, 1987; pp. 23-35.
64. Storb R, Doney K, Thomas ED, Appelbaum F, Buckner CD, Clift RA, Deeg HJ, Goodell BW, Hackman R, Hansen JA, Sanders J, Sullivan K, Weiden PL, Wither-

spoon RP: Marrow transplantation with and without donor buffy coat cells for 65 transfused aplastic anemia patients. Blood 1982;59:236-246.

65. Storb R, Prentice R, Sullivan KM, Shulman HM, Deeg HJ, Doney KC, Buckner CD, Clift RA, Witherspoon RP, Appelbaum FA, Sanders JE, Stewart PS, Thomas ED: Predictive factors in chronic graft versus host disease in patients with aplastic anemia treated by marrow transplantation from HLA-identical siblings. Ann Intern Med 1983;98:461-466.

66. Niederwieser D, Pepe M, Storb R, Loughran TP, Longton G for the Seattle Marrow Transplant Team: Improvement in rejection, engraftment rate and survival without increase in graft-versus-host disease by high marrow cell dose in patients transplanted for aplastic anaemia. Br J Haematol 1988;69:23-28.

67. Rodt H, Netzel B, Kolb HJ, Janka G, Rieder I, Belohradsky B, Haas RJ, Thierfelder S: Antibody treatment of marrow grafts in vitro: a principle for prevention of graft-versus-host disease. *Experimental Hematology Today*, edited by Baum SJ and Ledney GD. Springer-Verlag, New York 1979; pp. 197-206.

68. Prentice HG, Blacklock HA, Janossy G, Bradstock KF, Skeggs D, Goldstein G, Hoffbrand AV: Use of anti-T-cell monoclonal antibody OKT3 to prevent acute graft-versus-host disease in allogeneic bone marrow transplantation for acute leukemia. Lancet 1982;i:700-703.

69. Filipovich AH, McGlave PB, Ramsay NKC, Goldstein G, Warkentin PI, Kersey JH: Pretreatment of donor bone marrow with monoclonal antibody OKT3 for prevention of acute graft-versus-host disease in allogeneic histocompatible bone marrow transplantation. Lancet 1982;i:1266-1270.

70. Reisner Y, Kapoor N, Kirkpatrick D, Pollack MS, Cunningham-Rundles S, Dupont B, Hodes MZ, Good RA, O'Reilly K: Transplantation for severe combined immunodeficiency with HLA-A, B, D, DR incompatible parental marrow cells fractionated by soybean agglutinin and sheep red blood cells. Blood 1983;61:341-348.

71. Martin PJ, Hansen JA, Buckner CD, Sanders JE, Deeg HJ, Stewart P, Appelbaum FR, Clift R, Fefer A, Witherspoon RP, Kennedy MS, Sullivan KM, Flournoy N, Storb R, Thomas ED: Effects of in vitro depletion of T cells in HLA-identical allogeneic marrow grafts. Blood 1985;66:664-672.

72. Hervé P, Cahn JY, Flesch M, Plouvier E, Racadot E, Noir A, Couteret Y, Goldstein G, Bernard A, Lenys R, Bresson JL, Leconte des Floris R, Peters A: Successful graft-versus-host disease prevention without graft failure in 32 HLA-identical allogeneic bone marrow transplantations with marrow depleted of T cells by monoclonal antibodies and complement. Blood 1987;69:338-393.

73. Atkinson K, Biggs J, Cooley M, Farrelly H, O'Flaherty E, Raphael H, Ashby M, Concarmon A, Dodds A, Morgan G: A comparative study of T-cell depleted and non-depleted marrow transplantation for hematological malignancy. Aust N Z J Med 1987;17:16-23.

74. de Witte T, Hoogenhout J, de Pauw B, Holdrinet R, Janssen J, Wessels J, van Daal W, Hustinx T, Haanen C: Depletion of donor lymphocytes by counterflow centrifugation successfully prevents acute graft-versus-host disease in matched allogeneic marrow transplantation. Blood 1986;67:1302-1308.

75. Hale G, Bright S, Chumbly G, Trang Hoang, Metcalf D, Munro AJ, Waldmann H: Removal of T cells from bone marrow after transplantation: A monoclonal anti-lymphocyte antibody that fixed human complement. Blood 1983;62:873-882.

76. Mitsuyasu RT, Champlin RE, Gale RP, Ho WG, Lenarsky C, Winston D, Selch M, Elashoff R, Giorig JV, Wells J, Terasaki P, Billing R, Feig S: Treatment of donor bone marrow with monoclonal anti-T-cell antibody and complement for the prevention of graft-versus-host disease. Ann Intern Med 1986;105:20-26.

77. Kernan NA, Flomenberg N, Dupont B, O'Reilly R: Graft rejection in recipients of

T-cell-depleted HLA-nonidentical marrow transplants for leukemia. Transplantation 1987;43:842-847.

78. Atkinson K. Farrelly H, Colley M, O'Flaherty E, Downs K, Biggs K: Human marrow T cell dose correlates with severity of subsequent acute graft-versus-host disease. Bone Marrow Transplant 1987;2:51-79.

79. Atkinson K, Cooley M, Farrelly H, O'Flaherty E, Ashby M, Biggs J: CD4+ T cells appear capable of initiating graft-versus-host disease across non-major histocompatibility complex (MHC) barriers in man. Bone Marrow Transplant 1987;2:79-84.

80. Maraninchi D, Gluckman E, Blaise D, Guyotat D, Rio B, Pico JL, Leblond V, Michallet M, Dreyfus F, Ifrah N, Bordigoni A: Impact of T-cell depletion on outcome of allogeneic bone-marrow transplantation for standard-risk leukaemias. Lancet 1987; ii:175-178.

81. Atkinson K, Incefy GS, Storb R, Sullivan KM, Iwata T, Dardenne M, Ochs HD: Low serum thymic hormone levels in patients with chronic graft-versus-host disease. Blood 1982;59:1073-1077.

82. Witherspoon RP, Hersman J, Storb R, Ochs H, Goldstein AL, McClure J, Noel D, Weiden PL, Thomas ED: Thymosin fraction 5 does not accelerate reconstitution of immunologic reactivity after human marrow grafting. Br J Haematol 1983;55:595-608.

83. Gluckman E, Devergie A, Sohier J, Saurat JH: Graft-versus-host disease in recipients of syngeneic bone marrow. Lancet 1980; i:253-254.

84. Hess AD, Horwitz L, Beschorner WE, Santos GW: Development of graft-versus-host disease-like syndrome in cyclosporine-treated rats after syngeneic bone marrow transplantation. I. Development of cytotoxic T lymphocytes with apparent polyclonal anti-Ia specificity including autoreactivity. J Exp Med 1985;161:718-730.

85. Hood A, Vogelsang G, Black C, Farmer E, Santos GW: Acute graft-versus-host disease following autologous and syngeneic bone marrow transplantation. Arch Dermatol 1987;123:745-750.

86. Rappeport J, Reinherz E, Mihm M, Lopansii S, Parkman E: Acute graft-versus-host disease in recipients of bone marrow transplants from identical twin donors. Lancet 1979; ii:717-720.

87. Sakaguchi S, Sakaguchi N: Thymus and autoimmunity, transplantation of the thymus from cyclosporin A treated mice causes organ specific autoimmune disease in athymic nude mice. J Exp Med 1988;167:1479-1485.

88. MacDonald HR, Hengartner H, Pedrazzini T: Intrathymic deletion of self-reactive cells prevented by neonatal anti-CD4 antibody treatment. Nature 1988;335:174-176.

89. Jenkins MK, Schwartz RH, Pardoll DM: Effects of cyclosporine A on T cell development and clonal deletion. Science 1988;241:1655-1658.

90. Atkinson K, Storb R, Ochs HD, Goehle S, Sullivan KM, Witherspoon RP, Lum LG, Tsoi M-S, Sanders JE, Parr M, Stewart P, Thomas ED: Thymus transplantation after allogeneic bone marrow graft to prevent chronic graft-versus-host disease in humans. Transplantation 1982;33:168-173.

91. van Bekkum DW, Roddenburg J, Heidt PJ, van der Waaij D: Mitigation of secondary disease of allogeneic mouse radiation chimeras by modification of the intestinal microflora. J Natl Cancer Inst 1974;52:401-404.

92. van Bekkum DW, Knaan S: A role of bacterial microflora in development of intestinal lesions from graft versus host reactions. J Natl Cancer Inst 1977;58:787-789.

93. Truitt RL, Pollard M, Srivastaua KK: Allogeneic bone marrow chimerism in germ free mice. III. Therapy of leukemic AKR mice. Proceedings of the Society for Experimental Biology and Medicine 1974;146:153-158.

94. Ringden O, Paulin T, Lonnqvist B, Nilsson B: An analysis of factors predisposing to chronic graft-vs-host disease. Exp Hematol 1985;13:1062-1067.

95. Michallet M, Corront B, Bosson JL, Reiffers J, Marit G, Maraninchi D, Gaspart MH: Risk factors for GVHD: study of 157 patients from Bordeaux, Grenoble, Marseille. Bone Marrow Transplantation 1988;3;226.
96. Storb R, Thomas ED: Graft-vs-host disease in dog and man: The Seattle Experience. Immunol Rev 1985;88:215-238.
97. Moore RH, Cohen J: Passive immunisation with antiserum to _Escherichia coli_ J5 protects mice from the effects of "minor" graft versus host. Bone Marrow Transplant 1988;1(Suppl 1):80.
98. Vossen JM, Heidt PJ, Guiot HFL, Dooren LJ: Prevention of acute graft-versus-host disease in clinical bone marrow transplantation: Complete versus selective intestinal decontamination. In _Recent Advances in Germfree Research_, edited by Sasaki S. Tokai Univ. Press., Tokyo, 1981; pp. 573-577.
99. Storb R, Prentice RL, Buckner CD, Clift RA, Appelbaum F, Deeg HJ, Doney K, Hansen JA, Mason M, Sanders JE, Singer J, Sullivan KM, Witherspoon RP, Thomas ED: Graft-versus-host disease and survival in patients with aplastic anemia treated by marrow grafts from HLA-identical siblings. Beneficial effect of a protective environment. N Engl J Med 1983;308:302-307.
100. Gratama JW, Zwaan FE, Stijnen T, Weijers TF, Weiland HT, D'Amaro J, Hekker AC, The TH, De Gast GC, Vossen JM: Herpes-versus immunity and acute graft-versus-host disease. Lancet 1987; i:471-474.
101. O'Reilly RJ, Reich L, Gold J, Kirkpatrick D, Dinsmore R, Kapoor N, Condie R: A randomized trial of intravenous hyperimmune globulin for the prevention of cytomegalovirus infections following marrow transplantation: preliminary results. Transplant Proc 1983;15:1405-1411.
102. Winston DJ, Ho WG, Lin CH, Bartoni K, Budinger MD, Gale RP, Champlin RE: Intravenous immune globulin for prevention of cytomegalovirus infection and interstitial pneumonia after bone marrow transplantation. Ann Int Med 1987; 106:12-18.
103. Tutschka PJ, Copelan EA, Klein JP: Bone marrow transplantation for leukemia following a new busulfan and cyclophosphamide regimen. Blood 1987;70:1382-1388.
104. Deeg HJ, Cottler-Fox M, Cahill R, Lynch M, Spitzer TR: Decreased incidence of acute graft vs host disease (GVHD) and cytomegalovirus (CMV) infection with high dose intravenous immunoglobulin (IVIG), reduced dose methotrexate (MTX) and cyclosporine (CSP) after grafting. Bone Marrow Transplant 1989;4(Suppl. 2): 96.
105. Sullivan KM: Immunoglobulin therapy in bone marrow transplantation. Am J Med 1987;83:34-45.
106. Yamashita A, Hattori Y, Mri F, Kosaka A: Acquisition of graft-versus-host reactivity by immature thymocytes in the coexistence of activated macrophages. Transplantation 1982;33:80-86.
107. Guillen FJ, Ferrara J, Hancock W, Messadi D, Fonferko E, Burakoff SJ, Murphy GF: Acute cutaneous graft versus host disease to minor histocompatibility antigens in a murine model. Lab Invest 1986;55:35-42.
108. Ford WL, Deeg HJ: Bone marrow transplantation, with emphasis on GVH reactions. Transplant Proc 1983;15;1517-1519.
109. Elfenbein GJ, Anderson PN, Humphrey RL, Melleus GM, Sensenbrenner LL, Wands JR, Santos GW: Immune system reconstitution follow allogeneic bone marrow transplantation in man: a multi-parameter analysis. Transplant Proc 1976;8: 641-646.
110. Gale RP, Opelz G, Mickey MR, Graze PR, Saxon A, for the UCLA Bone Marrow Transplant Team: Immunodeficiency following allogeneic bone marrow transplantation. Transplant Proc 1978;10:223-227.

111. Reinherz EL, Parkman R, Rappeport J, Rosen FS, Schlossman S: Aberrations of suppressor T cells in human graft versus host disease. N Engl J Med 1979;300: 1061-1068.

112. De Bruin HG, Astaldi A, Leupers T, Van de Griend RJ, Dooren LJ, Schellekins PThA, Tanke HJ, Roos M, Vossen JM: T lymphocyte characteristics of bone marrow-transplanted patients. II. Analysis with monoclonal antibodies. J Immunol 1981;127:244-251.

113. Friedrich W, O'Reilly RJ, Koziner B, Gebhard DR Jr, Good RA, Evans RL: T lymphocyte reconstitution in recipients of bone marrow transplants with and without GVHD: imbalances of T cell subpopulations having unique regulatory and cognitive functions. Blood 1982;59:696-701.

114. Atkinson K, Hansen JA, Storb R, Goehle S, Goldstein G, Thomas ED: T cell subpopulations identified by monoclonal antibodies after bone marrow transplantation. I. Helper-inducer and cytotoxic-suppressor subsets. Blood 1982;59:1292-1298.

115. Lum LG: A Review: The kinetics of immune reconstitution after human marrow transplantation. Blood 1987;69:369-380.

116. Parkman R, Rappeport J, Rosen F: Human graft versus host disease. J Invest Dermatol 1980;74:276-279.

117. Tsoi M-S, Storb R, Weiden PL, Thomas ED: Studies on cellular inhibition and serum-blocking factors in 28 human patients given marrow grafts from HLA identical siblings. J Immunol 1977;118:1799-1805.

118. Tsoi M-S, Storb R, Weiden P, Santos E, Kopecky KJ, Thomas ED: Sequential studies of cell inhibition of host fibroblasts in 51 patients given HLA-identical marrow grafts. J Immunol 1982;128:239-242.

119. Shinohara N, Watanabe M, Sachs DH, Hozumi N: Killing of antigen-reactive B cells by class II-restricted, soluble antigen-specific CD8[+] cytolytic T lymphocytes. Nature 1988;336:481-484.

120. Shinohara N, Hozumi N, Watanabe M, Bluestone JA, Johnson-Leva R, Sachs DH: Class II antigen-specific murine cytolytic T lymphocytes (CTL). II. Genuine class II specificity of Lyt-2[+] CTl. J Immunol 1988;140:30-36.

121. Gratama J, Naipal A, Oyans P, Zwaan F, Verdonck L, de Witte T, Vossen JM, Bolhuis RL, de Gast GC, Jansen J: T lymphocyte repopulation and differentiation after bone marrow transplantation. Early shifts in the ratio between T4[+] and T8[+] T lymphocytes correlate with the occurrence of acute graft versus host disease. Blood 1984;63:1416-1423.

122. Tsoi M-S, Storb R, Dobbs S, Sullivan KM, Thomas ED: Suppressor cells in patients with HLA identical marrow grafts. In *Biology of Bone Marrow Transplantation*, edited by Gale RP, Fox CF. Academic Press, New York, 1980; pp. 119-125.

123. Tsoi M-S, Storb R, Dobbs S, Thomas ED: Specific suppressor cells in graft-host tolerance of HLA-identical marrow transplantation. Nature 1981;292:355-357.

124. Strober S, Palathumpat V, Schwadron R, Hertel-Wulff H: Cloned natural suppressor cells prevent lethal graft-vs-host disease. J Immunol 1987;138:699-703.

125. Holda JH, Maier T, Claman HN: Evidence that IFN-γ is responsible for natural suppressor activity in GVHD spleen and normal bone marrow. Transplantation 1988;45:772-777.

126. Lopez C, Sorell M, Kirkpatrick D, O'Reilly RJ, Ching C and the Bone Marrow Transplant Unit: Association between pre-transplant natural kill and graft-versus-host disease after stem-cell transplantation. Lancet 1979; ii:1103-1106.

127. Livnat S, Seigneuret M, Storb R, Prentice RL: Analysis of cytotoxic effector cell function in patients with leukemia or aplastic anemia before and after marrow transplantation. J Immunol 1980;124:481-490.

128. Lopez C, Kirkpatrick D, Livnat S, Storb R: Natural killer cells in bone marrow transplantation. Lancet 1980; ii:1025.

129. Dokhelar M-C, Wiels J, Lipinski M, Tetaud C, Devergie A, Gluckman E, Tursz T: Natural killer cell activity in human bone marrow recipients: early reappearance of peripheral natural killer activity in graft versus host disease. Transplantation 1981;31:61-65.

130. Peralvo J, Bacigalupo A, Pittaluga PA, Occhini D, Van Lint MT, Frassoni F, Nardelli E, Trasino A, Pantarotto M, Marmond AM: Poor graft function associated with graft-versus-host disease after allogeneic marrow transplantation. Bone Marrow Transplantation 1987;2:279-285.

131. Merritt CB, Mann DL, Rogentine GN: Cytotoxic antibody for epithelial cells in human graft versus host disease. Nature 1971;232:638-639.

132. Saurat J-H, Gluckman E, Bonnetblanc J-M, Didier-Jean L, Bussel A, Puissant A: Characteres cliniques et biolgiques des eruptions licheniennes apres greffe de moelle osseuse. Ann Dermatol Syphyligr 1975;102:521-525.

133. Ullman S, Spielvogel RL, Kersey JA, Goltz RW: Immunoglobulins and complement in skin in graft-versus-host disease. Ann Intern Med 1976;85:205.

134. Tsoi M-S: Immunological mechanisms of graft-versus-host disease in man. Transplantation 1982;33:459-464.

135. Jeannet M, Rubenstein A, Pelet B: Studies on non-HLA cytotoxic and blocking factor in a patient with immunological deficiency successfully reconstituted by bone marrow transplant. Tissue Antigens 1973;3:411-416.

136. Gluckman E, Andersen E, Lepage V, Dausset J: Non-HLA lymphocytotoxic antibodies during GVHD after bone marrow transplantation (BMT). Transplant Proc 1977;9:761-763.

137. Opelz G, Walker J, Gale RP: Detection of non-HLA antibodies in bone marrow transplant recipients. Transplant Proc 1978;10:963-964.

138. Warren RP, Storb R, Weiden PL, Su PJ, Thomas ED: Immunologic monitoring of marrow graft recipients following transplantation from HLA-identical siblings. Transplant Proc 1978;10:535-536.

139. Cheney RT, Sprent J: Capacity of cyclosporine to induce autograft-versus-host disease and impair intrathymic T-cell differentiation. Transplant Proc 1985;17:528-530.

140. Hess AD, Vogelsang GB, Heyd J, Beschorner WE: Cyclosporine-induced syngeneic graft-versus-host disease: Assessment of T-cell differentiation. Transplant Proc 1987;19:2683-2686.

141. deWaal Malefijt R, Leene W, Roholl PJM, Wormmeester J, Hoeben KA: T-cell differentiation within thymic nurse cells. Lab Invest 1986;55:25-34.

142. Jenkins MK, Schwartz RH, Pardoll DM: Effects of cyclosporine A on T cell development and clonal deletion. Science 1988;241:1655-1658.

143. Ferrara J, Marion A, Murphy G, Burakoff S: Acute graft-versus-host disease: Pathogenesis and prevention with a monoclonal antibody in vivo. Transplant Proc 1987;19:2662-2663.

144. Azogui O, Gluckman E, Fradelizi D: Inhibition of IL2 production after human allogeneic bone marrow transplantation. J Immunol 1983;131:1205-1208.

145. Shulman HM: Is graft-versus-host disease an alloimmune or autoimmune disorder? Clinical Aspects of Autoimmunity 1988;2:18-30.

146. Vogelsang GB, Hess AD, Berkman A, Tutschka P, Farmer E, Converse P, Santos GW: An in vitro predictive test for graft-versus-host disease in patients with genotypic HLA-identical bone marrow transplants. N Engl J Med 1985;313:645-650.

147. Bagot M, Cordonnier C, Tilkin FF, Heslan M, Vernan JP, Bubertret L, Levy JP: A possible predictive test for graft-versus-host disease in bone marrow graft recipi-

ents: The mixed epidermal cell-lymphocyte reaction. Transplantation 1986;41: 316-319.

148. Breatnach SM, Katz SI: Cell-mediated immunity in cutaneous disease. Hum Pathol 1986;17:161-167.

149. Deeg HJ: Ultraviolet irradiation in transplantation biology. Manipulation of immunity and immunogenicity. Transplantation 1988;45:845-851.

150. Granelli-Piperno A, Keane M, Steinman RM: Evidence that cyclosporine inhibits cell-mediated immunity primarily at the level of the T lymphocyte rather than the accessory cell. Transplantation 1988;46:53-60.

151. Spielberg H, June C, Cereb N, Nystrom-Rosander C, Deeg HJ: Differential sensitivity of human leukocyte subpopulations to ultraviolet light. Transplant Proc 1989;21:180-181.

152. Joseph LJ, Iwasaki T, Malek TR, Shearer GM: Interleukin 2 receptor dysfunction in mice undergoing a graft-vs-host reaction. J Immunol 1985;135:1846-1850.

153. Holda JH, Maier T, Claman HN: Natural suppressor activity in graft-vs-host spleen and normal bone marrow is augmented by IL 2 and interferon-γ. J Immunol 1986; 137:3538-3543.

154. Kupiec-Weglinski JW, Diamantstein T, Tilney NL, Strom TB: Therapy with monoclonal antibody to interleukin 2 receptor spares suppressor T cells and prevents or reverses acute allograft rejection in rats. Proc Natl Acad Sci 1986;83:2624-2627.

155. Henslee PJ, Byers VS, Jennings CD, Marciniak E, Thompson JS, MacDonald JS, Romond EH, Messino MJ, Scannon PJ: A new approach to the prevention of graft-versus-host disease using XomaZyme H65 following histo-incompatible partially T-depleted marrow grafts. Transplant Proc 1989;21:3004-3007.

156. Bellen DW, Graeven U, Schulz G, Grosse-Wilde H, Doxiadis I, Schaeffer UW, Quabeck K, Sayer H, Schmidt CG: Treatment of acute graft-versus-host disease after HLA-partially matched marrow transplantation with a monoclonal antibody (BMA031) against the T cell receptor. Onkologie 1988;11:56-58.

17

The Pathology of Acute Graft-vs.-Host Disease

Dale C. Snover
University of Minnesota Hospital
Minneapolis, Minnesota

I. INTRODUCTION

Acute Graft-vs.-Host Disease (GVHD) is manifested primarily by involvement of three organ systems: the skin, gastrointestinal tract, and liver. Histopathologically, it is characterized by infiltration of tissue by lymphoid cells and destruction of epithelium. The latter process may disrupt the usually protective cutaneous and mucosal barriers, facilitating infections which often lead to the demise of the patient. Therefore, early and accurate diagnosis and treatment of GVHD are essential to survival of the patient.

The use of biopsy in the diagnosis of GVHD varies among transplant centers based in large part on the value that the clinician places on histopathologic diagnosis. This, in turn, is in part a reflection of the accuracy of diagnosis provided by the pathologist. The skin, because of its accessibility, is the most commonly biopsied organ. However, the experience of several centers, including our own, is that the skin in many ways gives a less accurate reflection of the clinical status of the patient than the gastrointestinal (GI) tract (1). This is in part due to the relative nonspecificity of the characteristic histopathologic features of GVHD in the skin and perhaps to the common occurrence of isolated cutaneous GVHD. Therefore, gastrointestinal biopsy, most often of the rectum, is considered as or more important than skin biopsy in diagnosis.

As implied above, one role of biopsy in the management of the transplant patient is in establishing the *diagnosis* of GVHD. This is particularly true of the skin and GI tract where GVHD must be distinguished from other causes of skin rash, diarrhea, or upper GI complaints. Liver biopsy is less often used as a primary diagnostic tool for GVHD if there is unequivocal involvement of other organs since patients in the early posttransplant period are often poor candidates for biopsy because of the potential for bleeding. Liver biopsy is undertaken more often to rule out other causes of liver disease in patients treated for GVHD in whom the liver does not respond to therapy in concert with improvement in other organ involvement. Biopsy is also used to assess *severity* of GVHD.

Biopsies are graded based on degree of epithelial damage, although with the exception of severe disease this information appears to be of less value than clinical grading. Histologic grading is of some importance in providing the clinician with a sense of the security of diagnosis, however, since as the degree of damage increases, the accuracy of diagnosis increases as well.

II. SKIN

The clinical differential diagnosis for which skin biopsy is performed in the early posttransplant period includes GVHD, effect of cytoreductive radiation and chemotherapy, drug reactions, recurrent primary disease (e.g., cutaneous leukemic infiltrate), and cutaneous infections as may occur with disseminated fungal infections. In general, the diagnosis of infectious disease and malignant infiltrates does not present differential diagnostic difficulties, although it is possible that some viral infections may at times simulate GVHD (2).

Cutaneous acute GVHD is characterized by necrosis of epithelial cells of the basal layer, often accompanied by a mild lymphoid infiltrate (3,4). This latter point (i.e., the mildness of the lymphoid infiltrate) is a very important and often misunderstood aspect of the diagnosis. Although it is most probable that acute GVHD is a cell mediated process, due to the pancytopenia found in the early posttransplant period, lymphoid infiltration is often modest at best. Therefore, finding a lymphoid infiltrate is not a prerequisite for the diagnosis of GVHD in any organ. On the other hand, necrosis of epithelial cells is the sine qua non of the diagnosis (3).

Necrosis seen in cutaneous GVHD may take several forms. The earliest and most nonspecific form is simple hydropic or vacuolar degeneration of the basal layer (Figs. 1 and 2). This is seen most prominently at the tips of the rete ridges which is also the area with the greatest density of undifferentiated, presumably stem cells in the skin (Fig. 1) (5). With increased severity of disease, coagulated necrotic cells (dyskeratotic cells or apoptotic bodies) appear, often with attached lymphocytes ("satellitosis") (Fig. 2). These single necrotic cells are first seen in the basal layer, although with time they migrate to the surface. Continued damage may lead to separation of the epidermis from the dermis with the formation of vesicles or bullae and eventual desquamation (Figs. 3 and 4). In addition, in severe disease total necrosis of the epidermis may occur, leading to a picture of toxic epidermal necrosis (TEN) (Fig. 5).

In addition to these characteristic stages in the development of acute GVHD, other histologic variations may occur. Involvement of the adnexa may be seen, particularly of the hair follicles (Fig. 6). On rare occasions, acute GVHD may present as a folliculitis in which only the hair follicles are involved (6). Other occasional features which have no apparent clinical importance include purpura (extravasation of erythrocytes into the dermis) and perivascular lymphoid infiltration simulating a lymphoid vasculitis.

Acute cutaneous GVHD is graded based on degree of damage as described above (3). Grade 1 is characterized by hydropic degeneration alone and is a very nonspecific finding that is at best consistent with GVHD (Fig. 1). Grade 1 "GVHD" of the skin should be considered a nondiagnostic biopsy. Presence of coagulated necrotic cells indicates grade 2 disease, and is considered a much more diagnostic stage of disease (Fig. 2). Nevertheless, these changes may also be seen with some drug reactions and as a response to cytoreductive chemo- or radiation therapy (see below). Presence of small areas of subepidermal clefting rates a grade 3 designation and complete sloughing or TEN represent

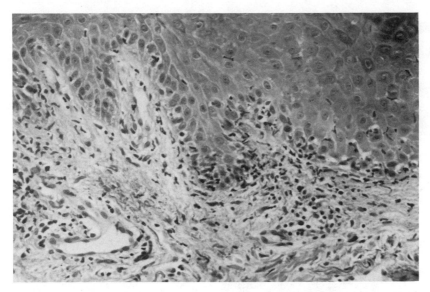

Figure 1 Grade 1 acute cutaneous graft-versus-host disease showing mild basal layer hydropic degeneration and lymphocytic infiltration affecting predominantly the tips of the rete ridges. There is also an accompanying sparse infiltrate in the upper dermis. (Hematoxylin and eosin ×192)

grade 4 disease (Figs. 3, 4, and 5). The clinical significance of histologic grading is not great, although grade 1 lesions need to be viewed with caution as to specificity, and grade 4 lesions are associated with poor prognosis due to the propensity for superinfection.

The differential diagnosis of the above-described changes will depend in part on the time posttransplant. In the first 20 days or so posttransplant, distinction of GVHD from the effects of cytoreductive chemoradiation therapy may be impossible (3). Essentially all of the features of acute GVHD can be caused by cytoreductive agents, although with the passage of time the effects diminish and, more importantly, evidence of active damage in the form of basal layer degeneration diminishes. In this context, it is important to remember the sequential nature of the changes of GVHD or other agents causing damage to the basal cells of the skin. If the damage is caused by a one-time event, such as chemoradiation, then one will see active damage only near the time of insult. However, the nonactive changes, in particular the presence of single necrotic cells and nuclear atypia, will persist until the involved cells migrate to the surface and are eliminated from the epidermis. Hence, a biopsy with numerous dyskeratotic cells but no basilar hydropic degeneration is more likely to result from previous cytoreduction than from ongoing GVHD (Fig. 7). In addition, cytoreductive agents tend to damage the epidermis diffusely, whereas GVHD may be more patchy. Therefore, patchiness may favor the latter diagnosis.

Distinction of GVHD from drug reaction may be extremely difficult. Features of some value are eosinophils seen in hypersensitivity reactions and marked vasculitis, seen more commonly in drug reactions. If the diagnosis is unclear, correlation with biopsy of other organs should be sought.

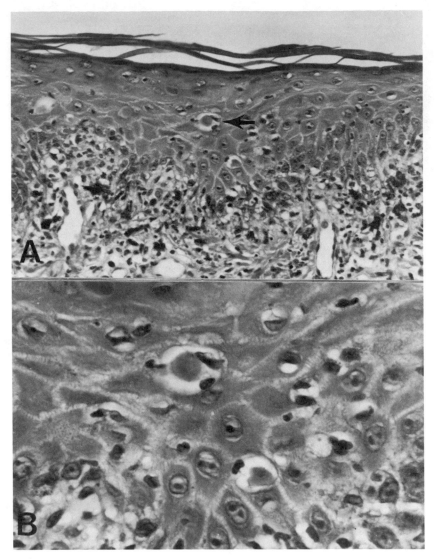

Figure 2 (A) Grade 2 acute cutaneous graft-versus-host disease. In addition to basal layer hydropic degeneration, several dyskeratotic cells are now apparent (arrow). (Hematoxylin and eosin ×192) (B) The dyskeratotic cells of graft-versus-host disease will often have attached lymphocytes, a feature termed "satellitosis." (Hematoxylin and eosin ×480)

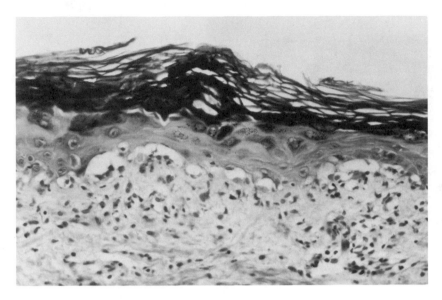

Figure 3   Grade 3 acute cutaneous graft-versus-host disease showing early clefting at the dermal-epidermal junction. (Hematoxylin and eosin ×192)

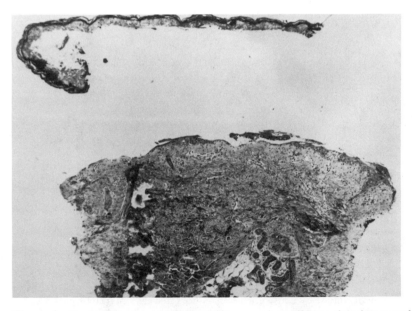

Figure 4   Grade 4 acute cutaneous graft-versus-host disease showing complete separation of the epidermis from the dermis. (Hematoxylin and eosin ×30)

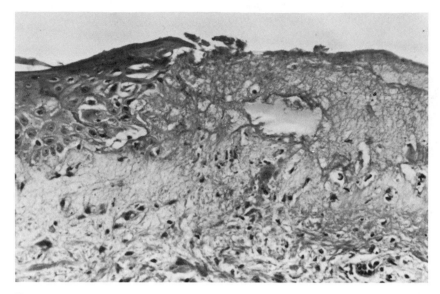

Figure 5 Grade 4 acute cutaneous graft-versus-host disease with a toxic epidermal necrosis-like picture. Note the sharply demarcated full thickness necrosis of the epidermis. (Hematoxylin and eosin ×192)

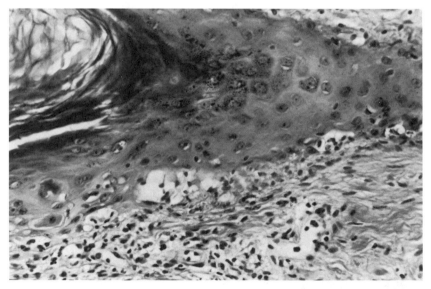

Figure 6 Follicular involvement by acute graft-versus-host disease. Marked hydropic degeneration of the follicular basal layer with occasional dyskeratotic cells and an associated lymphocytic infiltrate are noted. (Hematoxylin and eosin ×192)

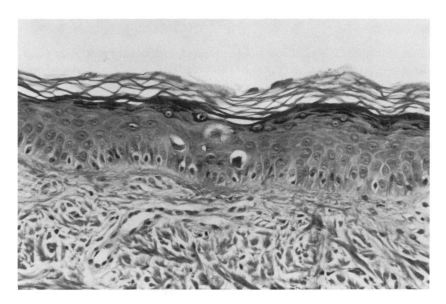

Figure 7 Biopsy of the skin taken early after transplantation showing the residual effects of cytoreductive therapy. Note the several dyskeratotic cells without basilar degeneration or associated infiltrate. (Hematoxylin and eosin ×192)

III. GASTROINTESTINAL TRACT

As in the skin, the clinical differential diagnosis for which gastrointestinal biopsy is performed includes GVHD, effects of cytoreductive therapy, and infectious disease, particularly with viral agents. Other less commonly encountered problems include pseudomembranous enterocolitis and recurrent malignancy. Histologic distinction of the latter two processes from GVHD is not difficult, but cytoreductive effect and viral infections can cause significant difficulties.

Acute GVHD of the gastrointestinal tract is characterized by necrosis of epithelial cells in the regenerating compartment of the particular organ biopsied (2,7). In the small and large intestine the crypt is primarily involved, whereas in the stomach the neck region is the major target. Esophagus is very rarely involved with acute GVHD, but when it is the basal layer appears to be the primary site of injury, as in the skin (4). The importance of recognition of the regenerating compartment as the area of attack is significant for several reasons. First, it provides possible insight into the pathogenesis of GVHD since it would appear that some special feature of the stem cell makes it the target (5,8). Determining the special features of these cells may provide data on molecular targets and specific cell of attack. More practically, it provides an area of focus for the pathologist to examine, i.e., the pathologist can save time and effort by examining this area first. As a corollary to this, it is imperative that the regenerative compartment be examined before a biopsy is interpreted as not showing evidence of GVHD. Specimens of rectum or duodenum that are sectioned tangentially so that the crypt region is not visible should have additional levels cut in order to see this region. If a specimen is so superficial that the crypts are not present, it is inadequate for diagnosis. It should be noted that necrosis of epithelial cells on the surface of the intestine, particularly in the colon, is a very nonspecific finding that may be related to normal migration and cell death and may also be related to the use of enemas as preparation for endoscopy (9).

Although the rectum is the most commonly biopsied of the gastrointestinal organs, it may not always accurately reflect the status of the entire GI tract (2). It has been our experience that symptomatology will vary with the segment of GI tract affected. Diarrhea is most often associated with rectal or duodenal disease, whereas nausea, vomiting, and upper abdominal pain are associated with positive gastric biopsies. In a series at the University of Minnesota, of 24 patients with gastrointestinal GVHD and biopsies of all three segments, rectal alone was positive in only 2, upper GI tract (stomach or duodenum) alone was positive in 11, and both areas were positive in 11. A reasonable approach to diagnosis in a patient with diarrhea is to biopsy the rectum first, and, if negative, then perform upper GI endoscopy and biopsy. In patients without diarrhea but with upper GI symptoms, it may be more expedient to biopsy the upper GI tract first.

The particular variant of necrosis which characterizes GI GVHD is the so-called "exploding crypt cell," recognized as a space within the epithelium filled with cellular and karyorrhexic nuclear debris (Fig. 8). These exploding crypt cells are larger and more easily identified in the rectum than in the stomach or small intestine. When present in sufficient numbers, they are nearly diagnostic of GVHD, with exceptions listed below. Of course, the definition of "sufficient numbers" is an elusive one. Clearly, if the majority of crypts contain such cells, there is no problem. However, the lower limit of sensitivity is not well defined. As a practical matter, if the necrotic cells can be detected on low or medium power evaluation of the specimen, then they are probably significant. If, on the other hand, they are detected only after careful high power search, then they should be viewed with caution. Biopsies with GVHD often contain crypt abscesses as well as the single necrotic cells, although crypt abscesses are nonspecific and of little

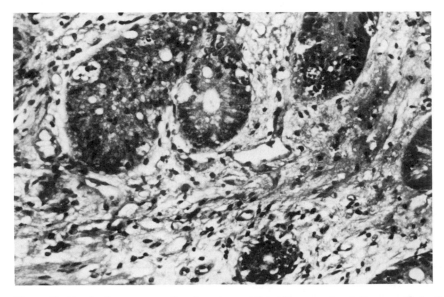

Figure 8 Exploding crypt cells of acute rectal graft-versus-host disease. Note the vacuoles containing cellular and nuclear debris. These "exploding crypt cells" are larger and more prominent in the rectum than in the duodenum or stomach. (Hematoxylin and eosin X75)

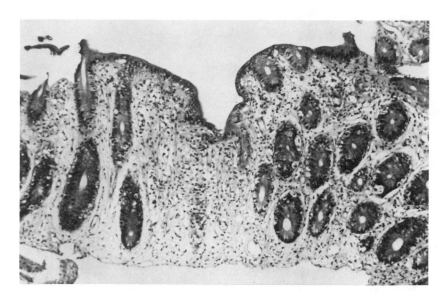

Figure 9 Grade 2 acute rectal graft-versus-host disease. Note the area of missing crypts along with visible cellular necrosis in the adjacent viable crypts. (Hematoxylin and eosin ×75)

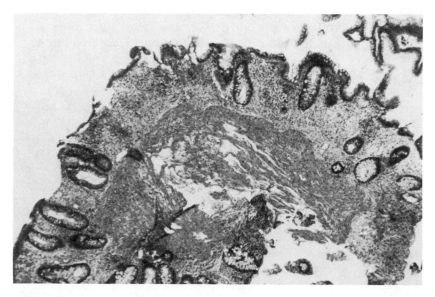

Figure 10 Grade 3 acute rectal graft-versus-host disease. There are several areas of missing crypts, one of which is approximately seven crypts in span. (Hematoxylin and eosin ×30)

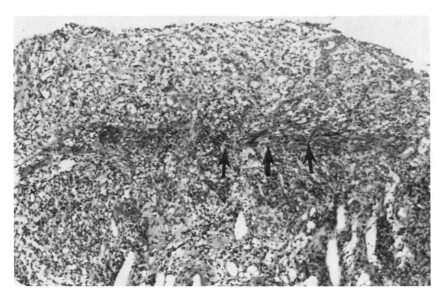

Figure 11 Grade 4 acute rectal graft-versus-host disease. The epithelium is completely absent although lamina propria is still present as evidenced by the muscularis mucosae (arrows). (Hematoxylin and eosin ×75)

diagnostic significance. Biopsies with GVHD may also contain abundant karyorrhexic debris in the lamina propria and in crypts without single cell necrosis. This debris is nonspecific although if present alone it should lead to a careful evaluation of additional levels of tissue for exploding crypt cells as well as cytomegalovirus (CMV) inclusions (10). Lymphocytic infiltration of the mucosa is usually very sparse in acute GI GVHD.

As destruction of epithelium increases with GVHD, crypts may be destroyed. Acute GVHD has been graded on the basis of degree of loss of crypts, a system first devised for the rectal biopsy (7). Biopsies with numerous exploding crypt cells but without crypt loss are grade 1 lesions. Loss of up to three contiguous crypts represents grade 2 and loss of four or more crypts without total sloughing is grade 3 (Figs. 9 and 10). Total sloughing represents grade 4, a very rare phenomenon and one in which the diagnosis of GVHD cannot actually be made on biopsy since there are no crypts left to demonstrate the diagnostic type of necrosis (Fig. 11). In such cases, the etiology of the sloughing is determined to be GVHD based on biopsies of other organs or previous GI biopsies. As in the skin, grading has little prognostic significance with the exception of grade 4, which leads to infectious complications. Our grading system represents a minor modification of the grading system proposed by Sale et al. (7) and includes a "consistent with but not diagnostic" category designed to accommodate those biopsies with a few rare exploding crypt cells but not enough to feel totally confident of the diagnosis. In addition, we have increased the range of acceptable grade 2 lesions by accepting cases with up to three contiguous missing crypts rather than the single missing crypt allowed by Sale et al. (7).

It should be noted that there are several artefactual causes of crypt loss that should not be mistaken for severe GVHD. Crypts are sometimes "squeezed" out of the biopsy in the process of obtaining the specimen, leading to crypt sheaths that appear empty

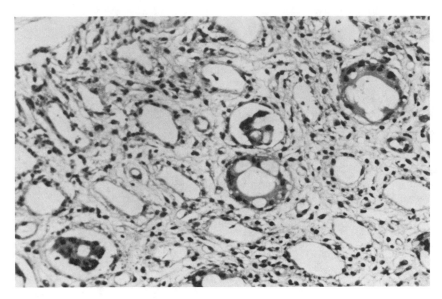

Figure 12 Artefactual loss of crypts caused by "squeezing" of the specimen. Note the absence of necrotic cells characteristic of graft-versus-host disease in the few remaining crypts. (Hematoxylin and eosin ×192)

(Fig. 12). In such a case the epithelium will often be found lying beside the major portion of tissue on the slide. Another cause of the appearance of missing crypts is the depleted lymphoid follicle. Normal GI tract contains mucosal or submucosal lymphoid follicles that are depleted by cytoreductive therapy, leaving a circular area devoid of crypts. These areas are recognizable by their circular character as well as by an associated defect in the muscularis mucosae. When in doubt about the cause of missing crypts, it is important to remember that crypts destroyed by GVHD are accompanied by other crypts in various stages of destruction, including intact crypts containing exploding crypt cells (Fig. 13). The other causes of "missing" crypts are not accompanied by these changes.

The differential diagnosis of the changes characteristic of GVHD in the GI tract includes effects of cytoreductive therapy and viral infection including, most importantly, CMV infection (10). We have also seen such changes in biopsies taken from patients with severe T-cell immunodeficiency taken prior to transplantation (11).

In the first 20 days posttransplant biopsies of the GI tract must be viewed with caution since cytoreductive therapy can mimick GVHD here as it does in the skin (7). One can sometimes suggest one diagnosis over the other based on the degree of active epithelial death (i.e., single cell necrosis) versus crypt loss and nuclear atypia. Biopsies with active destruction in the form of exploding crypt cells located deeply in the crypts are more likely to be GVHD; those with only nuclear atypia or necrotic cells above the level of the regenerating compartment more likely represent effects of cytoreductive therapy (Figs. 14 and 15).

In any GI biopsy with CMV inclusions, the diagnosis of GVHD cannot be made or ruled out since CMV often produces identical changes (10). The possibility that other viruses can produce similar changes has not been fully explored and should be considered possible if viruses are cultured from the biopsy specimen.

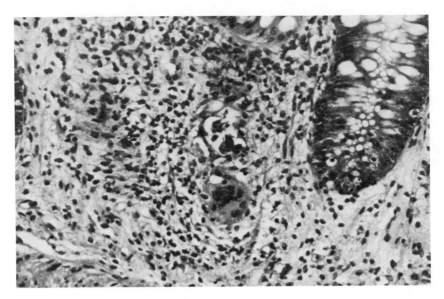

Figure 13 "True" crypt loss. Note, in addition to the space left by a completely destroyed crypts, the partly degenerated crypt as well as the presence of cellular necrosis in the adjacent intact crypt. (Hematoxylin and eosin ×192)

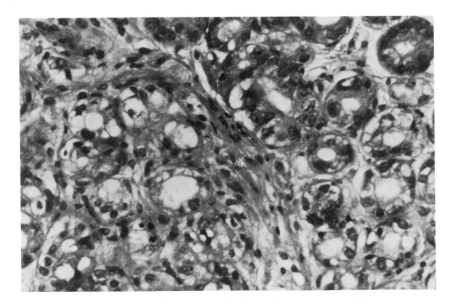

Figure 14 Damage to the gastric mucosa caused by cytoreductive therapy. The glands show nuclear pleomorphism and scattered karyorrhexic debris without exploding crypt cells. (Hematoxylin and eosin ×256)

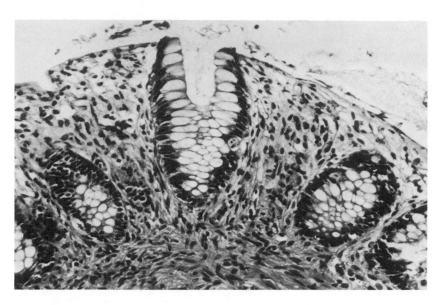

Figure 15   Rectal biopsy showing residual cytoreductive damage. A lonely exploding crypt cell is present in the midpoint of the crypt. (Hematoxylin and eosin ×192)

IV. LIVER

The liver has the widest range of possible diagnoses to consider in the biopsy taken in the first 100 days posttransplant. In the early posttransplant period, including the first 20 days, one may encounter liver disease that was preexisting at the time of transplantation. These include those caused by viral infections and drug reactions as well as residua of the primary disease process for which transplantation was undertaken (e.g., storage material in the case of transplantation for metabolic disease). In addition, cytoreductive therapy may lead to veno-occlusive disease or nodular regenerative hyperplasia (12-15). Following this, acute GVHD, infections including particularly those related to so-called opportunistic organisms and drug reactions, including toxicity due to hyperalimentation, become significant problems. The histologic differential diagnosis of GVHD, some forms of viral hepatitis and some drug reactions can be a major problem. Distinction of GVHD from veno-occlusive disease, nodular regenerative hyperplasia, viral infections with histologically identifiable agents such as cytomegalovirus and herpes simplex, and hyperalimentation toxicity are not problems in our experience.

The liver is the least often biopsied of the major organs that are susceptible to acute GVHD. The major reason for this is the often unacceptable risk of postbiopsy bleeding due to thrombocytopenia in the early posttransplant period. In point of fact, most patients with abnormal liver function tests and biopsy documented GVHD of the skin or GI tract will have hepatic GVHD, which will respond to therapy. However, it is our experience that apparent hepatic improvement will often lag behind improvement of the other organs. Therefore, biopsy of the liver is often taken after the patient has been treated for acute GVHD if liver function tests do not improve. This is done not so much to diagnose GVHD as to rule out other possible causes of liver disease such as concurrent CMV infection. Occasionally a patient will manifest predominantly hepatic GVHD with

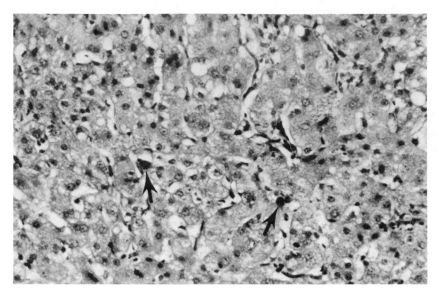

Figure 16 Early hepatic graft-versus-host disease showing a hepatitic picture with a sinusoidal lymphocytic infiltrate and occasional acidophil bodies (arrows). (Hematoxylin and eosin ×192)

minimal or no disease of other organs. In this case biopsy of the liver is undertaken for primary diagnostic purposes.

In hepatic GVHD the biliary epithelium, hepatocytes, and endothelial cells may all be the targets of attack (16,17). In early cases hepatocellular involvement may predominate, leading to a hepatitis-like picture that is difficult to distinguish morphologically from drug- or virally induced acute hepatitis (Fig. 16) (17). More characteristic, however, is portal inflammation with infiltration of lymphocytes into biliary epithelium causing damage or destruction of the interlobular ducts (Fig. 17). As in the other organs, the infiltrate may be sparse and is usually composed almost exclusively of lymphocytes. The bile duct damage is very similar to that seen in liver allograft rejection with loss of nuclei, stratification of nuclei, vacuolation of cytoplasm, and/or eventual loss of ducts. An uncommon but, in our experience, nearly diagnostic finding is the presence of lymphocytic infiltration of endothelium with endothelial damage (Fig. 18) (16). This is identical to the "endothelialitis" that is a diagnostic feature of allograft rejection, although it is a much rarer finding of GVHD (16,18). Reasons for this lack of endothelialitis include the possibility that GVHD is a different process from allograft rejection, that patients with GVHD are treated prior to biopsy, or that the small number of lymphocytes present make endothelialitis difficult to identify. The second of these possibilities seems likely since endothelialitis in allograft rejection is known to be very susceptible to immunosuppressive therapy (18). Endothelialitis has not been universally accepted as a diagnostic criterion (17). This may be due to differences in definition of the process. Simple attachment of a few lymphocytes to the endothelium is insufficient to diagnose "endothelialitis"; there must be evidence of damage to the endothelium.

Although the above-described changes will allow a diagnosis of hepatic GVHD in most cases, it is clear that difficulties in diagnosis exist as evidenced by the false positive

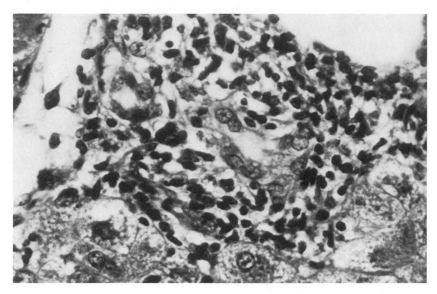

Figure 17 Typical acute hepatic graft-versus-host disease with a portal lymphocytic infiltrate and bile duct damage. Note the lymphocytes in the wall of the duct as well as ductal damage characterized by prominent nucleoli, irregular spacing of nuclei, loss of cells, and irregularity of the shape of the duct. (Hematoxylin and eosin X480)

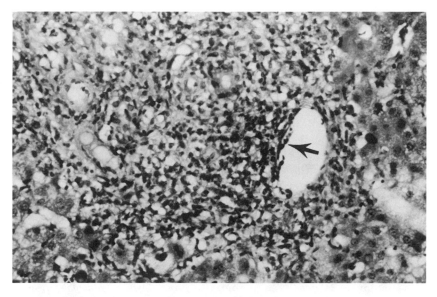

Figure 18 Acute hepatic graft-versus-host disease showing a portal lymphocytic infiltrate, bile duct damage, and portal vein endothelialitis (arrow). (Hematoxylin and eosin X192)

rate of approximately 15% reported in two studies (16,17). Grading of hepatic GVHD by quartile percentage of bile duct damage has been proposed but has not been shown to be of any prognostic significance (19). However, noting the degree of damage can be helpful in diagnosis. As a practical matter, if a biopsy shows minimal hepatocellular involvement and has more than 50% damaged bile ducts, it is most probably GVHD. On the other hand, if there is prominent hepatocellular damage and less than 50% of the ducts are damaged, it is more likely that another etiology is responsible for the damage. If there is both hepatocellular damage and greater than 50% bile duct damage, then neither process can be favored unless convincing endothelialitis is present.

V. OTHER ORGANS

Involvement of other organs by acute GVHD is an uncommon and somewhat controversial event. There is anecdotal evidence that acute pulmonary GVHD may occur, although the pathologic features remain to be defined. Beschorner et al. reported lymphocytic bronchitis to be characteristic of GVHD, although this finding was disputed by Hackman et al. (20,21). Our own experience would indicate that infiltration of the bronchial tree by lymphocytes may occur as part of GVHD but is not diagnostic. Interstitial pneumonitis can probably be caused by GVHD, although it too is obviously nonspecific. At the current time the diagnosis of pulmonary GVHD remains one of exclusion of other etiologies for an interstitial pneumonitis in a patient with documented GVHD of other organs.

Among other organs with reported acute GVHD are kidney and heart (22,23). However, these reports have not been confirmed in the more recent large experience and are somewhat doubtful (4). Even if true, they do not appear to represent a significant clinical problem requiring biopsy confirmation.

ACKNOWLEDGMENTS

The author acknowledges the clerical assistance of Ms. Sharon Leong in the preparation of the manuscript. This work was supported in part by Grant CA 21737 from the National Institutes of Health.

REFERENCES

1.   Sviland L, Pearson ADJ, Eastham EJ, Hamilton PJ, Proctor SJ, Malcolm AJ, and the Newcastle upon Tyne Bone Marrow Transplant Group: Histological features of skin and rectal biopsy specimens after autologous and allogeneic bone marrow transplantation. J Clin Pathol 1988;41:148-154.
2.   Snover DC, Weisdorf SA, Vercellotti GM, Rank B, Hutton S, McGlave P: A histopathologic study of gastric and small intestinal graft-versus-host disease following allogeneic bone marrow transplantation. Hum Pathol 1985;16:387-392.
3.   Sale GE, Lerner KG, Barker EA, Shulman HM, Thomas ED: The skin biopsy in the diagnosis of acute graft-versus-host disease in man. Am J Pathol 1977;89:621-625.
4.   Sale GE and Shulman HM, eds.: *The Pathology of Bone Marrow Transplantation.* Masson Publishing USA Inc., New York, 1984.
5.   Sale GE, Shulman HM, Gallucci BB, Thomas ED: Young rete ridge keratinocytes are preferred targets in cutaneous graft-versus-host disease. Am J Pathol 1985; 118:278-287.

6. Friedman KJ, LeBoit PE, Farmer E: Acute follicular graft-vs-host reaction: a distinct clinicopathological presentation. Arch Dermatol 1988;124:688-691.

7. Sale GE, Shulman HM, McDonald GB, Thomas ED: Gastrointestinal graft-versus-host disease in man. A clinicopathological study of the rectal biopsy. Am J Surg Pathol 1979;3:291-299.

8. Snover DC: Acute and chronic graft versus host disease: histopathological evidence for two pathogenetic mechanisms. Hum Pathol 1984;15:202-205.

9. Meisel JL, Bergman D, Graney D, Saunders DR, Rubin CE: Human rectal mucosa. Proctoscopic and morphological changes caused by laxatives. Gastroenterology 1977;72:1274-1279.

10. Snover DC: Mucosal damage stimulating acute graft-versus-host reaction in cytomegalovirus colitis. Transplantation 1985;39:669-670.

11. Snover DC, Filipovich AH, Ramsay NKC, Weisdorf SA, Kersey JH: Graft-versus-host-disease-like histopathologic findings in pre-bone marrow transplantation biopsies of patients with severe T-cell deficiency. Transplantation 1985;35:95-97.

12. Shulman HM, McDonald GB, Matthews D, Doney KC, Kopecky KJ, Gauvreau JM, Thomas ED: An analysis of hepatic venocclusive disease and centrilobular hepatic degeneration following bone marrow transplantation. Gastroenterology 1980;79:1178-1191.

13. Beschorner WE, Pino J, Boitnott JK, Tutschka PJ, Santos GW: Pathology of the liver with bone marrow transplantation. Effects of busulfan, carmustine, acute graft-vs-host disease and cytomegalovirus. Am J Pathol 1980;99:369-385.

14. McDonald GB, Sharma P, Matthews DE, Shulman HM, Thomas ED: Venocclusive disease of the liver after bone marrow transplantation: diagnosis, incidence and predisposing factors. Hepatology 1984;4:116-122.

15. Snover DC, Weisdorf SA, Bloomer J, McGlave P, Weisdorf D: Nodular regenerative hyperplasia: a possible cause of liver disease following bone marrow transplantation. Hepatology 1989;9:443-448.

16. Snover DC, Weisdorf SA, Ramsay NKC, McGlave P, Kersey JH: Hepatic graft versus host disease: a study of the predictive value of liver biopsy in diagnosis. Hepatology 1984;4:123-130.

17. Shulman HM, Sharma P, Amos D, Fenster LF, McDonald GB: A coded histologic study of hepatic graft-versus-host disease after human bone marrow transplantation. Hepatology 1988;8:463-470.

18. Snover DC, Freese DK, Sharp HL, Bloomer JR, Najarian JS, Ascher NL: Liver allograft rejection: an analysis of the use of biopsy in determining outcome of rejection. Am J Surg Pathol 1987;11:1-10.

19. Lerner KG, Kao GF, Storb R, Buckner CD, Clift RA, Thomas ED: Histopathology of graft-vs.-host reaction (GvHR) in human recipients of marrow from HL-A-matched sibling donors. Transplant Proc 1974;6:367-371.

20. Beschorner WE, Saral R, Hutchins GM, Tutschka PJ, Santos GW: Lymphocytic bronchitis associated with graft-vs-host disease in recipients of bone marrow transplants. N Engl J Med 1978;299:1030-1036.

21. Hackman RC and Sale GE: Large airway inflammation as possible manifestation of a pulmonary graft-versus-host reaction. Lab Invest 1981;44:26A.

22. Slavin RE and Woodruff JM: The pathology of bone marrow transplantation. Pathol Annu 1974;9:291-344.

23. Buja LM, Ferrans VJ, Graw RG: Cardiac pathologic findings in patients treated with bone marrow transplantation. Hum Pathol 1976;7:17-45.

18

Rationale and Influence of Cyclosporin A Donor Pretreatment

Peter Jacobs
University of Cape Town Leukaemia Centre and
Groote Schuur Hospital
Cape Town, Republic of South Africa

I. INTRODUCTION

Allogeneic bone marrow transplantation is the preferred form of treatment for aplastic anemia (1), lethal immunodeficiency and storage diseases (2), as well as acute (3,4) and chronic granulocytic leukemia (5). The initial, and often less than critical, enthusiasm for this procedure has been tempered by recognizing that substantial morbidity and mortality occur, with much of this attributable to GVHD. Paradoxically, since this latter unique immunologic entity may be associated with a beneficial antileukemic effect (6), attempts are being made to define its direct role, segregate associated but distinct mononuclear cell mechanisms, and then to harness and direct the way in which the specific effect or mechanism can be employed. Selective removal or functional impairment of subpopulations within the lymphocyte and monocyte fraction contained in the graft may vary cytolytic destruction of the skin, gastrointestinal tract, and biliary endothelium, while concurrently favoring the emergence of tolerance and varying degrees of immunologic reconstitution.

The basis for understanding these problems resides in a sequence of events that was recognized and described more than 30 years ago as the graft-vs.-host reaction (GVHR) (7-9), in which three essential components have been delineated. First, the host must be incapable of rejecting the foreign bone marrow; second, a degree of histoincompatibility must exist between donor and recipient; and third, the infused graft must be immunologically competent and contain T lymphocytes. There is evidence that the effects of T lymphocytes are mediated by cytokines (10-14), and conceivably GVHD can serve as a model for autoimmune diseases (15-17).

In the context of bone marrow transplantation, each of the three steps mediating GVHR is amenable to manipulation.

First, there is little difficulty in achieving a high percentage of graft acceptance. Generally transplant recipients are prepared by immunosuppressive chemotherapy alone or in combination with irradiation. Cyclosporin A, especially if used in combination with methotrexate, may have a graft-facilitating effect (18).

Second, absolute histocompatibility between donor and recipient should theoretically preclude the development of GVHD. However, and apparently in defiance of classical transplantation dogma, this entity may follow syngeneic (19) or autologous grafting (20). One explanation is that the conditioning regimens to which the recipient is exposed may bring about an imbalance between autoreactive lymphocytes and suppressor cells, and studies from humans and rodents support this concept (12). Among HLA-identical allogeneic transplant recipients, 30% to 50% develop GVHD (21).

Third, the composition of the graft can be modified to facilitate hematopoietic reconstitution and simultaneously to modulate the mononuclear cells mediating the immune response. This can be achieved in two different ways. Effector cells may be quantitatively impaired by ex vivo purging with a single monoclonal antibody, such as Campath-1 (22) or a cocktail (23), both of which may be directed against a relatively wide range of cells. Conversely, it may be more rational to select biological reagents that selectively remove the helper-inducer as opposed to the helper-suppressor subsets (24,25). However, there may be retarded immunologic recovery, leaving recipients susceptible to infection or recurrence of neoplastic disease (26). Accordingly, it is attractive to consider the alternative approach in which the entire spectrum of mononuclear cells in the graft is infused, but a qualitative or functional lesion is produced, the intensity of which can be titrated to damp down the emergence of GVHD, permitting the development of tolerance. One agent that can potentially function in this way is cyclosporin A. In bone marrow transplantation it has been employed with relatively limited success as the sole postgraft means of treating the recipient. Virtually no data are available on ex vivo incubation with the collected marrow. Alternatively, it can be used to pretreat the donor and the recipient, with subsequent reduction in dose to achieve the desired effect in the latter.

The present studies were aimed at establishing the feasibility of the latter approach in preventing acute GVHD and, concurrently, to document any risk to the donor of short-term exposure to this agent.

II. CYCLOSPORIN A

Cyclosporin A was discovered in early 1972 in the Research Laboratories of Sandoz Ltd in Basel. It is a hydrophobic cyclic peptide consisting of 11 amino acids with a molecular weight of 1203. The active compound is a fungal metabolite derived from cultures of *Cylindrocarpon lucidum* or *Trichoderma polysporum* (27). This agent has recently been extensively reviewed (28,29).

Available evidence localizes the action of cyclosporin A to the inductive phase of response in the immunocompetent cells as they encounter antigenic challenge. Cell division, by way of contrast, does not appear to be affected and, furthermore, no lymphocytotoxic effects are demonstrable. The reduction of lymphoblast numbers, which may be striking in vitro, probably reflects prevention of stimulation rather than elimination of blast cells by cytolytic mechanisms (30). Expressed in another way, the primary effect of this agent is directed against the earliest cellular events in the lymphocyte that follow mitogenic stimulation and finds expression by preventing transformation into the blast cell.

Cyclosporin A does not in all models lead to selective clonal deletion, but rather to the induction of a temporary suppressive state that is reversible when treatment is terminated (31,32). The availability of monoclonal antibodies may help resolve this difficulty. For example, CD4$^+$ T lymphocytes are now divisible into helper-suppressor, or CD4$^+$2H4$^+$, in contrast to helper-inducer, or CD4$^+$4B4$^+$, subpopulations (24,25).

III. EXPERIMENTAL STUDIES

A. Rabbits

New Zealand white (NZW) and R strain animals, having an average weight of 2 kg, were used throughout. They were individually housed and received an unrestricted supply of water, containing prophylactic sulphaquinoxaline sodium (Embazin, May and Baker, Dagenham, England), and a standard rabbit diet (Epol, Johannesburg) medicated with Amprolium (Merck and Company, Inc., USA). Temperature and weight were regularly charted. A full blood count and differential were carried out twice weekly. The biochemical profile was monitored regularly.

B. Radiation Technique

The rabbits were rendered aplastic by delivering 1200 cGy total body irradiation from a cobalt source placed 100 cm above the midplane of the prone but anesthetized animal. Radiation rates between 40 and 80 cGy/min were shown not to differ significantly. We have previously demonstrated (33) that uniform and irreversible aplasia is produced without unacceptable complications. Specifically, no gastrointestinal tract lesions were demonstrated. Furthermore, there was no difference between this technique and fractionating the radiotherapy, as suggested by others (34,35). In occasional animals unexplained death occurred within 24 hours after radiotherapy, ascribed to "radiation shock." In another series of experiments the alternative radiation dose rate at 8 cGy/min was examined, but this regimen was not found to be associated with less toxicity than the more rapid exposures.

In a series of controlled experiments, one or both of the femurs were shielded with lead, and in another group autologous reconstitution was undertaken to monitor both optimal rates of hematopoietic recovery and isolate possible complications of the radiotherapy and transplantation procedure itself.

C. Allogeneic Bone Marrow Transplantation

Thirty-six hours after completing lethal whole body irradiation, the animals underwent allogeneic bone marrow transplantation. Between 2 and 4 X 10^8 nucleated cells per kilogram were infused from R females into NZW males. Standard mixed lymphocyte cultures (36) to demonstrate nonidentity at the major histocompatibility complex were not uniformly successful. However, using a modified technique (37), antigenic disparity was demonstrated between the two strains; this was most striking when mitomycin-treated lymphocytes derived from the mesenteric lymph node were used as antigen and appendiceal lymphocytes as responding or target cells. Results at day 3 gave stimulation indices between 3.5 and 13.9. Even the latter technique does not produce absolutely uniform results, and we have subsequently demonstrated that mixed lymphocyte reaction, with minor modifications, can reliably predict histoincompatibility (Jacobs and Paulsen, unpublished).

D. Cyclosporin A Administration

Rabbits were given 10 mg/kg daily of cyclosporin A by intramuscular injection for 28 days following transplantation. Plasma levels were monitored by high-pressure liquid chromatography.

E. Results

1. Radiation Controls

Irradiated animals developed increasing pancytopenia, with platelet and granulocyte counts reaching their nadir between days 4 and 6 (Fig. 1), and all the rabbits died. Median survival (Fig. 2) was 6.8 days (SE ± 0.08; range 2-11 days).

Autopsy studies at intervals showed rapidly decreasing bone marrow cellularity, and death was uniformly due to infection, with widespread colonies of bacteria present in all organs. Minimal associated hemorrhage was present in the gastrointestinal tract of occasional rabbits. There was profound loss of lymphoid tissue throughout the gut, thymus and spleen (38).

2. Femoral Shielding and Autograft Rescue

In animals having one or both femora shielded, reduction in white cell and platelet counts were comparable to those observed in radiation controls, but peripheral values returned rapidly to reach normal by day 21 (Fig. 1). The bone marrow, when studied serially, showed clonal regeneration of the previously aplastic medullary spaces, and histology was normal by day 30.

In the autografted animals who received 2-4 X 10^8 nucleated cells/kg, peripheral blood values were indistinguishable from those observed with femoral shielding (Fig. 1). Median survival (Fig. 2) was not reached at any time during this study, and only an occasional death occurred.

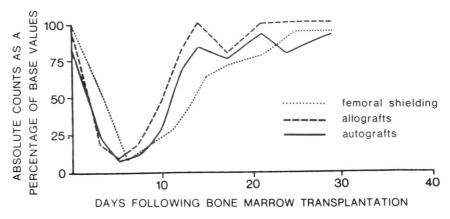

Figure 1 Peripheral blood granulocyte and platelet count. The fall in circulating levels and their subsequent return to normal is not statistically different in the three groups of animals. Data are expressed as a percentage of mean basal values and plotted against elapsed time in days. (Reproduced with permission of the Editors and Publishers of Experimental Hematology Today 1981, S. Karger AG, Basel.)

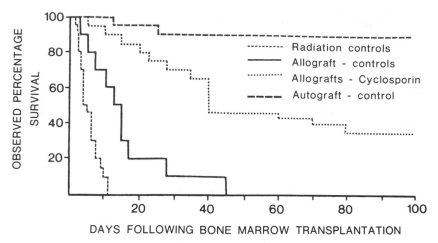

Figure 2 Observed survival in rabbit experimental studies. The median survival for irradiated controls was 6.8 days. Following allogeneic bone marrow transplantation without immunosuppressive agents, survival was 15 days and none were alive at 100 days, whereas in allografted animals receiving cyclosporin A, median survival was 40 days and 33% were alive and well at 100 days. The incidence of histologically proven GVHD in the allografted controls was 80% and in the cyclosporin A-treated animal this was below 25%. (Reproduced with permission of the Editors and Publishers of Experimental Hematology Today 1981, S. Karger AG, Basel.)

Anemia aggravated by repeated blood sampling was prevented by the use of microtechniques. In these animals, as opposed to radiation controls, daily oral prophylaxis with 10 ml trimethoprim combined with 50 mg sulphamethoxazole decreased deaths from infectious episodes and is routine practice in the animal transplantation program.

3. Allogeneic Bone Marrow Transplantation

In the allograft controls 2-4 X 10^8 nucleated cells/kg resulted in granulocyte and platelet reconstitution patterns in the peripheral blood that was comparable to that demonstrated by animals undergoing radiation with femoral shielding or after autografting (Fig. 1). The same findings were present with bone marrow on serial histologic studies.

Since the study was designed to examine the effect of cyclosporin A on the incidence and severity of GVHD, the rare animal dying before engraftment could be demonstrated was excluded from analysis.

The clinical findings in the allografted recipients were dramatically different from those in the autograft controls. Gross weight loss was the striking feature, and at day 40 respective values were 0.8 and 2.8 kg. There was, in addition, patchy but characteristic extensive hair loss. Diarrhea was a variable feature, with cultures generally being negative.

Survival of control animals (Fig. 2) was 10% at day 40 and 0% at day 100. The cause of death was typically infection in the respiratory tract, with nasal discharge of pus. Pneumonia was often present, with widespread destructive abscess formation being a feature. Histology of the skin, gastrointestinal tract, and liver were diagnostic of GVHD. In the skin, aggressor lymphocytes were present in the epidermis, and spongiosis was prominent, particularly at the dermoepidermal junction. In the gastrointestinal tract loss of glands and patchy to total mucosal denudation were most striking in the small bowel. The liver showed infiltration of lymphocytes, loss of the limiting plate and destruction of bile ducts by lymphocytes. Generalized lymphoid atrophy was evident in the spleen, lymph nodes, and thymus. These features were similar to those reported both in man (39) and in experimental animals.

4. Cyclosporin A-Treated Recipients

Two striking features were evident in these animals. First, they were uniformly in superior clinical condition, with weights not significantly different from autograft control animals. Hair distribution was normal and diarrhea was not present. The second was the markedly different survival rate between allografted controls and rabbits receiving cyclosporin A after bone marrow transplantation (Fig. 2). At day 40 10% of the allograft controls were alive compared to 44% of those receiving cyclosporin A. This difference was even more obvious at 100 days, when none of the controls survived but 33% of those that had been treated were alive and well, with normally functioning donor grafts.

Of particular note was the fact that the histologically recognizable features of GVHD, which characterized the allografted control animals, were present in only 25% of animals receiving cyclosporin A. Furthermore, in the latter group death due to typical GVHD was unusual and was often attributable to an incidental cause, such as perforated gastric ulcer. However, infection did occur and was most commonly due to bronchopneumonia and septicemia; it is presently not clear whether the latter may be unusual expressions of GVHD modified by cyclosporin A therapy.

5. Cyclosporin A Pretreatment of Donors and Recipients

In experiments where donors were pretreated for 7 days with cyclosporin A and the recipients continued to receive this agent for 28 days after transplantation, the survival curves (not shown in Fig. 2) were not statistically different from those where only the recipients were treated. Furthermore, examination of the tissues in this group and cause of death were also similar to the cyclosporin A-treated recipients.

F. Comments

Three points are relevant. First, in the cyclosporin A-treated allograft recipients, the death rate appeared to accelerate after day 28 when this agent was discontinued. It, therefore, remains possible that longer periods of drug administration are necessary. These findings are entirely compatible with the suggestion that the action of this unique immunosuppressive agent is not to produce lasting tolerance produced by selective clonal deletion, but is a transient phenomenon related to the presence of critical concentrations in the body (31,32). Furthermore, there are interesting parallels between this observation and those reported in a human transplantation study (40,41).

Second, in contrast to experience reported with a similar model (Speck, personal communication, 1980) biochemical disturbances or other gross toxicity attributable to the cyclosporin A were not found.

Third, and perhaps in partial explanation for the lack of major side effects in our animals, was the absence of significant concentrations of this agent in the plasma when examined by high pressure liquid chromatography. It remains possible, therefore, that the dosage administered may have been inadequate or the batch used had less biological activity than we had anticipated. This query is the subject of further study. Nevertheless, it can be concluded that there is an unequivocal and marked reduction in acute

GVHD and that striking prolongation in survival can be achieved with plasma concentration of cyclosporin A that may be lower or less critical than published evidence would suggest. Indeed, it remains to be proven that plasma levels are the most valid reflection for the immunosuppressive properties of this agent and concentration in cellular compartments or control by functional assays, such as mitogen response, may be more appropriate. Nevertheless, the measurements are clearly the best means currently available for monitoring patient compliance and drug absorption, and, therefore, to anticipate the development of toxicity.

IV. CLINICAL STUDIES

Difficulties exist in the prevention (42,43) or abrogation of GVHD (44,45), and while cyclosporin A is beneficial in a number of transplant situations (46), including marrow grafting (41,47), it is less than totally effective and appears approximately equivalent to methotrexate (48). It does not appear that the incidence or severity of the acute syndrome, with its high morbidity and mortality, or that of the chronic variant, with its relentless progression and mutilating side effects, can be eradicated with this agent alone. These observations raise the question that at least the acute disease might reflect transfer of immunocompetent lymphocytes with the graft and that such a situation might, theoretically at least, be amenable to donor pretreatment. In view of the limited side effects observed in animals and while recognizing that any responses in man may be different, it seemed appropriate to examine additional donor pretreatment with cyclosporin A in a clinical bone marrow transplantation program.

A. Materials and Methods

Fifty-one patients underwent allografting on a program approved by the Ethics and Research Committee of the University of Cape Town and Groote Schuur Hospital. Donors and recipients were fully informed and their participation required signed consent.

Initially, patients with refractory acute leukemia were offered the procedure but subsequently only those in consolidated complete remission or having severe acute aplastic anemia were considered eligible. Sibling donors compatible at the major histocompatibility complex and nonreactive with their recipients in the mixed lymphocyte culture were used.

Severe acute aplastic anemia was defined according to internationally accepted criteria (49) and patients were conditioned with 50 mg/kg of cyclophosphamide by intravenous injection on four consecutive days before transplantation (50). The patients with acute leukemia were treated with a combination of etoposide, cytosine arabinoside, and doxorubicin (51), after which they were conditioned with cyclophosphamide, 60 mg/kg on 2 consecutive days, and 1000 rads total body irradiation at a maximum exposure rate of 7 rad/min given 24 hours after the last dose of conditioning drug. All patients were managed in reverse isolation, and received hyperalimentation and such antibiotic and transfusion support as was appropriate.

Three different immunosuppressive regimens were evaluated in the course of this study (52). In group 1 (n = 23) cyclosporin A was not available, and following transplantation patients received only methotrexate (50). In group 2 (n = 8) cyclosporin A was commenced the day before infusion of the graft at an oral dose of 12.5 mg/kg twice a day for a week and then 6.25 mg/kg twice daily for the next week, after which adjustments were made to maintain plasma concentrations between 250 and 500 ng/mL by radioimmunoassay (53) at least once a week for the entire duration that patients received this immunosuppressive drug. In group 3 (n = 20) both donor and recipient commenced cyclosporin A on the same dosage schedule 2 weeks before transplantation; patients remained on this agent for the same duration as those in group 2. At all times, plasma concentrations were monitored and doses adjusted at least once every week to maintain levels in the same therapeutic range as in group 2.

Biochemical measurements of renal and hepatic function, as well as electrolyte status and acid-base balance, were measured on alternate days in donors and recipients. Any increase in creatinine or urea values, even while still in the normal range, was managed by small doses of oral furosemide, and failure to immediately reverse this trend required reduction in cyclosporin A dosage. In the donors, as well as in the recipients, these measurements were continued on an outpatient basis.

Acute (50) and chronic (54) GVHD were defined according to established criteria. Both syndromes were treated by continued administration of cyclosporin A; in the acute disease methylprednisolone was added; in the chronic form additional high-dose pulsed methylprednisolone (45) was initially used, followed by long-term corticosteroids and azathioprine. The dose of the two drugs was variable and started at 0.5 mg/kg and 2 mg/kg of lean body mass, respectively. Methylprednisolone was gradually reduced, whereas the dose of azathioprine remained constant; the efficacy of this two-drug combination on the clinical course of the chronic GVHD was constantly reviewed; average duration was generally in excess of 9 months.

B. Results

1. Methotrexate-Treated Patients

As shown in Table 1, these patients (group 1; n= 23) were treated with methotrexate for immunosuppression (50). Ten of the 23 patients (43%) developed classical severe acute GVHD within 6 weeks of transplantation, which was refractory to therapy and caused

Table 1 Incidence of Graft-vs.-Host Disease

Group	Graft-vs.-Host Disease		
	Acute	Acute, progressing to chronic	De novo chronic
1 (n = 23)	10	3	2
2 (n = 8)	2	0	3
3 (n = 20)	6	0	2

Group 1: posttransplant methotrexate only. Group 2: posttransplant cyclosporin A only. Group 3: donor and recipient cyclosporin A pretreatment and this agent continued after grafting in the recipient.

The incidence of acute GVHD was 43, 25, and 30%, respectively; $p > 0.05$.

Source: Reproduced with permission of the Editors and Publishers of the Scandanavian Journal of Haematology, Munksgaard International Publishers Ltd., Copenhagen, Denmark.

death in six patients. Of the remaining four patients one died of Budd-Chiari syndrome, which may have been related to the long period of prior intensive chemotherapy, and three progressed to chronic GVHD, of whom one is alive with disfiguring cutaneous lesions, one died from disseminated tuberculosis without evidence of GVHD, and the other died following a seizure but with severe skin lesions of GVHD; autopsy failed to reveal the cause of death.

Chronic GVHD arose de novo, that is, without any prior acute disease, in two patients (9%) and has been self-limiting in both.

2. Cyclosporin A-Treated Patients

These patients (group 2; n = 8) received cyclosporin A immunosuppression without donor pretreatment. Severe acute GVHD occurred in two patients (25%) and in both responded promptly to additional corticosteroids. One patient died from leukemic relapse and the second from a ruptured cerebral aneurysm.

Chronic GVHD without an antecedent acute episode occurred in three patients (38%). One died from disseminated fungal infection with poorly controlled cutaneous grade I GVHD. The other two developed minimal but characteristic skin lesions 3 months after discontinuing cyclosporin A. Both have responded to restarting cyclosporin A in conjunction with a single course of pulsed high-dose methylprednisolone.

3. Cyclosporin A-Treated Patients and Donors

These patients (group 3; n = 20) and their donors were pretreated with cyclosporin A for 2 weeks before transplantation. Six patients developed early GVHD (30%). In two this was mild and responded promptly and completely to corticosteroid therapy; one patient subsequently died from massive gastrointestinal tract hemorrhage and the second patient is currently well. In the other four patients the disease was also mild, being defined as grade I cutaneous changes, diarrhea less than 500 mL in 24 hours and without abnormality on liver biopsy. However, in none of these patients could this clinical syndrome be reversed on therapy and all died within 3 months—three from infection and one from massive hemorrhage from a duodenal ulcer.

4. Engraftment

Engraftment is defined as the time taken from transplantation to reach granulocyte counts of 0.5×10^9/L or a platelet count of 25×10^9/L. These findings were substantiated by a bone marrow aspiration and trephine biopsy, which showed greater than 15% of hematopoietic cell repopulation. The median time to achieve these criteria for the three groups was 21 days (range 9-26), 14 days (range 6-33), and 13 days (range 7-16), respectively.

Actuarially predicted survival curves (Fig. 3) show little difference for median survival, with a nonsignificantly higher plateau for patients in group 3.

5. Toxicity

In none of the donors did biochemical tests of renal function rise outside the normal range during the 2-week period of cyclosporin A administration. The donors were all fully reassessed, including biochemical measurements, before discharge and again within 1 month after discontinuing cyclosporin A therapy. Furthermore, in a separate series of individuals with severe acute aplastic anemia without a transplant option (55), cyclosporin A was used as the primary form of immunosuppression either singly or in combination with antilymphocyte globulin; in 12 individuals monthly follow-up for an average period

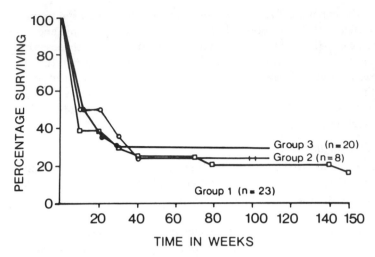

Figure 3 Survival of bone marrow transplantation patients. Actuarially predicted survival curves showed no significant difference between patients receiving methotrexate alone (group 1; n = 23), those in which recipients only received cyclosporin A (group 2; n = 8), and where donors and recipients received cyclosporin A pretreatment and the recipients, in the posttransplant period, continued with the same agent (group 3; n = 20). (Reproduced with permission of the Editors and Publishers of The Scandinavian Journal of Haematology, Munksgaard International Publishers Ltd, Copenhagen, Denmark.)

in excess of 9 months showed no late disturbances in biochemical tests of renal or hepatic function.

In recipients receiving cyclosporin A, transient elevation of blood urea and creatinine was seen in 50% of the patients in groups 2 and 3. Any increment in these biochemical measurements, despite their remaining within the normal range, was managed by treating the patient with 20-40 mg furosemide daily or twice a day. Failure to immediately reverse the trend required reduction in the dose of cyclosporin A being given. No examples of progressive deterioration or irreversible dysfunction were observed using this approach.

C. Comments

From these preliminary studies only three observations can be made. First, these overall results from bone marrow transplantation are less satisfactory than reported by others and those currently being achieved in our own program. This reflects the referral of patients during the early years of this program at a time when their clinical condition was poor, and, therefore, at least in those with aplastic anemia, extensive prior transfusions may have further compromised the outcome.

Second, and based on these results, it appears as though the administration of cyclosporin A to the recipients alone reduced the incidence of acute GVHD and improved the response to its management when additional methylprednisolone was required.

Third, the additional pretreatment of the donor, albeit the number of patients transplanted was small, had the further benefit of reducing the severity of clinical manifestations.

In both of the latter two groups, and particularly where donors were pretreated, it is noteworthy that meticulous monitoring of plasma levels and prompt management of changing hepatic biochemistry made it possible to use this agent without unacceptable morbidity.

Finally, in the clinical context, no beneficial effect from either cyclosporin A regimens could be demonstrated on de novo chronic GVHD.

V. SUMMARY AND CONCLUSIONS

The use of bone marrow transplantation in clinical practice is rapidly increasing. It is the preferred method of treatment in some instances and in others forms an integral part of current management programs, particularly in hematologic malignancies. A major deterrent to allografting is the morbidity and mortality associated with acute and chronic GVHD. The approach to this problem is not uniform. In patients with aplastic anemia, the objective is to eliminate this entity completely. Conversely, and perhaps paradoxically, in patients with leukemia there may be a need to retain a controlled level of GVHD in order to harness an associated and beneficial immunologic effect on preventing relapse (56). If this is to be achieved successfully, then a greater understanding of the various components of acute and chronic GVHD are needed so that these can be manipulated to selectively enhance those that lead to immunologic destruction of residual tumor cells and suppress cytotoxic processes that cause unwanted destruction of normal tissue. However, there remains controversy as to the relative contributions from cellular populations that directly mediate one or other events, in contrast to humoral mechanisms that reflects monocyte or lymphocyte activation. Indeed, it is not only possible but likely that both arms of the immune response mechanism may be acting in concert.

There are a number of new and novel approaches currently being examined that include the exposure of the graft to ultraviolet irradiation (57,58), selective depletion of a wide variety of cells with monoclonal antibodies having differing specificities, or variation in the posttransplant immunosuppressive regimens. Each of these have met with differing degrees of success, but none have uniformly led to the control of GVHD. In the quest for alternative regimens with less cytotoxic effects, cyclosporin A has been extensively studied. Although the induction of a qualitative lesion in T-helper lymphocytes was demonstrated in vitro and while initial in vivo studies were encouraging, frustratingly, much of the early promise has not been fulfilled. On the theoretical basis that the acute syndrome may be amenable to better control with longer periods of effector cell exposure to this unique biologic agent, donor pretreatment followed by the administration of cyclosporin A to the recipient was examined in both an experimental rabbit model and a clinical bone marrow transplantation program. The results of the former studies showed no clear-cut benefit over its administration to the recipient alone. In contrast, clinical studies, while limited by the historical nature of the trial design and the small number of patients entered, provided some evidence for a decrease in the incidence and severity with donor pretreatment which could be achieved without demonstrable morbidity.

It might reasonably be concluded, at a time when all possible means are being explored for the control of GVHD (59), that this schedule justifies further study. It can be hypothesized that manipulation of exposure time and titration of dosage would lend flexibility to modulating the acute and chronic forms of this unique phenomenon. Thus, additional donor pretreatment may have a role in retaining the beneficial antileukemic effects whilst concurrently preventing untoward damage to other organ systems in the recipient. Furthermore, with programs being rapidly expanded to include the use of mismatched siblings or phenotypically identical but unrelated donors, it also offers a wider choice in suppressing some of the very early events in the acute syndrome.

ACKNOWLEDGMENTS

We thank Dr. P. Hartman Stahelin and Professor Jean Borel for HPLC determination of cyclosporin A and Jackie Davies for help with preparation and typing of the manuscript. Some of these experimental and clinical studies have been previously reported and are reproduced in part with permission of the Editors and Publishers of The Scandinavian Journal of Haematology (1985;35:386-393, Munksgaard International Publishers, Ltd, Copenhagen, Denmark) and Experimental Hematology Today 1981 (pp. 37-96, S. Karger AG, Basel).

REFERENCES

1. Storb R, Thomas ED, Buckner CD, Appelbaum FR, Clift RA, Deeg HJ, Doney K, Hansen JA, Prentice RL, Sanders JE, Stewart P, Sullivan KM, Witherspoon RP: Marrow transplantation for aplastic anemia. Semin Hematol 1984;21:27-35.
2. Krivit W, Lipton ME, Lockman LA, Tsai M, Dyck PJ, Smith S, Ramsay NKC, Kersey J: Prevention of deterioration in metachromatic leukodystrophy by bone marrow transplantation. Am J Med Sci 1987;294:80-85.
3. Dinsmore R, Kirkpatrick D, Flomenberg N, Gulati S, Kapoor N, Brochstein J, Shank B, Reid A, Groshen S, O'Reilly RJ: Allogeneic bone marrow transplantation for patients with acute nonlymphocytic leukemia. Blood 1984;63:649-656.
4. Barrett AJ, Kendra JR, Lucas CF, Joss DV, Joshi R, Desai M, Jones KH, Phillips RH, Rogers TR, Tabara Z, Williamson S, Hobbs JR: Bone marrow transplantation for acute lymphoblastic leukaemia. Br J Haematol 1982;52:181-188.
5. Goldman JM, Gale RP, Horowitz MM, Biggs, JC, Champlin RE, Gluckman E, Hoffman RG, Jacobsen SJ, Marmont AA, McGlave PB, Messner HA, Rimm AA, Rozman C, Speck B, Tura S, Weiner RS, Bortin MM: Bone marrow transplantation for chronic myelogenous leukemia in chronic phase. Ann Intern Med 1988;108:806-814.
6. Weiden PL, Flournoy N, Thomas ED, Prentice R, Fefer A, Buckner CD, Storb R: Antileukemic effect of graft-versus-host disease in human recipients of allogeneic-marrow grafts. N Engl J Med 1979;300:1068-1073.
7. Simonsen M: The impact on the developing embryo and newborn animal of adult homologous cells. Acta Path Microbiol Scand 1957;40:480-500.
8. Billingham RE: The biology of graft-versus-host reactions. Harvey Lectures 1967; 89:621-635.
9. Seemayer TA, Gartner JG, Lapp WS: The graft-versus-host reaction. Hum Pathol 1983;14:3-5.
10 Piguet P-F, Grau GE, Allet B, Vassalli P: Tumor necrosis factor/cachectin is an effector of skin and gut lesions of the acute phase of graft-vs.-host disease. J Exp Med 1987;166:1280-1289.
11. Niederwieser D, Troppmaier J, Adolph G, Margreiter R, Huber C: Role of lymphokines in the induction of graft-versus-host disease. Exp Hematol 1985;13:131-132.
12. Parkman R: Clonal analysis of murine graft-vs-host disease. I. Phenotypic and functional analysis of T lymphocyte clones. J Immunol 1986;136:3543-3548.
13. Parkman R: Cyclosporine: GVHD and beyond. N Engl J Med 1988;319:110-111.

14. Weiss A, Imboden J, Hardy K, Manger B, Terhorst C, Stobo J: The role of the T3/ antigen receptor complex in T-cell activation. Ann Rev Immunol 1986;4:593-619.
15. Deeg HJ: The biology of chronic graft-versus-host disease. Exp Hematol 1985;13: 128-130.
16. Gale RP: Graft-versus-host disease. Immunol Rev 1985;88:193-214.
17. Barrett AJ: Graft-versus-host disease: A review. J Roy Soc Med 1987;80:368-373.
18. Storb R, Deeg HJ, Whitehead J, Appelbaum F, Beatty P, Bensinger W, Buckner CD, Clift R, Doney K, Farewell V, Hansen J, Hill R, Lum L, Martin P, McGuffin R, Sanders J, Stewart P, Sullivan K, Witherspoon R, Yee G, Thomas ED: Methotrexate and cyclosporine compared with cyclosporine alone for prophylaxis of acute graft versus host disease after marrow transplantation for leukemia. N Engl J Med 1986; 314:729-735.
19. Rappeport J, Mihm M, Reinherz E, Lopansri S, Parkman R: Acute graft-versus-host disease in recipients of bone-marrow transplants from identical twin donors. Lancet 1979; ii:717-720.
20. Hood AF, Vogelsang GB, Black LP, Farmer ER, Santos GW: Acute graft-vs-host disease. Arch Dermatol 1987;123:745-750.
21. Sullivan KM: Acute and chronic graft-versus-host disease in man. Int J Cell Cloning 1986;4:41-93.
22. Hale G, Cobbold S, Waldmann H: T cell depletion with CAMPATH-1 in allogeneic bone marrow transplantation. Transplantation 1988;45:753-759.
23. Autran B, Beaujean F, Pillier C, Kuentz M, Leblond V, Debre P, Bernard A, Binet JL, Duedari N, Vernant JP: T-cell depletion of bone marrow transplants: assessment of standard immunological methods of quantification. Exp Hematol 1987;15:1121-1127.
24. Morimoto B, Letvin NL, Distaso JA, Aldrich WR, Schlossman SF: The isolation and characterization of the human suppressor inducer T cell subset. J Immunol 1985; 134:1508-1515.
25. Morimoto C, Letvin NL, Boyd AW, Hagan M, Brown HM, Kornacki MM, Schlossman SF: The isolation and characterization of the human helper inducer T cell subset. J Immunol 1985;134:3762-3769.
26. Daley JP, Rozans MK, Smith BR, Burakoff SJ, Rappeport JM, Miller RA: Retarded recovery of functional T cell frequencies in T cell-depleted bone marrow transplant recipients. Blood 1987;70:960-964.
27. Borel JF, Feurer C, Gubler HU, Stahelin H: Biological effects of cyclosporin A: a new antilymphocytic agent. Agents and Actions 1976;6:468-475.
28. Jacobs P: Cyclosporin A. Current status, including the Cape Town experience. In *Immune Modulation Agents and Their Mechanisms*, edited by Fenichel RL, Chirigos MA. Marcel Dekker, Inc., New York, 1984;pp. 191-228.
29. Jacobs P, Novitzky N: Cyclosporin A in clinical perspective. In *Handbook of Immunotherapeutic Agents*, edited by Renoux G. Marcel Dekker, Inc., New York, in press.
30. Borel JF: Essentials of cyclosporin A. A novel type of antilymphocyte agent. TIPS 1980;2:146-149.
31. Leoni P, Garcia RC, Allison AC: Effects of cyclosporin A on human lymphocytes in culture. J Clin Lab Immunol 1978;1:67-72.
32. White DJG, Plumb AM, Pawelec G, Brons G: Cyclosporin A: An immunosuppressive agent preferentially active against proliferating T cells. Transplantation 1979; 27:55-58.
33. Parker JR, Taylor SP, Manuel G, Jacobs P: Bone marrow reconstitution using a block grafting technique. S Afr Med J 1976;50:577-579.
34. Piomelli S, Brooke MS: Studies on homologous bone marrow transplantation in irradiated rabbits. Blood 1961;17:579-596.

35. Porter KA, Murray JE: Long-term study of X-irradiated rabbits with bone-marrow homotransplants. J Nat Cancer Inst 1958;20:189-205.
36. Lancki DW, Tissot TG, Cohen C: Histocompatibility in the rabbit. Genetic control of rabbit mixed leukocyte culture reactivity. Transplantation 1979;27:79-86.
37. Ozer H, Jr and Waksman BH: The response of rabbit lymphocytes to mitogens and alloantigens: evidence for T cell heterogeneity. J Immunol 1974;113:1780-1792.
38. Jacobs P: Effect of cyclosporin A on the incidence of graft-versus-host disease (GVHD) and survival of rabbits following allogeneic bone marrow transplantation. In *Experimental Hematology Today 1981*, edited by Baum SJ, Ledney GD, Khan A. S. Karger, Basel, 1981; pp. 37-96.
39. Glucksberg H, Storb R, Fefer A, Buckner CD, Neiman PE, Clift RA, Lerner KG, Thomas ED: Clinical manifestations of graft-versus-host disease in human recipients of marrow from HLA-matched sibling donors. Tranplantation 1974;18:295-304.
40. Powles RL, Barrett AJ, Clink H, Kay HEM, Sloane J, McElwain TJ: Cyclosporin A for the treatment of graft-versus-host disease in man. Lancet 1978;2:1327-1331.
41. Powles RL, Clink HM, Spence D, Morgenstern G, Watson JG, Selby PJ, Woods M, Barrett A, Jameson B, Sloane J, Lawler SD, Kay HEM, Lawson D, McElwain TJ, Alexander P: Cyclosporin A to prevent graft-versus-host disease in man after allogeneic bone-marrow transplantation. Lancet 1980; i:327-329.
42. Editorial. Preventing graft-versus-host disease. Lancet 1980; ii:1343-1344.
43. Simonsen M: Induction and avoidance of graft-versus-host reactions: A review. J Roy Soc Med 1981;74:901-903.
44. Sullivan KM, Shulman HM, Storb R, Weiden PL, Witherspoon RP, McDonald GB, Schubert MM, Atkinson K, Thomas ED: Chronic graft-versus-host disease in 52 patients; adverse natural course and successful treatment with combination immunosuppression. Blood 1981;57:267-276.
45. Kendra J, Barrett AJ, Lucas C, Joshi R, Joss V, Desai M, Halil O, Rogers TR, Hobbs JR, Hugh-Jones K: Response of graft versus host disease to high doses of methyl prednisolone. Clin Lab Haemat 1981;3:19-26.
46. Morris PJ: Cyclosporin A. Transplantation 1981:32;349-354.
47. Barrett AJ, Kendra JR, Lucas CF, Joss DV, Joshi R, Pendharkar P, Hugh-Jones K: Cyclosporin A as prophylaxis against graft-versus-host disease in 36 patients. Br Med J 1982;285:162-166.
48. Storb R, Deeg HJ, Fisher L, Appelbaum F, Buckner CD, Bensinger W, Clift R, Doney K, Irle C, McGuffin R, Martin P, Sanders J, Schoch G, Singer J, Stewart P, Sullivan K, Witherspoon R, Thomas ED: Cyclosporine v methotrexate for graft-v-host disease prevention in patients given marrow grafts for leukemia: long-term follow-up of three controlled trials. Blood 1988;71:293-298.
49. Camitta BM, Thomas ED, Nathan DG, Santos G, Gordon-Smith EC, Gale RP, Rappeport JM, Storb R: Severe aplatic anemia: A prospective study of the effect of early marrow transplantation on acute mortality. Blood 1976;48:63-70.
50. Thomas ED, Storb R, Clift RA, Fefer A, Johnson FL, Neiman PE, Lerner KG, Glucksberg H, Buckner CD: Bone-marrow transplantation. N Engl J Med 1975;292:832-843, 895-902.
51. Dubovsky D, Kernoff L, Jacobs P: Rapid remission induction in adult acute non-lymphoblastic leukaemia. Europ J Cancer 1978;14:1179-1183.
52. Jacobs P: Cyclosporin A pretreatment of both donor and recipient undergoing allogeneic bone marrow transplantation. Scand J Haematol 1985;35:386-393.
53. Donatsch P, Abisch E, Homberger M, Traber R, Trapp M, Voges R: A radioimmunoassay to measure cyclosporin A in plasma and serum samples. J Immunoassay 1981; 2:19-32.
54. Shulman HM, Sullivan KM, Weiden PL, McDonald GB, Striker GE, Sale GE, Hackman R, Tsoi M, Storb R, Thomas ED: Chronic graft-versus-host syndrome in man.

A long-term clinicopathologic study of 20 Seattle patients. Am J Med 1980;69:204–217.

55. Jacobs P, Wood L, Martell R: Cyclosporin A in the treatment of severe acute aplastic anaemia. Br J Haematol 1985;61:267-272.

56. Kohler PC, Hank JA, Minkoff DZ, Sondel PM: Clinical adoptive chemoimmunotherapy with allogeneic alloactivated HLA-haploidentical lymphocytes: controlled induction of graft-versus-host reactions. Cancer Immunol Immunother 1988;26:74-82.

57. Ullrich SE: Suppression of graft rejection and the induction of graft-v-host disease by explsure to UV radiation. Transplantation Proc 1988;10:302-304.

58. Atkinson K, Weller P, Ryman W, Biggs J: PUVA therapy for drug-resistant graft-versus-host disease. Bone Marrow Transplantation 1986;1:227-236.

59. Bortin MM: Bone marrow transplantation in leukemia using family donors other than HLA-identical siblings: A preliminary report from the International Bone Marrow Transplant Registry. Transplantation Proc 1987;21:2629-2631.

19

T-Cell Depletion for the Prevention of Graft-vs.-Host Disease

Paul J. Martin
Fred Hutchinson Cancer Research Center
University of Washington School of Medicine
Seattle, Washington

Nancy A. Kernan
Memorial Sloan-Kettering Cancer Center
New York, New York

I. INTRODUCTION

The ability to prevent Graft-vs.-Host Disease (GVHD) by removing T cells from donor marrow has been demonstrated in numerous experimental models. Impetus for testing this approach for preventing GVHD in clinical trials came from the development of a variety of methods for selective depletion of T cells in human marrow. Data from animal models indicated that the need for posttransplant immunosuppression could be entirely circumvented by T-cell depletion. This led to the anticipation that the risks of mucositis, delayed engraftment, renal impairment, infections, and other complications could be diminished by avoiding the necessity of GVHD prophylaxis with methotrexate, cyclosporine, antithymocyte globulin, prednisone, or cyclophosphamide. It was hoped that more effective GVHD prevention would lead to improved survival.

Initially, there were few data from animal experiments to indicate that T-cell depletion could lead to complications. Early enthusiasm for this approach in man was reflected by the widespread testing in many centers. More than 800 T-cell-depleted marrow transplants were carried out worldwide during the 6-year period between 1981, when the initial reports were published, and the end of 1986 (1). Data from these studies have confirmed the expectation of decreased incidence and severity of GVHD but have also led to recognition of the problems of increased graft failure and leukemic relapse and delayed immune reconstitution. This recognition has indicated the need for greater understanding of the immunobiology of marrow transplantation, particularly in terms of the relationship between engraftment, GVHD, and immunologic control of malignant cells.

This chapter will not attempt a comprehensive review of data from clinical trials of T-cell-depleted marrow transplantation. Emphasis will be placed, instead, on providing a perspective on what has been learned from human trials. Of possibly greater importance, this chapter will help to delineate what has not been, and perhaps cannot be, learned from clinical studies. The discussion will largely be confined to results and interpretation of human studies, since other chapters in this volume are focused on animal studies.

II. METHODS OF T-CELL DEPLETION

Marrow aspirated for human transplantation typically contains on the order of 10^{10} nucleated cells (2), of which approximately 10% or 10^9 represent mature T cells, depending on the amount of blood coaspirated with marrow. Marrow obtained directly from cadaveric vertebral bodies contains 4-5-fold fewer T cells (3). Patients transplanted with unmodified marrow generally receive on the order of 10^7 T cells/kg recipient body weight. Initially it was not known how much depletion of T cells would be required in order to prevent GVHD in man, and efforts were, therefore, made to develop methods that could achieve a maximum degree of depletion without damage to hematopoietic progenitors.

Both antibody-based and physical methods have been used for depletion of T cells in human marrow. Anti-T-cell antibodies have been employed alone (4-6), together with homologous or heterologous complement (7-14), conjugated to immunotoxins (15,16), or combined with immunomagnetic beads (17). With sufficient preclinical development and testing, most antibody-based methods are capable of at least 2 log depletion of T cells. Among methods that do not rely on antibody, counterflow centrifugal elutriation (18,19) and density gradient fractionation (20) exploit physical differences to separate T cells and hematopoietic stem cells. Highly efficient removal of T cells and enrichment of hematopoietic progenitors in human marrow can be achieved by differential agglutination with soybean lectin followed by rosetting with sheep erythrocytes (21-24).

A variety of antibodies and combinations of antibodies have been used in different clinical trials. The most extensive experience worldwide has been with the rat IgM monoclonal antibody CAMPATH-1 (25), which recognizes a heterogeneous 23-30 kDa glycoprotein expressed by all lymphocytes and monocytes (26). Other trials have employed antibodies that recognize antigens with a more restricted pattern of expression specific for T cells. (See Ref. 1 for summary and Refs. 27-29 for descriptions of T-cell antigens.) These include CD2, which represents the E-rosette receptor, CD3, which is noncovalently associated with the antigen receptor of T cells, CD5, which represents the human equivalent of murine Lyt-1 (also expressed by a small subpopulation of B lymphocytes), CD6 (a 120 kDa molecule of undefined function) and CD7 (a 41 kDa molecule of undefined function). Antibodies against T-cell subset antigens such as CD4, CD8, and CD28 have also been tested either alone (30) or as components of mixtures.

Evaluation of various marrow treatment methods has required the development of suitable assays for enumerating residual T cells (31-36). E-rosetting assays can be very sensitive, but many CD2-specific antibodies interfere with rosette formation. Mitogen-stimulated proliferation measured as ^{3}H-thymidine incorporation lacks sensitivity because of the high background proliferation of marrow cells (37). Under optimal conditions, indirect immunofluorescence and flow cytometry can reliably detect T cells at levels of approximately 0.1% (32), but this method does not provide information about the functional competence of residual cells. Mitogen stimulation and short-term culture of treated marrow can improve the sensitivity of immunofluorescent methods and can provide a semiquantitative measure of the number of residual T cells (32). Limiting dilution analysis represents the assay method best able to provide a highly sensitive and quantitative measure of functional T cells remaining after marrow treatment. Limiting dilution assays to enumerate cells capable of proliferating in response to PHA and IL-2 (32-34) or Con A and IL-2 (35) have been described by several investigators. More recently, assays for cells capable of producing IL-2 in response to PHA or Con A and assays for cells capable of developing cytotoxic activity have also been described (35-36).

In vitro assays do not provide insight regarding the clinical utility of various methods, nor do they indicate which cell surface antigen(s) would serve as the best target(s) for T-cell depletion. Too little is known about the effects of different T-cell subtypes to predict optimal depletion strategies based solely on in vitro depletion data. Nonetheless, the interpretation of clinical outcome always requires enumeration and functional assessment of T cells remaining in treated marrows.

III. EFFECTS ON GVHD

Initially it was reported that treatment of marrow with a murine IgG2a anti-CD3 antibody alone was sufficient to prevent GVHD (4), but this finding was not confirmed in subsequent studies (5,6). Thus, it appeared that in vivo mechanisms such as complement-mediated lysis, antibody-dependent cell-mediated cytotoxicity and reticuloendothelial clearance were inadequate to eliminate the antibody-coated T cells in marrow transplant recipients. In vitro testing has indicated that most murine anti-T-cell antibodies do not lyse human T cells with human serum as a source of complement. Certain rat antibodies such as CAMPATH-1, however, show highly efficient complement-mediated lysis in the presence of human serum (38). Variation in ability to mediate complement-dependent lysis reflects not only the species and isotype-specific interaction between antibody and human complement components (39,40), but also other factors such as the cell surface density of antigen expression and the valency of antibody binding (41).

Most studies with monoclonal antibodies have employed in vitro procedures to assure destruction of T cells before infusion of marrow into the recipient. This has the advantage of allowing the number of viable T cells remaining in the graft to be estimated. In clinical studies in which 2 log depletion of T cells was achieved by in vitro marrow treatment, there was approximately a 10% incidence of clinically significant acute GVHD among durably engrafted patients transplanted with HLA-identical marrow even when no posttransplant immunosuppression was administered (1,20,25). This contrasts with a GVHD incidence of at least 80% when posttransplant immunosuppression is omitted in patients given unmodified marrow (42). Thus it appears that as many as 10^5 HLA-identical donor T cells/kg recipient body weight can generally be tolerated with a minimal risk of acute GVHD in patients given no posttransplant immunosuppression. Studies in which only 1 log depletion of T cells was achieved showed correspondingly higher rates of acute GVHD (20). In some studies, clinically significant acute GVHD was not seen in patients who received HLA-identical marrow containing less than 10^5 T cells/kg (43,44), but other investigators have reported acute GVHD in patients receiving as few as 4×10^3 T cells/kg (45). Technical differences between assays for enumerating residual viable T cells remaining in the marrow after treatment and additional in vivo elimination of T cells with certain treatment methods may account for some of the variation in estimates of the number of T cells required to cause GVHD.

The extent of T-cell depletion required to prevent GVHD probably depends on multiple factors already known to affect the risk of GVHD in patients transplanted with

unmodified marrow (46). These include recipient age, parity of the donor, the underlying diagnosis and preparative regimen, the amount of posttransplant immunosuppression, and the type of reverse isolation and antimicrobial prophylaxis. HLA genetic disparity between the donor and recipient probably represents the single factor having
greatest influence on GVHD risk (47). Attempts to employ T-cell depletion for HLA-
mismatched marrow transplantation have generally been discouraging since either acute
GVHD or graft rejection has been encountered in as many as 50% of the patients (23).
To some extent, these results may reflect the greater degree of T-cell depletion required
to prevent GVHD in the setting of HLA disparity. With a sufficient degree of depletion
(3.0-3.5 logs), the incidence of clinically significant acute GVHD in HLA-haploidentical
recipients can be reduced to 10% or less (48). As an alternative approach some investigators have begun to use T-cell depletion as an adjunctive measure together with conventional posttransplant immunosuppression for GVHD prevention (19). It has not yet
been shown that survival can be improved with this type of approach.

    There is relatively little published information concerning the effects of T-cell de-
pletion on chronic GVHD, although the incidence in some studies appears to be lower
than might have been expected with conventional marrow transplantation (19,25,45,48,
49). These findings are noteworthy because conventional posttransplant immunosuppressive regimens have had little impact on chronic GVHD (50-52).

IV. GRAFT FAILURE

In virtually all clinical studies, the use of T-cell-depleted marrow for allogeneic transplantation has been complicated by an increased incidence of graft failure (9,10,12-16,
19,20,23,25,30,48,49,53). At least three patterns of graft failure have been recognized:
(1) failure of initial engraftment, (2) prompt initial engraftment followed by the subsequent development of pancytopenia and marrow aplasia, and (3) late graft failure associated with cytogenetic but not morphologic evidence of relapse. In the latter group it is
possible that the recurrent leukemia was responsible for suppression of hematopoiesis.
More likely, leukemic cells present in small numbers merely became evident after the
graft failed for other reasons. The incidence of graft failure has varied widely among
different centers and in different patient populations. For patients with HLA-identical
donors, the incidence has ranged from less than 5% (19) to more than 60% (45,54). At
least four factors may contribute to this variation: patient selection, the pretransplant
immunosuppressive regimen, the method and extent of T-cell depletion, and the small
size of most studies. When results from different studies are pooled, it appears that graft
failure occurs in approximately 10% of patients transplanted with T-cell-depleted HLA-
identical marrow and in approximately 30% of those transplanted with HLA-mismatched
marrow (1). These estimates would be somewhat higher after actuarial correction for
early death.

    Possible explanations for the increased incidence of graft failure fall in two general
categories that are not mutually exclusive: (1) procedures for removal of T cells may
cause inadvertent stem cell loss or damage, and (2) T cells may in some way contribute
to allogeneic marrow engraftment. Circumstantial evidence has suggested that stem cell
damage did not represent the predominant cause of graft failure, at least in some studies.
First, no correlation has been reported between the risk of graft failure and the numbers
of nucleated cells or committed hematopoietic progenitors in the treated marrow. Second, in many patients, graft failure occurred after initial engraftment had been well estab-

lished. Stem cell damage would ordinarily be expected to manifest itself as failure of initial engraftment. Third, T-cell depletion has not been associated with graft failure after autologous transplantation or after second allogeneic marrow transplantation where T cells in the host are of donor origin (Martin et al., unpublished). These observations do not exclude stem cell damage as a contributory cause of graft failure. In vitro assays for committed hematopoietic progenitors may not reflect the number of pluripotent hematopoietic stem cells responsible for sustained engraftment. Marrow treatment could conceivably have limited the self-renewal capacity of stem cells or caused a differential toxic effect on the least mature stem cells required for durable engraftment without affecting more mature stem cells required for initial engraftment. Finally, it is well recognized that fewer stem cells are required for autologous engraftment than for allogeneic engraftment. Thus, autologous transplantation with the usual number of marrow cells does not represent a stringent test for stem cell damage. Reliable assessment of stem cell damage as a possible cause of graft failure will require a direct assay for measuring pluripotent hematopoietic stem cell number and function.

In some studies, risk factors associated with graft failure have been identified by retrospective analysis. Three reports showed an inverse relationship between the risk of graft failure and the amount of pretransplant cytoreduction and immunosuppression achieved by increased total body irradiation (TBI) (45,54,55). However, a randomized prospective trial indicated no benefit of adding 600 rads total lymphoid irradiation to a conditioning regimen of cyclophosphamide and 1000 rads single exposure TBI (56). One study showed a fivefold increased hazard of graft failure in patients with acute leukemia compared to those with chronic myelogenous leukemia (CML) (45), while another study demonstrated a strikingly increased risk of graft failure in patients with male donors (57). Neither finding has yet been confirmed (25). Pretransplant transfusion has been associated with graft rejection in aplastic patients transplanted with unmodified marrow (58), but associations between pretransplant transfusion and graft failure after T-cell-depleted marrow transplantaton have not been found (10,45,57). Graft failures have occurred in untransfused males, suggesting that transfusion-induced sensitization cannot account for the entire problem, although it may represent a contributory factor. Even though the p values seen for certain associations may appear to exclude fortuity, it is very difficult to gain any truly meaningful clues about possible causes of graft failure from retrospective analyses of risk factors, particularly when the various studies have inconsistent results. If such associations are accepted as biologically relevant, then it must be concluded that the causes of graft failure are not uniform in different studies.

Some clues have come from careful in vitro studies of lymphoid cells in patients with graft failure. Lymphoid cells circulating at the time of graft failure generally have a $CD2^+$, $CD3^+$, $CD8^+$, HLA-DR$^+$ cell surface phenotype but do not express the CD25-associated IL-2 receptor after in vitro mitogen stimulation (59-64). Cells of similar phenotype have also been identified in patients with poorly functioning autologous grafts (B. Torok-Storb, personal communication). These results suggest that certain regulatory abnormalities in T cells can be associated with graft failure, but it is not at all clear whether the T-cell regulatory abnormalities are a cause of graft failure or whether the poorly functioning graft is a cause of T-cell regulatory abnormalities. Host lymphocytes with antidonor cytotoxic activity have been identified in the blood of patients with graft failure after T-cell-depleted HLA-mismatched marrow transplantation (59-62). In some cases, it was possible to show that these cells had specificity for donor HLA antigens, indicating that the effectors were T lymphocytes (59,61). In general, however, it has not been possible to detect direct antidonor cytotoxic activity in lymphocytes from patients with graft failure after T-cell-depleted HLA-identical marrow transplantation (62-64). As a different approach, hematopoietic progenitors have been tested as targets for cytotoxic activity or suppression. One group found that cells from patients with graft failure before day 29 showed specific suppression of HLA-identical donor CFU—GM but not BFU—E (63,64). Cells from patients with graft failure at later time points did not show this suppression. Another group reported nonspecific suppression of CFU—GM but, again, not BFU-E (60). Similar results were seen when culture supernates from patients cells were tested. The inconsistency of results might reflect technical differences in the assay systems or might indicate the involvement of multiple mechanisms contributing to graft failure. Interpretations must be made with caution since in vitro results do not necessarily reflect causal mechanisms of graft failure in vivo.

Other clinical observations in trials of T-cell depletion may offer some insight regarding causes of graft failure. At least four studies have noted a high incidence of mixed lymphoid and mixed hematopoietic chimerism in patients transplanted with T-cell-depleted marrow compared to similar patients transplanted with unmodified marrow (45,65-67). In keeping with these observations, it has been possible to recover viable host cells after administration of the conditioning regimen but before infusion of the marrow (68,69). In general, the proportion of persisting host lymphoid cells was much higher than the proportion of host myeloid cells. The host lymphoid cells persisted in some patients for more than a year after transplantation. It was noteworthy that some of the patients with persisting mixed lymphoid chimerism had perfectly functioning donor hematopoietic grafts, indicating little relationship between mixed lymphoid chimerism and the risk of graft failure (45). Increased persistence of host myeloid and lymphoid cells could reflect the smaller numbers of stem cells and lymphoid cells in T-cell-depleted marrow. Alternatively, donor T cells may help to eliminate residual host hematopoietic stem cells and lymphoid cells that survive the preparative regimen.

Clinical trials of T-cell depletion are continuing in many centers despite the problem of graft failure. Previous studies have indicated that the risk of graft failure is unaffected by posttransplant immunosuppression with methotrexate, cyclosporine, or the combination of cyclosporine plus methotrexate, or by the omission of posttransplant immunosuppression (45). The use of more intensive pretransplant immunosuppression, larger numbers of marrow cells in the graft and less complete removal of T cells represent the empirical approaches currently under most active investigation as possible ways of avoiding graft failure. Attempts to employ more intensive pretransplant immunosuppression generally cause increased toxicity that may offset any possible benefits (12). The use of monoclonal antibodies for this purpose may offer an attractive alternative to increased doses of chemotherapy or radiation (70,71). Attempts to obtain larger amounts of marrow may increase the risk of complications for the donor and may disproportionately increase the number of T cells due to the blood coaspirated with the marrow. Less complete removal of T cells may require the adjunctive use of posttransplant immunosuppression, thus negating one of the major benefits potentially to be gained by T-cell depletion.

As a new approach, the use of lymphokines to promote growth of donor hematopoietic stem cells in vitro before transplantation or in vivo after transplantation is also being explored as a method for avoiding graft failure. These studies follow from the concept that factors elaborated by T cells are directly or indirectly responsible for sustaining hematopoietic function after marrow transplantation and that graft failure after T-cell depletion is caused by deficiency of one or more lymphokines. Empirical trials in appropriate animal models are needed to test the validity of this concept and to identify the relevant factor(s). It also remains to be determined whether the T cells that facilitate engraftment are distinct from those that cause GVHD. In patients given marrow transplants for treatment of aplastic anemia, it has been observed that GVHD precludes rejection and rejection precludes GVHD, giving rise to the concept of "reciprocal interference" between host-vs.-graft (HVG) and graft-vs.-host (GVH) reactions (72, 73). This concept has been supported by observations that certain transplant variables such as transfusion-induced sensitization of the donor or host, the degree of pretransplant immunosuppression, the number of lymphocytes in the graft, the sex of the donor, and degee of host gut decontamination influence HVG and GVH reactions in reciprocal ways. However, it does not follow from this relationship that GVHD is either necessary or sufficient to avoid rejection or that graft facilitation and GVHD represent one and the same activity of donor lymphoid cells.

V. LEUKEMIC RELAPSE

Data suggesting an increased incidence of leukemic relapse in patients transplanted with T-cell-depleted marrow were first reported in a prospective randomized study of patients with acute leukemia in remission or chronic myelogenous leukemia (CML) in various phases, but the trend in this study was not statistically significant even when patients with graft failure and cytogenetic but not morphologic evidence of relapse were classified as having relapsed (14). More convincing evidence came from retrospective studies which found an increased relapse rate in patients transplanted with T-cell-depleted marrow during the chronic phase of CML compared to similar historical patients transplanted with unmodified marrow (25,74,75).

Two retrospective multivariate analyses have confirmed an increased relapse hazard associated with T-cell depletion in CML patients (76,77). The relative risk of relapse after transplantation during chronic phase was estimated to be approximately fivefold higher in recipients of T-cell-depleted marrow compared to recipients of unmodified marrow (76), and the corresponding relative risk after transplantation during accelerated phase was estimated at 18 (77). Separate analyses of patients with and without clinically evident acute or chronic GVHD confirmed an increased risk of relapse associated with T-cell depletion in all subgroups. Thus, decreased GVHD produced by T-cell depletion could not in itself entirely account for the increased relapse risk. Neither retrospective study of CML was able to detect an effect of T-cell depletion on relapse-free survival despite the marked impact of T-cell depletion on relapse risk. At least in chronic phase patients, it appeared that the increased risks of relapse and graft failure associated with T-cell depletion had been offset by decreased GVHD-related mortality. Further follow-up will be required in order to assess the long-term effects and ultimate impact of T-cell depletion.

There are limitations to the interpretation of data from these two multivariate analyses. In neither study were the T-cell-depleted transplants concurrent with the conventional transplants. In both studies, there were differences between the respective patient groups, but none of the differences was found to account for the markedly increased risk of relapse in patients given T-cell-depleted marrow. Inability to exclude a causal relationship between T-cell depletion and increased relapse risk in this type of retrospective analysis cannot be interpreted as proof of such a relationship. Nonetheless, the concordant findings of both studies add to the growing evidence for an association between T-cell-depletion and relapse in CML patients. Mechanisms for this association could well be identical to those responsible for the increased mixed hematopoietic chimerism seen after T-cell depletion (45,65-67), since in CML, hematopoiesis originates from a clonal population of pluripotent stem cells that has largely replaced its normal counterpart (78). It is of interest that no relationship between unmanipulated marrow cell dose and relapse risk was found in the study of chronic phase patients despite a 30-fold range from the lowest to the highest values (76). This observation argues against the idea that the increased relapse (and increased mixed hematopoietic chimerism) associated with T-cell depletion might be related to a smaller number of stem cells in the graft (25). Overall, the data best fit the hypothesis that donor T cells help to eliminate residual malignant and normal host hematopoietic stem cells.

The association between T-cell depletion and increased relapse risk may not apply uniformly to all studies of CML. In the future, it might be possible to identify subgroups of patients for whom T-cell depletion has a minimal or undetectable adverse effect. It is also possible that improved pretransplant cytoreductive regimens may reach a level of efficacy that does not require antileukemic activity from donor T cells in order to prevent relapse. Finally, it should not be inferred from the data in patients with CML that T-cell depletion is likely to be associated with an increased relapse risk in patients with other hematologic malignancies. Preliminary analyses have indicated no detectable adverse effect in patients with acute nonlymphoblastic leukemia or acute lymphoblastic leukemia (79).

VI. IMMUNOLOGIC RECONSTITUTION

Transplantation of syngeneic, autologous, or allogeneic marrow is followed by a period of immunodeficiency that is frequently complicated by life-threatening infections. It is well documented that GVHD and its treatment can further delay or inhibit immune recovery (80,81). On the other hand, it is unknown to what extent initial immune reconstitution depends on mature T cells in the graft, particularly in older individuals with impaired thymic function. Thus, at the initiation of clinical trials, it was unclear how depletion of mature T cells from allogeneic donor marrow would affect the duration of immunodeficiency after transplantation. Recent reports have indicated that T-cell depletion has had a minimal effect on the kinetics of immune reconstitution whether recipients received marrow depleted of T cells by treatment with monoclonal antibodies plus complement (82-87) or by soybean lectin agglutination and E-rosetting (88). However, analysis of immune recovery following T-cell-depleted transplatation has been limited, while the tempo of reconstitution following allogeneic unmodified marrow transplantation has been well documented by in vitro studies (89-91).

Hematopoietic and immune recovery have been compared concurrently in recipients of HLA-identical marrow depleted of T cells by soybean lectin agglutination and E-rosetting and in recipients of unmodified marrow (88). In this study and in other reports (82,84), natural killer cells were the first lymphoid subset to recover in all recipients irrespective of the type of transplant, with initial recovery occurring between 2 and 3 weeks after transplantation. Phenotypic analysis of blood leukocytes indicated that the total number of lymphocytes was slightly higher in conventional marrow recipients during the first month. Thereafter, patients with chronic GVHD had a lymphocytosis, while recipients of T-cell-depleted marrow remained normal, consistent with the absence of chronic GVHD. Lymphocytes predominantly had a CD3$^+$, CD8$^+$ phenotype with the number of CD4$^+$ cells remaining well below normal in both groups of patients throughout the first 6 months. The number of CD4$^+$ cells began to increase at 7-9 months in recipients of T-cell-depleted marrow. T-cell function measured by proliferative response to phytohemagglutinin recovered to the normal range at 4-6 months after conventional transplantation and at 10-12 months after T-cell-depleted transplantation.

In this study, as well as in other reports (82,87,92-94), the number of circulating B lymphocytes recovered to the normal range by the second month and exceeded normal levels after 7 months. Similarly, responses to *Staphylococcus aureus* were normal in both groups of patients by 2-3 months posttransplant. In fact, by 4 months the responses were higher than normal and remained elevated for at least 18 months. In vitro assays showed that normal levels of IgM production were achieved in both groups of patients by 4-6 months posttransplant. However, the time to achieve normal IgG production differed in the two groups of patients: recipients of conventional grafts reached normal production at 7-9 months, while recipients of T-cell-depleted grafts did not recover until 13-15 months.

Removal of mature T cells from the marrow graft did not affect the rate of recovery of lymphoid cells but did affect the regeneration of in vitro T-cell-dependent functions. Further evidence for T-cell-functional impairment has come from limiting dilution assays that enumerate precursors for helper, cytotoxic and proliferative T lymphocytes (95). During the first 180 days, precursor frequencies for cytotoxic T cells and proliferating T cells were lower in patients transplanted with T-cell-depleted marrow than in patients transplanted with unmodified marrow. After the first 6 months, the precursor frequencies for these cells were similar in the two groups, but still well below normal values. T-cell depletion did not have a statistically significant effect on the precursor frequency for helper T cells, but only limited data were available. Other factors such as age and GVHD did not detectably affect the results.

Despite the in vitro observations described above, there is little reported evidence to suggest an increased risk of infectious complications in durably engrafted recipients of T-cell-depleted marrow. Two groups, however, have suggested that the incidence of Epstein-Barr virus-associated lymphoproliferative syndromes (EBV-LPS) may be increased in recipients of T-cell-depleted marrow (96,97). In one study, the occurrence of EBV-LPS appeared to be associated with T-cell depletion of marrow from HLA-mismatched donors (96). In the other study, the EBV-LPS occurred in recipients of T-cell-depleted HLA-identical marrow (97). By multivariate proportional hazards analysis, the relative risk for EBV-LPS was estimated to be sevenfold greater in recipients of HLA-identical T-cell-depleted marrow compared to recipients of unmodified marrow. EBV-specific cytotoxic T lymphocytes are believed to represent the primary mechanism for controlling the proliferation of EBV-infected B lymphocytes (98). Thus, the increased incidence of EBV-LPS after T-cell-depleted transplantation may correspond with the impaired reconstitution of cytotoxic precursors observed during the first 6 months (95).

VII. CONCLUSIONS

Clinical trials evaluating T-cell depletion of donor marrow have clearly indicated both the benefits and the drawbacks of this method for preventing GVHD. Unfortunately, these studies have provided little insight concerning mechanisms for the detrimental effects associated with this procedure. For this reason, the clinical trials reported to date have not suggested approaches likely to solve the problems of increased graft failure and leukemic relapse and delayed immune reconstitution. Although most trials have employed methods aimed at global T-cell depletion, it should be recognized that GVHD is initiated by the relatively small subset of cells that are specifically alloreactive against host histocompatibility antigens. The extent to which these same cells are necessary for engraftment and antileukemic activity remains unknown. If separate populations are responsible for these different functional activities, then efforts should be focused on developing methods for depleting the subset(s) specifically involved in causing GVHD. On the other hand, if a single subset is responsible for all three effects, then alternative methods must be developed for assuring adequate engraftment and eliminating residual malignant cells if T-cell depletion of donor marrow is used to prevent GVHD.

ACKNOWLEDGMENT

The authors' investigations were supported by Grants CA18029, CA29548, CA22507, CA23766, and CA08748 awarded by the National Cancer Institute, Department of Health and Human Services, and by contract N00014-82-K-0660 from the Office of Naval Research, Department of Defense. We thank Dr. Mary Horowitz for providing unpublished information. We especially thank Alison Wiegmann for assistance in preparation of the manuscript.

REFERENCES

1. Gale RP: T cells, bone marrow transplantation and immunotherapy: Use of monoclonal antibodies, in *Immune Interventions in Disease*, Fahey JL (moderator), Ann Intern Med 1987;106:257-274.
2. Thomas ED, Storb R: Technique for human marrow grafting. Blood 1970;36:507-515.
3. Lucas PJ, Quinones RR, Moses RD, Nakamura H, Gress RE: Alternative donor sources in HLA-mismatched marrow transplantation: T cell depletion of surgically resected cadaveric marrow. Bone Marrow Transplantion 1988;3:211-220.
4. Prentice HG, Blacklock HA, Janossy G, Bradstock KF, Skeggs D, Goldstein G, Hoffbrand AV: Use of anti-T cell monoclonal antibody OKT3 to prevent acute graft-versus-host disease in allogeneic bone-marrow transplantation for acute leukemia. Lancet 1982;i:700-703.
5. Filipovich AH, McGlave PB, Ramsay NKC, Goldstein G, Warkentin PI, Kersey, JH: Pretreatment of donor bone marrow with monoclonal antibody OKT3 for prevention of acute graft-versus-host disease in allogeneic histocompatible bone-marrow transplantion. Lancet 1982;i:1266-1269.
6. Martin PJ, Hansen JA, Thomas ED: Preincubation of donor bone marrow cells with a combination of murine monoclonal anti-T-cell antibodies without complement does not prevent graft-versus-host disease after allogeneic marrow transplantation. J Clin Immunol 1984;4:18-22.
7. Reinherz EL, Geha R, Rappeport JM, Wilson M, Penta AC, Hussey RE, Fitzgerald KA, Daley JF, Levine H, Rosen FS, Schlossman SF: Reconstitution after transplantation with T-lymphocyte-depleted HLA haplotype-mismatched bone marrow for severe combined immunodeficiency. Proc Natl Acad Sci USA 1982;79:6047-6051.

8. Prentice HG, Janossy G, Price-Jones L, Trejdosiewicz LK, Panjwani D, Graphakos S, Ivory K, Blacklock HA, Gilmore MJML, Tidman N, Skeggs DBL, Ball S, Patterson J, Hoffbrand AV: Depletion of T lymphocytes in donor marrow prevents significant graft-versus-host disease in matched allogeneic leukaemic marrow transplant recipients. Lancet 1984; i:472-475.

9. Waldmann H, Hale G, Cividalli G, Weshler Z, Manor D, Rachmilewitz EA, Polliak A, Or R, Weiss L, Samuel S, Brautbar C, Slavin S: Elimination of graft-versus-host disease by in vitro depletion of alloreactive lymphocytes with a monoclonal rat anti-human lymphocyte antibody (Campath-1). Lancet 1984; ii:483-486.

10. Martin PJ, Hansen JA, Buckner CD, Sanders J, Deeg HJ, Stewart P, Appelbaum FR, Clift R, Fefer A, Witherspoon RP, Kennedy MS, Sullivan KM, Flournoy N, Storb R, Thomas ED: Effects of in vitro depletion of T cells in HLA-identical allogeneic marrow grafts. Blood 1985;66:664-672.

11. Hervé P, Flesch M, Cahn JY, Racadot E, Plouvier E, Lamy B, Rozenbaum A, Noir A, Leconte Des Floris R, Peters A: Removal of marrow T cells with OKT3-OKT11 monoclonal antibodies and complement to prevent graft-versus-host disease. Transplantation 1985;39:138-143.

12. Sondel PM, Bozdech MJ, Trigg ME, Hong R, Finlay JL, Kohler PC, Longo W, Hank JA, Billing R, Steeves R, Flynn B: Additional immunosuppression allows engraftment following HLA-mismatched T cell-depleted bone marrow transplantation for leukemia. Transplant Proc 1985;17:460-461.

13. Trigg ME, Billing R, Sondel PM, Exten R, Hong R, Bozdech MS, Horowitz SD, Finlay JL, Moen R, Longo W, Erickson C, Peterson A: Clinical trial depleting T lymphocytes from donor marrow for matched and mismatched allogeneic bone marrow transplants. Cancer Treatment Rep 1985;69:377-386.

14. Mitsuyasu RT, Champlin RE, Gale RP, Ho WG, Lenarsky C, Winston D, Selch M, Elashoff R, Giorgi JV, Wells J, Terasaki P, Billing R, Feig S. Treatment of donor bone marrow with monoclonal anti-T cell antibody and complement for the prevention of graft-versus-host disease: A prospective, randomized, double-blind trial. Ann Intern Med 1986;105:20-26.

15. Filipovich AH, Vallera DA, Youle RJ, Haake R, Blazar BR, Arthur D, Neville D, Ramsay NK, McGlave P, Kersey JH: Graft-versus-host disease prevention in allogeneic bone marrow transplantation from histocompatible siblings. Transplantation 1987;44:62-69.

16. Martin PJ, Hansen JA, Torok-Storb B, Moretti L, Press O, Storb R, Thomas ED, Weiden PL, Vitetta ES. Effects of treating marrow with a CD3-specific immunotoxin for prevention of acute graft-versus-host disease. Bone Marrow Transplantation 1988;3:437-444.

17. Vartdal F, Albrechtsen D, Ringden O, Kvalheim G, Lea T, Bosnes V, Gaudernack G, Brinchmann J, Ugelstad J: Immunomagnetic treatment of bone marrow allografts. Bone Marrow Transplantation 1987;2(Suppl.2):94-98.

18. DeWitte T, Hoogenhout J, De Pauw B, Holdrinet R, Janssen J, Wessels J, van Daal W, Hustinx T, Haanen C: Depletion of donor lymphocytes by counterflow centrifugation successfully prevents acute graft-versus-host disease in matched allogeneic marrow transplantation. Blood 1986;67:1302-1308.

19. Wagner JE, Donnenberg AD, Noga SJ, Cremo CA, Gao IK, Yin HJ, Vogelsang GB, Rowley S, Saral R, Santos GW: Lymphocyte depletion of donor bone marrow by counterflow centrifugal elutriation: Results of a phase I clinical trial. Blood 1988; 72:1168-1176.

20. Lowenberg B, Wagemaker E, van Bekkum DW, Sizoo W, Sintnicolaas K, Hendriks W, Hagenbeen A: Graft-versus-host disease following transplantation of "one log" versus "two log" T-lymphocyte depleted bone marrow from HLA-identical donors. Bone Marrow Transplantation 1986;1:133-140.

21. Reisner Y, Kapoor N, Kirkpatrick D, Pollack MS, Dupont B, Good RA, O'Reilly RJ: Transplantation for acute leukaemia with HLA-A and B nonidentical parental marrow cells fractionated with soybean agglutinin and sheep red blood cells. Lancet 1981; ii:327-331.

22. Reisner Y, Kapoor N, Kirkpatrick D, Pollack MS, Cunningham-Rundles S, Dupont B, Hodes MZ, Good RA, O'Reilly RJ: Transplatation for severe combined immunodeficiency with HLA-A,B,D,DR incompatible parental marrow cells fractionated by soybean agglutinin and sheep red cells. Blood 1983;61:341-348.

23. O'Reilly RJ, Collins NH, Kernan NA, Brochstein J, Dinsmore R, Kirkpatrick D, Siena S, Keever C, Jordan B, Shank B, Wolf L, Dupont B, Reisner Y: Transplantation of marrow depleted T cells by soybean lectin agglutination and E-rosette depletion: Major histocompatibility complex-related graft resistance in leukemic transplant patients. Transplant Proc 1985;17:455-459.

24. Matthay KK, Wara DW, Ammann AJ, Ablin AR, Cowan MJ: Mismatched bone marrow transplantation using soybean agglutinin processed T-cell depleted marrow, in Progress in Bone Marrow Transplantation, edited by Gale RP and Champlin RE. Alan R Liss, Inc., New York, 1987; pp. 343-351.

25. Hale G, Cobbold S, Waldmann H: T cell depletion with Campath-1 in allogeneic bone marrow transplantation. Transplantation 1988;45:753-759.

26. Cobbold S, Hale G, Waldmann H: Non-lineage, LFA-1 family, and leukocyte common antigens: new and previously defined clusters, in Leucocyte Typing III, White Cell Differentiation Antigens, edited by McMichael AJ. Oxford University Press, Oxford, 1987; pp. 788-803.

27. Bernard A, Boumsell L, Hill C: Joint report of the First International Workshop on human leucocyte differentiation antigens by the investigators of the participating laboratories, in Leucocyte Typing, edited by Bernard A, Boumsell L, Dausset J, Milstein C, Schlossman SF. Springer-Verlag, New York 1984; pp. 9-142.

28. Haynes BF: Summary of T cell studies performed during the Second International Workship and conference on human leukocyte differentiation antigens, in Leukocyte Typing II, Vol. 1, edited by Reinherz EL, Haynes BF, Nadler LM, Bernstein ID. Springer-Verlag, New York, 1986; pp. 3-30.

29. McMichael AJ, Gotch FM: T-cell antigens: new and previously defined clusters, in Leucocyte Typing III, White Cell Differentiation Antigens, edited by McMichael AJ. Oxford University Press, Oxford, 1987; pp. 31-62.

30. Maraninchi D, Mawas C, Guyotat D, Reiffers J, Vernant JP, Gratecos N, Hirn J, Novakovitch G: Selective depletion of marrow-T cytotoxic lymphocytes (CD8) in the prevention of graft-versus-host disease after allogeneic bone-marrow transplantation. Transplant International 1988;1:91-94.

31. Knott LJ, Levinsky RJ, Newland A, Jones HM, Linch DC: Bone marrow T-cell colony-forming cells: studies of their origin and use in monitoring T cell-depleted bone marrow grafts. Clin Exp Immunol 1985;62:561-569.

32. Martin PJ, Hansen JA: Quantitative assays for detection of residual T cells in T-depleted human marrow. Blood 1985;65:1134-1140.

33. Kernan NA, Flomenberg N, Collins NH, O'Reilly RJ, Dupont B. Quantitation of T lymphocytes in human bone marrow by a limiting dilution assay. Transplantation 1985;40:317-322.

34. Rohatiner A, Gelber R, Schlossman SF, Ritz J. Depletion of T cells from human bone marrow using monoclonal antibodies and rabbit complement. Transplantation 1986;42:73-80.

35. Rozans MK, Smith BR, Emerson S, Crimmins M, Laurent G, Reichert T, Burakoff SJ, Miller RA: Functional assessment of T cell depletion from bone marrow prior to therapeutic transplantation using limiting dilution culture methods. Transplantation 1986;42:380-387.

36. Irlé C, Kaestli M, Aapro M, Chapuis B, Jeannet M. Quantity and nature of residual bone marrow T cells after treatment of the marrow with Campath-1. Exp Hematol 1987;15:163–170.
37. Sharp TG, Sachs DH, Fauci AS, Messerschmidt GL, Rosenberg SA. T cell depletion of human bone marrow using monoclonal antibody and complement-mediated lysis. Transplantation 1983;35:112–120.
38. Hale G, Bright S, Chumbley G, Hoang T, Metcalf D, Munro AJ, Waldmann H: Removal of T cells from bone marrow for transplantation: a monoclonal antilymphocyte anti-antibody that fixes human complement. Blood 1983;62:873–882.
39. Cobbold SP, Thierfelder S, Waldmann H: Immunosuppression with monoclonal antibodies. A model to determine the rules for effective serotherapy. Molecular Biology and Medicine 1984;1:285–304.
40. Kummer U, Thierfelder S, Hoffmann-Fezer G, Schuh R: In vivo immunosuppression by pan-T cell antibodies relates to their isotype and to their Clq uptake. J Immunol 1987;138:4069–4074.
41. Cobbold SP, Waldmann H: Therapeutic potential of monovalent monoclonal antibodies. Nature 1984;308:460–462.
42. Sullivan KM, Deeg HJ, Sanders J, Klosterman A, Amos D, Shulman H, Sale G, Martin P, Witherspoon R, Appelbaum FR, Doney K, Stewart P, Meyers J, McDonald GB, Weiden P, Fefer A, Buckner CD, Storb R, Thomas ED: Hyperacute graft-versus-host disease in patients not given immunosuppression after allogeneic marrow transplantation. Blood 1986;67:1172–1175.
43. Kernan NA, Collins NH, Juliano L, Cartagena T, Dupont B, O'Reilly RJ: Clonable T lymphocytes in T cell-depleted bone marrow transplants correlate with development of graft-versus-host disease. Blood 1986;68:770–773.
44. Atkinson K, Farrelly H, Cooley M, O'Flaherty E, Downs K, Biggs J: Human marrow T cell dose correlates with severity of subsequent acute graft-versus-host disease. Bone Marrow Transplantation 1987;2:51–57.
45. Martin PJ, Hansen JA, Torok-Storb B, Durnam D, Przepiorka D, O'Quigley J, Sanders J, Sullivan KM, Witherspoon RP, Joachim Deeg H, Appelbaum FR, Stewart P, Weiden P, Doney K, Buckner CD, Clift R, Storb R, Thomas ED: Graft failure in patients receiving T cell-depleted HLA-identical allogeneic marrow transplants. Bone Marrow Transplantation 1988;3:445–456.
46. Gale RP, Bortin MM, vanBekkum DW, Biggs JC, Dicke KA, Gluckman E, Good RA, Hoffmann RG, Kay HEM, Kersey JH, Marmont A, Masaoka T, Rimm AA, van Rood JJ, Zwaan FE: Risk factors for actue graft-versus-host disease. Br J Haematol 1987;67:397–406.
47. Beatty PG, Clift RA, Mickelson EM, Nisperos B, Flournoy N, Martin PJ, Sanders JE, Storb R, Thomas ED, Hansen JA. Marrow transplantation from related donors other than HLA-identical siblings. N Engl J Med 1985;313:765–771.
48. O'Reilly RJ, Kernan N, Cunningham I, Brochstein J, Collins N, Laver J, Castro-Malaspina H, Flomenberg N, Gulati S, Emanuel D, Bordignon C, Keever C, Shank MB: Soybean lectin agglutination and E-rosette depletion for removal of T-cells from HLA-identical and non-identical marrow grafts administered for the treatment of leukemia, in *T-Cell Depletion in Allogeneic Bone-Marrow Transplantation*, edited by Martelli MF, Grignani F, Reisner Y. Ares-Serono Symposia, Rome, Italy, 1988; pp. 123–129.
49. Maraninchi D, Blaise D, Rio B, Leblond V, Dreyfus F, Gluckman E, Guyotat D, Pico JL, Michallet M, Ifrah N, Bordigoni A: Impact of T-cell depletion on outcome of allogeneic bone marrow transplantation for standard-risk leukaemias. Lancet 1987; ii:175–178.

50. Storb R, Deeg HJ, Pepe M, Appelbaum FR, Anasetti C, Beatty P, Bensinger W, Berenson R, Buckner CD, Clift R, Doney K, Longton G, Hansen JA, Hill R, Loughran T, Martin PJ, Singer J, Sanders J, Stewart P, Sullivan K, Witherspoon R, Thomas ED: Methotrexate and cyclosporine versus cyclosporine alone for prophylaxis of graft-versus-host disease in patients given HLA-identical marrow grafts for leukemia: Long-term followup of a controlled trial. Blood 1989;73:1729-1734.

51. Storb R, Deeg HJ, Pepe M, Doney K, Appelbaum FR, Beatty P, Bensinger W, Buckner CD, Clift R, Hansen JA, Hill R, Longton G, Anasetti C, Martin PJ, Loughran T, Sanders J, Singer J, Stewart P, Sullivan K, Witherspoon R, Thomas ED: Graft-versus-host disease prevention by methotrexate combined with cyclosporine compared to methotrexate alone in patients given marrow grafts for severe aplastic anemia: Long-term followup of a controlled trial. Br J Haematol 1989; in press.

52. Sullivan KM, Storb R, Witherspoon RP, Weiden PL, Anasetti C, Appelbaum FR, Beatty P, Buckner CD, Deeg HJ, Doney K, Fisher L, Loughran TP, Martin PJ, Meyers J, McDonald GB, Sanders JE, Shulman H, Stewart P, Thomas ED: Deletion of immunosuppressive prophylaxis after marrow transplantation increases hyperacute graft-versus-host disease but does not influence chronic graft-versus-host disease or relapse in patients with advanced leukemia. Clinical Transplantation 1989;3:5-11.

53. Hervé P, Cahn JG, Flesch M, Plouvier E, Racadot E, Noir A, Couteret Y, Goldstein G, Bernard A, Lenys R, Bresson JL, Leconte des Floris R, Peters A: Successful graft-versus-host disease prevention without graft failure in 32 HLA-identical allogeneic bone marrow transplantations with marrow depleted of T cells by monoclonal antibodies and complement. Blood 1987;69:388-393.

54. Patterson J, Prentice HG, Brenner MK, Gilmore M, Janossy G, Ivory K, Skeggs D, Morgan H, Lord J, Blacklock HA, Hoffbrand AV, Apperley JF, Goldman JM, Burnett A, Gribben J, Alcorn M, Pearson C, McVickers I, Hahn IM, Reid C, Wardle D, Gravett PJ, Bacigalupo A, Robertson AG: Graft rejection following HLA matched T-lymphocyte depleted bone marrow transplantation. Br J Haematol 1986;63:221-230.

55. Guyotat D, Dutou L, Erhsam A, Campos L, Archimbaud E, Fiere D: Graft rejection after T cell-depeleted marrow transplantation: Role of fractionated irradiation. Br J Haematol 1987;65:499-507.

56. Ganem G, Kuentz M, Beaujean F, Lebourgeois J, Vinci G, Cordonnier C, Vernant JP: Additional total-lymphoid irradiation in preventing graft failure of T-cell depleted bone marrow transplantation from HLA-identical siblings. Transplantation 1987;45:244-248.

57. Kernan NA, Bordignon C, Collins NH, Castro-Malaspina H, Cunningham I, Brochstein J, Shank B, Flomenberg N, Dupont B, O'Reilly RJ: Graft failures following SBA⁻E⁻ T-cell depleted marrow transplants for leukemia: Clinical features and results of secondary transplants, in *T-Cell Depletion in Allogeneic Bone-Marrow Transplantation*, edited by Martelli MF, Grignani F, Reisner Y. Ares-Serono Symposia, Rome, Italy, 1988; pp. 169-172.

58. Storb R, Prentice RL, Thomas ED: Marrow transplantation for treatment of aplastic anemia. An analysis of factors associated with graft rejection. N Engl J Med 1977;296:61-66.

59. Sondel PM, Hank JA, Trigg ME, Kohler PC, Finlay JL, Blank J, Meisner L, Borcherding W, Hong R, Steeves R, Billing R, Flynn B, Bozdech MJ: Transplantation of HLA-haploidentical T cell-depleted marrow for leukemia: Autologous marrow recovery with specific immune sensitization to donor antigens. Exp Hematol 1986; 14:278-286.

60. Bunjes D, Heit W, Arnold R, Schmeiser T, Wiesneth M, Carbonell F, Porzsolt F, Raghavachar A, Heimpel H: Evidence for the involvement of host-derived OKT8-positive T cells in the rejection of T-depleted, HLA-identical bone marrow grafts. Transplantation 1987;43:501-505.

61. Kernan NA, Flomenberg N, Dupont B, O'Reilly RJ: Graft rejection in recipients of T-cell depleted HLA-nonidentical marrow transplants for leukemia. Transplantation 1987;43:842-847.

62. Sandell L, Johnson G, Przepiorka D, Torok-Storb B: Phenotype and function of T-cells associated with marrow graft failure and rejection, in *T-Cell Depletion in Allogeneic Bone-Marrow Transplantation*, edited by Martelli MF, Grignani F, Reisner Y. Ares-Serono Symposia, Rome, Italy, 1988; pp. 49-56.

63. Bordignon C, Kernan NA, Keever CA, Cartagena T, Benazzi E, Burns J, Flomenberg N, Dupont B, O'Reilly RJ: Graft failures following SBA⁻E⁻T-cell depleted marrow transplants for leukemia: in vitro correlates, in *T-Cell Depletion in Allogeneic Bone-Marrow Transplantation*, edited by Martelli MF, Grignani F, Reisner Y. Ares-Serono Symposia, Rome, Italy 1988; pp. 57-60.

64. Bordignon C, Kernan NA, Keever CA, Small TN, Collins NH, Burns J, Flomenberg N, Dupont B, O'Reilly RJ: Graft failures following T-cell depleted grafts for leukemia: Emergence of host T-lymphocytes (CD3+ CD8+) with donor-specific reactivity. Blood 1987;70(suppl. 1):303a.

65. Bretagne S, Vidaud M, Kuentz M, Cordonnier C, Henni T, Vinci G, Goossens M, Vernant JP: Mixed blood chimerism in T cell-depleted bone marrow transplant recipients: Evaluation using DNA polymorphisms. Blood 1987;70:1692-1695.

66. Bertheas MF, Maraninchi D, Lafage M, Fraisse J, Blaise D, Stoppa AM, Michel G, Brizard CP, Gaspard MH, Novakovitch G, Mannoni P, Viens P, Carcassonne Y. Partial chimerism after T-cell depleted allogeneic bone marrow transplantation in leukemic HLA-matched patients: A cytogenetic documentation. Blood 1988;72:89-93.

67. Schouten HC, Sizoo W, van't Veer MB, Hagenbeek A, Lowenberg B: Incomplete chimerism in erythroid, myeloid and B lymphocyte lineage after T cell-depleted allogeneic bone marrow transplantation. Bone Marrow Transplantation 1988; 3: 407-412.

68. Butturini A, Seger RC, Gale RP: Recipient immune-competent T-lymphocytes can survive intensive conditioning for bone marrow transplantation. Blood 1986;68: 948-956.

69. Kedar E, Or R, Naparstek E, Zeira E, Slavin S: Preliminary characterization of functional residual host-type T lymphocytes following conditioning for allogeneic HLA−matched bone marrow transplantation (BMT). Bone Marrow Transplantation 1988;3:129-140.

70. Fischer A, Blanche S, Veber F, Delaage M, Mawas C, Griscelli C, Le Deist F, Lopez M, Olive D, Janossy G: Prevention of graft failure by an anti-HLFA-1 monoclonal antibody in HLA-mismatched bone marrow transplantation. Lancet 1986; ii: 1058-1061.

71. Waldmann H, Hale G, Cobbold S: The immunobiology of bone marrow transplantation, in *Leucocyte Typing III, White Cell Differentiation Antigens*, edited by McMichael AJ. Oxford University Press, Oxford, 1987; pp. 932-937.

72. Vriesendorp HM, Wagemaker G, van Bekkum DW: Engraftment of allogeneic bone marrow. Transplant Proc 1981;13:643-648.

73. Gale RP, Reisner Y: Graft rejection and graft-versus-host disease: Mirror images. Lancet 1986; i: 1468-1470.

74. Apperley JF, Jones L, Hale G, Waldmann H, Hows J, Rombos Y, Tsatalas C, Marcus RE, Goolden AWG, Gordon-Smith EC, Catovsky D, Galton DAG, Goldman JM:

Bone marrow transplantation for patients with chronic myeloid leukaemia: T cell depletion with Campath-1 reduces the incidence of graft-versus-host disease but may increase the risk of leukaemic relapse. Bone Marrow Transplantation 1986;1:53-66.

75. Papa G, Arcese W, Mauro FR, Bianchi A, Alimena G, De Felice L, Isacchi G, Pasqualetti D, Malagnino F, Purpura M, Givelli G, Mandelli F: Standard conditioning regimen and T-depeleted donor bone marrow for transplantation in chronic myeloid leukaemia. Leuk Res 1986;10:1469-1475.

76. Goldman JM, Gale RP, Horowitz MM, Biggs JC, Champlin RE, Gluckman E, Hoffmann RG, Jacobsen SJ, Marmont AM, McGlave PB, Messner HA, Rimm AA, Rozman C, Speck B, Tura S, Weiner RS, Bortin MM: Bone marrow transplantation for chronic myelogenous leukemia in chronic phase: Increased risk for relapse associated with T cell-depletion. Ann Intern Med 1988;108:806-814.

77. Martin PJ, Clift RA, Fisher LD, Buckner CD, Hansen JA, Appelbaum FR, Doney KC, Sullivan KM, Witherspoon RP, Storb R, Thomas ED: HLA-identical marrow transplantation during accelerated-phase chronic myelogenous leukemia: Analysis of survival and remission duration. Blood 1988;72:1978-1984.

78. Fialkow PJ, Jacobson RJ, Papayannopoulou T: Chronic myelocytic leukemia: Clonal origin in a stem cell common to the granulocyte, erythrocyte, platelet and monocyte/macrophage. Am J Med 1977;63:125-130.

79. Ringdén O, Horowitz MM for the Advisory Committee of the International Bone Marrow Transplant Registry: Graft-versus-leukemia reactions in humans. Transplant Proc 1989;21:2989-2992.

80. Noel DR, Witherspoon RP, Storb R, Atkinson K, Doney D, Mickelson EM, Ochs HD, Warren RD, Weiden PL, Thomas ED: Does graft-versus-host disease influence the tempo of immunologic recovery after allogeneic human bcne marrow transplantation? An observation on 56 long-term survivors. Blood 1978;51:1087-1105.

81. Paulin T, Ringdén O, Nilsson R, Lonnqvist B, Gahrton G: Variables predicting bacterial and fungal infections after allogeneic marrow engraftment. Transplantation 1987;43:393-398.

82. Ault KA, Antin JH, Ginsburg D, Orkin SH, Rappeport JM, Keohan ML, Martin P, Smith BR: Phenotype of recovering lymphoid cell populations after marrow transplantation. J Exp Med 1985;161:1483-1502.

83. Janossy G, Prentice HG, Grob JP, Ivory K, Tidman N, Grundy J, Marie Favrot, Brenner MK, Campana D, Blacklock HA, Gilmore MJML, Patterson J, Griffiths, PD, Hoffbrand AV: T lymphocyte regeneration after transplantation of T cell depleted allogeneic bone marrow. Clin Exp Immunol 1986;63:577-586.

84. Rooney CM, Wimperis JZ, Brenner MK, Patterson J, Hoffbrand AV, Prentice HG: Natural killer cell activity following T-cell depleted allogeneic bone marrow transplantation. Br J. Haematol 1986;62:413-420.

85. Wimperis JZ, Prentice HG, Karayiannis P, Brenner MK, Reittie JE, Griffiths PD, Hoffbrand AV: Transfer of a functioning humoral immune system in transplantation of T-lymphocyte depleted bone marrow. Lancet 1986; i:339-343.

86. Parreira A, Smith J, Hows JM, Smithers SS, Apperley J, Rombus Y, Goldman JM, Gordon-Smith EC, Catovsky D. Immunological reconstitution after bone marrow transplant with Campath-1 treated bone marrow. Clin Exp Immunol 1987;67:142-150.

87. Wimperis JZ, Brenner MK, Prentice HG, Thompson EJ, Hoffbrand AV. B cell development and regulation after T cell-depleted marrow transplantation. J Immunol 1987;138:2445-2450.

88. Keever CA, Small TN, Flomenberg N, Heller G, Pekle K, Black P, Pecora N, Kernan NA, O'Reilly RJ: Immune reconstitution following bone marrow transplantation: Comparison of recipients of T cell-depleted marrow with recipients of conventional marrow grafts. Blood 1989;73:1340-1350.

89. Witherspoon RP, Lum LG, Storb R: Immunologic reconstitution after human marrow grafting. Semin Hematol 1984;21:2-10.
90. Martin PJ, Hansen JA, Storb R, Thomas ED: Human marrow transplantation: An immunological perspective, in *Advances in Immunology*, Vol. 40. Academic Press, Inc., Orlando, FL, 1987; pp. 379-438.
91. Lum LG: The kinetics of immune reconstitution after human marrow transplantation. Blood 1987;69:369-380.
92. Brenner MK, Wimperis JZ, Reittie JE, Patterson J, Asherson GL, Hoffbrand AV, Prentice HG: Recovery of immunoglobulin isotypes following T cell depleted allogeneic bone marrow transplantation. Br J Haematol 1986;64:125-132.
93. Brenner MK, Reittie JE, Grob J-P, Wimperis JZ, Stephens S, Patterson J, Hoffbrand AV, Prentice HG: The contribution of large granular lymphocytes to B cell activation and differentiation after T-cell-depleted allogeneic bone marrow transplantation. Transplantation 1986;42:257-261.
94. Antin JH, Ault KA, Rappeport JM, Smith BR: B lymphocyte reconstitution after human bone marrow transplantation. Leu-1 antigen defines a distinct population of B lymphocytes. J Clin Invest 1987;80:325-332.
95. Daley JP, Rozans MK, Smith BR, Burakoff SJ, Rappeport JM, Miller RA: Retarded recovery of functional T cell frequencies in T cell-depleted bone marrow transplant recipients. Blood 1987;70:960-964.
96. Shapiro RS, McClain K, Frizzera G, Gaji-Peczalska KJ, Kersey JH, Blazar BR, Arthur DC, Patton DF, Greenberg JS, Burke B, Ramsay NKC, McGlave P, Filipovich AH. Epstein-Barr virus associated B cell lymphoproliferative disorders following bone marrow transplantation. Blood 1988;71:1234-1243.
97. Zutter MM, Martin PJ, Sale GE, Shulman HM, Fisher L, Thomas ED, Durnam DM: Epstein-Barr virus lymphoproliferation after bone marrow transplantation. Blood 1988;72:520-529.
98. Rickinson AB: Cellular immunological responses to the virus infection, in *The Epstein-Barr Virus: Recent Advances*, edited by Epstein MA, Achong BG. Wiley, New York, 1986; pp. 75-126.

20

Immunosuppressive Drugs for the Prevention of Acute Graft-vs.-Host Disease

Eliane Gluckman
Hôpital Saint Louis
Paris, France

I. INTRODUCTION

Graft-vs.-Host Disease (GVHD) results from an interaction of donor T lymphocytes which contaminte the marrow inoculum with recipient antigens. The main targets are the epidermal basal cells, the small interlobular bile ducts, and intestinal crypt cells. The consequence is necrosis and destruction of the target organs. GVHD is always associated with a profound immunodeficiency, which causes various opportunistic infections, the major cause of mortality after marrow transplantation. GVHD is largely due to HLA and non-HLA histocompatibility differences between donor and recipient. GVHD also increases with age (1). Similarly, the sex of the donor is an important variable: immunized female donors for male recipients increased the relative risk of GVHD to 2.9 (p < 0.0001). Other factors include infections before transplant, herpes virus infection before and after transplant, lack of gut decontamination and isolation in laminar air flow rooms, multiple previous transfusions, transfusion of nonirradiated blood after transplant, underlying diagnosis, type of conditioning, degree of chimerism, and type of GVHD prophylactic regimen (2,3). The risk of chronic GVHD increases with age, transfusions of donor nonirradiated leukocytes after transplantation, and previous acute GVHD (4).

Two in vitro tests have been described for prediction of GVHD before transplant (5,6). In the skin explant test, the recipient's irradiated lymphocytes are used to sensitize the donor lymphocytes before transplant. The donor's lymphocytes are then cocultured with recipient's skin explants. Histological changes of GVHD are seen in positive explants and are predictive in 85% (5). Bagot et al. (6) used a mixed culture between donor lymphoid cells and recipient epidermal cells isolated from suction blisters to predict GVHD. The reproducibility of these tests has not yet been routinely demonstrated, and additional studies are necessary.

Another difficulty in analyzing the results of preventive treatment of GVHD is related to the accuracy and reproducibility of GVHD diagnosis and grading. A recent IBMTR survey showed good consistency in reporting no or mild GVHD (grades 0-1), and moderate to severe GVHD (grades II-IV) but difficulties in differentiating between grades (1). For this reason, many reported statistics include grade I GVHD in the no GVHD group. This may be misleading as patients with grade I GVHD (at least 25% of patients) have an increased incidence of chronic GVHD and opportunistic infections compared to the no GVHD group. Furthermore, GVHD grade I patients frequently require additional immunosuppression with corticosteroids. The same is true with grade II GVHD, which should be differentiated from grades III-IV, which are often resistant to high dose corticosteroids and have a higher probability of being fatal.

The endpoints for evaluation of the efficacy of treatment for GVHD should be incidence, maximum grade, impact on overall survival, and impact on the causes of death. The causes of death are often difficult to assess because of the simultaneous presence of various complications. They can be divided into disease-related deaths (relapse, for example), conditioning or toxicity-related death (veno-occlusive disease of the liver, idiopathic interstitial pneumonitis), or transplant-related deaths (GVHD, infection). For the purpose of analysis, many investigators have separated the causes of mortality into primary cause of death (for example, CMV infection) and contributory cause of death (for example, GVHD).

Overall, the reported incidence of GVHD of grades II-IV is 40-60% in many studies; it is the main cause of death in 20-30% of patients. These numbers have not changed significantly in recent years, and the general impact of various preventive treatments on survival is not readily apparent. Various immunosuppressive drugs have been used alone or in combination to prevent GVHD. Most of the data have been accumulated with cyclosporin A and methotrexate (MTX) given either alone or in combination in patients given HLA-identical sibling transplants. The concept of GVHD prophylaxis is accepted worldwide for patients not receiving T-cell-depleted bone marrow.

II. METHOTREXATE

Studies in dogs conditioned with 920 rads of total body irradiation and given marrow grafts from DLA-identical littermates showed more than 90% disease-free survival in dogs given MTX after grafting compared to a 55% incidence of acute GVHD, and only 45% survival in dogs not given postgrafting immunosuppression (7). Based on these animal studies, the Seattle team developed a regimen of GVHD prophylaxis consisting of intravenous MTX administered at 15 mg/m^2 on day 1 and 10 mg/m^2 on days 3, 6, and 11 and weekly thereafter until day 102 (8). Three studies have compared MTX prophylaxis to no immunosuppression. One study found no difference in incidence and severity of acute GVHD in patients who did or did not receive MTX; however, MTX treated patients appeared to have a higher incidence of GVHD than expected for patient age (9,10). Different results were obtained by the Seattle team (11) who selected a group of 16 young patients with high risk leukemia to be given no immunosuppression after BMT in the hope of reducing leukemic relapse by augmenting the graft-vs.-leukemia effect. This group was compared to a similar group of patients receiving standard MTX. Patients not given immunosuppression had a 100% incidence of hyperacute GVHD compared to 25% in patients given MTX (p < 0.0001). Relapse-free survival was similar in both groups but the authors concluded that deleting immunosuppression was associated with frequent and severe acute GVHD, infectious complications, and occasional poor graft function.

As already discussed, results with MTX prophylaxis vary considerably, the lowest incidence of GVHD reported being 18% (12) and the highest 56% (13). Both results were extracted from two randomized studies comparing MTX to another regimen published by the same center. These discrepancies can be related to the relatively small number of patients involved in the study and differences in patient age. This intracenter variation points to the value of large registry reports which give a general overview of the overall incidence of GVHD after MTX. The International Bone Marrow Transplant Registry (IBMTR) acute GVHD study reported that the incidence of moderate to severe GVHD in 2036 patients transplanted for aplastic anemia or leukemia was 45% ± 2%, and the actuarial probability at 6 months was 46% ± 2%. Forty-eight percent of the patients who developed moderate to severe GVHD died with this complication. Overall, GVHD was a primary or contributory cause of death in 22% of patients in the study. The incidence of GVHD in 1235 patients who received MTX was 44% ± 3%, and did not differ from the cyclosporin A (CsA) -treated group (1).

The toxicity of MTX is usually limited to transient mucositis and some delay of engraftment. One IBMTR study showed that MTX was one of the factors which increased the risk of interstitial pneumonitis (14), an observation not confirmed by others (15).

III. CYCLOSPORIN A

CsA was introduced for GVHD prevention in marrow transplant recipients in 1978. It has remarkable immunosuppressive activity in vitro and in vivo. However, most controlled randomized studies comparing MTX and CsA have failed to show any improvement of survival or incidence of acute or chronic GVHD. Faster rates of engraftment and a decrease in mucosistis and other transplant-related complications have, however, been observed in CSA-treated patients (16). Ten years after the first clinical trials many questions still remain unsolved: optimal dose and duration of treatment, monitoring, and management of CsA-related toxicity are still being investigated.

A. Optimal Dose and Duration of Treatment

CsA is usually started on the day prior to marrow infusion and continued for at least 6 months after transplantation. Because of gastrointestinal problems following conditioning, it is usually given i.v. by continuous infusion or divided in two or three one-hour infusions for at least 3 weeks, and then given orally every 12 hours. The inital dose varies from 2 mg/kg to 20 mg/kg i.v. Subsequently, it is usually adjusted according to CsA levels and renal function.

Pharmacokinetic studies have shown substantial variability of absorption and metabolism of CsA. Using a test dose technique, Lokiec et al. have described the intravenous and oral pharmacokinetic profile of CsA (17). Tables 1 and 2 show the CsA pharmacokinetic parameters obtained in children and adults, respectively. In both groups, and for all parameters, there were differences in individual sensitivity to the drug represented by large standard deviations of the means. The volume of the central compartment (Vc) which indicated distribution and tissue binding of CsA varied from 0.3 to 5.6 L/kg for children, and from 0.2 to 17 L/kg for adults. The results of the second half-life, which indicates CsA elimination from the plasma, varied even more

Table 1 CSA Pharmacokinetic Parameters in Children

C_{max} = 3,870 ± 3,400 ng/mL (536-16,430 ng/mL)
First half-life = 0.45 ± 0.38 h (0.08-1.75 h)
Second half-life = 10.1 ± 12.6 h (1.15-72.7 h)
First slope = 2.69 ± 1.95 L/h (0.40-8.66 L/h)
Second slope = 0.17 ± 0.15 L/h (0.01-0.60 L/h)
Plasma clearance = 31 ± 24 mL/min/kg (6-88 mL/min/kg)
Vc = 2.4 ± 2.6 L/kg (0.3-5.6 L/kg)
Vdss = 21.2 ± 35.2 L/kg (0.8-93.1 L/kg)

than Vc. In children this half-life ranged from 1.15 to 72.7 hours giving a 1:63 ratio, and in the adult group it ranged from 1.30 to 38.6 hours giving a 1:53 ratio. The results of CsA clearance have also shown large individual variations indicating a different plasma disappearance from case to case (for further details see Chapter 00). According to these results, our group performed systematically an individual pharmacokinetic profile prior to transplant in order to determine the optimal dose which should be given to obtain plasma levels of 100-200 ng/ml measured by RIA. The calculation of the CsA dose to be administered to the patient was based on the formula Q = Cl X C X 24, where Q was the dose to be administered to the patient to obtain a plasma level of 100 ng/ml CsA, Cl was the plasma clearance, and C was the required plasma level; 24 indicates that Q was calculated for a 24-hour continuous IV infusion.

In a series of 109 consecutive patients, the initial mean daily i.v. dose of CsA was 1.9 mg/kg with a range varying from 0.3 mg/kg to 10.5 mg/kg. The initial dose rapidly declined to a mean of 1.4 mg/kg. The mean oral dose given on day 21 was 1.2 mg/kg with a variation from 0 to 6.75 mg/kg. This decline of the dose administered reflected the high frequency of toxicity related to the accumulation of the drug during the first weeks. A correct prediction of plasma levels was usually achieved during the first week with a mean plasma level of 100 ± 14.2 ng/ml. During the first month, the mean plasma level remained around 100 ng/ml with large individual variations from 32 to 840 ng/ml. At 12 weeks, as the dose of CsA was slowly decreased, the mean trough level was 64 ± 75 ng/ml, and the mean peak level 113 ± 87 ng/ml. Overall, during the first month of treatment, 30 patients had a plasma level below 75 ng/ml, 35 between 75 and 140 ng/ml, and 23 above 140 ng/ml. In 88 patients, GVHD was graded 0 in 13 patients, I in 51 patients, II in 10 patients, and III-IV in 14 patients. The median date of appearance

Table 2 CSA Pharmacokinetic Parameters in Adults

C_{max} = 6,790 ± 5,200 ng/mL (2,010-23,600 ng/mL)
First half-life = 0.45 ± 0.27 h (0.06-2.44 h)
Second half-life = 6.49 ± 5.37 h (1.30-38.6 h)
First slope = 2.36 ± 1.93 L/h (0.48-11.6 L/h)
Second slope = 0.16 ± 0.10 L/h (0.02-0.53 L/h)
Plasma clearance = 14 ± 11 mL/min/kg (2-79 mL/min/kg)
Vc = 1.0 ± 1.6 L/kg (0.2-17.0 L/kg)
Vdss = 4.4 ± 4.2 L/kg (0.2-26.4 L/kg)

was 15 days, with only 5% of GVHD appearing after day 35. There was no correlation between GVHD and CsA plasma levels (p = 0.2), although there was a trend toward a higher frequency of GVHD in the low plasma level group.

Renal toxicity was defined as a rise of creatinine to ⩾1.13 mg/dl (100 μmol/L). Creatinine was found to be abnormal after transplant in 15 of 100 cases; 13 patients had a normal creatinine throughout the posttransplant course, and 72 patients had a transient rise of creatinine. There was a correlation between CsA plasma levels and a rise of creatinine (p = 0.05). Liver abnormality was defined as a rise of transaminases by a factor of >2, and a rise of alkaline phosphatase of more than 250 I.U. Fifty-three of 100 patients had abnormal liver function studies before transplant, 7 remained normal after transplantation, and in 40 patients liver abnormalities appeared after transplantation without correlation with CsA plasma levels (p = 2). Overall, 81 patients had no or mild toxicity, and the treatment was never interrupted, 26 patients (24%) had a transient or permanent interruption of CsA. In 6 cases, interruption was because of severe liver failure, in 5 cases because of renal failure, and in 13 cases because of the association of renal and liver failure.

Other signs of intolerance were observed, including most commonly a sensation of burning pain in the extremities, nausea, vomiting, and tremor. Hypertension was observed in 60% of patients; it usually responded to specific therapy and never led to an interruption of CsA.

Tallman et al. (19) compared two intravenous infusion schedules: CsA given once daily over 12-18 hours in intravenous lipids, and CsA given twice daily as a one-hour i.v. infusion. All patients received the same dose of 3 mg/kg/day. Both the absolute and actuarial risks of developing renal dysfunction and acute GVH were similar. However, the continuous i.v. infusion group experienced less hypertension, paresthesias, and flushing.

In our study including 133 patients with acute leukemia, chronic granulocytic leukemia and severe aplastic anemia, CsA was associated with an incidence of grades II-IV GVHD of 35%, an incidence of chronic GVHD of 45%, and a 2-year actuarial survival of 55.4%. A Cox multivariate analysis showed that the initial diagnosis was the main prognostic factor. GVHD grades II-IV was observed in 45% of patients transplanted for severe aplastic anemia, and in 25% of patients transplanted for leukemia (p = 0.02). Chronic GVHD was observed in 17% and 5% of patients, respectively. This difference was not explained by other factors known to increase the risk of GVHD such as age or donor sex.

The above study was aimed at obtaining constant plasma levels with minimal toxicity. Other investigators prefer to use a standard dose, usually 3-5 mg/kg i.v. on day 1, and adjusted subsequently to CsA plasma levels and to renal toxicity. The initial oral dose, usually beginning on day 21, is 6.25 mg/kg every 12 hours. Thereafter, the dose is reduced or the drug withheld in case of renal failure. This treatment is continued for 3 months to one year and slowly tapered.

B. Drug Interactions

Many adverse drug interactions have been described. In our series of patients, some of these drugs were systematically used. Ketoconazole is known to increase CsA toxicity. For this reason, all preliminary pharmacokinetic studies were performed while the patients were on ketoconazole for at least 48 hours. The combined use of ketoconazole with CsA explains why the doses used were lower than those usually reported in the literature. Other drugs systematically used in our patients for prevention of infection such as acyclovir or the quinolone pefloxacine were not found to interact with the metabolism of CsA. Some patients received i.v. antibiotics for treatment of infection. Among these antibiotics, aminoglycosides, macrolides, cotrimoxazole, and amphotericin B have been described to increase the renal toxicity of CsA. In our series, aminoglycosides were associated with renal toxicity in 37 of 62 treatments (59%), macrolides in 13 of 35 treatments (35%), cotrimoxazole in 3 of 28 treatments (10%), and amphotericin B in 10 of 60 treatments (16%). Therefore, aminoglycosides seem to be the most toxic drug. For this reason, their use has been completely abandoned in the treatment of nondocumented infections (18).

Numerous investigators have reported drug interactions with CsA. An increase in CsA concentrations was observed not only with ketoconazole (22), but also diltiazem (23), danazol, norethisterone (24), and high dose methylprednisolone (25). A reduced CsA concentration occurs after rifampicin, phenytoin, phenobarbital (26), and erythromycin (27,28). The nephrotoxic agents that have been shown to potentiate the nephrotoxic effect of CsA include aminoglycosides, diltiazem, amphotericin B (29), melphalan, and cotrimoxazole (30).

C. Drug Monitoring

The importance of monitoring the CsA plasma or blood levels has not been clearly demonstrated. Many authors agree that very high plasma levels (above 500 ng/ml) correlate with increased renal toxicity. We have shown a trend toward an increased incidence of acute GVHD in patients with CsA plasma levels below 75 ng/ml, and an increased rate of renal dysfunction and hypertension in the group of patients with plasma CsA levels above 200 ng/ml (20). This correlation was not significant in a second study and was expressed only as a trend (18). Yee et al. showed that the trough CsA concentration for a given week was significantly associated with the risk of GVHD developing during the following week (21). The relative risks were 0.7 for every increase of 100 ng/ml in CsA concentration and 1.0, 0.6, 0.2 for concentrations of less than 100, 100 to 199 and 200 or more ng/ml respectively (p = 0.01). These data indicate that low CsA concentrations can be a cause of treatment failure and that concentrations should be monitored in recipients of marrow transplants. This may be true but difficult to adapt to daily patient care because it is not rare to observe renal impairment with low CsA plasma levels. New methods of monitoring or the ability to detect the nephrotoxic metabolites of CsA may improve the safety of the drug.

D. Toxicity

The most disturbing side effect of CsA is nephrotoxicity, which is usually reversible upon dose reduction and is most easily monitored by following serum creatinine levels (31-33).

Reversible central nervous toxicity has been noted and may be aggravated by CsA-induced hypomagnesemia (34-36) or by hypocholesterolemia as described in liver transplant patients (37). Paresthesias may be severe enough to lead to the interruption of drug administration. Seizures are often found in children; they are not always associated with hypertension. Hypertension has been reported in 23-60% of CsA-treated patients. Its mechanism is not well known but may be related to hypomagnesemia and is usually easily controlled by standard antihypertensive therapy (38-40). Other side effects include tremor, anorexia, nausea, vomiting, hirsutism, and gum hypertrophy.

E. Impact on Survival

The effect of CsA on prevention of GVHD and survival has been extensively studied. Overall, both retrospective and prospective randomized studies comparing MTX to CsA have failed to show any improvement of survival and incidence of GVHD in patients transplanted for hematological malignancies. The reported incidence of grades II-IV GVHD in patients treated with CsA alone varies from 28 to 54% (41-46). Storb et al. (15) reported a long-term followup of three randomized studies comparing MTX to CsA for prevention of GVHD. This study involved 179 patients transplanted for acute nonlymphoblastic leukemia in first complete remission, chronic granulocytic leukemia in chronic or accelerated phase, and leukemia in advanced stage. CsA and MTX were comparable regarding the likelihood of acute and chronic GVHD, interstitial pneumonitis, leukemic relapse, and long-term survival. These findings agree with those of two controlled trials comparing MTX and CsA that were reported from Stockholm (46) and Sydney (43). The IBMTR reported the same incidence of GVHD in the groups of patients treated with CsA or MTX (1). In severe aplastic anemia, CsA may be beneficial in patients conditioned with cyclophosphamide alone because it decreases both the incidence of acute and chronic GVHD and also the incidence of rejection (42). In an IBMTR study on aplastic anemia, patients treated with MTX had a higher relative risk of rejection (RR:3.1 (p = 0.02)), of acute GVHD (RR:1.2), and of interstitial pneumonitis (RR:2.4). Survival was better in the CsA group, with a 2-year probability of survival at 2 years of 82% as compared to 65% in the MTX-treated group (47).

Some investigators have described an increase of leukemic relapses in CsA-treated patients, an observation that still requires confirmation.

IV. COMBINED IMMUNOSUPPRESSION: CSA AND "SHORT" MTX

The combination of CsA and short-course MTX seems to be more successful than either drug alone and is now extensively used worldwide. In experimental studies in dogs, Deeg et al. showed that the survival rate of dogs given DLA nonidentical unrelated marrow was increased from 6% with CsA or MTX alone to 35% with the combination (48), and that of recipients of DLA haploidentical littermate marrow from 8 to 70% (49). On the basis of these results Storb et al. (50) performed a prospective randomized study, in a series of 46 patients with severe aplastic anemia, comparing standard MTX to CsA combined with MTX, given at doses of 15 mg/m^2 i.v. on day 1, and 10 mg/m^2 on days 3, 6, and 11 postgrafting. There was a significant reduction in the cumulative incidence of grade II to IV acute GVHD, with 18% incidence in the MTX/CsA group compared to 53% in the CsA group (p = 0.012). The actuarial survival at 2 years was 82% in the MTX/CsA group and 60% in the MTX group (p = 0.062). There was no difference in the incidence of chronic GVHD.

A second study performed by the same team compared MTX/CsA alone in 93 patients with acute nonlymphoblastic leukemia in first remission or chronic granulocytic leukemia in chronic phase (51). A significant reduction in the cumulative incidence of grades II to IV acute GVHD was observed in patients who received MTX/CsA (33%), as compared to those receiving CsA alone (54%) (p = 0.014). The actuarial survival rates in the two groups at 1.5 years were 80% and 50%, respectively (p = 0.062). These results were confirmed in other nonrandomized studies showing a significant reduction of GVHD with the combination of MTX/CsA compared to historical controls (18,52). In most of these studies, the followup was too short to determine the effect of this treatment on chronic GVHD, long-term survival, and leukemic relapses.

One of the major concerns is that of the well-known inverse relationship between GVHD and leukemic relapse, illustrated by the increased probability of relapse in twin transplants, in patients without GVHD, and more recently in patients receiving T-cell-depleted marrow. Leukemic relapse has apparently been seen more often in patients with chronic granulocytic leukemia, and less in acute nonlymphoblastic leukemia; patients with acute lymphoblastic leukemia seem to have an intermediate risk. It is not known, as yet, if an improvement of immunosuppression for prevention of GVHD will increase the number of relapses. A study performed by the Toronto team (53) compared a group of patients treated with MTX and prednisone to a group treated with MTX/CsA. This study confirmed the diminution of acute GVHD, and the improvement of survival in the MTX/CsA group. However, there was a significantly increased relapse rate in the MTX/CsA group, which was more pronounced in patients with chronic granulocytic leukemia in first chronic phase: there were 6/13 cytogenetic and clinical relapses in the MTX/CsA group compared to 1/22 in the MTX/prednisone group (p = 0.01). In all disease categories, relapses occurred significantly earlier in the group receiving MTX/CsA. The Seattle team did not confirm this increased relapse rate in a series of 129 patients with chronic granulocytic leukemia in chronic phase receiving either MTX, CsA, or MTX/CsA. The only predictor of survival was the interval from diagnosis to transplant (54).

V. OTHER COMBINATIONS

In two studies comparing MTX to MTX + ATG prophylaxis, there was no difference between ATG + MTX and MTX alone in terms of GVHD and survival (55,56). The Minnesota team reported that when ATG was combined with MTX and prednisone, the incidence of GVHD was decreased from 48% in patients receiving MTX alone to 21% in the combined therapy group. There was no significant difference in survival between the two groups, and the incidence of chronic GVHD was the same. Thus, it appeared that ATG did not offer any additional benefit for GVHD prophylaxis.

The addition of prednisone to CsA or MTX has been studied by two groups. In a study performed at the Baltimore transplant unit, patients were randomized to receive either cyclophosphamide and prednisone or CsA and prednisone (57). The probability of developing acute GVHD was 0.68 in the cyclophosphamide/prednisone group and 0.32 in the CsA/prednisone group, and the probability of survival in the former was only half that in the latter. Similar results have been reported by the City of Hope transplant team (58), whose patients were randomized to receive MTX/prednisone or CsA/prednisone. In the MTX group 47% of patients developed GVHD while 28% of patients in the CsA group developed GVHD. There was a better survival in the CsA group. In both studies, despite the decrease of acute GVHD, there was no effect on chronic GVHD.

VI. NEW APPROACHES

This review has shown that attempts at preventing GVHD by various immunosuppressive drugs have been largely unsatisfactory, since as many as 30% of patients receiving a genotypically HLA-identical bone marrow transplant will die directly or indirectly from this complication. This problem is more critical in the case of matched unrelated or mismatched bone marrow transplants, where it has been shown that the risk of GVHD increases with the number of HLA antigen disparities.

As discussed in Chapter 19, the use of monoclonal anti-T-cell antibodies in vitro or in vivo results in a substantial reduction in the incidence of GVHD. This, approach, however, has resulted in an increased incidence of engraftment failure and impaired immunoreconstitution. New immunosuppression agents or new derivatives of CsA should also be tested, but these compounds have not yet been entered in clinical trials. Clearly, additional studies utilizing novel approaches are needed.

ACKNOWLEDGEMENT

To the physicians and nurses of the Bone Marrow Transplant Unit, and to the secretarial help of Mrs. Poulet.

REFERENCES

1. Gale RP, Bortin MM, Van Bekkum DW, Biggs JG, Dicke KA, Gluckman E, Good RA, Hoffmann RG, Kay HEM, Kersey JH, Marmont A, Masaoka T, Rimm AA, Van Rood JJ, Zwaan FE: Risk factors for acute graft versus host disease. Brit J Haematol 1987; 67:397-406.

2. Bross DS, Tutschka PJ, Farmer ER, Beschorner WE, Braine HG, Mellits ED, Bias WB, Santos GW: Predictive factors for acute graft versus host disease in patients transplanted with HLA identical bone marrow. Blood 1984;63:1265-1270.

3. Shulman HM, Sullivan KM, Weiden PL, McDonald GB, Striker GE, Sale GE, Hackman R, Tsoi M, Storb R, Thomas ED: Chronic graft versus host syndrome in man. A long term clinico-pathologic study for 20 Seattle patients. Amer J Med 1980,69:204-218.

4. Storb R, Pentice RL, Sullivan KM, Shulman HM, Deeg HJ, Doney KC, Buckner CD, Clift RA, Witherspoon RP, Appelbaum FA, Sanders JE, Stewart PS, Thomas ED: Predictive factors in chronic graft versus host disease in patients with aplastic anemia treated by marrow transplantation from HLA identical siblings. Ann Int Med 1983;98:461-466.

5. Vogelsang GB, Hess AD, Berkman A, Tutschka P, Farmer E, Converse P, Santos GW: An in vitro predictive test for graft versus host disease in patients with genotypic HLA identical bone marrow transplants. N Engl J Med 1985;313:645-650.

6. Bagot M, Cordonnier C, Tilkin FF, Heslan M, Vernant JP, Dubertret L, Levy JP: A possible predictive test for graft versus host disease in bone marrow graft recipients: the mixed epidermal cell-lymphocyte reaction. Transplantation 1986; 41:316-319.

7. Storb R, Epstein RB, Graham TC, Thomas ED: Methotrexate regimens for control of graft versus host disease in dogs with allogeneic marrow grafts. Transplantation 1970,9:240-246.

8. Thomas ED, Storb R, Clift RA, Fefer A, Johnson FL, Neiman PE, Lerner KG, Glucksberg H, Buckner CD: Bone marrow transplantation. N Engl J Med 1975; 292:832-843.

9. Elfenbein G, Graham-Pole J, Weiner R, Goedert T, Gross T: Consequences of no prophylaxis for acute graft versus host disease after HLA identical bone marrow transplantation. Blood 1987;Suppl. 1,305.

10. Lazarus HH, Coccia PF, Herzig RH, Graham-Pole J, Gross S, Strandjord S, Gordon

E, Cheung N-KV, Warkentin PI, Spitzer TR, Warm SE. Incidence of acute graft versus host disease with and without methotrexate prophylaxis in allogeneic bone marrow transplant patients. Blood 1984;64:215-220.

11. Sullivan KM, Deeg HJ, Sanders J, Klosterman A, Amos D, Shulman H, Sale G, Martin P, Witherspoon R, Appelbaum F, Doney K, Stewart P, Meyers J, McDonald GB, Weiden P, Fefer A, Buckner CD, Storb R, Thomas ED: Hyperacute graft vs host disease in patients not given immunosuppression after allogeneic marrow transplantation. Blood 1986;67:1172-1175.

12. Weiden PL, Doney K, Storb R, Thomas ED: Anti-human thymocyte globulin for prophylaxis of graft versus host disease: a randomized trial in patients with leukemia treated with HLA identical sibling matched grafts. Transplantation 1979;27:227-230.

13. Deeg HJ, Storb R, Thomas ED, Flournoy N, Kennedy MS, Banaj M, Appelbaum FR, Bensinger WI, Buckner CD, Clift RA, Doney K, Fefer A, McGuffin R, Sanders JE, Singer J, Stewart P, Sullivan KM, Witherspoon RP: Cyclosporine as prophylaxis for graft versus host disease: a randomized study in patients undergoing marrow transplantation for acute nonlymphocytic leukemia. Blood 1985;65:1325-1334.

14. Weiner RS, Bortin MM, Gale RP, Gluckman E, Kay HEM, Kolb HJ, Martz AJ, Rimm AA: Interstitial pneumonitis after bone marrow transplantation. Assessment of risk factors. Ann Int Med 1986;104:168.

15. Storb R, Deeg HJ, Fischer L, Appelbaum F, Buckner CD, Bensinger W, Clift R, Doney K, Irle C, McGuffin R, Martin P, Sanders J, Schoch G, Singer J, Stewart P, Sullivan K, Witherspoon R, Thomas ED: Cyclosporine vs. methotrexate for graft vs. host disease prevention in patients given marrow grafts for leukemia: long term follow-up of three controlled trials. Blood 1988;71:293-298.

16. Atkinson K, Biggs JC, Ting A, Concannon AJ, Dodds AJ, Pun A: Cyclosporin A is associated with faster engraftment and less mucositis than Methotrexate after allogeneic bone marrow transplantation. Brit J Haematol 1983;53:265-270.

17. Lokiec F, Fischer A, Gluckman E: A safer approach to the clinical use of Cyclosporine: the predose calculation. Transplant Proc 1986;18,Suppl.5:194-199.

18. Gluckman E, Devergie A. Lokiec F: Use of Cyclosporine for prevention of graft versus host disease after allogeneic bone marrow transplantation. Transplant Proc 1988;20:461-469.

19. Tallman MS, Nemunaitis JJ, McGuire TR, Yee GC, Hughes TE, Almgren JD, Appelbaum FR, Higano CS, McGuffin RW, Singer JW, Thomas ED: Comparison of two intravenous Cyclosporine infusion schedules in marrow transplant recipients. Transplantation 1988;45:810-812.

20. Gluckman E, Lokiec F, Devergie A: Pharmacokinetic monitoring of Cyclosporine A in allogeneic bone marrow transplant. Transplant Proc 1985;17:500-501.

21. Yee GC, Self SG, McGuire TR, Carlin J, Sanders JE, Deeg HJ: Serum Cyclosporine concentration and risk of acute graft versus host disease after allogeneic marrow transplantation. N Engl J Med 1988;319:65-70.

22. Diererink H, Moller J: Ketoconazole and Cyclosporine. Lancet 1982;II:1218.

23. Pochet JM, Pirson Y: Cyclosporin-Diltiazem interaction. Lancet 1986;I:979.

24. Ross WB, Roberts D, Griffin PJA, Salaman JR: Cyclosporine interaction with danazol and norethesterone. Lancet 1986;I:330.

25. Ost C, Klintmalm G, Ringden O: Mutual interaction between Prednisolone and Cyclosporine in renal transplant patients. Transplant Proc 1985;17:1232.

26. Duncan JI, Whiting PH, Simplson JG, Thomson AW: Alleviation of Cyclosporine mediated nephrotoxicity by Phenobarbitone during the suppression of graft versus host reactivity. Transplant Proc 1986;18:650-651.

27. Martell R, Heinrichs D, Stiller CR, Jenner M, Keown PA, Dupre J: The effects of erythromycin in patients treated with cyclosporine. Ann Int Med 1986;104:660-661.

28. Murray BM, Edwards L, Morse GD, Kohli RQ, Venuto RC: Clinically important interaction of Cyclosporine and erythromycin. Transplantation 1987;43:602-603.

29. Kenned MS, Deeg HJ, Siegel M, Crowley JJ, Storb R, Thomas ED: Acute renal toxicity with combined use of Amphotericin B and Cyclosporine after marrow transplantation. Transplantation 1983;35:211-215.

30. Thompson JF, Chalmers DHK, Hunnisett AGW, Wood RFM, Morris PJ: Nephrotoxicity of trimethoprim and cotrimoxazole in renal allograft recipients treated with Cyclosporine. Transplantation 1983;36:204-206.

31. Gluckman E, Devergie A, Lokiec F, Poirier O, Baumelou A: Nephrotoxicity of Cyclosporine A in bone marrow transplantation. Lancet 1981;II:144-145.

32. Shulman H, Striker G, Deeg HJ, Kennedy M, Storb R, Thomas ED: Nephrotoxicity of Cyclosporin A after allogeneic marrow transplantation: glomerular thrombosis and tubular injury. N Engl J Med 1981;305:1392-1394.

33. Yee GC, Kennedy MS, Deeg HJ, Leonard TM, Thomas ED, Storb R: Cyclosporine associated renal dysfunction in marrow transplant recipients. Transplant Proc 1984; 17:196-201.

34. Thompson CB, June CH, Sullivan KM, Thomas ED: Association between Cyclosporin neurotoxicity and hypomagnesemia. Lancet 1984;II:1116-1119.

35. June CH, Thompson CB, Kennedy MS, Nims J, Thomas ED: Profound hypomagnesemia and renal magnesium wasting associated with the use of Cyclosporine for marrow transplantation. Transplantation 1985;39:620-623.

36. Atkinson K, Biggs J, Darveniza P, Boland J, Concannon A, Dodds A: Cyclosporine associated central nervous system toxicity after allogeneic bone marrow transplantation. Transplantation 1984;38:34-36.

37. De Groen PC, Aksamit AJ, Rakela J, Forbes GS, Krom RAE: Central nervous system toxicity after liver transplantation. The role of Cyclosporine and cholesterol. N Engl J Med 1987;317:861-866.

38. Loughran TP, Deeg HJ, Dahlberg S, Kennedy MS, Storb R, Thomas ED: Incidence of hypertension after bone marrow transplantation among 112 patients randomized to either Cyclosporine or Methotrexate as graft versus host disease prophylaxis. Brit J Haematol 1985,59:547-554.

39. Lustig S, Stern N, Lee DBN, Berger ME, Eggena P, Balabanian NI, Golub MS: Mechanisms of Cyclosporine A hypertension. Transplant Proc 1987;19:1262-1264.

40. June CH, Thompson CB, Kennedy MS, Loughran JP, Deeg HJ: Correlation of hypomagnesemia with the onset of Cyclosporine associated hypertension in marrow transplant patients. Transplantation 1986;41:47-51.

41. Vogelsang GB, Hess AD, Santos GW: Acute graft versus host disease clinical characteristics in the Cyclosporine era. Medicine 1988;67:163-174.

42. Hows J, Harris R, Palmer S, Gordon-Smith EG: Immunosuppression with Cyclosporin A in allogeneic bone marrow transplantation for severe aplastic anaemia: preliminary studies. Brit J Haematol 1981;48:227-236.

43. Biggs JC, Atkinson K, Gillett E, Downs K, Concannon A, Dodds A: A randomized prospective trial comparing Cyclosporine and Methotrexate given for prophylaxis of graft versus host disease after bone marrow transplantation. Transplant Proc 1986; 18:253-255.

44. Storb R, Deeg HJ, Thomas ED, et al.: Marrow transplantation for chronic myelocytic leukemia: a controlled trial of Cyclosporine versus Methotrexate for prophylaxis of graft versus host disease. Blood 1985;66:698-702.

45. Storb R, Deeg HJ, Thomas ED, Appelbaum FR, Buckner CD, Cheever MA, Clift RA, Doney KC, Flournoy N, Kennedy MS, Loughran TP, McGuffin RW, Sale GE, Sanders JR, Singer JW, Stewart PS, Sullivan KM, Witherspoon RP: Marrow transplantation for chronic myelocytic leukemia: a controlled trial of Cyclosporine versus Methotrexate for prophylaxis of graft versus host disease. Blood 1985;66:698-702.

46. Ringden O, Backman L, Lonnquist B, Heimdahl A, Lindholm A, Bolme P, Gahrton G: A randomized trial comparing use of Cyclosporin and Methotrexate for graft versus host disease. Prophylaxis in bone marrow transplant recipients with haematologic malignancies. Bone Marrow Transplant 1986;1:41-51.

47. Gluckman E, Horowitz M, Esperou H, Devergie A: Influence of conditioning and prophylaxis of graft versus host disease on the results of bone marrow transplantation for severe aplastic anemia. Recent advances in bone marrow transplantation, UCLA Symposia on molecular and cellular biology. (Eds. R Pgale, RE Champlin), Alan R. Liss, New York; 1989; 1-8.

48. Deeg HJ, Storb R, Weiden PL, Raff RF, Sale GE, Atkinson K, Graham TC, Thomas ED: Cyclosporin A and Methotrexate in canine marrow transplantation. Engraftment, graft versus host disease and induction of tolerance. Transplantation 1982; 34:30-35.

49. Deeg HJ, Storb R, Appelbaum FR, Kennedy MS, Graham TC, Thomas ED: Combined immunosuppression with Cyclosporine and Methotrexate in dogs given bone marrow grafts from DLA haplo identical littermates. Transplantation 1984;37:62-65.

50. Storb R, Deeg HJ, Farewell V, Done K, Appelbaum F, Beatty P, Bensinger W, Buckner CD, Clift R, Hansen J, Hill R, Longton G, Lum L, Martin P, McGuffin R, Sanders J, Singer J, Stewart P, Sullivan K, Witherspoon R, Thomas ED: Marrow transplantation for severe aplastic anemia: Methotrexate and Cyclosporine for prevention of acute graft versus host disease. Blood 1986;68:119-125.

51. Storb R, Deeg JH, Whitehead J, Appelbaum F, Beatty P, Bensinger W, Buckner CD, Clift R, Doney K, Farewell V, Hansen J, Hill R, Lum L, Martin P, McGuffin R, Sanders J, Stewart P, Sullivan K, Witherspoon R, Yee G, Thomas ED: Methotrexate and Cyclosporine compared with Cyclosporine alone for prophylaxis of acute graft versus host disease after marrow transplantation for leukemia. N Engl J Med 1986; 314:729-735.

52. Tollemar J, Ringden O, Heimdahl A. Lonnquist B, Sundberg B: Decreased incidence and severity of graft versus host disease in HLA matched and mismatched marrow recipients of Cyclosporine and Methotrexate. Transplant Proc 1988;20,Suppl 3: 470-479.

53. Meharchand JM, Fyles GM, Minden MD, Curtis JE, Lockwood G, Tpitchler D, Messner HA: Acute graft versus host disease and relapse rate in allogeneic bone marrow transplant recipients receiving prophylaxis with Cyclosporine A and Methotrexate in comparison to Methotrexate and Prednisone. Experimental Hematol 1988; 16:517 (abstract).

54. Clift RA, Buckner CD, Storb R, Thomas ED: Transplantation regimens for chronic myelogenous leukemia (CML) in chronic phase (CP). Experimental Hematol 1988; 16:501 (abstract).

55. Doney KC, Weiden PL, Storb R, Thomas ED: Failure of early administration of antithymocyte globulin to lessen graft versus host disease in human allogeneic marrow transplant recipients. Transplantation 1981;31:141-143.

56. Ramsay NK, Kersey JH, Robinson LL, McGlave PB, Woods WG, Krivit W, Kin TH, Goldman AI, Nesbit ME: A randomized study of the prevention of acute graft versus host disease. N Engl J Med 1982;306:293-397.

57. Santos GW, Tutschka PJ, Brookmeyer R, Saral R, Beschorner WE, Bias WB, Braine HG, Burns WH, Farmer ER, Hess AD, Kaizer H, Mellits D, Sensenbrenner L, Stuart

R, Yeager A: Cyclosporine plus methyl prednisolone versus Cyclophosphamide plus methyl prednisolone as prophylaxis for graft versus host disease: a randomized double blind study in patients undergoing allogeneic marrow transplantation. Clin Transplantation 1987;1:21-28.

58. Forman SJ, Blume KG, Krance RA, Miner PJ, Metler GE, Hill LR, O'Donnell MR, Nademanee AP, Snyder DS: A prospective randomized study of acute graft versus host disease in 107 patients with leukemia. Methotrexate/Prednisone versus Cyclosporine/Prednisone. Transplant Proc 1987;21:2605-2607.

21

Gnotobiotic Measures for the Prevention of Acute Graft-vs.-Host Disease

Jaak M. Vossen
University Hospital
Leiden, The Netherlands

Peter J. Heidt
Radiobiological Institute TNO
Rijswijk, The Netherlands

I. INTRODUCTION

The effectiveness of gnotobiotic measures for the prevention of delayed-type Graft-vs.-Host Disease (GVHD) in experimental models of allogeneic bone marrow transplantation (BMT) led several groups of clinical investigators to apply such measures to allogeneic BMT in man. The experimental data underlying the efforts to employ methods for protective isolation against exogenous microbial contamination and to try to eliminate endogenous microorganisms residing in the gastrointestinal (GI) tract of children and adults receiving a bone marrow graft are summarized in Table 1, as far as they are relevant to the prevention of acute GVHD.

Acute GVHD in the MHC-matched donor-recipient combination in man, the symptoms of which usually start between one and 7 weeks after allogeneic BMT, is the equivalent of the experimental delayed-type GVHD as seen in the MHC-mismatched donor-recipient combination in the mouse. Any variable which may affect the development of delayed-type GVHD can only be studied in that MHC-mismatched model because the GvH-inducing potential of rodent bone marrow is very low due to its low content of mature T lymphocytes, i.e., less than 2% of nucleated bone marrow cells (1). In contrast, bone marrow aspirate of primates, including man, contains 20-40% of mature T lymphocytes, and consequently has a high GVHD-inducing potential, even in the MHC-matched allogeneic donor-recipient combination. In dogs, bone marrow aspirates contain a number of mature T lymphocytes in between that of rodents and primates (2). The composition of the bone marrow graft with respect to number (and maybe specific immune competence) of mature T lymphocytes should be taken into consideration, when extrapolating data from animal models to man. The number of T lymphocytes grafted has a major impact on the risk to provoke GVHD in man, and depleting the graft of T lymphocytes has an obvious beneficial effect in this respect.

Table 1 Data on the Effect of Gnotobiotic Measures for the Prevention of Delayed-
Type GVHD in Animal Models

Experimental model	Protective isolation	Effect on delayed-type GvHD		
		MHC-matched	MHC-mismatched	Ref.
Germfree mice	SPI[a]	n.d.	+	3,4
Completely decontaminated mice	SPI[a]	n.d.	+	4-6
Selectively decontaminated mice	SPI[a]			
associated with CRF[b]		n.d.	+	4
associated with conventional anaerobes[c]		n.d.	–	7
Selectively decontaminated dogs	PPI[d]			
associated with conventional anaerobes[c]		+	n.d.	8
Completely decontaminated monkeys	SPI[a]	n.d.	+[e]	9,10

[a]SPI: strict protective isolation.

[b]CRF: "colonization resistance flora," obtained from a SPF-mouse colony and composed largely of spore-forming gram-positive anaerobic bacteria, mainly different *Clostridium spp.* (11).

[c]Conventional anaerobes: wild-type anaerobic intestinal microflora.

[d]PPI: partial protective isolation.

[e]Mismatched either for class I or class II MHC antigens, grafted with 1 log T-cell-depleted bone marrow.

n.d. = not done.

Besides the relative number of mature T lymphocytes in the graft, there is at least one other variable which has an effect on the risk of developing delayed-type GVHD in animal models, i.e., the composition of the intestinal microflora of the recipient. From the data in Table 1 it can be concluded that absence or complete elimination of GI tract microflora in mice prevents the development of delayed-type GVHD in MHC-mismatched recipient mice effectively. This effect can be abrogated by adding mature T lymphocytes, e.g., from the spleen, to the graft (12). In addition, the duration of absence or suppression of the gut microflora was found to be critical; these conditions were required from about 10 days before (13) until about 40 days after BMT (14). A similar beneficial effect on the occurrence of GVHD was observed when recipient mice were only selectively decontaminated of their facultative anaerobic microorganisms, leaving the strict anaerobic part of their endogenous microflora intact (4). However, the composition of the residing strict anaerobic gut microflora seems to limit the effectiveness of this approach: success was achieved in cases where the anaerobic gut microflora was composed mainly of gram-positive microorganisms, as obtained by decontaminating specific pathogen-free animals in strict protective isolation. Recent observations showed that the beneficial effect was no longer observed when recipient mice kept under conventional conditions and harbouring a wild-type anaerobic intestinal flora were used as graft recipients following selective gastrointestinal decontamination (GID) (7). In dogs, obtained from a breeding colony for experimental animals (TNO-Zeist, The Netherlands) and maintained under conditions of partial protective isolation, a beneficial effect of the suppression of the facultative anaerobic GI tract microflora on the development of delayed-type GVHD was observed-

(8). A similar effect was seen in completely decontaminated rhesus monkeys, kept in strict protective isolation and grafted with 1 log T-cell-depleted partially MHC-mismatched bone marrow cells (see Table 1).

Based on the data obtained in animal experiments we treated all children (n = 89), suffering from either bone marrow failure (severe aplastic anemia, myelodysplastic syndrome, Fanconi's anemia), leukemia (acute nonlymphoblastic leukemia (ANLL), acute lymphoblastic leukemia (ALL), chronic myelogenous leukemia (CML)), or non-Hodgkin lymphoma (NHL), and admitted consecutively from end-1971 until end-1988 to our department for BMT, under conditions of strict protective isolation, using different regimens for gastrointestinal decontamination in succession. Here we report on the retrospective evaluation of these gnotobiotic measures for the prevention of acute GVHD in these children. Extensive data on bacterial and fungal infections, and on GVHD, both acute and chronic, of the first 65 cases are presented elsewhere (15).

II. PATIENTS AND METHODS

A. Patients

All 89 children and adolescents grafted consecutively from end-1971 until end-1988 for bone marrow failure, leukemia, or NHL were included in this retrospective evaluation. For all but two patients an HLA genotypically identical sibling was available for bone marrow donation. The two exceptions were one 9-year-old girl, grafted for ALL in third remission, whose sibling donor was genotypically haploidentical, phenotypically one-locus mismatched at HLA-A and mixed-lymphocyte-culture (MLC) negative, and one 7-year-old girl, grafted for ANLL in second remission, whose sibling donor was MHC-class I genotypically identical, but MHC class II haploidentical (and MLC reactive) due to crossing over. The patients were classified into three groups, because of major differences in the antimicrobial gastrointestinal decontamination regimens, and additionally of minor modifications in the drugs used following BMT for the suppression of GVHD. The three groups of patients, whose characteristics are given in Table 2, correspond chronologically to different time periods, i.e., end-1971-1977 (first part of group I), 1977-1982 (group II), 1982-1986 (second part of group I), and 1986 to end-1988 (group III).

B. Bone Marrow Transplantation

All patients received bone marrow grafts following the usual pretreatment regimens, i.e., either cyclophosphamide (50 mg/kg/day X 4) alone or cyclophosphamide (idem) plus procarbazine (15 mg/kg/day X 3) and rabbit antithymocyte globulin (2 mg/kg/day X 3), or cyclophosphamide (idem) plus total body irradiation (TBI, 400 cGy, high dose rate, in one session) for children with severe aplastic anemia and Fanconi's anemia. Cyclophosphamide (60 mg/kg/day X 2) plus TBI (700-800 cGy, high dose rate, in one session, depending on age) was given for leukemia, NHL, and myelodyplastic syndrome. From the six children with Fanconi's anemia, five were grafted before mid-1980 (belonging to groups I and II). They received 50 mg cyclophosphamide/kg/day X 4, whereas the Fanconi's anemia patient in group III received a reduced dose of cyclophosphamide, 5 mg/kg/day X 4. Thirty-eight patients of group I received methotrexate for GVHD prophylaxis until day +102 after BMT (16), and six received cyclosporin A (2 mg/kg/day in continuous i.v. infusion for ≥ two months, followed by 6 mg/kg/day orally until at least

Table 2 Patient Characteristics

	Group I	Group II	Group III
Number of patients	44	21	24
Age (years) range	1-17	< 1-16	1-18
median	10	10	9
Sex M/F	23/21	12/9	14/10
Diagnosis SAA	11	12	1
Fanconi	2	3	1
MDS	2	1	3
ANLL	9	5	6
ALL	19	0	9
NHL	0	0	3
CML	1	2	1
Patients evaluable for acute GvHD	40	18	23

SAA = severe aplastic anemia; Fanconi = Fanconi's anemia; MDS = myelodysplastic syndrome; ANLL = acute non-lymphoblastic leukemia; ALL = acute lymphoblastic leukemia; NHL = non-Hodgkin's lymphoma; CML = chronic myelogenous leukemia.

6 months after BMT). All recipients of group II received methotrexate. Seven recipients of group III received methotrexate, three cyclosporin A, and the other 14 a combination of methotrexate (at day +1, +3, +6, and +11) and cyclosporin A (17).

C. Gnotobiotic Measures and Surveillance Cultures

All recipients of bone marrow grafts were maintained in strict protective isolation using laminar down flow isolators (18) and nursed using aseptic techniques and sterilization of food, beverages, and other items brought into the isolator (19). The isolation period started 2 weeks before BMT and lasted until 2-3 months after BMT, except when continuation of intensive therapy under protective isolation was needed, e.g., further parenteral nutrition and immunosuppressive therapy for severe gut GVHD. Antimicrobial drugs administered orally for complete gastrointestinal decontamination of patients in group I, selective gastrointestinal decontamination of patients in group II, and complete gastrointestinal decontamination of patients in group III are indicated, together with their daily dosages, in Table 3. Young children below the age of 2 years received half of the indicated dosages. The drugs were administered in four divided doses per day, except for co-trimoxazole, which was given twice daily. After complete gastrointestinal decontamination was discontinued, recontamination of the GI tract was performed by oral gavage of lyophylized cultures of *Lactobacillus acidophilus, Bifidobacterium bifidum*, and *Streptococcus thermophilus* (Biogarde®) and an anaerobic human-derived donor flora (20,21). When during the early period after BMT children were unable to swallow the drugs for complete gastrointestinal decontamination due to nausea and vomiting, the suppression of the gut microflora was continued by i.v. administration of co-trimoxazole and cefamandole in usual therapeutical dosages; this was only done in children of group III. Also, i.v. 5-flucytosine treatment was added to the oral administration of amphotericin B in individual cases of group III, when elimination of yeasts from the gut had not been successful, in order to suppress the further growing of these microorganisms.

Table 3 Antimicrobial Drugs for Complete and Selective Gastrointestinal Decontamination (daily dose)

Group I		Group II		Group III	
neomycin	2000 mg	nalidixic acid	90 mg[a,b]	gentamicin	800 mg
polymyxin B	2000 mg	co-trimoxazole	12/60 mg[a,b]	cephaloridin	2000 mg
cephaloridin	2000 mg	neomycin	15 mg[a]	amphotericin B	2000 mg
amphotericin B	2000 mg	polymyxin B	20 mg[a]		
		amphotericin B	2000 mg		

[a]per kg body weight.

[b]Used only in a limited number of patients.

Surveillance cultures from skin, nose, and throat swabs and samples of feces were performed twice weekly during the entire observation period, i.e., from 7 days before until 40 days after BMT. Culturing was focused at all aerobic and facultative anaerobic bacteria, yeasts, and fungi. After discontinuation of gastrointestinal decontamination, surveillance culturing was continued once weekly until discharge.

D. Evaluation of the Study

Gastrointestinal decontamination was considered successful when during the whole observation period, i.e., from day −7 to day +40, target microorganisms could not be cultured from more than two consecutive fecal samples. Target microorganisms were all bacteria, yeasts, and fungi in case of complete gastrointestinal decontamination, and gram-negative facultative anaerobic bacteria, e.g., *Enterobacteriaceae, Pseudomonas aeruginosa*, staphylococci, yeasts, and fungi in case of selective GI decontamination. GVHD was diagnosed by clinical symptoms and graded for severity according to Thomas et al. (22). In all cases of ⩾grade II GVHD, the diagnosis was confirmed by histology of skin, gut, or liver biopsies. Patients were considered at risk for GVHD when they survived for at least 50 days, had a proven engraftment of donor hematopoietic cells, and were not grafted with bone marrow from an identical twin donor; patients who developed acute GVHD before day +50 and died before that date were included into the evaluation. The probability of developing acute GVHD of ⩾grade II in children of the three different groups was estimated by actuarial survival curves and tested for possible significant differences by the Lee-Desu logrank test.

III. RESULTS

Four children of group I (two with no engraftment, one with syngeneic donor, one who died on day +15), three of group II (all three early deaths on days +1, +12, and +16, respectively), and one of group III (death on day +23) were not evaluable for the occurrence of acute GVHD. Figure 1 depicts the cumulative incidence of ⩾grade II acute GVHD in the evaluable children of the three different groups; it was 17.5% for group I, 50% for group II, and 4% for group III. Differences between group I and group II as well as between group III and group II were significant ($p < 0.05$). The difference between groups I and III was not significant. From this it can be concluded that complete gastrointestinal decontamination was superior to selective gastrointestinal decontamination in

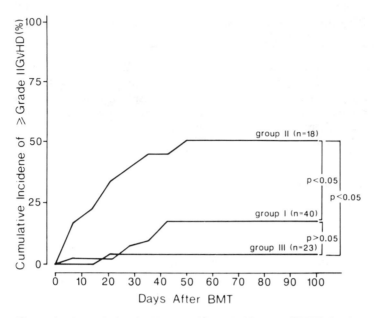

Figure 1 Cumulative incidence of ≥grade II acute GVHD in three groups of pediatric patients receiving an allogeneic bone marrow graft (for characteristics of patients of groups I, II, and III, see Table 2 and text).

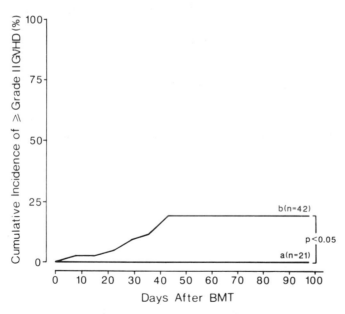

Figure 2 Cumulative incidence of ≥grade II acute GVHD in children grafted with allogeneic bone marrow under conditions of strict protective isolation and complete gastrointestinal decontamination (a: successful gastrointestinal decontamination (n = 21); b: unsuccessful gastrointestinal decontamination (n = 42)).

preventing ≥grade II acute GVHD in the children under study. Acute GVHD was the ultimate cause of death, either alone or in association with infectious complications, in two of seven cases in group I, five of nine cases in group II, and in no case in group III. The relative number of children with successful complete gastrointestinal decontamination, assessed as indicated above, was considerably lower than the relative number with successful selective gastrointestinal decontamination, i.e., 11 of 40 (27.5%) in group I, 10 of 23 (43.5%) in group III, and 14 of 18 (78%) in group II. The major reason for failure of gastrointestinal decontamination was persistence of *Candida albicans* in the GI tract, which occurred in 30-70% of the fecal cultures of the unsuccessful cases. In order to determine whether a successful complete gastrointestinal decontamination offered an additional advantage in preventing ≥grade II acute GVHD, its cumulative incidence was compared in children of groups I and III combined and then analyzed according to either success or failure of gastrointestinal decontamination. As can be seen from Figure 2, none of 21 children with successful complete gastrointestinal decontamination developed ≥grade II acute GVHD, whereas the cumulative incidence was 9% in the nonsuccessful group of 42 children ($p < 0.05$).

IV. DISCUSSION

This study on the possible effect of gastrointestinal decontamination on the development of acute GVHD was not prospectively randomized, but its results gain in weight because all children grafted with bone marrow for bone marrow failure, leukemia, or NHL in a single transplantation center were included. The principal conclusion which can be drawn from the data is that complete decontamination as compared to selective decontamination, of pediatric recipients of a T-cell replete bone marrow allograft effectively prevents the occurrence of ≥grade II acute GVHD. The cumulative incidence of GVHD was 17.5% in patients of group I and 4% in patients of group III, which is considerably lower than the 39 ± 4% for the age group 0.6 to 14.4 years reported in a recent evaluation of the International Bone Marrow Transplant Registry (23).

Studies performed by others on the possible effect of complete decontamination on acute GVHD gave controversial results: a reduction in the incidence of GVHD was reported by Mahmoud et al. (24) and Schmeiser et al. (25), but not by Leblond et al. (26) and Skinhøj et al. (27). Storb et al. (28) reported such an effect in recipients suffering from severe aplastic anemia, but not in recipients with leukemia (29). This discrepancy may either be due to the use of less strict criteria for the definition of success of complete decontamination or to too short a period of actual suppression of the gut microflora. Indeed, in the MHC-mismatched mouse BMT-model the effect on GVHD was only observed when the gut microflora had been eliminated from day −10 (13) until about day +40 (14).

Failures of complete decontamination were due to regrowth of microorganisms in the GI tract, mainly as a consequence of poor compliance due to nausea and vomiting in the early posttransplantation period. This involved especially *Candida albicans*. Replacing orally administered nonabsorbable antimicrobial drugs by temporary protection by systemic antimicrobial drugs administered i.v. (e.g., children in group III) most probably resulted in an improvement of the success rate of complete decontamination from 27.5 to 43.5%.

In the future, we will attempt to further increase the success rate of complete suppression of the gut microflora by the use of systemic antimicrobial drugs, excreted in considerable amounts as active substances in the bile, and by the administration of more active antimycotic drugs. However, the greater success rate of complete decontamination in children in group III cannot be the only reason for the efficient prevention of ≥grade II acute GVHD. In the 13 unsuccessfully decontaminated children, only a single case of GVHD was observed. A possible explanation for this very low incidence of GVHD may be that 14 of 23 children received the combination of methotrexate and cyclosporin A as GVHD prophylaxis, which was shown to be superior to cyclosporin A alone (17) and which is probably also superior to methotrexate alone. Cyclosporin A and methotrexate have comparable preventive effects for GVHD when used as single drugs (30).

In experimental animals, three parameters are of major importance for the possible development of acute GVHD: (1) MHC disparity between donor and recipient, (2) numbers of mature T lymphocytes in the graft, and (3) degree of suppression of the recipient's gut microflora. In an outbred species such as man, with a wild-type anaerobic gut microflora, the GVHD-inducing potential of a T-lymphocyte rich bone marrow graft in the MHC-matched donor-recipient combination can successfully be abrogated by complete decontamination, not by selective decontamination. A 2-3 log T-lymphocyte depletion of the bone marrow also has a clear effect on the prevention of GVHD in the MHC-matched donor-recipient combination (see Chapter 19), but may be associated with a considerable incidence of failure of engraftment, thus requiring an intensification of the conditioning regimen. In the patient population under study only 2 of 89 cases failed to achieve engraftment following the usual pretreatment for BMT. Both children suffered from severe aplastic anemia and had received multiple blood transfusions before BMT. They were pretreated with cyclophosphamide alone in the early transplantation era, i.e., end-1971 and beginning-1975. One must weigh the possible adverse effects of additional cytoreductive or immunosuppressive treatment in T-lymphocyte-depleted BMT, e.g., unacceptable late effects of more intensive irradiation on growth and development of children, a higher frequency of secondary malignancies, and a delay or defect of immunological reconstitution, against the advantages of such a BMT procedure.

In the MHC-mismatched donor-recipient combination in human BMT, T-lymphocyte depletion of the graft may be advantageous in preventing hyperacute GVHD. This type of GVHD disease resembles early-onset "acute-type" GVHD in experimental animals, a type of GVHD which cannot be mitigated by gnotobiotic measures (4,12). For BMT in man it is neither known how many T lymphocytes are acceptable in a bone marrow graft of a mismatched donor, nor to what extent donor and recipient may be disparate with respect to MHC antigens, in order for gnotobiotic measures in the host to have a modulatory effect on acute GVHD. The preclinical model of BMT in rhesus monkeys offers an excellent tool to study the fine tuning of all relevant variables, i.e., MHC-disparity, number of T lymphocytes in the graft, degree of suppression of the host microflora, and intensity of conditioning regimen, in order to obtain an optimum combination of conditions for success for BMT in man (31).

The mechanism by which complete suppression of the gut microflora in the bone marrow graft recipient has a clear beneficial effect on the occurrence of acute GVHD, as shown in this study, is still unknown. The most plausible explanation is that gnotobiotic measures either hamper or slow down the activation of T lymphocytes grafted into the recipient. This activation may either be a nonspecific one, for example, via IL-1 secretion by macrophages, resulting in a chain reaction of other lymphokines such as IL-2 and interferon-gamma, or a specific one via recognition of specific epitopes in association with the host MHC background. Some support for a possible nonspecific stimulation of the immune system after BMT comes from the finding of a significant difference between fecal concentrations of endotoxins in a small number of children incorporated into this study, i.e., six completely (mean concentration of 53.5 ng/g) versus seven selectively (mean concentration of 1360 ng/g) decontaminated children (32). Also, other macromolecular microbial substances, penetrating via the GI tract mucosa, may exert a polyclonal stimulation of the donor's immune competent cells. Similarly, the presence of EBV-infected cells in the recipient may generate a polyclonal T-lymphocyte activation in EBV-nonimmune donor cells, contributing to the development of GVHD (33). Besides a nonspecific immune stimulation, there is experimental evidence for a specific activation of donor T lymphocytes by bacterial antigens, cross-reacting with tissue antigens of the gut epithelium, resulting in intestinal lesions of GVHD as described by Van Bekkum and Knaan (34) using an elegant model of fetal gut transplants under the skin of grafted mice. Other indirect evidence comes from the finding of an increased GVHD-inducing potential of parous or transfused female donors for male recipients, indicating that previous (allo-) immunization of women may enhance a T-lymphocyte-mediated alloimmune response directed against tissues of the male graft recipient (23). There is also some indication that grafting cells from a bone marrow donor immune for HSV increases the risk of developing GVHD (33). This may be interpreted as a rapid activation of specific immune competent T lymphocytes, resulting in a response against cells of the graft recipient. The relationship between viral infections and GVHD is further described in Chapter 25.

ACKNOWLEDGMENT

The medical staff and other personnel of the BMT-unit for children at Leiden, Dr. H. F. L. Guiot and co-workers, and Dr. J Hermans are gratefully acknowledged for their contributions.

REFERENCES

1. Bekkum DW van, de Vries MJ: *Radiation Chimeras*. Academic Press, New York; 1967.
2. Bekkum DW van, Wagemaker G, Vriesendorp HM: Mechanisms and avoidance of Graft-versus-Host-Disease. Transpl Proc 1979;XI:189-195.
3. Jones JM, Wilson R, Bealmear PM: Mortality and gross pathology of secondary disease in germfree mouse radiation chimeras. Radiat Res 1971;45:577-580.
4. Bekkum DW van, Roodenburg J, Heidt PJ, van der Waaij D: Mitigation of secondary disease of allogeneic mouse radiation chimeras by modification of the intestinal microflora. J Natl Cancer Inst 1974;52:401-404.
5. Heit H, Wilson R, Fliedner TM, Kohne E: Mortality of secondary disease in antibiotic treated mouse radiation chimeras. In *Germfree Research: Biological Effects of Gnotobiotic Environment*, edited by Heneghan JB. Academic Press, New York, 1973; pp. 477-483.
6. Truitt RL, Winter M, Winter S: Application of germfree techniques to the treatment of leukemia in AKR mice by allogeneic bone marrow transplantation. In *The Handbook of Cancer Immunology, Immunotherapy*, volume 5, edited by Waters H. Garland STPM Press, New York and London, 1978; pp. 432-452.
7. Heidt PJ: unpublished observation.
8. Vriesendorp HM, Heidt PJ, Zurcher C: Gastrointestinal decontamination of dogs treated with total body irradiation and bone marrow transplantation. Exp Hematol 1981;9:904-916.

9.   Wagemaker G, Heidt PJ, Merchav S, van Bekkum DW: Abrogation of histocompati-
     bility barriers to bone marrow transplantation in rhesus monkeys. In *Experimental
     Hematology Today*, edited by Baum SD, Ledney GD, Thierfelder S. Karger, Basel,
     1982; pp. 111-118.

10. Heidt PJ, Wagemaker G, van Bekkum DW: Influence of gastrointestinal decontami-
     nation on graft-versus-host disease and infections in rhesus monkeys after (partially)
     mismatched allogeneic bone marrow transplantation. Submitted for publication.

11. Wensinck F, Ruseler-van Embden JGH: The intestinal flora of colonization resis-
     tant mice. J Hyg Camb 1971;69:413-420.

12. Heidt PJ, Wagemaker G, Knaan-Shanzer S, van Bekkum DW: Two distinct types of
     late onset graft-versus-host disease after bone marrow transplantation in lethally
     irradiated mice. Transplantation 1981;32:263-264.

13. Truitt RL: Allogeneic marrow transplantation in experimental leukemia: influence
     of microbial status at time of transplant. Abstract no. 8, 17th Annual Meeting
     of the Association for Gnotobiotics, New York; 1979.

14. Bekkum DW van; Bone marrow transplantation. Transpl Proc 1977;IX:147-154.

15. Vossen JM, Heidt PJ, van den Berg H, Gerritsen EJA, Hermans J, Dooren LJ: Pre-
     vention of infection and graft-versus-host disease by suppression of the intestinal
     microflora in children treated with allogeneic bone marrow transplantation. Eur J
     Clin Microbiol Infect Dis (in press).

16. Storb R, Epstein RB, Graham TC, Thomas ED: Methotrexate regimens for control
     of graft-versus-host disease in dogs with allogeneic marrow grafts. Transplantation
     1970;9:240-246.

17. Storb R, Deeg HJ, Whitehead J, Appelbaum F, Beatty P, Bensinger W, Buckner CD,
     Clift R, Doney K, Farewell V, Hansen J, Hill R, Lum L, Martin P, McGuffin R,
     Sanders J, Stewart P, Sullivan K, Witherspoon R, Yee G, Thomas ED: Methotrex-
     ate and cyclosporine compared with cyclosporine alone for prophylaxis of acute
     graft versus host disease after marrow transplantation for leukemia. N Engl J Med
     1986;14:729-735.

18. Waaij D van der, Vossen JM, Korthals-Altes C: Patient isolators designed in the
     Netherlands. In *Germfree Research. Biological Effect of Gnotobiotic Environ-
     ment*, edited by Heneghan JB. Academic Press, New York, 1973; pp. 31-36.

19. Vossen JM, van der Waaij D: Reverse isolation in bone marrow transplantation:
     ultra-clean room compared with laminar flow technique. I. Isolation systems.
     Eur J Clin Biol Research 1972;17:457-461.

20. Vossen JM, van der Waaij D: Recolonization after decontamination: clinical ex-
     periences. In *Airborne Transmission and Airborne Infection*, edited by Hers JFP,
     Winkler KC. Oosthoek, Utrecht, 1973; pp. 549-553.

21. Heidt PJ, van der Waaij D, Vossen JM, Hendriks WDH: Recontamination following
     antibiotic decontamination: restoration of colonization resistance. Microecol Ther
     1981;11:71-82.

22. Thomas ED, Storb R, Clift RA, Fever A, Johnson FL, Neiman PE, Lerner KG,
     Glucksberg H, Buckner CD: Bone marrow transplantation. N Engl J Med 1975;
     292:895-902.

23. Gale RP, Bortin MM, van Bekkum DW, Biggs JC, Dicke KA, Gluckman E, Good
     RA, Hoffmann H, Kay EM, Kersey JH, Marmont A, Masaoka T, Rimm AA, van
     Rood JJ, Zwaan FE: Risk factor for acute graft-versus-host disease. Brit J Haema-
     tol 1987;67:397-406.

24. Mahmoud HK, Schaefer UW, Schüning F, Schmidt CG, Bamberg M, Haralambie E,
     Linzenmeier G, Hantschke D, Grosse-Wilde H, Luboldt W, Richter HJ: Laminar
     air flow versus barrier nursing in marrow transplant recipients. Blut 1984;49:375-
     381.

25. Schmeiser T, Kurrle E, Arnold R, Heit W, Krieger D, Kubanek B, Heimpel H: Application of antimicrobial prophylactic treatment to the prevention of infection and graft-versus-host disease in allogeneic bone marrow transplantation (BMT). Exp Haematol 1984;12(Suppl 15):105-106.

26. Leblond V, Belanger C, Dreyfus F, Brunet F, Gabarre J, Asselain B, Binet JL: Interest of laminar air flow for prevention of GVHD and infections in BMT for leukaemia and lymphoma. Bone Marrow Transpl 1987;2(Suppl 1):181.

27. Skinhøj P, Jacobsen N, Høiby N, Faber V, and the Copenhagen Bone Marrow Transplant Group: Strict protective isolation in allogeneic bone marrow transplatation; effect on infectious complications, fever and graft versus host disease. Scand J Infect Dis 1987;19:91-96.

28. Storb R, Prentice RL, Buckner CD, Clift A, Appelbaum F, Deeg J, Doney K, Hansen JA, Mason M, Sanders JE, Singer J, Sullivan KM, Witherspoon RP, Thomas ED: Graft-versus-host disease and survival in patients with aplastic anemia treated by marrow grafts from HLA-identical siblings. N Engl J Med 1983;308:302-307.

29. Storb R, Thomas ED: Graft-versus-host disease in dog and man: the Seattle experience. Immunol Rev 1985;88:215-238.

30. Storb R, Deeg HJ, Fisher L, Appelbaum F, Buckner CD, Bensinger W, Clift R, Doney K, Irle C, McGuffin R, Martin P, Sanders J, Schoch G, Singer J, Stewart P, Sullivan K, Witherspoon R, Thomas ED: Cyclosporine v methotrexate for graft-v-host disease prevention in patients given marrow grafts for leukemia: long-term follow-up of three controlled trials. Blood 1988;71:293-298.

31. Wagemaker G: Problems and prospect of histoincompatible bone marrow transplantation studied in rhesus monkeys. In *Minimal Residual Disease in Acute Leukemia 1986*, edited by Hagenbeek A, Löwenberg B. Martinus Nijhoff Publishers, Dordrecht/Boston/Lancaster, 1986; pp. 363-373.

32. Heidt PJ, Timmermans CPJ, van den Hout Y, Vossen JM: Endotoxin concentrations in the faeces of completely and selectively decontaminated children treated with bone marrow transplantation for leukaemia or severe aplastic anemia. In *Gnotobiology and Its Applications*. Lyon: Fondation Marcel Mérieux, 1988; pp. 178-180.

33. Gratama JW, Stijnen T, Weiland HT, Hekker AC, de Gast GC, Zwaan FE, Weijers TF, D'Amaro J, The TH, Vossen JMJJ: Herpes-virus immunity and acute graft-versus-host disease. Lancet 1987; i:471-474.

34. Bekkum DW van, Knaan S: Role of bacterial flora in development of intestinal lesions from graft versus host reaction. J Natl Cancer Inst 1977;58:787-790.

22

Immunogenetic Factors Relevant to Human Acute Graft-vs.-Host Disease

Patrick G. Beatty
Fred Hutchinson Cancer Research Center
University of Washington School of Medicine
Seattle, Washington

Patrick Hervé
Bone Marrow Transplant Unit
Hôpital Jean Minjoz
Besançon, France

I. INTRODUCTION

The genetic elements most likely responsible for significant human acute Graft-vs.-Host Disease (GVHD) can be divided into four categories as shown in Table 1: minor histocompatibility antigens, "traditional" HLA alleles (HLA-A, B, DR, DQ), microvariants of traditional HLA alleles, and other MHC region loci (HLA-C, E, tumor necrosis factor, etc.). The table summarizes how each of six possible patient-donor pairs are expected to be matched for each of these four categories. This chapter will analyze available clinical data in the context of this table to dissect the relative impact of each particular category of disparity upon the incidence of human GVHD.

II. MINOR HISTOCOMPATIBILITY LOCI

Minor histocompatibility loci encode for those antigens important to alloreactivity which are not located within the major histocompatibility complex (MHC) on chromosome 6. Their importance to human alloactivation in vivo is most simply demonstrated by comparing the incidence of GVHD in patients receiving grafts from genotypically identical twins (incidence < 1%) to the incidence of GVHD in patients receiving grafts from siblings genotypically identical for the MHC (incidence = 10-40%; line 1 vs. line 2 in Table 1). This increment is ascribable to presumed disparity with respect to minor histocompatibility antigens (minor-HA).

      The best understood minor HA locus in humans is located on the Y chromosome and encodes the H-Y antigen. For over 10 years it has been recognized that the H-Y antigen is capable of eliciting a strong cytolytic T-cell response restricted by HLA class I antigens (1,2). Anti-H-Y proliferative T-cell clones restricted by HLA class II antigens have also been described (3). The relevance of the H-Y antigen in marrow grafting is indicated

Table 1 Immunogenetic Factors Relevant to Acute Graft-vs.-Host Disease

	A. Minor-HA loci	B. Traditional HLA	C. HLA micro-variants	D. Non-HLA MHC	Risk of AGVHD ≥ III
1. Identical twin	+++	+++	+++	+++	< 1%
2. HLA genotypically identical sibling	+++/−	+++	+++	+++	20
3. HLA 1/2 genotypically, 1/2 phenotypically =	+++/−	+++/++	+++/+	+++/+	20
4. HLA 1/2 genotypically =, 2/3 phenotypically =	+++/−	+++/(++,++,−)	+++/(+,+,−)	+++/+	50
5. Unrelated HLA phenotypically matched for 6/6 antigens	−	++	+	+	30
6. Unrelated phenotypically matched for 5/6 antigens	−	(5/6:++),(1/6:−)	(5/6:+),(1/6:−)	+/−	60

+++: genotypically identical

++: phenotypically identical.

+: random, with a possibility of increased chance of phenotypic matching due to linkage disequilibrium.

−: completely random.

/ : designates two haplotypes.

by a higher incidence of GVHD in female-to-male grafts, particularly if the female donor had been previously pregnant (relative risks 2.9 and 2.0, respectively; p < 0.001) (4). This differential impact of the sex of the donor has also been seen in renal allografts, with shorter survival of male grafts compared to female grafts when transplanted into female patients (5).

H-Y is not the only relevant minor-HA locus, as there is a significant risk of GVHD in those cases where H-Y is irrelevant, such as female patients receiving either male or female grafts, and males receiving male grafts. Attempts to define other loci are in progress, using T-cell clones as typing reagents, in vitro T-cell antifibroblast assays, and genomic mapping.

Goulmy (6) has generated panels of HLA-restricted cytolytic T-cell clones capable of recognizing minor HA. These clones were generated by harvesting peripheral blood lymphocytes from patients after HLA genotypically identical sibling marrow grafting, then restimulating them with cryopreserved pretransplant patient cells. As the responder and stimulator are genotypically identical for their respective MHCs, these donor-anti-patient clones likely recognize minor HA. A series of these clones was used to prospectively type HLA-matched sibling patient-donor combinations undergoing marrow grafting. If patient and donor cells differed in their phenotypes as detected by these clones, 6 of 8 (75%) developed acute GVHD, as opposed to 22 of 36 (61%) matched patients. Obviously, much larger numbers of patients need to be analyzed before firm conclusions can be drawn. Widespread application of typing with anti-HA clones is limited by the difficulty of generating and maintaining them. This technical problem is magnified by the necessity of generating a panel of clones for each HA allele. All clones so far identified as recognizing a minor-HA antigen are restricted by an HLA class I allele. Thus, it is necessary to generate a clone for every possible minor-HA class I allele combination which might be encountered. Efforts to date have therefore focused upon generating clones restricted by common HLA alleles such as HLA-A2.

Similar studies of other minor-HA systems have proven unsuccessful in linking mismatch for a particular locus with risk of GVHD. Elkins (7) and Warren (8) each describe systems, "W1" and "5" respectively, neither of which correlates with risk for GVHD. Both studies demonstrate an apparent low degree of polymorphism for these loci, resulting in few informative patient-donor pairs for analysis. Thus, a small contribution of risk might be undetected. Furthermore, humans may resemble mice and possess numerous relatively nonpolymorphic loci, with each locus nevertheless contributing a small degree of risk (9).

An alternative approach does not require generation of a typing panel, but rather directly measures the strength of the antiminor HA response in vitro. Vogelsang (10) described the destruction of cultured patient skin by sensitized donor cells. A pretransplant punch biopsy of patient skin was incubated with presensitized donor-versus-patient lymphocytes, then examined histologically for evidence of lesions characteristic of GVHD. In the 32 patients studied, 16 of 18 with positive tests developed grade II or greater GVHD, while only 3 of 14 with negative tests developed GVHD. The minor HA target antigen(s) in the skin of the primed lymphocytes are not known.

A direct approach to localizing significant minor-HA loci was taken by de Gast (11). Five hundred and forty-three HLA genotypically matched patient-donor combinations were studied for expression of a series of 22 polymorphic blood genetic markers. These markers were chosen on the basis of their known localization to particular chromosomes throughout the genome. Disparity for any of three of the markers (rhesus, MNSs, and acid phosphatase) correlated with development of GVHD, with a mismatch for all three markers resulting in an additive risk. Analysis of cases with both patient homozygosity and sharing of one allele with the donor indicated that none of these three loci were themselves the minor-HA, but rather were tightly linked genetically. As further marker loci are defined (12), it may prove possible to use such linkage analysis methods to identify and clone these minor-HA loci.

None of the latter three approaches to minor-HA has allowed identification of a specific minor HA locus. Indeed, it is not clear that the loci putatively detected by each method are the same. As none of the methods is absolutely predictive of GVHD, it is possible each identifies a different locus (loci). A comparison of the three methods in the same group of patients would be of interest.

III. TRADITIONAL HLA (HLA-A, B, DR, DQ)

The major histocompatibility complex (MHC) in man has long been thought to contain those loci most important to the clinical alloimmune response. For this reason, most early marrow grafts were from HLA genotypically identical sibling donors. If a family study of HLA inheritance established that the patient and donor were indeed haploidentical for MHC, it could be presumed that they were genotypically identical for all loci within the region, not just HLA. With the development of modern molecular biology techniques, knowledge of the detailed genetic structure of the human MHC has dramatically expanded (Fig. 1). From 1950 to 1980, serologic techniques were refined to identify and localize the HLA-A,B,C and DR loci. More recently, the loci of the class II region have been mapped and characterized. Similarly, new loci are being identified in the class I region. As long as marrow transplantation was limited to patients transplanted from an HLA genotypically identical sibling, the complexity of the MHC could be disregarded. Since fewer than 35% of patients have an HLA genotypically identical sibling, several transplant centers began exploring the use of relatives who share one HLA haplotype with the patient and differ variably on the nonshared HLA haplotype (Table 1, lines 3 and 4). By comparing line 2 with line 4, we see the average expected disparity for minor-HA is the same: all the differences are within the MHC. The increase in risk of GVHD due to such disparity is substantial, from 20% for patients receiving grafts from matched siblings to approximately 50% for patients receiving grafts from one locus mismatched relatives. Although there was a strong correlation between GVHD risk and HLA disparity, if the disparity was limited successful transplants could often be carried out. Data both from Seattle (13) and from groups at the Hammersmith Hospital (14) and the International Bone Marrow Transplant Registry (15) indicate that for one locus mismatched patients in remission, there is an increased GVHD risk but no difference in survival when compared to similar patients transplanted from HLA matched siblings. Surprisingly, there was a minimal differential impact of HLA class I (HLA-A or -B) disparity versus HLA class II (HLA-D) disparity (16). The risk of GVHD in both groups was similarly increased in patients receiving grafts from HLA-matched siblings. Of interest is a differential impact by different GVHD prophylactic regimens on class I and class II mismatched patients. For instance, preliminary data from Seattle show that a change from a 100-day course of methotrexate alone to a combination of an 11-day course of methotrexate plus cyclosporine had a substantial and significant impact upon the incidence of severe GVHD in class I, but not class II, mismatched patients (17).

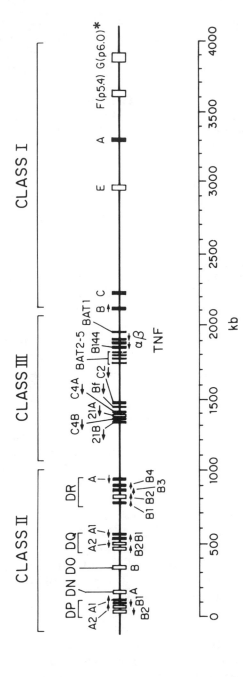

Figure 1 The major histocompatibility complex in man. (*Order of F and G not determined.)

Within groups of patients mismatched for a single locus, risk for GVHD can be determined based on whether the mismatched alleles share some structural homology. For instance, it is possible to identify a group of patients who are at lower risk for GVHD if their mismatched alleles fall within a serologically defined cross-reactive group or split (18).

Thus, in order to define the risk for particular patient-donor combinations incompatible for HLA, it is necessary to consider the number of mismatched loci, which loci differ, the form of GVHD prophylaxis employed, and the relative homology of the particular mismatched alleles.

IV. MICROVARIANTS OF TRADITIONAL HLA

It has recently become clear that previous definitions of phenotypic identity for HLA are imprecise, as microvariants of the traditional alleles have been identified. In 1982 Biddison described a series of antigen-specific HLA-A2 restricted T-cell clones capable of lysing some cells bearing HLA-A2, but not others, implying polymorphism within HLA-A2 (19). Later it was proven that these functional differences could be attributed to slight differences in amino acid sequences (20-22). Similar observations have been made for HLA-B7 and HLA-B27 (23-28). Many of these variants are resolvable on one-dimensional isoelectric focusing (1D-IEF) gels. In 1987 the Tenth International Histocompatibility Workshop described 34 HLA-A 1D-IEF alleles among 18 serologically defined HLA-A alleles (29). For example, there were five distinct 1D-IEF alleles of the serologically defined HLA-A2 allele. Similarly, there were 52 HLA-B 1D-IEF alleles among 37 serologically defined HLA-B alleles, with the maximum 7 alleles of HLA-B27. This likely represents an underestimation of the polymorphism as a relatively limited cell panel was used and it is likely some amino acid polymorphisms may not be readily resolvable on IEF.

A comparison of lines 2 and 3 in Table 1 demonstrates the potential clinical relevance of these variants. In both cases patient and donor share one HLA haplotype and have a similar likelihood of genetically sharing minor-HA alleles (assuming the patient and donor in line 3 are first-degree relatives). The patient-donor combination in line 2 is genotypically matched for their second haplotypes, whereas the pair in line 3 is only phenotypically matched for HLA-A,B, and DR. Thus, they would be expected to differ for both microvariants (column C) and non-HLA MHC (column D). Data from Seattle indicate no difference in the incidence of GVHD between these two groups (13). Given the limited number of clinical observations, it is difficult to determine which one of two possible factors is responsible for this similarity. Perhaps there were few "mismatches" for HLA microvariants in the data set, either because most alleles may have a dominant allele within ethnic groups or because particular microvariants may be in linkage disequilibrium with the other HLA loci (which by definition were phenotypically matched). Alternatively, these microvariants may have no clinical significance given current GVHD prophylactic regimens. It is unlikely there will be enough patient-donor combinations in which half phenotypic-half genotypic identity for HLA will be present to allow dissection of the relevant genetic elements. More likely, the question of clinical relevance of the microvariants ultimately will be answered by careful immunogenetic analysis of large numbers of unrelated patient-donor combinations. However, that analysis will be complicated not only by non-HLA MHC differences but also by presumed minor-HA differences. Thus, many pairs need to be studied to provide sufficient numbers of informative differences for adequate statistical power.

V. OTHER MHC LOCI

Within the MHC region are several loci whose relevance to the alloimmune response is unknown. HLA-C has been recognized since 1970, but no clinical data are available to judge its role in the development of GVHD in humans. A clue to its possible relevance is the demonstration that skin from transgenic mice expressing human HLA-Cw3 was rapidly rejected by normal, otherwise syngeneic nontransgenic mice. Furthermore, mouse cells expressing HLA-Cw3 were capable of being recognized by cytolytic T cells (30). Other class I loci are even less well defined. Orr described 17 class I-like genes within the MHC, three of which have sequences that appear to have the potential for transcription and expression (31). One of these, HLA-E, was sufficiently well described to receive a WHO designation in 1987. Two others, provisionally designated p5.4 and p6.0, are less well understood. It is not yet clear what degree of polymorphism, if any, is present at these loci, or whether their alleles can provoke an alloimmune response.

As the HLA region is further explored, new loci are described. For instance, five HLA-B-associated transcripts (BATS), corresponding to five genes located between HLA-B and the class III complement components, have been cloned (32). At present nothing is known about the nature of the putative proteins encoded by these loci. In the same region are the genes encoding tumor necrosis factor (TNF) alpha and beta (33). Although TNF appears to have a role in the effector phase of the alloresponse, there is as yet no evidence that they function as classic histocompatibility antigens. Before determining the relevance of any of these loci, it will be necessary to develop reagents capable of detecting polymorphisms at each locus. The most useful clinical data for studying the relevance of these loci will come from unrelated, HLA-matched patient-donor combinations. The group needs to be large enough for a multivariate analysis which controls for possible microvariants of the traditional HLA alleles and for differences in minor-HA.

REFERENCES

1. Goulmy E, Termijtelen A, Bradley BA, van Rood JJ: Alloimmunity to human H-Y. Lancet 1976; ii: 1206.
2. Goulmy E, Termijtelen A, Bradley BA, van Rood JJ: Y-antigen killing by T cells of women is restricted by HLA. Nature 1977;266:544-545.
3. Mickelson EM, Beatty PG, Storb R, Hansen JA: Immune responses in an untransfused patient with aplastic anemia: analysis of cytolytic and proliferative T cell clones. Human Immunol 1984;10:189-201.
4. Bortin MM, for the Advisory Committee of the International Bone Marrow Transplant Registry: Acute graft-versus-host disease following bone marrow transplantation in humans: prognostic factors. Transplant Proc 1987;19:2655-2657.
5. Goulmy E, Bradley BA, Lansbergen Q, van Rood JJ: The importance of H-Y incompatibility in human organ transplantation. Transplantation 1978;25:315-319.
6. Goulmy E: Minor histocompatibility antigens in man and their role in transplantation. In *Transplantation Reviews*, vol. 2, edited by Morris PJ, Tilney NL. W. B. Saunders & Company, 1988; pp. 29-53.
7. Elkins WE, Pierson GR, Storb R: Study of a human minor alloantigen in relation to clinical graft-versus-host disease. Bone Marrow Transplantation 1987;1 :397-403.
8. Warren RP, Storb R, Nguyen DD, Thomas ED: Failure to demonstrate an involvement of human leukocyte group 5 antigens in graft-versus-host disease and marrow graft rejection. Transplantation 1977;24:89-91.

9. Rammensee HG, Klein J: Polymorphism of minor histocompatibility genes in wild mice. Immunogenetics 1983;17:637-647.

10. Vogelsang GB, Hess AD, Berkman AW, Tutschka PJ, Farmer ER, Converse PJ, Santos GW: An in vitro predictive test for graft versus host disease in patients with genotypic HLA-identical bone marrow transplants. N Engl J Med 1985;313:645-650.

11. De Gast GC, Beatty PG, Anderson JE, Amos D, Sullivan KM, Mickelson EM, de Lange G, Thomas ED, Hansen JA: Identification of genetic loci linked to putative 'minor' non-HLA antigens involved in GVHD in HLA-identical marrow transplantation. Bone Marrow Transplantation 1986;1(Suppl 1):149.

12. White R, Leppert M, Bishop DT, Barker D, Berkowitz J, Brown C, Callahan P, Holm T, Jerominski L: Construction of linkage maps with DNA markers for human chromosomes. Nature 1985;313:101-105.

13. Beatty PG, Clift RA, Mickelson EM, Nisperos B, Flournoy N, Martin PJ, Sanders JE, Stewart P, Buckner CD, Storb R, Thomas ED, Hansen JA: Marrow transplantation from related donors other than HLA identical siblings. N Engl J Med 1985; 313:765-771.

14. Hows JM, Yin JL, Marsh J, Jones L, Apperley JF, James DCO, Smithers S, Batchelor JR, Goldman JH, Gordon-Smith EC: Histocompatible unrelated volunteer donors compared with HLA non-identical family donors in marrow transplantation for aplastic anemia and leukemia. Blood 1986;68:1322-1328.

15. Ash RC, Casper J, Menitove J, Chitambar C, Hansen R, Lum L, Lawton C, Murray K, Hunter J, Anderson T, Camitta B: Evolving role of the closely HLA-matched unrelated donor: HLA matching considerations for alternative donor transplantation. In *Bone Marrow Transplantation: Current Controversies*, edited by Gale RP, Champlin RE. Alan R. Liss, New York, 1989; pp. 629-640.

16. Beatty PG, Anasetti C, Thomas ED, Hansen JA: Marrow transplantation from relatives other than HLA identical siblings. In *Bone Marrow Transplantation: Current Controversies*, edited by Gale RP, Champlin RE. Alan R. Liss, New York, 1989; pp. 619-624.

17. Beatty PG, Hansen JA, Thomas ED: Differential efficacy of cyclosporin in the prevention of acute graft-versus-host disease in patients receiving class II as opposed to class I incompatible marrow grafts. Hum Immunol 1988;23a:80.

18. Beatty PG, Nisperos B, Mickelson E, Thomas ED, Hansen JA: Correlation between acute graft vs. host disease and matching for public class I epitopes in patients receiving one-locus incompatible haploidentical bone marrow transplants. Hum Immunol 1986;17a:150.

19. Biddison WE, Krangel MS, Strominger JL, Ward FE, Shearer GM, Shaw S: Virus-immune cytotoxic T cells recognize structural differences between serologically indistinguishable HLA-A2 molecules. Hum Immunol 1980;3:225.

20. Spits H, Breuning M, Ivanyi P, de Vries JE: Definition of four HLA-A2 subtypes by CML typing and biochemical analysis. Immunogenetics 1982;17:609.

21. Krangel MS, Biddison WE, Strominger JL: Comparative structural analysis of HLA-A2 antigens distinguishable by cytotoxic T lymphocytes: variants M7 and DR1. Biochemistry 1983;21:6313.

22. Mattson DH, Handy DE, Bradley DA, Coligan JE, Cowan EP, Biddison WE: DNA sequences of the genes that encode the CTL-defined HLA-A2 variants M7 and DK1. Immunogenetics 1987;26:190-192.

23. Taketani S, Krangel MS, Spits H, de Vries J, Strominger JL: Structural analysis of an HLA-B7 antigen variant detected by cytotoxic T lymphocytes. J Immunol 1984; 13:816-821.

24. Choo SY, Antonelli P, Nisperos B, Nepom GT, Hansen JA: Six variants of HLA-B27 identified by isoelectric focusing. Immunogenetics 1986;23:24-29.

25. Bruer-Vriesendorp BS, Neefjes JC, Huis B, van Seventer GA, Ploegh HL, Ivanyi P: Identification of new B27 subtypes (B27C and B27D) prevalent in Oriental populations. Hum Immunol 1986;16:163-168.
26. Van Seventer GA, Huis B, Melief CJM, Ivanyi P: Fine specificity of human HLA-B7-specific cytotoxic T-lymphocyte clones. I. Identification of HLA-B7 subtypes and histotopes of the HLA-B7 crossreacting groups. Hum Immunol 1986;16:375.
27. Breuning MH, Lucas CJ, Bruer BS, Engelsma MY, de Lange GG, Dekker AJ, Biddison WE, Ivanyi P: Subtypes of HLA-B27 detected by cytotoxic T lymphocytes and their role in self-recognition. Hum Immunol 1982;5:259.
28. Vega MA, Wallace L, Rojo S, Bragado R, Aparicio P, Lopez de Castro JA: Deliniation of functional sites in HLA-B27 variant Wewak I defined by cytotoxic T lymphocytes. J Immunol 1985;135:3323.
29. Yang SY: Nomenclature for HLA-A and HLA-B alleles detected by ID-IEF gel electrophoresis. In *Immunology of HLA*, volume 1, edited by Dupont B. Springer-Verlag Inc., New York, 1989; pp. 54-57.
30. Dill O, Kievits F, Koch S, Ivanyi P, Hammerling GJ: Immunological function of HLA-C antigens in HLA-Cw3 transgenic mice. Proc Natl Acad Sci USA 1988;85: 5664-5668.
31. Koller BH, Geraghty D, Orr HT, Shimizu Y, DeMars R: Organization of the human class I major histocompatibility complex genes. Immunological Research 1987; 6:1-10.
32. Spies T, Blanck G, Bresnahan M, Sands J, Strominger JL: A new cluster of genes within the human major histocompatibility complex. Science 1989;243:214-217.
33. Carroll MC, Katzman P, Alicot EM, Koller BH, Geraghty DE, Orr HT, Strominger JL, Spies T: Linkage map of the human major histocompatibility complex including the tumor necrosis factor genes. Proc Natl Acad Sci USA 1987;84:8535-8539.

23

Graft-vs.-Host Disease After Bone Marrow Transplantation from Donors Other Than HLA-Identical Siblings

Patrick Hervé and Jean-Yves Cahn
Bone Marrow Transplant Unit
Hôpital Jean Minjoz
Besançon, France

Patrick G. Beatty
Fred Hutchinson Cancer Research Center
University of Washington School of Medicine
Seattle, Washington

I. INTRODUCTION

Allogeneic and autologous bone marrow transplantation (BMT) can provide long-term disease-free survival when used as therapy for a variety of lethal disorders. Unfortunately, the majority of patients requiring high-dose chemo-radiotherapy followed by BMT lack a HLA-identical sibling, and indications for autologous rescue are restricted (acute leukemias in first or second complete remission if the first relapse does'nt occur too early, lymphomas, and solid tumors). The possibility to extend BMT to a larger group of patients has been investigated by different teams to explore the real impact of major histocompatibility complex (MHC) identity using HLA-incompatible related donors as well as phenotypically identical unrelated donors, for patients with potentially lethal hematologic or immunologic disorders.

Results have shown that donors other than genotypically identical siblings may be used successfully for severe combined immunodeficiency disease (SCID), aplastic anemia, or leukemia, but with a higher incidence of lethal GVHD and graft failure than after HLA-identical BMT. For these reasons, different approaches to limit treatment-related mortality have been developed.

II. HISTORICAL ASPECTS

The first attempts to perform human BMT were made during the decade ending in the early 1960s. At that time, little was known about human MHC and supportive care facilities were still very limited. These trials were almost uniformly unsuccessful except for transplants between identical twins. Owing to the limited availability of typing techniques then, most of the BMTs performed must have been non-HLA identical.

The first successful HLA-identical BMT using an HLA genotypically identical sibling was published in 1968, and with time, genotypically HLA-identical BMT became a successful therapeutic approach to lethal hematologic or immunologic disorders, and within 10 years acquired an established and expanding place (1,2).

Following such encouraging results and so as to expand the number of potential donors, two different approaches have been investigated: HLA-nonidentical BMT using family donors and phenotypically unrelated BMT.

Early attempts to transplant HLA haplotype disparate bone marrow into patients with SCID consistently either failed to engraft or produced fatal GVHD (3).

In the late 1970s, various teams published some successful BMTs in hematologic malignancies, aplastic anemia, or SCID, but associated with a high incidence of severe GVHD or poor graft function and rejection. However the rate of graft failure has varied from one team to another (4,5).

After 1980, several teams developed various techniques for producing a T-cell depletion of the graft by means of either soybean lectin agglutination and rosette formation or with monoclonal antibodies (6-10).

As in animal models and allogeneic BMTs, T-cell-depleted transplants led to a significant decrease in the incidence of severe GVHD, but failure to engraft durably became an increasingly important problem and several consecutive transplantations were sometimes required to achieve durable engraftment because of host's resistance. At the same time, Powles et al. developed an alternative approach using cyclosporine in the posttransplant period on the basis of the encouraging results obtained for GVHD prophylaxis with HLA-identical transplantation (69).

In 1985, P. Beatty et al. demonstrated that mismatched transplants using related donors with disparity at only one locus without modifying the conditioning regimen could lead to a survival probability not statistically different than with genotypically identical siblings (12). The number of patients receiving grafts from donors who were incompatible at two or three loci was too low to allow for a statistical analysis of survival. In the same period, teams from the Sloan-Kettering and Madison Institutes investigated other approaches to HLA nonidentical BMT using T-cell depletion and more intensive preparative regimens associated or not with additional immunosuppression (11,13). However, toxicities due to additional therapy, the risk of subsequent infections, and B-cell lymphoproliferative diseases represented problems.

Another approach developed during the same period consisted in using phenotypically matched unrelated donors or, in some cases, partly matched donors (14-16).

The time and cost involved in establishing donor programs explain the fact that to date, too few series have been reported in sufficient detail. In 1973, the first record of an unsuccessful attempt to use an unrelated donor for severe aplastic anemia appeared (17). Then a few cases of SCID and other congenital disorders were published between 1975 and 1977 with encouraging results (18). In 1980 Hansen reported the first leukemic patient to receive an HLA phenotypically matched donor graft not developing acute GVHD and resulting in good engraftment (19). Then several donor registries were developed between 1980 and 1985, especially in England and in the United States (20). Between 1985 and 1988, the first series of patients were published (14,21).

III. GVHD AND MISMATCHED BONE MARROW TRANSPLANTATION

In fully matched situations, despite successive improvements in GVHD prophylaxis (see Chapter 20), GVHD remains a major cause of morbidity and mortality (22,23). There is a high variability in the GVHD incidence within and between institutions. Acute GVHD occurs in 20-80% of recipients of HLA-identical sibling marrow transplants. According to the IBMTR study, the reason for this variability is unclear and probably reflects the impact of several risk factors which act differently depending on the patient's status and GVHD prophylaxis. (Differences in the diagnosis and grading of GVHD can explain this variability from one team to another.) We can expect that the use of MHC-mismatched BMT would lead to an increased risk of severe GVHD occurrence. Likewise, we can assume that the predictive risk factors which were previously well known in situations of matched donors (24) should combine their effects with the impact of immunogenetic disparity between the donor and the recipient. (In fact, according to the published data, the respective impacts of each predictive factor involved in matched BMTs remain controversial.)

Two major problems are related to the use of mismatched BMT: poor graft function, graft rejection and increased incidence and severity of GVHD. As a corollary we note a great susceptibility of those patients whose status is complicated by infection, especially of viral etiology. Rejection and GVHD are both influenced by the same factor: HLA antigen incompatibility.

A. Predictive Factors

Three factors emerge which can influence the outcome of a mismatched BMT (24,25).

1. Influence of *immunogenetic disparity* between the donor and the recipient (see Chapter 22).

2. Influence of *sex-mismatching*: in the HLA-matched situation, it has been shown that the combination female → male graft has a higher incidence of GVHD (53% versus 42% in male → female). If the female donor is alloimmunized (previous pregnancies) there is a 66% incidence of GVHD versus 39% for female → female. The relative risk was 2.9 (p < 0.0001). One should be aware of this risk factor when selecting donors prior to mismatched bone marrow transplantation, especially if the marrow inoculum is not T-cell depleted.

3. *Age*: in man, increasing age correlates with a higher incidence of GVHD (relative risk 1.6; p < 0.001). The observation that the majority of the mismatched marrow transplant recipients are young is not fortuitous (most of them are less than 30 years of age). Currently, the tendency is to propose a mismatched BMT to young patients only. Obviously, in mismatched situations, the presence of a single major risk factor will be associated with an increased risk for severe GVHD, although until now published data on the incidence of GVHD in mismatched BMTs have taken into account HLA disparity only. If these three main factors are associated, there is a cumulative risk, and probability of developing GVHD can reach 90% after mismatched BMT.

Numerous other controversial risk factors for GVHD have been reported by individual BMT centers. Such factors might contribute to an increased GVHD incidence following mismatched BMT:ABO matching, prophylaxis protocols against GVHD, the bone marrow cell dose, the patient's performance status prior to BMT, donor antibodies to herpes simplex virus, HLA-DP incompatibility, splenectomy prior to BMT, TBI protocols (source, dose, dose rate, fractionation), HLA antigens, decontamination and protective environmental measures, trimethoprim-sulfamethoxazole treatment. (For the most part the possible interactions of these "risk factors" with GVHD have not obtained the consensus from the majority of BMT centers.) According to IBMTR data the estimated probability of GVHD occurring after *matched* BMT is 16% in the absence of any of the adverse risk factors. With all the main risk factors the relative risk of GVHD is 5.4 times higher.

Predictive in vitro models of acute GVHD have been developed using HLA-identical siblings (26,27). Even if such models are not useful in HLA-mismatched situations, they could be informative when a phenotypically identical unrelated donor is proposed.

B. GVHD Prophylaxis by T-Cell Depletion

A number of agents has been used to prevent GVHD after matched BMT both in animals and in man. Agents classified as modulators of the immune response are analyzed elsewhere (Chapter 20). Acute GVHD remains the major lethal complication after mismatched BMT in spite of the progressive improvements being achieved in GVHD prophylaxis. Owing to the encouraging results of marrow T-cell-depletion techniques in matched situations, several pilot studies have been initiated in the mismatched setting.

1. Methods of T-Cell Depletion (TCD)

We know that GVHD is initiated by mature donor T lymphocytes in the graft (28-30) although previous work has failed to detect any correlation between the number of T cells infused and subsequent GVHD in recipients of unmanipulated marrow transplants from HLA-identical sibling (31). Nevertheless, depletion methods which result in the elimination of T lymphocytes from the bone marrow appear a priori as the best method to abrogate GVHD in HLA-disparate marrow graft recipients. Numerous experimental models suggest that it is necessary to use pan-T MAbs to remove the helper and cytotoxic T-cell subsets (29). The different techniques of T-cell depletion are reviewed elsewhere (Chapter 19).

In HLA incompatibility cases, problems arising from the application of T-cell depletion are manyfold:

What is the critical T-cell dose in mismatched BMT? Would it be necessary to be more
   effective than in matched situations and have less than 0.3% T cells?
Is post-BMT immunoprophylaxis necessary to achieve GVHD prevention? (acute GVHD
   is possible in the murine model when 0.1% of T cells remain in the inoculum.)
Is there a T-cell-depletion method better adapted to mismatched BMT?

Much remains to be learned about T-cell depletion (TCD) as a means for GVHD prophylaxis. The analysis of 406 patients from 10 teams who received a T-cell-depleted HLA-matched marrow inoculum showed a 16.2% graft failure incidence (versus <5% in 1106 patients receiving unmanipulated marrow) and a 10.3% incidence of grade II-IV acute GVHD (versus 41% with unmanipulated marrow) (32). The graft failure incidence varied from one technique to another: 5.2% with the elutriation method (34) and 27.6% with the utilization of a cocktail of eight monoclonal antibodies inducing a drastic T-cell depletion (33). At present there is a growing consensus recognizing the low incidence of GVHD after T-cell depletion. In some published series there is a total absence of GVHD higher than grade II (9,32,35).

2. Critical T-Cell Dose

In matched situations the optimal level of T-cell reduction is still an open question. Using limiting dilution analysis, Atkinson et al. have shown that the infusion of $\leqslant 10^5$ T cells/kg is associated with minimal GVHD rates, if any (36). On the other hand, the infusion of more than 1×10^6 T cells/kg caused significant GVHD. In the same way, Eierman et al. (37) showed that $< 1 \times 10^5$ T cells infused per kg did not induce significant GVHD.

In SCID patients using haploidentical marrow grafts the critical T-cell dose range is 10^4-10^5 T cells/kg, with a difference in terms of GVHD incidence between immunocompetent and incompetent hosts. When an immunoincompetent host received more than 10^5 T cells/kg, little or no GVHD was observed while with an immunocompetent host the threshold was 10^5 T cells/kg (38).

Löwenberg et al. (39) compared two methods of T-cell depletion. The first one utilized a discontinuous albumin gradient which removed 90% (1 log) of the original T-cell population (5/9 GVHD). The second one employed rosetting with sheep red blood cells and removed 99% (2 logs) of the T cells (0/9 GVHD). In the Sloan-Kettering series the degree of T-cell depletion achieved by the soybean agglutinin and E-rosetting methods was sufficient to abrogate GVHD in HLA-disparate marrow graft recipients (40).

To avoid the variability in T-cell-depletion levels from one manipulation to another, one can add back a fixed low number of peripheral blood T cells after T-cell depletion (2×10^5/kg) to create a balance between residual donor and host clonogenic T cells (see Chapter 30). Poynton et al. (41) used this technique in six patients (three haplo identical family donors, three unrelated donors). Engraftment occurred in all patients. In our institution, we have used the same approach in four patients receiving either mismatched marrow (two patients) or matched marrow (two patients). One patient experienced grade III GVHD while another achieved an autologous reconstitution (unpublished data).

The main question is to know whether the threshold doses for matched and mismatched grafts are likely to be in the same order of magnitude. When compiling the overall data available from the literature a 10^5 T cell/kg limit seems to be critical for the prevention of GVHD.

C. Problems Related to T-Cell Depletion

1. Graft Failure

The low incidence of GVHD following T-cell depletion is obtained at the cost of increased graft failure (nontake, rejection, poor engraftment, autologous reconstitution) and relapse rates, especially in BMTs performed for chronic myelogenous leukemia (33, 42). In reference to matched BMT, there is no evidence that T-cell depletion is associated with improvement in survival (32). Indiscriminate removal of T cells is based on the fact that GVHD across both major and minor histocompatibility barriers involves helper T cells and cytolytic T cells alike (43). It is obvious now that the presence of some T cells is desirable. Elutriation could be the most suitable method for infusing sufficient numbers of T cells into the host in matched situations (34). Under conditions of mismatching, the number of residual viable T cells is probably too high (0.64×10^6/kg range 0.2-1.6), although no data are available concerning the possibility of combining elutriation with a post-BMT MTX + CSP regimen.

In situations where fully matched related donors are involved, T depletion results in a high rate of graft failures (10-20%). In a multicenter study including 441 patients who had received Campath-1 T-depleted grafts, Hale et al. (35) reported 14.4% engraftment failures, and 3% poor graft function. With regimens including total lymphoid and total body irradiation 11% graft failures were observed. With HLA nonidentity the incidence reached 15-30%. Some definite interactions do exist between T depletion and such factors as the patient's pregrafting chemotherapeutic and radiotherapeutic regimen, chimerism (complete or mixed), and the occurrence of relapse.

Published data compiled by seven different teams illustrate the high frequency with which mixed chimerism is found: 63.5% among 118 patients assessed who received T-depleted grafts, as opposed to 20.7% among 251 patients engrafted with unmanipulated marrow (44-47).

The host-vs.-graft reaction (HVGR) is a determinant for the quality of engraftment. The residual host lymphocyte population (up to 20%) is made up of "radio-resistant" lymphocytes (T-cell, B-cell, and NK-cell subsets) surviving for many months even following 1400 cGy irradiation of the recipient.

Recent studies have shown host lymphocytes do persist following a course of cyclophosphamide + TBI, thus proving insufficient in itself in eradicating all of the recipient's cells (48-53). Sondel et al. (54), working with a mixed lymphocyte culture, have reported recipient-derived cytotoxic lymphocytes which exhibited in vivo sensitization against donor antigens. Kernan et al. (55) have characterized the nature of the cells present at the time of graft rejection in five HLA-incompatible graft recipients, by means of phenotypic and functional analysis. In all instances, rejection was associated with the emergence of host-derived T cells (CD8$^+$) with specific antidonor cytotoxicity. In one patient, the specific target of the cytotoxic lymphocytes was a donor HLA-B7 antigen. The radio-resistance (up to 1500 cGy) of sensitized T cells has often been demonstrated in animal models.

Bourque et al. have shown that post-PHA and IL-2 stimulation residual T lymphocytes were able to give rise to T colonies in 41% of the 46 cases that were assessed following preparation for grafting (48). Chemotherapy combined with TBI was more effective in eradicating the cells than a preparation protocol excluding irradiation (21% versus 63% of residual T-cell colonies).

CD8$^+$ cytotoxic lymphocytes and NK cells could be responsible for the rejection process. Moulinier et al. have shown relative radio- and chemoresistance in a population of T cells carrying the gamma- and delta-chain of the T-cell receptor for the antigen which might be involved in the rejection process (52). The CD16$^+$ population of NK cells seems to be stable from day −7 to day +1 (day 0 = grafting day). The Creteil team has studied the residual T cells (T3$^+$) in 11 patients subjected to pretransplantation conditioning with chemo- and radiotherapy. The residual cells manifested an inhibition of donor granulocyte-monocyte and erythrocyte stem cell proliferation (30-60%), whereas blood cell samples taken prior to pretransplantation treatment had no inhibitory effect whatsoever. The authors hypothesize that a possible soluble factor present in the residual cell culture supernatant would be capable of preventing the growth of colonies originating from different subjects. The addition of an anti-tumor necrosis factor monoclonal antibody could prevent such inhibition (53).

In a primate preclinical model, Reisner et al. demonstrated the presence of clones of radio-resistant T cells originating from the bone marrow graft recipient (56). On the other hand, Slavin's team could not observe any apparent correlation between graft failure and in vitro residual T-cell precursor proliferation (57). Although the transplants were carried out under HLA-compatible conditions, most of these observations are applicable to HLA-incompatible situations, where engraftment failure and rejection rates are higher. In mismatched situations, precise identification of the residual immunocompetent cells is essential if one is to achieve progress in defining the best type of immunosuppression conducive to complete chimerism. Petz et al. have recently shown better engraftment to occur in patients receiving T-depleted HLA-identical grafts, when the total irradiation dose was increased (46).

It is of general consensus that the characteristics of the irradiation protocol (total dose, dose rate, single or fractionated dose) prior to T-depleted transplants are critical in determining the transplantation outcome (49,58).

Several experimental models have sought to determine the minimal irradiation dose required for achieving stable TCD engraftment. Engraftment was not observed with an irradiation dose equal to or lower than 2×5 Gy, whereas an irradiation dose equivalent to 2×6 Gy promoted successful engraftment in all cases. Gassman et al. (50) have emphasized the importance of the time lapsed between TBI administration and grafting. With longer periods of time separating these two events, chances for obtaining successful TCD engraftment are higher. The authors advocate carrying out TBI prior to chemotherapy, on the basis that radio-resistant T cells are liable to persist for a limited period of time following irradiation. The TBI + cyclophosphamide sequence has been put into practice in several institutions (11,59). It is of the utmost importance that we should discern the conjugated mechanisms behind graft rejection, in order to be able to choose from new therapeutic strategies, whether these be an adaptation of the combined chemo- and radiotherapy, or the utilization of rejection effector-specific monoclonal antibodies. The selection of monoclonal antibodies depends upon the presumed mechanisms responsible for graft rejection. The postulated effector cells are of two types: T cells and NK cells. In one murine model, Lyt-2^+ cells are instrumental in mediating rejection; however, in vivo monoclonal antibody-induced immunosuppression suggests that Lyt-2^+ and Lyt-3^+ cells might play a role in this phenomenon (29). Moreover, even in the absence of T-cell depletion, performing mismatched BMT may expose one to higher rates of graft failure. In this respect, the Seattle group has evaluated the risk factors involved in graft rejection (14.6%) among 296 HLA-incompatible transplantation patients, using a control group of 930 HLA-identical transplantation patients (2.2% rejections, $p < 0.0001$) (60). The authors have identified several risk factors, such as positive cross-matching between donor and recipient (49% rejections vs. 12% when negative); the HLA-B and -D incompatibility grade; relapsing leukemias (19% vs. 9.5% when in complete remission); presence of residual host T lymphocytes (detected in 11 patients out of 14 who had graft rejection). The inducing role of viral infections (cytomegalovirus) on rejection has often been discussed, although it has not been proven.

2. Relapse of Leukemia

T depletion enhances relapse rates, particularly following BMT for chronic myelogenous leukemia (42,61). Two randomized studies have brought forth evidence of increased rates of relapse following TCD. The Prentice group (62), as well as Slavin's (57) and DeWitte's teams (34), have not observed any rise in the incidence of relapse in the course of acute leukemia. Several hypotheses (which have not been proven) are proposed to explain the difference noted in the incidence of relapse from one series to another: TBI protocols; factors determining prognosis; utilization or nonutilization of cyclosporin A following grafting; methods of T-depletion.

Although no final conclusion can be drawn from the literature so far as acute leukemia is concerned, the same does not hold true for chronic myelogenous leukemia. Goldman's team clearly reports a high rate of relapse, both of the isolated cytogenetic

Table 1 B-Cell Lymphoproliferative Disorders (BLPD) Following Bone Marrow Transplantation: Clinical Features

No. of patients	Diagnosis	BLPD incidence		TCD	HLA disparity	EBV	Outcome	Ref.
		No.	%					
2475	Leukemia SAA	15	0.6	no	6/15(40%)	13/13 EP	13/15 deaths	Seattle (63)
506	Leukemia SCID	8	1.6	yes	6/8(75%)	7/8	7/8 deaths	Minneapolis
239	SCID non-SCID	18	7.5	yes	16/18(88%)	16/18	12/18 deaths	EBMTG (64)
117	Leukemia	5	4.2	yes	3/5(60%)	NA	5/5 deaths	Besancon (unpublished data)
76	Leukemia	8	10.5	yes	6/8(75%)	NA	7/8 deaths	Wisconsin (13, 70)
Total: 3413		54	4.8%	39/54 (72%)	37/54 were mismatched (68.5%)	36/38 EP (94.7%)	44/54 deaths (81.5%)	

EP: evaluable patients.

and cytogenetic/hematologic type, following TCD BMT (41). With the present state of knowledge, TCD-HLA genotypically identical transplantation for this indication is not acceptable. Under conditions of HLA incompatibility, however, one may expect a more effective eradication of the leukemic clones, provided intensified pregrafting preparation protocols are applied, possibly associated with the administration of biological response modifiers (for example, monoclonal antibodies). As will be discussed further, during the course of chronic leukemias where the donor is an HLA-phenoidentical unrelated individual, cytogenetic relapse occurs both more frequently and more rapidly.

3. B-Cell Lymphoproliferative Disorders (BCLD)

In a recent study carried out on 2475 BMTs, Zutter et al. (63) reported a 0.6% overall incidence rate (i.e., 15 cases). A risk factor was identified for 13 cases (in vivo monoclonal antibody, T depletion, HLA disparity). This therapeutic complication caused death in 13 of 15 patients. The role of EBV virus was demonstrated in all of the 13 patients who were assessed. Eighty percent of the cases involved polyclonal proliferation. Donor cells were implicated in 10 cases of 12 that were studied. In most of the series including cases of HLA-incompatible transplantation, a high incidence of BCLD was found (Table 1). In a study relating to the overall incidence of BCLD among patients transplanted for congenital disorders (12.8%), lymphoproliferative diorders occurred 16 times following transplantation of HLA disparate grafts (64). Shapiro et al. reported a 24% incidence of BCLD, most of which were fatal, following T-depleted BMT performed under conditions of HLA incompatibility (against a 0 of 47 following TCD BMT from HLA identical donors, and a 1 in 424 following non-TCD transplantation using HLA-identical donors) (65).

Our own experience shows an 11.5% incidence of BCLD following HLA-incompatible grafting vs. 2% in our HLA-identical, T-depleted series (unpublished data).

IV. BONE MARROW TRANSPLANTATION USING DONORS OTHER THAN HLA-IDENTICAL SIBLINGS

A. Mismatched BMT from Related Donors

In reviewing the literature, we will differentiate between mismatched BMTs performed for hematologic malignancies and those carried out during the course of nonmalignant diseases.

1. Hematologic Malignancies

A total of 632 patients is included in Table 2. An overall analysis of the 9 series studied allows for the following observations:

0 to 1 HLA antigen disparity was noted in 47.5%, and 2 to 3 HLA antigen disparities in 52.5%.

70% of the cases were not T depleted and showed a mean incidence of acute GVHD of 71.6% (range: 37–90%), with a high proportion of severe (grade III-IV) patterns. In the TCD group 26% had acute GVHD grade II for the most part. The severity of the graft-vs.-host reaction did not consistently correlate with the degree of HLA disparity.

The mean incidence of graft failure was 20.5% (range: 6.8-30%). In 4 of 5 series where bone marrow had been T depleted, the relapse rate approximated 30%.

One must be careful when analyzing the overall survival of 32% (range: 17-51), these figures seem somewhat artificial in view of the heterogeneity of the clinical status

Table 2 Clinical Characteristics of Mismatched Bone Marrow Transplantation for Leukemia Using Family Donors

No. of patients	HLA disparity	T-cell depletion	Graft failure (%)	GVHD II-IV (%)	Overall survival (%)	Ref.
250	0-1 ≠ (145) 2-3 ≠ (105)	no	6.8	37-90	20-40 according to the HLA disparity	Seattle (66)
141	0-1 ≠ (61) 2-3 ≠ (80)	yes (40%)	28	70 (TCD−) 23 (TCD+)	43.5	EBMTR (67)
59	0-1 ≠ (31) 2-3 ≠ (28)	yes (54%)	32	70 (TCD−) 28 (TCD+)	30.5	GEGMO (68)
52	0-1 ≠ (17) 2-3 ≠ (35)	yes	30	8.5	15	MSKCC (11)
35	1 ≠ (11) 2-3 ≠ (24)	no	28	80	31	Royal Marsden Hosp. (69)
26	0-1 ≠ (11) 2-3 ≠ (15)	yes	15	30	26	Besancon (59)
31	1 ≠ (17) 2-3 ≠ (14)	no	9.6	55	51	Copenhagen (71)
21	N.A.	yes	30	43	21	Wisconsin (70)
17	0-1 ≠ (7) 2-3 ≠ (10)	no (but 4)	5.8	90	47	Munich (99)
Total: 632	300 0-1 ≠ (47.5%) 332 2-3 ≠ (52.5%)	192 TCD + (30%) 440 TCD − (70%)	20.5% (6.8-32)	71.6 (TCD−) 26.5 (TCD+)	32.7 (15-51)	

encountered: the pretransplantation protocols; the methods of GVHD prevention; the distribution of HLA disparities from one series to another, and, more particularly, different follow up periods. Late infection-related complications can occur beyond 6 months post-BMT.

GVHD together with bone marrow graft rejection stands out in the evolution of HLA-incompatible transplantation. Depending on the team, prevention of these complications has varied: standard prophylaxis programs identical to those used for HLA identical grafts (12) versus intensification of the conditioning regimen + TCD (11,13,21,38, 59) which may be responsible for an increase of toxic or infectious complications.

A more detailed analysis of some of the clinical series will enable us to oversee better the factors which interact to influence the evolution of HLA-incompatible grafting for hematologic malignancies.

The Seattle series included 250 patients with HLA-nonidentical related BMT (12, 66). Patients received a GVHD-prophylaxis preparation protocol identical to that usually applied for HLA-identical transplantation. In this way, the real impact of HLA disparity on the evolution of allografts could be appraised. The 250 patients were genotypically HLA identical to their donors for one haplotype, while certain disparities existed on the second haplotype. (Parents were donors for 116 patients; full siblings were available for 113, and the remaining 21 received transplants from other related donors.)

A very significant difference existed in the incidence of acute GVHD between genotypically HLA-identical donors and donors HLA disparate for the unshared haplotype, either at one or several loci. With one disparate antigen, the incidence of acute GVHD was 62%; when two disparate antigens were involved, the incidence was 72%, and 96% with three disparate antigens. For comparison, the acute GVHD rate was 58% in the series, which included genotypically identical transplant recipients. Whenever there was a three-loci disparity, the GVHD occurred earlier than with HLA-identical grafts. With a one-locus disparity, the overall incidence of grades II-IV GVHD was comparable to that in HLA-identical recipients. The MTX + CSP combination proved more effective in preventing GVHD than did MTX alone, when the difference concerned one antigen only. On the contrary, no significant advantage of the combination was noted for 12 antigenic disparities.

In the group of 117 patients with a one-locus disparity, graft failures occurred in 2.5% of the cases and poor graft function was found in 20%. In the group of 83 patients with two-loci disparities, the graft failure and poor graft function occurred in 15.6% and 22%, respectively. It is noteworthy that among the 22 transplanted patients who had three disparate antigens, not a single case of graft failure was detected, and poor graft function occurred in 10%.

In this large series, it appears that the probability of survival is similar (40%) both for those patients with a one-locus disparity and those of comparable clinical status receiving genotypically identical grafts, even though GVHD incidence was significantly higher in the former group of patients. With a two-antigen mismatch, survival was below 20% (p = 0.001). The group was too small to allow for a statistical comparison of three-antigen mismatched transplants.

The European study reported 242 cases of mismatched BMT (12% phenotypically identical; 33% with a one-antigen disparity; 29% and 26% with two- and three-antigen disparities, respectively) (67). The fact that this study was retrospective explains the great heterogeneity in terms of clinical status, pregrafting preparation programs, and GVHD prevention. A more uniform, 141-patient group was culled from this series (C.

Irlé, manuscript in preparation). The incidence of GVHD rose concomitantly with the number of HLA disparities. Although the overall GVHD incidence was 49%, it was 70% in the non-T-depleted group and 23% in the T-depleted group. MLR results did not predict incidence rates of severe forms of GVHD.

Forty patients manifested graft failure (28%); the difference was significant and was related to T depletion: 53% graft failures with TCD (the majority of the patients were pretreated with cyclophosphamide + TBI) vs. 13% with unmanipulated marrow (p < 0.001). In this series, graft rejections occurred in 8.8% of patients with GVHD grades II-IV and in 46% with minimal or no GVHD. Although this difference was not significant, survival was improved in the non-TCD group (56%) as compared to the TCD group (31.5%). Independently from T depletion, in the presence of a negative MLR, survival was 45% at 36 months, compared to 23% with a positive MLR. Fifty-five percent of the patients died from causes directly related to transplantation: 35% of infection-related complications (19% bacterial or fungal, 10% CMV, and 6% interstitial pneumonitis); 13% of the patients died from hemorrhagic complications.

In a French series of 59 patients which excluded subjects transplanted at Besançon, we noted 32% graft failures and a 9.3% incidence of severe (grades III-IV) GVHD in the TCD group vs. 55.5% with unmanipulated marrow. The frequency of early deaths was 10% with a standard pregrafting preparation regimen vs. 48% when the latter was intensified. Mortality in case of infection-related complications was identical to that found in the European series (33.8%) (68).

One may want to emphasize certain facts from the single-center reports concerned with smaller series. In the Royal Marsden series (69) including 35 patients, 45% had received a graft disparate for three antigens. Most of them had received a standard preparation treatment, while cyclosporin A had been the only GVHD prophylaxis used. Acute GVH reactions were observed in 80% and were fatal in six instances. A capillary leak syndrome was observed in 34% (14% in the European series). Thirty-one percent of patients were alive at 2.5-4.5 years following BMT (those less than 19 years of age had a 53% probability of survival vs. 0% for those older than 30 years). The Memorial Sloan-Kettering Cancer Center reports a series of 52 leukemic patients (prepared by hyperfractionated TBI) who received T-depleted (soybean + E-rosetting) grafts. Of 48 patients assessed, 16 (30%) rejected their grafts, while among 35 who had complete hematologic reconstitution only 3 (8.5%) developed >grade II GVHD. Fifty-four percent of the 35 patients died of infection-related problems. Among seven patients surviving (14.4%) only four had achieved complete remission (8.3%) (11,38).

In our institution, 20 of 26 patients received an intensive preparative protocol (TAM), and three of the four failures observed (15%) occurred with TAM. In all instances the marrow had been T-depleted. Three cases (11%) of severe GVHD were noted. No relationship could be demonstrated between HLA disparity and the occurrence of GVHD. The survival rate was 19% (deaths were mostly linked to infections, particularly of viral etiology and the occurrence of two lymphoma cases) (59).

Data collected by the Madison group show some differences (13,70): 21 patients given cyclophosphamide + TBI or high dose cytosine arabinoside + TBI preparation received pan-T (CD2)-depleted grafts; 24% had graft failure. Among 14 evaluable patients, 6 (43%) presented with severe GVHD leading to early infection-related death in 52%. Five patients (21%) are surviving in complete remission.

In a series including 31 patients with leukemia prepared with cyclophosphamide + TBI, the Copenhagen team showed a strong influence of age on patient survival: 0 survivor in the over-20 age group (n = 6) versus 16 survivors in patients less than twenty years of age (n = 25). No apparent difference existed in relation to the incidence of GVHD (55%), or MHC class I and class II related graft failures (71).

2. Nonmalignant Diseases (Table 3)

Congenital Disorders (Inborn Errors)

The European Registry (EBMTG) reports 75 mismatch transplantation cases for SCID (n = 57), combined immunodeficiency (n = 11), Wiskott-Aldrich syndrome (n = 5), and osteopetrosis (n = 2). Most often, the donor was a parent, i.e., haploidentical. Among SCID patients, 40 had not received any preparation treatment, while the others had been given TBI, chemotherapy or both (64,72). Among the 57 SCID patients, the overall incidence of GVHD was 28% (3.5% only had >grade II); engraftment was obtained in 82.6%. Survival was correlated to T depletion, 57% with T-depleted grafts (n = 46), 18% for non-T-depleted patients (n = 11; p < 0.001). Successful engraftment rates were 75%, 55.5%, and 60.5% with one, two, or three disparate antigens, respectively. For non-SCID patients probability of survival was 29% (47% in HLA-identical situations). In an earlier Sloan-Kettering series including 35 children with SCID grafted with HLA-mismatched non-T-depleted allografts, overall survival was 30% vs. 56% with HLA-identical transplants. Moderate or severe GVHD was noted in half of the patients (73). In a second series, 35 children (cumulative data derived from six centers) received HLA-mismatched, T-depleted grafts: 29 (82%) are surviving without GVHD and 28 achieved complete reconstitution of T-cell-mediated immunity. B-cell-mediated immunity was established more slowly (10/26 children assessed) (11).

In a recent series including 23 children with SCID given parental HLA-mismatched T-depleted marrow, O'Reilly et al. have shown that 21 children achieved lasting engraftment following one (n = 16) or two (n = 7) allotransplants (18 children had received no TCD prior to their first transplantation). Two children only (8%) developed a limited cutaneous GVH reaction. No clinical manifestations of chronic GVHD were noted. Among the 23 childen, 16 (69%) are surviving with either partial or complete T-cell reconstitution (38).

Bone Marrow Aplasia (Severe Aplastic Anemia)

With HLA-identical transplantation the incidence of graft rejection approximates 40% in transfused patients when the preparation protocol consists only of high doses of cyclophosphamide without irradiation. If either TBI or thoraco-abdominal irradiation is added to chemotherapy, a decrease in rejection rates can be observed, although complications related to toxicity are increased.

The first results obtained for HLA-incompatible grafts have been disappointing (74). In Seattle, 17 patients were prepared with traditional treatments for HLA mismatched allografting (12 patients with one disparate antigen; 3 with two different antigens, and 2 with phenotypically identical grafts). Eleven instances of graft rejection, and four cases of lethal GVHD were observed. The only two patients who survived (11%) received phenotypically identical grafts. Whenever TBI was included in the pregrafting preparation protocol, engraftment was improved (2/3 patients survived for longer than one year after transplant) (4,75).

On the other hand, the Minneapolis team transplanted six children with aplastic anemia with HLA-mismatched grafts following preparation consisting either of cyclophosphamide + TBI or cyclophosphamide + TLI. Failure of engraftment occurred in three cases, and severe GVHD in two (33%). Only one child is currently alive (7,76).

Table 3 Clinical Characteristics of Mismatched Bone Marrow Transplantation for Nonmalignant Diseases Using Family Donors

No. of patients	Diagnosis	HLA disparity	TCD	Graft failure (%)	GVHD II-IV (%)	Overall survival (%)	Ref.
57	SCID	2-3 ≠ mostly	yes (80%)	17.4	28	57 (TCD+) 18 (TCD−)	EBMT (64)
24	SCID	3 ≠ (20)	yes	8.4	9	71	MSKCC (11)
17	SAA	0-1 ≠ (12) 2-3 ≠ (5)	no	53	44	12	Seattle (75)
16	SCID (11) non-SCID (5)	3 ≠ (15)	yes	25	12.5	50	Wisconsin (100)
6	SAA	NA	no	50	33	16	Minnesota (76)
10	SAA	0-1 ≠ (7) 2 ≠ (3)	no but 4	33	43	40	London (77)

Table 4 Clinical Characteristics of Bone Marrow Transplantation Using Unrelated Volunteer Donors

No. of patients	Diagnosis	HLA disparity	TCD	Intensified preparative regimen	Graft failure (%)	GVHD II-IV (%)	Infectious complic. (%)	Overall survival (%)	Ref.
68	Leukemia (54) SAA (10) SCID (2) others (2)	matched (19) partially mismatched (49)	no but 7	various	8	58	36	39	EBMTR (79)
40	Leukemia (36) SAA (4)	partially mismatched	no	yes	5	47.5	72	15	Iowa (14)
28	Leukemia	matched	yes	yes	0	33	NA	57	Wisconsin (78)
14	SAA (11) Leukemia (3)	matched (6) partially mm (8)	yes (50%)	no	38	77	7	28	Hammersmith (77)
16	Leukemia	matched	yes	yes	6.2	25	6.2	73	(21)
9	Leukemia	matched	no	no	0	78	33	22	Seattle (66)
8	Leukemia	matched (3) partially mm (5)	no	yes	0	87	37	50	Minneapolis (43)

Hows et al. (77) reported one series including 10 patients with severe aplasia (of whom 5 had Fanconi's anemia). Most of the patients were prepared with cyclophosphamide + ATG, while those with Fanconi's anemia received cyclophosphamide + TBI (at lowered doses). In 5 of 10, a family donor phenotypically identical was found. Three rejections occurred, and 43% of patients developed >grade II GVHD) (40% of the grafts were T-depleted). Four patients are surviving with complete hematologic reconstitution.

B. Marrow Transplantation From Full Matched or Partially Mismatched Unrelated Volunteer Donors

Results from six published series including 183 patients are summarized in Table 4 (14,21,43,66,72-79). As has been pointed out previously, malignant hematologic diseases represent the most frequent indication (84%) for bone marrow transplantation. In 55% of cases HLA phenotypical identity was present. The graft was T-depleted in 32% of the cases (using mostly monoclonal antibody).

Pregrafting preparation regimens were intensified for over half of the patients using varying protocols which typically included high doses of cytosine arabinoside as the additional chemotherapeutic (14,78). The Iowa Center series (14) deserves being analyzed in some detail. It included 40 patients (36 leukemias with poor prognosis) who had received non-T-depleted marrow transplants from unrelated, partially mismatched donors (42% had negative mixed lymphocyte cultures; 67% differed for one or two HLA-antigens, and 7.5% for three antigens). Preparation consisted of high-dose cytosine arabinoside with cyclophosphamide and TBI (1200 rads). Engraftment was achieved in 38 leukemic patients. Two graft failures were observed among four patients with aplastic anemia. Grades II-IV GVHD developed in 47.5% of the 32 patients assessed (including 37.5% grades III-IV). Major complications responsible for the death of 29 patients were infection-related. Six patients survive (15%), 5 of them with chronic GVHD.

With non-T-depleted grafts, the incidence of GVHD is high, even when the donor is phenotypically HLA-identical (70% to 80% occur in moderate or severe forms).

The Madison series (70) using an intensified preparation regimen (high-dose cytosine arabinoside + cyclophosphamide + TBI) recorded successful engraftment in all instances, and with T-depleted marrow obtained a GVHD incidence (grade II for the most part) as low as 33%. Overall survival (57%) was encouraging. Fourteen patients from Hammersmith's historical series (11 with bone marrow aplasia) received grafts from unrelated donors; these grafts differed either by one class II antigen (n = 7) or by one class I antigen (n = 8). For T-depleted grafts performed in 7 cases out of 14, grade II-IV GVHD was observed in 77%. Given the large number of aplastic anemia patients, a high incidence of graft failure could be observed (38%). The 4 surviving patients (28%) achieved satisfactory hematologic reconstitution (77). In a more recent series, the same group reported 16 patients with CML who all received fully matched grafts (21). Preliminary findings seem quite encouraging. With strongly intensified preparative regimens and TCD, a single case of graft failure was observed, while GVHD occurred in 25% of cases. The overall survival rate for a follow up period averaging 7 months was 73%. Unfortunately, data collected more recently over longer observational periods bring forth evidence of late infection-related complications occurring in 31% cases and leukemic relapse. Overall survival declined to 50%, disease-free survivors making up 28% of this figure (unpublished data).

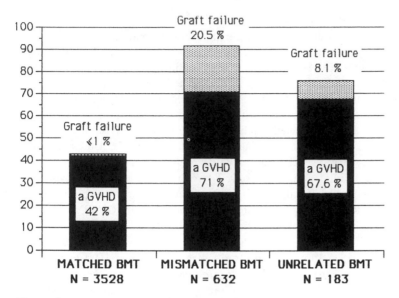

Figure 1   Rates of occurrence of acute GVHD and graft failure between matched (from family or unrelated donors) and mismatched allografting.

C. Comments

Figure 1 shows schematically the varying incidence of acute GVHD and graft failure noted between matched and mismatched family donor allografts, as well as allografts (mostly matched) from unrelated donors.

1. Mismatched BMT from Related Donors

On the basis of the 800 American and European series cases (83% malignant hematologic diseases), which exhibited a strong heterogeneity in terms of clinical status, preparation protocols, anti-GVHD prophylaxis and HLA disparity, one can identify four major specific complications: a high incidence (75-90%) of acute GVHD, often occurring early and with severe manifestations (grades III-IV), engraftment failures (nontake, rejection, autologous reconstitution, and poor graft function) which showed a frequency strongly linked with the preparation protocol used; early or late infections, especially of viral etiology, responsible for the death of more than half the patients, and lastly, occurrence of lymphoproliferative diseases in 15%-25% of cases, depending on the series (80). In mismatch situations, T depletion is effective in preventing severe forms of GVHD, however, it causes the frequency of graft failure to rise, and it is sometimes responsible for relapse (CML), thereby improving in no way the overall survival (61).

Given the high incidence of early deaths, the duration of the follow up period, which was less than 12 months in many cases, and the frequency of very advanced, poor prognosis disease which often had motivated the use of mismatched transplants, it is difficult to analyze the relapse rates in these series. On the other hand, in SCID the good results of mismatched BMT are undeniable (64,72). T-cell depletion is effective with a significant impact on survival.

2. BMTs from Unrelated Volunteer Donors

Nearly 200 cases have already been reported in the literature. Hematologic diseases represent three quarters of the cases. The complications noted with partially mismatched grafts are equivalent to those observed in mismatched situations when the donor is a family member, although the frequency of lethal infection-related complications seems to be particularly high. The incidence of acute GVHD in the absence of TCD, even with perfectly HLA-identical grafts, is similar to that which can be observed in HLA-incompatible family transplants. In HLA phenotypically identical situations, one will require some tests for determining the expected risk of having severe forms of GVHD. Under these circumstances, Vogelsang's or Bagot's technique are worth evaluating (26,27). The assessment of limiting dilutions of alloreactive cytotoxic T-lymphocyte precursors for volunteer donors has been proposed by Kaminski et al. (82). Such systems might potentially prove useful for the selection of donor to circumvent the risk of severe GVHD.

In looking for HLA phenotypically identical unrelated donors, one must be aware of the polymorphism of the HLA system, which is much greater than is suggested by the alleles identified so far (20,83). Should the splits or subgroups found in HLA alleles be taken into account? If we were to agree to include a mismatched antigen or a higher proliferation response index in mixed lymphocyte cultures (10-20%), the number of potential donors could increase.

V. PREVENTION OF COMPLICATION AFTER HLA-INCOMPATIBLE BMT

All published data show the great frequency of complications, often lethal, which are associated with HLA-incompatible bone marrow transplants. Such observations stress the "experimental" aspect of this type of transplantation, in which standard preparation regimens and conventional methods of GVHD prophylaxis are often insufficient, if not ineffective in preventing graft failures and severe forms of GVHD. It appears that the future of HLA-incompatible transplantation depends upon innovative protocols, especially in matters of prevention, and treatment for acute GVHD, graft failure, induced lymphoma, and infection-related complications (Fig. 2).

A. Prevention and Treatment of Acute GVHD

T depletion, which is considered to be the most effective method in that it made it possible to perform incompatible marrow transplants, can only be recommended provided that one has the means to prevent engraftment failure and relapse (most importantly, in CML).

One should explore the methods of cell depletion through immunophysical technique, as well as define the minimal T-cell dose. Combining elutriation with the infusion, to the donor, of irradiated buffy coat cells should be discussed in mismatched or phenotypically identical unrelated situations (84).

As animal models indicate (29), real progress will be achieved when phenotypic and functional *identification* of those T cells specifically responsible for GVH reactions will be possible. Their eradication from the graft via monoclonal antibodies should not be a major obstacle considering the diversity of monoclonal antibodies available.

The cyclosporin A (long-term treatment) and methotrexate (short-term treatment) combination therapy has presently become the "standard" protocol regularly in use, es-

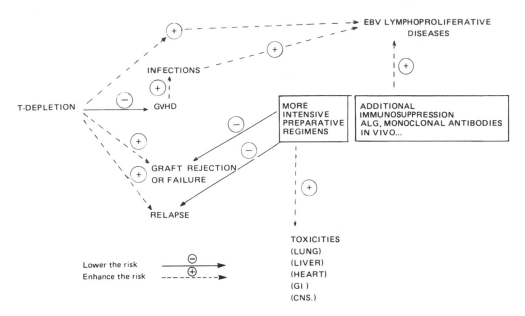

Figure 2 Diagram of key problems in bone marrow transplantation using donors other than HLA-identical siblings.

pecially in phenotypically identical unrelated programs (66). Current treatment of acute GVHD refractory to corticosteroids calls for the administration of monoclonal antibodies in vivo (Table 5). The specificity of the antibody may apply to the CD8$^+$ cells, all T cells (pan T), or the receptor for IL-2 on activated T-cells (85). In our own experience, we have utilized anti-IL-2-R(B-B10) antibodies (81) in 18 patients presenting with acute corticosteroid-resistant GVHD (12 had received HLA-identical grafts and 6 had HLA-incompatible grafts). The maximum GVHD score was grade II in 7 patients, grade III in 9 patients, and grade IV in 2. Patients were injected with 5 mg of B-B10 daily for 10 days. No signs of intolerance were observed. In 11 cases (61%), acute GVHD was completely eradicated. These were 7 grade II and 4 grade III cases (9 matched, 2 mismatched). In three instances (16%), improvement was clearly noted (2 grade III and 1 grade IV case, 2 mismatched and 1 matched), and finally, four patients (22%) showed no improvement (3 grade III, 1 grade IV, 2 mismatched and 2 matched). As far as graft failures are concerned, treatment with monoclonal antibody had been instituted late in two out of three cases (>40 days after GVHD onset). Among the 11 responders, GVHD recurred three times (86). Further studies will be necessary to appraise the value of prolonged therapy administered more or less discontinuously, in preventing GVHD recurrences upon cessation of treatment. It would seem that the utilization of this type of monoclonal antibody is promising for GVHD therapy, even in mismatched situations, provided it is administered early. The question to be asked will concern the possibility of monoclonal antibody prophylaxis of GVHD as early as day 0 (grafting day), especially in mismatched situations. The effect of such immunotherapy on the reconstitution of immunity, as well as on the frequency of infection-related complications will have to be analyzed.

Table 5 Treatment of Acute Graft-vs.-Host Disease with Monoclonal Antibody In Vivo

MAb	Target cells	BMT context	No. of patients	Response (%)	Ref.
B-B10 (IgG1)	Il-2 R + cells	matched and mismatched	13	84	Hervé et al. (86,104)
Campath 2 (Ig G2b)	CD7 + cells	matched and mismatched	3	66	Morgan et al. (101)
X 8 (IgG2)	CD8 + cells	matched	23	80	Gluckman et al. Unpublished data
A 50 (IgG2)	CD5 + cells	matched and mismatched	18	61	Pico et al.
X 8 (IgG2)	CD8 + cells	mismatched			Unpublished data
Ricin-A chain Immunotoxin (Xomazyme R H65)	CD5 + cells	matched and mismatched	10	40[a]	Byers et al. (87)
Campath - IG	T and B cells	matched	28	100[a]	Hale et al. (35)
BMA 031 (IgG2b)	Human T cell receptor CD3	mismatched	3	66	Beelen et al. (102)
10.2 (IgG2a)	CD5 + cells	matched	15	40	Martin et al. (8,103)
35.1 (IgG2a)	CD2 + cells				

[a] Lack of data.

Other monoclonal antibodies have been suggested for the treatment of acute GVHD refractory to corticosteroids. Results are given in Table 5. The first studies were carried out in HLA—identical recipients with findings varying depending on the study. Nevertheless, the timing of treatment after the onset of GVHD undoubtedly influences the efficacy of immunotherapy. The Boston group has demonstrated the efficacy in vivo of an anti-T12 antibody in the early phase of posthaploidentical grafting severe acute GVHD in SCID patients receiving grafts that had been depleted by using the same anti-T12 (2).

A CD5-ricin chain A immunotoxin has been proposed for use in GVHD by the Minneapolis group (87), which yielded a 50% rate of response: most of these favorable results were obtained when the treatment had been started in the early phase of the disease. We do not have sufficient information concerning the impact of in vivo pan-T-cell antibodies on the reconstitution of immunity, nor of the incidence of infection-related complications. We already stressed their role in the occurrence of BCLD.

In HLA-mismatched marrow transplant settings, taking into consideration the results obtained in HLA-matched situations, one can make the following recommendations regarding the use of monoclonal antibody in the treatment of acute GVHD. Monoclonal antibodies must be used in the early phase (less than 10 days), at effective dosages for sufficiently long periods of time, followed by a discontinuous treatment, in order to avoid early GVHD recurrences. A study of the pharmacokinetics of circulating antibody should be carried out for each patient; moreover, it is necessary that the latter be tested for alloimmunization with respect to the murine antibody (antiisotype, antiidiotype) three weeks following the last injection day.

Systematic in vivo prophylaxis against GVHD with monoclonal antibody may be argued against in HLA identical situations. Can we expect the same to be true in nonidentical or unrelated fully matched settings, knowing the frequency with which severe forms of GVHD occur when non T-depleted grafts are used? With such monoclonal antibodies as the anti-IL2-R, prevention of GVHD could be used starting as early as day 0 within controlled study programs.

B. Prevention of the Host-vs.-Graft Reaction

Monoclonal antibody can be used in vivo in another situation, i.e., during graft failures following T depletion of the graft and in HLA-incompatible situations. Two possibilities are offered to the investigator: either to utilize in vivo antibodies specific to the immunocompetent cells which survived the preparation course of chemotherapy and irradiation, or to intensify the latter.

1. Monoclonal Antibodies Directed at Residual Host Immunocompetent Cells

In one experimental model, Cobbold et al. (88) have noted suppression of the allo-reactivity mechanisms through controlling immune responses in vivo. In H2-incompatible situations in the mouse, the eradication of L3T4$^+$ cells (equivalent to human CD4$^+$ cells) and of Lyt-2$^+$ cells (equivalent to human CD8$^+$ cells) by using specific antibodies in vivo suppresses the rejection phenomenon. Both lymphocyte populations are independently capable of rejecting marrow transplants. However, L3T4$^+$ cells seem more effective than Lyt-2$^+$ cells in inducing rejection.

The clinical use of antibodies directed against cells which are thought to be implicated in BMT rejection has been suggested in HLA-different transplantation settings, or after T-depletion of the graft. One of the most interesting pilot studies has dealt with the utilization of anti-LFA1 alpha-chain antibodies (CD11) during mismatched transplants performed for severe combined immunodeficiency (SCID) and acute leukemias (89). Among the 48 patients treated *prophylactically* with this antibody, engraftment was observed in 74% (in one control group which was not treated with anti-LFA1 antibodies, functional grafts developed only in 20% of cases). Although such results seem indisputable as far as congenital diseases are concerned they are contested by other studies which used the same anti-LFA1 antibody, or an anti-LFA1 beta-chain (CD18) antibody, and were carried out in TCD HLA-identical transplantation settings during the course of acute leukemia (90). The authors have noted that the frequency of graft failure was similar to that found with the use of antibody. In other clinical studies, Campath-1 G (35) and anti-IL-2-R (81) were proposed. Clinical data are all too fragmentary to yield any information. Other preclinical studies have been concerned with antibodies directed against class II antigens (91) or NK cells presumably implicated in the rejection reaction (92,93). In the dog, this type of monoclonal antibody was capable of inducing engraftment in 7/10 animals versus 3/36 for controls. In one murine model, Tiberghien et al. have confirmed the impact of anti-asialo GM-1 antibodies on the engraftment of histologically incompatible transplants (94).

2. Intensification of the Radio-Chemotherapeutic Preparative Regimen

Although it is a priori more advantageous to introduce antibodies in the preparation protocol (tolerance, specificity), their availability for clinical use is often a problem and their real effectiveness remains to be proven. Increasing the total TBI dose, supplementing it with TLI, and using additional chemotherapy to the standard protocol can induce superior host immunosuppression. In this respect, many suggestions have been brought forth, aiming at enhancing immunosuppression. About 10 different protocols have been proposed, with a marked preference either for increasing the total TBI dose (1400-1500 rads) (96), or for supplementing the standard cyclophosphamide + TBI regimen with high dose cytosine arabinoside (12-36 g/m^2) (95,13). The incidence of early deaths directly traceable to the preparation therapy has varied from 14 to 30%. In another series including about ten patients, the TBI + cytosine arabinoside + cyclophosphamide combination ended up with 80% early deaths. With the TAM (TBI, high dose cytosine arabinoside and melphalan) protocol which was initiated in our institution, the incidence of early deaths in a 50-patient multicenter pilot study was 14.6% (97). The intensification of the preparation regimen and the expected immunosuppressive result must be balanced against increased nonmarrow toxicity. The latter consideration tends to make high-dose cytosine arabinoside, introduced by the Madison group, the more appealing one.

The irrefutable usefulness of TLI (600-700 rads) + TBI combinations in experimental models (57,58) remains controversial in clinical trials following T depletion of the grafts or in mismatched situations.

The third problem raised is a possible increase of the rate of T-depletion-related relapse, conceivably due to an elimination of the GVL effect. Data collected from published clinical series to date are not conclusive. Many suggestions have been made. The irradiation protocols could be modified so as to act more suppressively on residual disease, by increasing the total dose, accelerating the dose rate (>7 rads/min), using single fractions or boosts of high energy electrons to the chest wall according to the Sloan-Kettering protocol (11), or introducing additional chemotherapy.

Certain factors may increase the chances of relapse: post-BMT immunosuppression, and delayed engraftment due to host antigraft alloreactivity allowing host cells (including leukemic ones) to repopulate the bone marrow. It is clear that donor T cells implicated in GVL can act directly on leukemic cells via cytotoxicity.

VI. CONCLUSION

Clearly, in situations of HLA incompatibility, GVHD graft rejection or relapse are closely linked and all the protocols proposed for the treatment and the prevention of GVHD must be adapted to this reality. In HLA-incompatible (family donor) or phenotypically identical (unrelated) situations, a protocol for the prophylaxis and treatment of acute GVHD might be worked out on the basis of the present state of knowledge as well as on certain hypotheses to combine:

1. more selective partial T depletion, i.e., through the reintroduction in the T-depleted inoculum of viable T cells (the dose having to remain below a currently poorly defined critical threshold);
2. optimal B-cell depletion in the graft when the donor is positive for EBV;
3. intensified radio-chemotherapeutic protocols via additional chemotherapy such as cytosine arabinoside (upper limit of the tolerated dose to be determined in relation of the age of the recipient);
4. treatment of recipient with in vivo monoclonal antibodies specific for residual, radio-resistant immunocompetent cells, prior to grafting.

Given the partial T depletion, prophylaxis against GVHD with CSP and methotrexate is necessary; possibly this should be *quickly* followed by monoclonal antibodies directed against effector T cells for the GVH reaction. The feasibility and efficacy of such a protocol still have to be proven in experimental BMTs.

In order to promote better engraftment following T depletion, or in mismatching, the usefulness of incubating donor marrow with recombinant growth factors, such as GM-CSF, is under investigation (98).

REFERENCES

1. Clift RA, Hansen JA, Thomas ED, Buckner CD, Sanders JE, Mickelson EM, Storb R, Johnson FL, Singer JW, Goodell BW: Marrow transplantation from donors other than HLA identical siblings. Transplantation 1979;28:235-242.
2. Reinherz EL, Geha R, Rappeport JM, Wilson M, Penta AC, Hussey RE, Fitzgerald KA, Daley JF, Levine H, Rosen FS, Schlossman SF: Reconstitution after transplantation with T-lymphocyte-depleted HLA haplotype-mismatched bone marrow for severe combined immunodeficiency. Proc Natl Acad Sci USA 1982;79;6047-6051.
3. Bortin MM, Rimm AA: Severe combined immunodeficiency disease: characterization of the disease and results of transplantation. JAMA 1977;238:591-600.
4. Clift RA, Storb R: Histoincompatible bone marrow transplants in humans. Ann Rev Immunol 1987;5:43-64.
5. Hansen JA, Clift RA, Beatty PG, Mickelson EM, Nisperos B, Martin PJ, Thomas ED: Marrow transplantation from donors other than HLA genotypically identical siblings. In *Recent Advances in Bone Marrow Transplantation*, edited by Gale RP, Champlin R. Alan R. Liss, Inc., New York, 1983; pp. 739-756.
6. Delfini C, Polchi P, Izzi T, Nicolini G, Paradisi O, Lucarelli G: Bone marrow donors other than HLA genotypically identical siblings for patients with Thalassemia. Exp Hematol 1985;13:1197-1200.

7. Filipovich AM, Ramsay NKC, Arthur DC, McGlave P, Kim T, Kersey JH: Allo-geneic bone marrow transplantation with related donors other than MLC-matched siblings, and the use of antithymocyte globulin, prednisone and methotrexate for prophylaxis of graft-versus-host disease. Transplantation 1985;39:282-285.

8. Martin PJ, Hansen JA, Remlinger K, Torok-Storb B, Storb R, Thomas ED: Mono-clonal anti-human T-cell antibodies for the prevention and treatment of graft-versus-host disease. In *Recent Advances in Bone Marrow Transplantation*, edited by Gale RP. Alan R. Liss Inc., New York 1983; pp. 313-329.

9. Poynton CH; T-cell depletion in bone marrow transplantation. Bone Marrow Transplant 1988;3:265-280.

10. Reisner Y, Kapoor N, Kirkpatrick D, Pollack MS, Cunningham-Rundles S, Dupont B, Hodes MZ, Good RA, O'Reilly RJ: Transplantation for severe combined im-munodeficiency with HLA-A, B, D, DR incompatible parental marrow cell frac-tionated by soybean agglutinin and sheep red blood cells. Blood 1983;61:341-348.

11. O'Reilly RJ, Keever C, Kernan NA, Brochstein J, Collins N, Flomenberg N, Laver J, Emanuel D, Dupont B, Cunningham I, Castro-Malaspina H, Gulati S: HLA non-identical T-cell depleted marrow transplants: a comparison of results in patients treated for leukemia and severe combined immunodeficiency disease. Transplant Proc 1987;19:55-60.

12. Beatty PG, Clift RA, Mickelson EM, Nisperos BB, Flournoy N, Martin PY, Sanders JE, Stewart P, Buckner CD, Storb R, Thomas ED, Hansen JA: Marrow transplan-tation from related donors other than HLA-identical siblings. N Engl J Med 1985; 313:765-771.

13. Trigg ME, Sondel PM, Billing R, Finally JL, Peterson A, Hong R, Friedrich S, Shahidi N: Mismatched bone marrow transplantation in children with hematologic malig-nancy using T-lymphocyte depleted bone marrow. J Biol Resp Modif 1985;4:602-612.

14. Gingrich R, Ginder GD, Goeken NE, Howe CWS, Wen BC, Hussy DH, Fyfe MA: Allogeneic marrow grafting with partially mismatched unrelated marrow donors. Blood 1988;71:1375-1381.

15. O'Reilly RJ, Dupont B, Pahwa S, Grimes E, Smithwick EM, Pahwa R, Schwartz S, Hansen JA, Siegal F, Sorell M, Svejgaard A, Jersild C, Thomsen M, Platz P, L'Esper-ance P, Good RA: Reconstitution in severe combined immunodeficiency by trans-plantation of marrow from an unrelated donor. N Engl J Med 1977;297:1311-1318.

16. Storb R, Weiden PL, Graham TC, Lerner KG, Thomas ED: Marrow grafts between HLA-identical and homozygous unrelated dogs. Transplantation 1977;24:165-174.

17. Speck B, Zwaan FE, Van Rood JJ, Eernisse JG: Allogeneic bone marrow transplan-tation in a patients with aplastic anemia using a phenotypically HLA-identical un-related donor. Transplantation 1973;16:24-28.

18. Horowitz SD, Groshong T, Bach FH, Hong R, Yunis EJ: Treatment of severe com-bined immunodeficiency with bone marrow from an unrelated mixed-leucocyte-culture-nonreactive donor. Lancet 1975;2:431-433.

19. Hansen JA, Clift RA, Thomas ED, Buckner CD, Storb R, Giblett ER: Transplanta-tion of marrow from an unrelated donor to a patient with acute leukemia. N Engl J Med 1980;303:565-567.

20. Eckman MH, Sonnenberg FA, Jacoby I, Pauker SG: HLA matched donor registries for bone marrow transplants. Int J Technol Assess Health Care 1986;2:507.

21. Mackinnon S, Arthur CK, Apperley JF, Hows JM, Batchelor JR, Brookes P, Hale G, Waldmann H, Goldman JM: Histocompatible unrelated volunteer donors for BMT in patients with chronic myeloid leukemia. Bone Marrow Transplant 1988;3(Suppl 1): 176-177.

22. Santos GW, Hess AD, Vogelsang GB: Graft-versus-host reactions and disease. Im-munol Rev 1985;88:169-192.

23. Van Bekkum DW: Graft-versus-host disease. In *Bone Marrow Transplantation: Biological Mechanisms and Clinical Practice*, edited by Van Bekkum DW, Löwenberg R. Marcel Dekker, New York, 1985; pp. 147-212.

24. Bortin MM; Factors influencing the risk of acute Graft versus Host Disease in man. In *Progress in Bone Marrow Transplantation*, edited by Gale RP, Champlin R. UCLA symposia on molecular and cellular biology, Alan R. Liss Publisher, New York, 1987; pp. 243-264.

25. Ringden O, Nilsson B: Death by graft-versus-host disease associated with HLA mismatch, high recipient age, low marrow cell dose, an splenectomy. Transplantation 1985;40:39-44.

26. Bagot M: Mixed epidermal cell-lymphocyte culture. A predictive test for GVHD in bone marrow recipients. Path Biol 1988;36:293-295.

27. Vogelsang GB, Hess AD, Berkman AW, Tutschka PJ, Farmer ER, Converse PJ, Santos GW: An in vitro predictive test for graft-versus-host disease in patients with genotypic HLA-identical bone marrow transplants. N Engl J Med 1985;313:645-650.

28. Korngold R, Sprent J: Lethal graft-versus-host disease following bone marrow transplantation across minor histocompatibility barriers in mice: prevention by removing mature T-cells from marrow. J Exp Med 1978;148:1687-1698.

29. Korngold R, Sprent J: T-cell subsets and graft-versus-host disease. Transplantation 1987;44:335-339.

30. Vallera DA, Soderling CCB, Kersey JH: Bone marrow transplantation across major histocompatibility barriers. in mice. Treatment of donor grafts with monoclonal antibodies directed against Lyt determinants. J Immunol 1982;128:871-875.

31. Jansen J, Goselink HM, Beenhof WFJ: The impact of the composition of the bone marrow graft on engraftment and GVHD. Exp Hematol 1983;11:967-973.

32. Hervé P: Prevention of the graft-versus-host disease by T-cell depletion in allogeneic bone marrow transplants. Presse Med 1987;16:2019-2025.

33. Martin PJ, Hansen JA, Torok-Storb B, Durnam D, Przepiorka D, O'Quigley J, Sanders J, Sullivan KM, Witherspoon H, Deeg J, Appelbaum FR, Stewart P, Weiden P, Doney K, Buckner CD, Clift R, Storb R, Thomas ED: Graft failure in patients receiving T-cell depleted HLA-identical allogeneic marrow transplants. Bone Marrow Transplant 1988;3:445-456.

34. De Witte T, Hoogenhout J, De Pauw B, Holdrinet R, Janssen J, Wessels J, Van Daal W, Hustinx T, Haanen C: Depletion of donor lymphocytes by counterflow centrifugation successfully prevents acute graft versus host disease in matched allogeneic marrow transplantation. Blood 1986;67:1302-1308.

35. Hale G, Waldmann H: Campath-1 for prevention of graft-versus-host disease and graft rejection. Summary of results from a multi-centre study. Bone Marrow Transplant 1988;3(Suppl 1):11-14.

36. Atkinson K, Farrell H, Cooley M, O'Flaherty E, Down K, Biggs J: Human marrow T-cell dose correlates with severity of subsequent acute GVHD. Bone Marrow Transplant 1987;2:51-57.

37. Eiermann TH, Friedrich W: The critical T-cell dose causing graft-versus-host disease in T-cell depleted haploidentical BMT. Bone Marrow Transplant 1988;3(Suppl 1):210-211.

38. O'Reilly RJ, Kernan NA, Cunningham I, Brochstein J, Castro-Malaspina H, Laver J, Flomengerg N, Emanuel D, Galati S, Keever C, Collins NH, Bordignon C: Allogeneic transplants depleted of T-cells by soybean lectin agglutination and E rosette depletion. Bone Marrow Transplant 1988;3(Suppl 1):3-5.

39. Löwenberg B, Wagemaker G, Van Bekkum DW, Sizoo W, Sintnicolaas K, Hendriks WDH, Hagenbeek A: Graft-versus-host disease following transplantation of "one

log" versus "two log" T-lymphocyte-depleted bone marrow from HLA-identical donors. Bone Marrow Transplant 1986;1:133-140.

40. O'Reilly RJ, Brochstein J, Collins N, Keever C, Kapoor N, Kirkpatrick D, Kernan N, Dupont B, Burns J, Reisner Y: Evaluation of HLA-haplotype disparate parental marrow grafts depleted of T-lymphocytes by differential agglutination with a soybeam lectin and E-rosette depletion for the treatment of severe combined immunodeficiency. Vox Sang 1986;51:81-86.

41. Poynton CH: Mismatched family and unrelated donors for bone marrow transplantation using fixed low numbers of T-cells. Bone Marrow Transplant 1988;3(Suppl 1):223.

42. Goldman JM, Gale RP, Horowitz MM, Biggs JC, Champlin RE, Gluckman E, Hoffmann RG, Jacobsen SJ, Marmont AM, McGlave PB, Messner HA, Rimm AA, Rozman C, Speck B, Tura S, Weiner RS, Bortin MM: Bone marrow transplantation for chronic myelogenous leukemia in chronic phase. Increased risk for relapse associated with T-cell depletion. Ann Intern Med 1988;108:806-814.

43. McGlave P, Scott E, Ramsay N, Arthur D, Blazar B, McCullough J, Kersey J: Unrelated donor bone marrow transplantation therapy for chronic myelogenous leukemia. Blood 1987;70:877-881.

44. Bertheas MF, Maraninchi D, Lafage M, Blaise D, Stoppa AM, Michel G, Brizard CP, Gaspart MH, Novakovitch G, Mannoni P, Viens P, Carcassonne Y: Partial chimerism after T-cell depleted allogeneic bone marrow transplantation in leukemic HLA-matched patients: a cytogenetic documentation. Blood 1988;72:89-93.

45. Bretagne S, Vidand M, Kuentz M, Cordonnier C, Henni T, Vinci G, Goossens M, Vernant JP: Mixed blood chimerism in T-cell depleted bone marrow transplant recipients: evaluation using DNA polymorphisms. Blood 1987;70:1692-1695.

46. Petz LD, Yam P, Wallace RB, Stock AD, de Lange G, Knowlton RG, Brown VA, Donis-Keller H, Hill LR, Forman SJ, Blume KG: Mixed hematopoietic chimerism following bone marrow transplantation for hematologic malignancies. Blood 1987; 70:1331-1337.

47. Schattenberg A, De Witte T, Vet J, Salden M, Hustinx Th, Van Dijk B: Mixed chimerism after allogeneic transplantation with lymphocyte-depleted bone marrow. Bone Marrow Transplant 1988;3(Suppl 1):152.

48. Bourgue F, Maraninchi D, Olive D, Lopez M, Stoppa AM, Blaise D, Mercier P, Carcassonne Y: Incidence and characterization of residual host lymphocytes after various conditioning regimen to bone marrow transplantation. Bone Marrow Transplant 1988;3(Suppl 1):199-200.

49. Ferrara JL, Michaelson J, Burakoff SJ, Mauch P: Engraftment following T-cell depleted bone marrow transplantation. Transplantation 1988;45:948-952.

50. Gassman W, Kolszynski M, Wottge HU, Müller-Ruchholtz W: Demonstration of strong classic immune reactivity after total body irradiation for bone marrow transplantation. Implications for human T-depleted bone marrow transplantation. Transplant Proc 1987;19:2687-2688.

51. Kedar E, Or R, Naparstek E, Zeira E, Slavin S: Preliminary characterization of functional residual host-type T lymphocytes following conditioning for allogeneic HLA-matched bone marrow transplantation. Bone Marrow Transplant 1988;3:129-140.

52. Moulinier-Chapuis F, Autran B, Leblond V, Dombret H, Hercend T, Binet JL, Debre P: Analysis of residual lymphoid cells after pre BMT conditioning regimen. Bone Marrow Transplant 1988;3(Suppl 1):129.

53. Vinci G, Henri A, Kuentz M, Cordonnier C, Ganem G, Breton-Gorius J, Vernant JP: Recipient radioresistant T lymphocytes inhibit donor haematopoiesis in vitro. Bone Marrow Transplant 1988;3(Suppl 1):201-202.

54. Sondel PM, Hank JA, Trigg ME, Kohler PC, Finlay JL, Blank J, Meisner L, Borcherding W, Hong R, Steeves R, Billing R, Flynn B, Bozdech MJ: Transplantation of

HLA-haploidentical T-cell depleted marrow for leukemia: autologous marrow recovery with specific immune sensitization to donor antigens. Exp Hematol 1986; 14:278-286.

55. Kernan NA, Flomenberg N, Dupont B, O'Reilly RJ: Graft rejection in recipients of T-cell depleted HLA-non identical marrow transplants for leukemia. Identification of host-derived antidonor allocytoxic lymphocytes. Transplantation 1987;43: 842-847.

56. Reisner Y, Ben-Bassat I, Dover D, Kaploon A, Schwartz E, Ramot B: A primate pre-clinical model for bone marrow transplantation: definitive proof for host radio resistant clonable T-cells. Exp Hematol 1985;13:321 (abstract).

57. Slavin S, Naparstek E, Cividalli G, et al: The use of Campath-1 for prevention of graft versus host disease (GVHD) and total lymphoid irradiation (TLI) for abrogation of host resistance to T-cell depleted allografts. In *Progress in Bone Marrow Transplant*, edited by Gale RP and Champlin R. Alan R. Liss, New York, 1987; p. 399.

58. Blazar BR, Soderling CB, Robinson LL, Vallera DA: Short course total lymphoid irradiation combined with total-body irradiation to facilitate engraftment of T-cell depleted marrow across a major histocompatibility barrier in mice. Transplantation 1988;46:324-327.

59. Cahn JY, Hervé P, Flesch M, Plouvier E, Racadot E, Vuillier J, Montcuquet P, Noir A, Rozenbaum A, Leconte des Floris R: Marrow transplantation from HLA nonidentical family donors for the treatment of leukaemia: a pilot study of 15 patients using additional immunosuppression and T-cell depletion. Brit J of Haematol 1988; 69:345-349.

60. Anasetti C, Amos D, Beatty PG, Martin PJ, Hansen JA, Thomas ED: Risk factors for graft rejection of marrow from HLA-haploidentical donors. Blood 1987;70:301a.

61. Henslee PJ, Thompson JS, Romond EH, Doukas MA, Metcalfe M, Marshall ME, Mac Donald JS: T-cell depletion of HLA and haplo-identical marrow reduces graft-versus-host-disease but it may impair a graft-versus leukemia effect. Transplant Proc 1987;19:2701-2706.

62. Prentice HG, Hermans J, Zwaan FE: Relapse risk in allogeneic BMT with T-cell depletion of donor marrow. Bone Marrow Transplant 1988;3(Suppl 1):30-32.

63. Zutter MM, Martin PJ, Sale GE, Shulman HM, Fisher L, Thomas ED, Durnam DM: Epstein-Barr virus lymphoproliferation after bone marrow transplantation. Blood 1988;72:520-529.

64. Fischer A, Griscelli C, Friedrich W, Kubanek B, Levinsky R, Morgan G, Vossen J, Wagemaker G, Landais P: Bone marrow transplantation for immunodeficiencies and osteopetrosis: European Survey. Lancet 1986;2:1080-1083.

65. Shapiro RS, McClain K, Frizzera G, Gajl-Peczalska KJ, Kersey JH, Blazar BR, Arthur DC, Patton DF, Greenberg JS, Burke B, Ramsay NKC, McGlave P, Filipovich AH: Epstein-Barr virus associated B cell lymphoproliferative disorders following bone marrow transplantation. Blood 1988;71:1234-1243.

66. Hansen JA, Beatty PG, Anasetti C, Clift RA, Martin PJ, Sanders J, Sullivan K, Buckner CD, Storb R, Thomas ED: Treatment of leukemia by marrow transplantation from donors other than HLA genotypically identical siblings. In *Progress in Bone Marrow Transplantation*, edited by Gale RP, Champlin R. Alan R Liss Inc, New York, 1987; pp. 667-675.

67. Irlé C, D'Amaro J, Van Rood JJ: Bone marrow transplantation from other than HLA-identical siblings. Bone Marrow Transplant 1988;3(Suppl 1):37-38.

68. Hervé P, Vernant JP, Maraninchi D, Reiffers J, Bordigoni P, Harousseau JL, Michalet M, Attal M: Mismatched bone marrow transplantation in 83 patients with hematological malignancies: a GEGMO study. Bone Marrow Transplant 1988;3(Suppl 1):178-179.

69. Powles R, Pedrazzini A, Crofts M, Clink H, Millar J, Bhattia G, Perez D: Mismatched family bone marrow transplantion. Sem Hematol 1984;21:182-187.

70. Trigg ME, Billing R, Sondel PM, Exten R, Hong R, Bozdech MJ, Horowitz SD, Finlay JL, Moen R, Longo W, Erickson C, Peterson A: Clinical trial depleting T-lymphocytes from donor marrow for matched and mismatched allogeneic bone marrow transplants. Cancer Treat. Reports 1985;69:377-386.

71. Nielsen L, Moller J, Platz P, Jacobsen N: Thirty-seven cases of mismatch BMT in Copenhagen. Bone Marrow Transplant 1988;3(Suppl 1):174-175.

72. Fischer A, Landair P: Bone marrow transplantation for immunodeficiencies and osteopetrosis. Bone Marrow Transplant 1988;3(Suppl 1):46-47.

73. O'Reilly RJ, Brochstein J, Dinsmore R, Kirkpatrick D: Marrow transplantation for congenital disorders. Sem Hematol 1984;21:188-221.

74. Doney K, Dahlberg SJ, Monroe D, Storb R, Buckner CD, Thomas ED: Therapy of severe aplastic anemia with anti-human thymocyte globulin and androgens: the effect of HLA-haplo-identical marrow infusion. Blood 1984;63:342-348.

75. Storb R, Thomas ED, Appelbaum F, Clift RA, Deeg J, Doney K, Hansen JA, Prentice RL, Sanders JE, Singer JW, Shulman H, Stewart PS, Sullivan KM, Dahlberg SJ, Buckner CD, Witherspoon H: Marrow transplantation for severe aplastic anemia: the Seattle experience. In *Aplastic Anemia: Stem Cell Biology and Advances in Treatment*, Alan R. Liss, New York, 1984; pp. 297-313.

76. Filipovich AH: Progress in broadening the uses of marrow transplantation: donor availability. Vox Sang 1986;51:95-103.

77. Hows JM, Yin JL, Marsh J, Swirsky D, Jones L, Apperley JF, James DCO, Smithers S, Batchelor JR, Goldman JM, Gordon-Smith EC: Histocompatibility unrelated volunteer donors compared with HLA non identical family donors in marrow transplantation for aplastic anemia and leukemia. Blood 1986;68:1322-1328.

78. Ash RC, Menitove J, Casper J, Chitambar C, Hansen R, Bratonow N, Lum L, Anderson T, Bunin N, Camitta B, Truitt DR, Hunter J, Aster R: Successful allogeneic marrow transplantation utilizing HLA-closely matched unrelated donors. Blood 1987;70(Suppl 1):1011 (abstract).

79. Zwaan FE: The use of donors other than HLA–identical siblings in bone marrow transplantation–A workshop summary. In *Progress in Bone Marrow Transplantation*, edited by Gale RP, Champlin R. UCLA Symposia on molecular and cellular biology, Alan R. Liss, New York, 1987; pp. 677-687.

80. Bortin MM, Horowitz MM, Rimm AA: Bone Marrow transplantation: the difficulties ahead. Exp Hematol Today, Springer-Verlag, New York-Berlin-Heidelberg-Tokyo, 1987; pp. 134-140.

81. Wijdenes J, Clément C, Morel-Fourrier B, Béliard R, Hervé P, Peters A: A monoclonal antibody against the human IL-2 receptor with high inhibitory activity on IL-2 induced proliferation of T-cells, experimental and clinical results. In *Cellular Basis of Immunomodulation*, edited by Kaplan JG, Green DR. Alan R. Liss, New York, 1988; in press.

82. Kaminski E, Sharrock C, Hows J, Ritter M, Arthur C, McKinnon S, Batchelor JR: Frequency analysis of cytotoxic T-lymphocyte precursors—possible relevance to HLA-matched unrelated donor bone marrow transplantation. Bone Marrow Transplant 1988;3:149-155.

83. Van Rood JJ, Zwaan FE, Willemze R: The unrelated bone marrow donor. Bone Marrow Transplant 1988;3:371-377.

84. Gratwohl A, Tichelli A, Würsch A, Dieterle A, Lori A, Thomssen Ch, Baldomero H, De Witte T, Nissen C, Speck B: Irradiated donor buffy coat and T-cell depleted bone marrow transplantation. Bone Marrow Transplant 1988;3(Suppl 1):203.

85. Ferrara JL, Marion A, McIntyre JF, Murphy GF, Burakoff SJ: Amelioration of acute

GVHD due to minor histocompatibility antigens by in vivo administration of anti-L2 receptor antibody. J of Immunol 1986;137:1874-1877.

86. Hervé P, Widjenes J, Bergerat JP, Milpied N, Gaud C, Bordignoni P: In vivo treatment of acute GVHD with a monoclonal antibody specific for the IL-2 receptor (B-B10). Lancet 1988;2:1012.

87. Byers V, Blazar NB, Antin J, Henslee P, Fay J, Mischak R, Scannon P: Anti-pan-T lymphocyte monoclonal antibody-ricin A chain immunotoxin in initial therapy in acute graft versus host disease. Exp Hematol 1988;16,6:518 (abstract).

88. Cobbold SP, Martin G, Qin S, Waldmann H: Monoclonal antibodies to promote marrow engraftment and tissue graft tolerance. Nature 1986;323:164-167.

89. Fischer A, Griscelli C, Blanche S, Le Desist F, Veber F, Lopez M, Delaage M, Olive D, Mawas C, Janossy G: Prevention of graft failure by an anti-HLFA-1 monoclonal antibody in HLA-mismatched bone marrow transplantation. Lancet 1986;2:1058-1061.

90. Baume D, Kuentz M, Pico JL, Beaujan F, Cordonnier C, Vernant JP, Hayat M, Bernard A: Failure of a CD18/anti-LFA1 monoclonal antibody infusion to prevent graft rejection in leukemic patients receiving T-depleted allogeneic bone marrow transplantation. Transplantation 1989;47:472-474.

91. Deeg HJ, Sale GE, Storb R, Graham TC, Schuening F, Appelbaum FR, Thomas ED: Engraftment of HLA-non identical bone marrow facilitated by recipient treatment with anti-class II monoclonal antibody and methotrexate. Transplantation 1987; 44:340-345.

92. Murphy WJ, Kumar V, Bennett M: Rejection of bone marrow allografts by mice with severe combined immune deficiency (SCID): evidence that natural killer cells can mediate the specificity of marrow graft rejection. J Exp Med 1987;165:1212-1216.

93. Schuening F, Storb R, Goehle S, Meyer J, Graham TC, Deeg HJ, Appelbaum FR, Sale GE, Graf L, Loughran T: Facilitation of engraftment of HLA-non identical marrow by treatment of recipients with monoclonal antibody directed against marrow cells surviving radiation. Transplantation 1987;44:607-613.

94. Tiberghien P, Wine JW, Alvord WG, Longo DL, Reynolds C: Depletion of natural killer activity in lethally irradiated recipients prior to bone marrow transplantation reduces the amount of bone marrow cells necessary for survival (submitted).

95. Bolwell BJ, Cassileth PA, Gale RP: High dose cytarabine: a review. Leukemia 1988;2:253-260.

96. Dickinson AM, Sviland L, Carey P, Reid MM, Hamilton PJ, Pearson AJ, Proctor SJ: Prevention of graft-versus-host-disease by ex-vivo T-cell depletion reduction in graft failure with augmented total body irradiation. Leukemia 1988;2:300-303.

97. Cahn JY, Hervé P, Souillet G, Bordigoni P, Flesch M, Plouvier E, Pico J, Benz-Lemoine E, Reiffers J, Bergerat JP, Lutz P, Colombat P, Lanino E: The TAM protocol as conditioning regimen prior to BMT for high-risk acute leukaemias: a multicentre study of 48 patients. Bone Marrow Transplant 1988;3(Suppl 1):187.

98. Blazar BR, Widmer MB, Soderling CCB, Urdal DL, Gillis S, Robison LL, Vallera DA: Augmentation of donor bone marrow engraftment in histoincompatible murine recipients by granulocyte/macrophage colony-stimulating factor. Blood 1988;71: 320-328.

99. Bender-Götze Ch, Haas RJ, Kolb HJ, Rieber E, Walter JU: Bone marrow transplantation from donors other than HLA—identical siblings: the Munich experience. Bone Marrow Transplant 1988;3(Suppl 1):186.

100. Moen RC, Horowitz SD, Sondel PM, Borcherding WR, Trigg ME, Billing R, Hong R: Immunologic reconstitution after haploidentical bone marrow transplantation for immune deficiency disorders: treatment of bone marrow cells with monoclonal antibodies CT-2 and complement. Blood 1987;70:664-669.

101. Morgan G, Strobel S, Hale G, Waldmann H, Levinsky RJ: Treatment of acute GVHD with an anti-CD7 monoclonal antibody (Campath-2). Bone Marrow Transplant 1987;2(Suppl 1):167.

102. Beelen DW, Graeven U, Schulz G, Grosse-Wilde H, Quabeck K, Sayer H, Schaefer UW, Schmidt CG: Primary treatment of acute graft-versus-host disease with a monoclonal antibody (BMA031) against the human T-cell receptor. Bone Marrow Transplant 1988;3(Suppl 1):219.

103. Remlinger K, Martin PJ, Hansen JA, Doney KC, Smith A, Deeg HJ, Sullivan K, Storb R, Thomas ED: Murine monoclonal anti-cell antibodies for treatment of steroid resistant acute GVHD. Human Immunol 1984;9:21-36.

104. Hervé P, Wijdines J, Bugerat JP, Bordigoni P, Milpied N, Cahn JY, Clément C, Béliard R, Mozel-Fourrier B, Racadot E, Troussard X, Gaud C, Attal M, Klcft H, Peters A. Treatment of corticosteroid resistant acute GVHD by in vivo administration of anti IL-2 receptor monoclonal antibody (B-B10). Blood (in press Feb. 1990).

24

Syngeneic and Autologous Graft-vs.-Host Disease

Joel M. Rappeport
Yale University School of Medicine
New Haven, Connecticut

I. INTRODUCTION

As defined extensively throughout this book, Graft-vs.-Host Disease (GVHD) is a clinical syndrome affecting primarily the skin, liver, and gastrointestinal tract. This reaction is characterized by histopathologic criteria which are suggestive, but not pathognomonic for the diagnosis (1,2). Thus, it is the clinical syndrome along with the pathologic patterns which lead to the diagnosis of the GVHD. The disorder has been subdivided into acute and chronic forms which have distinctive clinical manifestations and pathologic histologies. The primary clinical setting in which GVHD occurs is bone marrow transplantation. However, other clinical settings have also been implicated and include blood transfusions in the immunosuppressed recipient and maternal transplacental transfusions to immunosuppressed fetuses (3-6).

The pathophysiologic prerequisites for GVHD were initially formulated by Billingham in 1966 (7): (1) immunologically competent cells must be engrafted in the recipient, (2) the immunologic state of the recipient must be such that the engrafted cells cannot be rejected, and (3) the engrafted cells recognize foreign transplantation antigens in the recipient to which they mount an immunologic reaction, resulting in the GVHD syndrome. Experimental work demonstrated that the greater the disparity between the histocompatibility antigens of the donor and the recipient the greater the frequency of GVHD and the more severe the disease. The syndrome was not limited to disparities for major histocompatibility complex antigens, but could also result from minor histocompatibility antigenic differences.

Experience in human bone marrow transplantation, although not as rigorously controlled, also confirmed in principle these requirements for the development of GVHD. In recipients of HLA complex disparate bone marrow transplants, the incidence and severity of GVHD was increased. Virtually all recipients of unmanipulated haploidentical transplants developed fatal GVHD. Even among recipients of histocompatible transplants a significant number demonstrated clinical and histopathologic findings of GVHD, and in 40-60% of these patients the reaction was clinically relevant. These findings suggested a role for as yet undefined minor histocompatibility antigens in human GVHD.

Analysis of clinical data suggested that other factors are also involved in GVHD. Many studies have reported an increased incidence of severe acute and chronic GVHD in older recipients (8). Infections with herpesviruses also seem to be associated with an increased incidence of GVHD (9,10). Several other factors not linked to immunologic disparity but associated with increased GVHD are less well defined. There is convincing evidence that GVHD is mediated by donor T lymphocytes, and the probability of developing GVHD may depend upon the number of T cells infused (11).

II. SYNGENEIC MARROW TRANSPLANTATION AND GVHD

A. Genetic Considerations

A human syngeneic bone marrow transplant is a transplant between identical twins. By definition there should be no genetic differences between donor and recipient. Thus, the requirement for the development of GVHD that a foreign antigen be recognized by the engrafted donor lymphocyte in the recipient is not fulfilled. Based on this supposition, patients given identical twin bone marrow transplants for the treatment of aplastic anemia are generally not given immunosuppressive treatment pregrafting. Failure to achieve engraftment in some of these transplants has been explained on the basis of an autoimmune disorder which caused the original aplasia and which was still active after donor marrow infusion. Similarly, patients given syngeneic marrow grafts are not given prophylactic immunosuppression for the prevention of GVHD.

It is important to emphasize, however, that monozygosity of human twins can generally not be proven, rather, nonidentity is demonstrated. Each individual is tested for a variety of genetic markers inherited from parents who are heterozygous for known alleles; each of two twins has an equal likelihood of inheriting either one of the two different alleles. For example, a parent who has the erythrocyte genotype A/O has a 50% chance of providing either gene (A or O) to an offspring. With each determined identity (for heterozygous parental genes) between twins, the statistical likelihood of the twins being identical increases. If a single difference is documented then identity is disproven, i.e., the twins are fraternal. With conventional methods one could generally arrive at a 90-99% probability of twins being identical. This was in general the result of testing antigens of the HLA complex, erythrocyte antigenic markers and enzymes, and gamma globulin allotypes. The development of methodology to analyze DNA sequence polymorphism has allowed the analysis of a large amount of genetic material, providing the ability to analyze many potential DNA differences between twins and arrive at an extremely high probability of identity.

B. Clinical Studies

1. GVHD Limited to the Skin

In 1979 we reported the occurrence of a clinical and pathologic syndrome consistent with cutaneous acute GVHD in three recipients of syngeneic bone marrow transplants (12). All three patients had received their transplants for the treatment of leukemia following preparation with cytosine arabinoside, cyclophosphamide, and single dose total body irradiation. Maculopapular skin rashes appeared between 7 and 17 days following transplantation and lasted for 5 to 28 days. Skin biopsies revealed loss of polarity, vacuolization at the dermo-epidermal junction, and lymphocytic infiltration. Both the clinical picture and biopsy material were consistent with acute GVHD. Two of the patients had had normal skin biopsies following the preparation regimen but prior to the onset of cutaneous eruptions. Of interest was the fact that no clinical evidence of either hepatic or gastrointestinal GVHD was noted, although biopsies were not performed. Chronic GVHD did not develop in these patients.

The identical twin bone marrow transplant experience at Brigham and Women's Hosptial/Children's Hospital Bone Marrow Transplantation Program includes 10 patients. One young patient with aplastic anemia had no evidence of GVHD. Among nine patients transplanted for hematologic malignancies, five developed both clinical and pathologic findings consistent with acute cutaneous GVHD. Three had grade I severity and two grade II. Two of these patients had acute nonlymphocytic leukemia, two acute lymphocytic leukemia, and one chronic myelogenous leukemia. Among the four patients without acute GVHD, one had acute nonlymphocytic leukemia, one acute lymphocytic leukemia, one chronic myelogenous leukemia, and one non-Hodgkin's lymphoma. All patients had received identical preparative regimens. Four of the five patients receiving single dose total body irradiation were among those who developed GVHD, while only one of four patients receiving fractionated irradiation developed GVHD. Two of the five patients with GVHD had a concurrent bacterial infection, and one had a concurrent cytomegalovirus infection. In no cases was a definitive diagnosis of either hepatic or gastrointestinal GVHD made, and none developed chronic GVHD. Subsequent reports confirmed those observations (13). One 31-year-old male received a syngeneic bone marrow transplant for chronic myelogenous leukemia. A GVHD-like picture began on day 8, and the cutaneous reaction was accompanied by diarrhea, liver function abnormalities, and fever. This syndrome responded to corticosteroid therapy. A skin biopsy was consistent with stage 3 acute GVHD. The patient subsequently developed a cytomegalovirus infection.

In 1987 Hood et al. reported the development of an acute GVHD syndrome in syngeneic transplant recipients (15). Of nine recipients of syngeneic transplants, two developed a widespread cutaneous eruption with abnormal skin biopsies consistent with GVHD 2 and 3 weeks post bone marrow transplantation, respectively. In one patient a biopsy was still abnormal 34 days posttransplant. Two other patients had histologic GVHD without a rash 2 and 4 weeks posttransplant, respectively.

In an earlier analysis Sale and co-workers attempted to differentiate skin biopsy findings in patients with presumed acute GVHD from those in patients given chemoradiotherapy only (14). This blinded analysis also included patients who had undergone either syngeneic or autologous transplants. Epidermal cytologic atypia, dyskeratosis and satellitosis of mononuclear cells around degenerating epidermal cells was noted in both allogeneic transplant recipients with GVHD and in syngeneic and autologous transplant recipients. Of 13 skin biopsies obtained from syngeneic transplant recipients in the first 2 weeks following bone marrow transplant, four were consistent with stage 2 acute GVHD, and two of nine biopsies obtained more than 2 weeks posttransplant were diagnosed as stage 2 GVHD. The ability to distinguish the two groups of patients was extremely limited, and agreement among three pathologists was observed in only 31%. The conclusions were that a clinocopathologic correlation was necessary to establish the diagnosis of acute GVHD. At least for the first 2-3 weeks posttransplant, nonspecific cytotoxic effects were difficult to distinguish from GVHD. A definitive diagnosis should include pathologic material from the liver and gastrointestinal tract. As indicated above, the authors of this study did not consider the possibility of syngeneic or autologous GVHD in those patients but rather attributed histologic findings to radiochemotherapy effects.

2. GVHD Involving Other Organs

In 1988 Einsele and co-workers reported the occurrence of an acute GVHD-like syndrome in three of nine recipients of syngeneic transplants and the possibility of GVHD in another four patients (16). In addition to cutaneous manifestations, hepatic or gastrointestinal abnormalities or both consistent with GVHD were noted in six patients. Three patients required immunosuppressive therapy with corticosteroids or cyclosporine. The onset of the manifestations of GVHD coincided with the establishment of hematopoietic engraftment, and findings persisted for as long as 4 months posttransplant. While previous reports were limited to patients undergoing transplantation for hematologic malignancies, this report included one patient with aplastic anemia who received a transplant from an identical twin following cyclophosphamide preparation. A note of caution is indicated, however, since only two of five skin biopsies were histologically indistinguishable from GVHD, although negative biopsies were obtained coincident with the resolution of the rash or after institution of therapy.

III. AUTOLOGOUS MARROW GRAFTS AND GVHD

The occurrence of a GVHD-like syndrome in recipients of supposed identical twin transplants raised major questions about the conventional dogma of the pathophysiological requirements for GVHD. The question arose as to whether these donor/recipient pairs were truly syngeneic. In 1981 Thien et al. described a patient with chronic myelogenous leukemia in blast crisis, who, following marrow-ablative therapy, received an autograft of previously stored chronic phase peripheral blood cells (17). Both skin and gastrointestinal biopsies were consistent with GVHD, as were abnormal liver function tests. A virtually identical case was observed at our own institution (unpublished observations). These observations of a GVHD-like syndrome in autologous transplantation eliminated the question of undetected genetic disparity in presumed syngeneic transplants.

In a retrospective analysis, Hood and co-workers studied 96 autologous transplant recipients, and noted the development of maculopapular rashes consistent with the clinical diagnosis of acute GVHD in seven patients (15). The rashes developed 3-58 days following bone marrow infusion. Only one of the patients concurrently had liver function abnormalities, and three patients had mild, otherwise unexplained diarrhea. Skin biopsies were consistent with stages 1 and 2 acute GVHD. Ten patients were followed prospectively with serial skin biopsies, two had biopsies consistent with stage 2 acute GVHD without clinically apparent disease. Four patients required systemic corticosteroid therapy which resulted in prompt resolution of the clinical syndrome.

Sviland and co-workers reported a prospective study of the histological features of skin and rectal biopsies after autologous and allogeneic marrow transplantation (18). Thirteen recipients of autologous and 18 recipients of allogeneic marrow had skin biopsies before transplant and at 4 weeks and 6 months after transplant. In addition biopsies were obtained when clinically suspected cutaneous lesions developed. Rectal biopsies were obtained 4 weeks posttransplant. In nine recipients of autologous marrow available for study, no clinical manifestations of GVHD were noted. Seven patients had basal cell vacuolation, and three patients had evidence of spongiosis and eosinophilic bodies in early skin biopsies. Seven patients had evidence of dermal lymphocytic infiltration, but no epidermal infiltrates were noted. Of four patients studied 6 months following transplant, two had persistent basal cell vacuolation.

According to previously described criteria, therefore, four patients had cutaneous findings consistent with grade I acute GVHD, and three patients had findings of grade II GVHD. Among nine patients who underwent rectal biopsies 4 weeks following autologous marrow infusion, no evidence of single cell necrosis was noted. However, among 30 patients studied prior to transplant, 18 had basal cell vacuolation, 11 spongiosis, and 4 eosinophilic bodies. Whether all of these patients transplanted for malignant disorders had previusly received cytotoxic therapy was not clearly indicated; nor was the time interval since such therapy. In contrast, among the 13 allogeneic recipients studied post-transplant, 9 had suspected cutaneous GVHD. Only one patient had diarrhea, and none had hepatic changes consistent with GVHD. Three patients had findings consistent with stage 1 GVHD, eight stage 2 GVHD, and two stage 3 GVHD. Of 13 rectal biopsies obtained in this group, 6 demonstrated single cell necrosis consistent with acute GVHD. The conclusion of this study was that findings of pathologic stages 1 and 2 acute GVHD are nonspecific and that rectal biopsies were more specific. However, not all patients suspected of having acute GVHD on other grounds had positive rectal biopsies. Of note is the fact that in neither case reports nor larger studies did chronic GVHD develop by either clinical or histopathologic criteria.

IV. MECHANISMS OF AUTOLOGOUS AND SYNGENEIC GVHD

The findings described above have led to much speculation concerning the pathophysiologic processes involved in GVHD. Whether all reported cases truly represent a GVHD-like syndrome is not certain. However, even a single case would raise the same questions about the mechanisms involved.

A. Incidental Events

There may be several simple explanations for the development of GVHD after autologous or syngeneic transplantation.

1. Transfusions

GVHD-like reactions may result from transfusions of nonirradiated blood into a severely immunosuppressed patient. However, in almost all situations discussed here, the transfusion records have been reviewed and it appears that all blood products were irradiated. Furthermore, transfusion-induced GVHD has usually been severe and often lethal.

2. Chemoradiotherapy Effect

Skin rashes and histopathologic changes can be the result of cytotoxic changes secondary to the preparative chemoradiation therapy (see above), suggesting that stages 1 and 2 findings are nonspecific cutaneous changes. Although this is possible, it would then raise the question as to whether mild stage 1 or moderate stage 2 GVHD exist at all, even in allogeneic marrow transplants. Clearly, the actual incidence would be less than currently reported. In support of such a concept would be the observation of similar findings pre-transplant as noted by Sviland and colleagues (18). Second, with a single exception, the

GVHD-like syndrome has been reported only in patients undergoing transplantation for malignant disorders. Although preparative regimens have varied, and although normal biopsies have been obtained in some patients subsequent to the preparative regimen but prior to the development of a GVHD-like syndrome, this might suggest that the usually more intensive conditioning regimen given to patients with malignant disorders might modify host cells in a way which would cause them to appear foreign to the infused (untreated) cells.

3. T-Cell Tropism

A major histopathologic difference between the mild GVHD-like reaction and more severe GVHD has been the absence of epidermal mononuclear cell infiltration. However, in one study of the cutaneous histopathology in allogeneic marrow transplants, T cell purging of the donor marrow was associated with a decreased incidence of epidermal lymphocytic infiltrates suggesting the number of lymphocytes available may influence the findings (19). Analysis of the reports on syngeneic and autologous GVHD also reveals a conspicuous infrequency of hepatic and gastrointestinal involvement in comparison to allogeneic GVHD. Conceivably T lymphocytes responsible for GVHD have a predilection for the skin. These questions can only be resolved in a prospective manner involving patients with autologous and syngeneic marrow transplantation.

4. Infections

Clinical bone marrow transplantation is often complicated by infections requiring the administration of antibiotics. Many of these infections, particularly those caused by herpesviruses, may be associated with cutaneous eruptions. In allogeneic transplants there is evidence that severe acute and chronic GVHD are seen more frequently in patients with cytomegalovirus infections (10,20). Prior exposure of the donor and recipient to Epstein-Barr virus infections and herpes simplex have also been associated with an increased incidence of acute GVHD (9). A number of recipients of either syngeneic or autologous transplants that have been reported had herpesvirus infections at approximately the time when the GVHD-like reaction occurred. In six nontransplant patients with documented cytomegalovirus enterocolitis, GVHD-like pathology with single cell necrosis was noted (21), in all six patients inclusion bodies were noted pathologically. However, in no cases of reported syngeneic or autologous GVHD have viral inclusions been noted in the biopsy material.

5. Drugs

Similarly, the occurrence of a drug eruption, particularly in a patient with a disordered immune system, might be difficult to identify. An increased incidence of cutaneous drug eruptions has been noted in other immunoregulatory disorders including acquired hypogammaglobulinemia, chronic lymphocytic leukemia, and others, and virtually all patients who developed syngeneic or autologous GVHD have been on systemic antibiotics.

B. Immune Mechanism

Other possible explanations of autologous and syngeneic GVHD have to consider the basic pathophysiological processes involved in the reaction. Clearly, if the Billingham concept is correct and represents the only criteria by which GVHD can occur, the reports of GVHD-like reactions in syngeneic and autologous transplant recipients may represent an entirely different process resulting in the same manifestations. It may be caused by altered self antigens or, as strongly suggested by animal experiments, by a failure to eliminate T cells with receptors for self antigens.

1. Lymphokines

It has been shown in a murine model that antibodies to tumor necrosis factor prevented histopathologic changes of acute GVHD suggesting the possibility that lymphokines may be nonspecifically involved in the development of GVHD (22). Vogelsang and co-workers have recently reported a model using recipient skin explants incubated with donor lymphocytes to predict the development of GVHD following transplantation (23). It was noted that areas of skin not directly exposed to donor lymphocytes also developed findings consistent with GVHD, again suggesting that either specific or nonspecific lymphokine production is involved in the development of a GVHD-like syndrome. It has also been shown in HLA-matched transplants that only 50% of patients with GVHD have T lymphocytes cytotoxic to host fibroblasts (24). Often these cells were not detectable for at least one month after the development of acute GVHD. Possibly both direct cellular activity and nonspecific lymphokine effects are operative in GVHD.

2. Antiviral Immunity

As described above, it appears that the incidence of GVHD is increased in patients with active herpesvirus infections, particularly CMV. In a murine model CMV infection also appeared to augment GVHD (25). This effect is likely due to the development and stimulation of natural killer cells directed initially against CMV infected cells (26,27). IL-2 production in response to the infection (or other antigens) could result in a secondary GVHD-like reaction. Other foreign antigens in the recipient include, for example, histocompatibility antigens on infused random blood products. The infusion of LAK cells and recombinant IL-2 in patients with malignancies has resulted in a GVHD-like syndrome including a cutaneous rash, diarrhea, and liver function abnormalities (28,29). It is possible that the lymphokines have a direct effect which results in GVHD or, as will be discussed later, initiate an autoreactive disorder.

3. Leukemia-Associated Antigens

The initiating antigen need not be foreign as with a viral infection or after transfusion. As noted in allogeneic bone marrow transplants for malignancies, there is evidence that relapse is inversely related to the presence of GVHD (30). Ex vivo T-cell depletion of the bone marrow has decreased the incidence of GVHD but has resulted in a higher incidence of recurrent leukemia, particularly in chronic myelogenous leukemia (31), supporting the concept of a graft-vs.-leukemia effect. Whether this reaction is the same or separable from GVHD is currently unclear. Conversely, whether a graft-vs.-leukemia effect can produce GVHD is also unclear. As pointed out, however, syngeneic GVHD has only been observed in one case of aplastic anemia, with all other cases being seen in patients with malignancies. It is conceivable that in recipients of syngeneic transplants a leukemia-associated antigen, foreign to the donor, is recognized, initiating a nonspecific release of lymphokines either directly producing GVHD or activating autoreactive cells which secondarily produce GVHD. With such a hypothesis the classic concepts of GVHD would still hold but would need to be modified to include the nonspecific effects of lymphokine production.

4. T-Lymphocyte Imbalance

A final explanation of true acute GVHD in recipients of syngeneic and autologous transplants would dictate a major change in our understanding of the criteria necessary for the development of GVHD. In this situation, the host would not be required to have recognizably different histocompatibility antigens to which the donor immune system normally reacted. Instead, a true autoimmune reaction would develop as a result of an immunologic imbalance during the recapitulation of ontogeny of the immune system posttransplant. In 1979 Reinherz and co-workers, utilizing heteroantiserum directed against T-lymphocyte membrane antigens, reported an imbalance in the recovering immune system following marrow transplantation in those patients who developed acute or chronic GVHD (32). In three patients who developed acute GVHD there was an absence of suppressor/cytotoxic cells, with a relative increase in helper cells. The reappearance of suppressor/cytotoxic cells occurred with the cessation of acute GVHD. One of the three patients studied was the recipient of a syngeneic bone marrow transplant. The infused bone marrow had a normal ratio of short-lived suppressor cells and long-lived helper cells. During recovery of the immune system an imbalance existed until the engrafted marrow began to produce new suppressor cells. Until then the existing imbalance created an autoreactive condition of appropriate self-tolerance.

Subsequent studies utilized monoclonal antibodies directed against T-lymphocyte maturation and differentiation antigens. Friedrich et al. studied 24 recipients of allogeneic bone marrow transplants with monoclonal antibodies anti-leu 2 (CD8) and anti-leu 3 (CD3) (33). The ratio of suppressor/cytotoxic T cells (CD8$^+$) to helper cells (CD3$^+$) was elevated in nearly all patients early in the posttransplant course. In patients without GVHD the ratios returned to normal after the first month, whereas in patients with acute GVHD the abnormal ratios persisted. This imbalance, however, was exactly the opposite of that described by Reinherz and colleagues.

Gratama and co-workers evaluated the ratios of helper/suppressor cells early in the posttransplant period in 24 recipients of allogeneic transplants and 11 autologous transplants (34). Lymphoid reconsitution was faster with autologous transplants, probably in part due to the fact that no GVHD prophylaxis was utilized. The first cells noted were helper cells (CD4$^+$) resulting in an initial imbalance. However, suppressor/cytotoxic cells (CD8$^+$) reappeared 4-7 days later with a marked proliferation resulting in an excess of CD8$^+$ cells. Of 10 patients with the most marked CD4/CD8 inversion, 9 developed severe acute GVHD, while less severely abnormal ratios in 14 patients resulted in acute GVHD in only two situations. While one could suggest that this imbalance was the immunologic response to GVHD rather than the cause, the severe imbalances were detected prior to the onset of the clinical reaction in most patients. In autologous patients studied, the absolute lymphocyte count and CD4$^+$ cells became normal much faster than in the allogeneic situation. The imbalance noted early in autologous recipients might explain the development of a GVHD-like reaction, and the subsequent rapid normalization could explain the limited nature of the disorder. In another study by Anderson et al., however, the abnormal CD4/CD8 ratios in recipients of anti-B1 purged autologous transplants persisted for periods up to 3 years posttransplant (35).

Utilizing more sophisticated technology, several unusual lymphocyte phenotypes have recently been identified (36,37). Suppressor/cytotoxic cells appeared to be a composite of at least two populations: the CD8 antigen could be identified on both T cells and NK cells. Analysis of DNA sequence polymorphisms confirmed the donor origin of these cells (38).

5. NK Cells

Utilizing a functional assay, Lopez and co-workers noted a correlation between the presence, pretransplantation, of NK activity and the development of GVHD (39), an observation not confirmed by other studies (40). In a murine model GVHD was prevented by administration of a monoclonal antibody against NK cells (41). The expansion of NK cells in the presence of IL-2 leading to LAK cells showed that NK cells may expand and be activated not only by the presence of specific targets, but also by nonspecific lymphokines. Another study showed that both CD4$^+$ and CD8$^+$ cells posttransplant co-expressed the NK markers Leu7 and CD11b (42). These apparently abnormal cell populations deserve further study.

C. Animal Models

Interesting models of syngeneic and autologous GVHD have recently been described (43-45). Cyclosporine has been used to prevent and treat acute allogeneic GVHD in both murine models and man. The drug appears to be immunosuppressive through inhibition of the activation of cytotoxic T cells and NK cells as well as decreasing the production of IL-2. Rats undergoing either syngenic or autologous marrow transplantation and treated with cyclosporine developed GVHD upon cessation of the drug. This syndrome was associated with the development of cytotoxic T cell directed at Ia, and a loss of Ia$^+$ cells from the thymus. Shielding of the thymus during the preparative regimen prevented the development of GVHD. Conversely, neonatally thymectomized animals also develop a GVHD-like disorder (46). Damage to the thymus, the presence of cyclosporine or both appear to inhibit differentiation of thymocytes into mature CD4$^+$8$^-$ or CD4$^-$8$^+$ T-cell receptor $\alpha\beta$ + T cells and to interfere with the deletion of cells expressing self-reactive T-cell receptor specificities (47). Similar alterations might be responsible for "self-reactivity" and a GVHD-like syndrome in patients given syngeneic or autologous marrow grafts.

V. CONCLUSIONS

From a clinical point of view the syndrome of acute GVHD in recipients of syngeneic and autologous bone marrow transplantation has little relevance in that it occurs infrequently and is rarely of major clinical significance. However, its potential importance in the understanding of the pathophysiology of allogeneic GVHD cannot be underestimated. Clearly, both human and animal experience would indicate that in the majority of instances the presence of the classic conditions as described by Billingham results in GVHD. However, it is possible that other contributing factors might also result in this reaction. The imbalance of the reconstituting immune system could produce autoreactivity or autoimmunity. Understanding these processes might also lead to a better understanding of other autoimmune disorders.

REFERENCES

1. Glucksberg H, Storb R, Fefer A, Buckner CD, Nieman PE, Clift RA, Lerner KG, Thomas ED: Clinical manifestations of graft-versus-host disease in human recipients of marrow from HLA-matched sibling donors. Transplantation 1974;18: 295-304.

2. Lerner KG, Kao GF, Storb R, Buckner CD, Clift RA, Thomas ED: Histopathology of graft-versus-host reaction (GVHR) in human recipients of marrow from HLA-matched sibling donors. Transplant Proc 1974;6:367-371.
3. Brubaker BB: Human posttransfusion graft-versus-host disease. Vox Sang 1983;45: 401-420.
4. Weiden P: Graft-v-host disease following blood transfusions. Arch Intern Med 1984; 144:1557-1558.
5. Dinsmore RE, Straus DJ, Pollack MS, Woodruff JM, Garrett TJ, Young CW, Clarkson BD, Dupont B: Fatal graft-versus-host disease following blood transfusion in Hodgkin's disease documented by HLA typing. Blood 1980;55:831-834.
6. Parkman R, Mosier D, Umansky I, Cochran W, Carpenter CB, Rosen FS: Graft-versus-host disease after intrauterine and exchange transfusions for hemolytic disease of the newborn. N Engl J Med 1974;290:359-363.
7. Billingham RE: The biology of graft-versus-host reactions. Harvey Lect 1966-1967; 62:21-78.
8. WeidenP and the Seattle marrow transplant team: Graft-versus-host disease in alloggeneic marrow transplantation, in *Biology of Bone Marrow Transplantion,* edited by Gale RP and Fox CF. Academic Press, New York, 1980; p. 37.
9. Gratama JW, Stijnen T, Weiland HT, Hekker AC, deGast GC, Zwaan FE, Weijers TF, D'Amaro J, Vossen TH, Vossen JMJJ: Herpes-virus immunity and acute graft-versus-host disease. Lancet 1987,1:471-474.
10. Vilmer E, Mazeron MC, Rabian C, Azoqui O, Devergie A, Perol Y, Gluckman E: Clinical significance of cytomegalovirus viremia in bone marrow transplantation. Transplantion 1985;40:30-35.
11. Kernan NA, Collins NH, Julano L, Cartagena T, Dupont B, O'Reilly RJ. Clonable T lymphocytes in T cell-depleted bone marrow transplants correlate with development of graft-v-host disease. Blood 1986;68:770-773.
12. Rappeport JM, Mihm M, Reinherz EL, Lopansri S, Parkman R: Acute graft-vs.-host disease in recipients of bone marrow transplants from identical twin donors. Lancet 1979;2:717-720.
13. Gluckman E, Devergie A, Sohier J, Saurat JH: Graft-versus-host disease in recipients of syngeneic bone marrow. Lancet 1980;1:253-254.
14. Sale GE, Lerner KG, Barker EA, Shulman HM, Thomas ED: The skin biopsy in the diagnosis of acute graft-versus-host disease in man. A J Path 1977;89:621-632.
15. Hood AF, Vogelsang GB, Black LP, Farmer ER, Santos GW: Acute graft-vs-host disease, development following autologous and syngeneic bone marrow transplantation. Arch Dermatol 1987;123:745-750.
16. Einsele H, Ehninger G, Schneider EM, Kruger GFR, Vallbracht A, Dopfer R, Schmidt H, Waller HD, Muller CA: High frequency of graft-versus-host-like syndromes following syngeneic bone marrow transplantation. Transplantation 1988;45:579-585.
17. Thein SL, Goldman JM, Galton DAG. Acute "graft-versus-host disease" after autografting for chronic granulocytic leukemia in transformation. Ann Intern Med 1981; 94:210-211.
18. Sviland L, Pearons ADJ, Eastham EJ, Hamilton PJ, Proctor SJ, Malcolm AJ, and the Newcastle Upon Tyne Bone Marrow Transplant Group: Histological features of skin and rectal biopsy specimens after autologous and allogeneic bone marrow transplantation. J Clin Pathol 1988;41:148-154.
19. Elliott CJ, Sloane JP, Sanderson KV, Vincent M, Shepherd V, Powles R: The histological diagnosis of cutaneous graft versus host disease: relationship of skin changes to marrow purging and other clinical variables. Histopathology 1987;11:145-155.
20. Persson U, Myrenfors P, Ringden O, Sundberg B, Larsson P, Gunnar S: T lymphocyte subpopulations in bone-marrow-transplanted patients in relation to graft-versus-

host disease and cytomegalovirus-induced infection. Transplantation 1987;43:663-668.

21. Snover DC: Mucosal damage simulating acute graft-versus-host reaction in cytomegalovirus colitis. Transplantation 1985;39:669-670.

22. Piguet PF, Grau GE, Aller B, Vassalli P: Tumor necrosis factor/cachectin is an effector of skin and gut lesions of the acute phase of graft-vs.-host disease. J Exp Med 1987;166:1280-1289.

23. Vogelsang GB, Hess AD, Berkman AW, Tutschka PJ, Farmer ER, Converse PJ, Santos GW: An in vitro predictive test for graft versus host disease in patients with genotypic HLA-identical bone marrow transplants. N Engl J Med 1985;313:645-650.

24. Tsoi M-S, Storb R, Weiden PL, Thomas ED: Studies on cellular inhibition and serum-blocking factors in 28 human patients given marrow grafts from FHLA identical siblings. J Immunol 1977;118:1799-1805.

25. Grundy JE, Shanley JD, Shearer GM: Augentation of graft-versus-host reaction by cytomegalovirus infection resulting in interstial pneumonitis. Transplantation 1985;39:548-553.

26. Bowden RA, Day LM, Amos DE, Meyers JD: Natural cytotoxic activity against cytomegalovirus-infected target cells following marrow transplantation. Transplantation 1987,44:504-508.

27. Hokland M, Jacobsen N, Ellegaard J, Hokland P: Natural killer function following allogeneic bone marrow transplantation. Very early reemergence but strong dependence of cytomegalovirus infection. Transplantation 1988;45:1080-1084.

28. Lotze MT, Matory YL, Ettinghausen SE, Rayner AA, Sharrow SO, Seipp CA, Custer MC, Rosenberg SA: In vivo administration of purified human interluekin 2. II. Half life, immunologic effects and expansion of peripheral lymphoid cells in vivo with recombinant IL 2. J Immunol 1985;135:2865-2875.

29. Gaspari AA, Lotze MT, Rosenberg SA, Stern JB, Katz SI: Dermatologic changes associated with interleukin 2 administration. JAMA 1987;258:1624-1629.

30. Weiden PL, Sullivan KM, Flournoy N, Storb R, Thomas ED, and the Seattle Marrow Transplant Team: Antileukemic effect of chronic graft-versus-host disease. N Engl J Med 1981;304:1529-1533.

31. Goldman JM, Gale RP, Horowitz MM, Biggs JC, Champlin RE, Gluckman E, Hoffmann RG, Jacobsen SJ, Marmont AM, McGlave PB, Messner HA, Rimm AA, Rozman C, Speck B, Tura S, Weiner RS, Bortin MM: Bone marrow transplantation for chronic myelogenous leukemia in chronic phase. Increased risk for relapse associated with T-cell depletion. Ann Intern Med 1988,108:806-814.

32. Reinherz EL, Parkman R, Rappeport JM, Rosen FS, Schlossman SF: Aberrations of suppressor T cells in human graft-versus-host disease. N Engl J Med 1979;300:1061-1068.

33. Friedrich W, O'Reilly RJ, Kaziner B, Gebhard DF, Good RA, Evans RL: T-lymphocyte reconstitution in recipients of bone marrow transplants with and without GVHD: Imbalances of T-cell subpopulations having unique regulatory and cognitive function. Blood 1982,59:696-701.

34. Gratama JW, Naipal A, Oljans P, Zwaan FE, Verdonck LF, deWitte T, Vossen JM, Bolhuis RLH, de Gast GC, Jansen J: T lymphocyte repopulation and differentiation after bone marrow transplantation. Early shifts in the ratio between T4+ and T8+ T lymphocytes correlate with the occurrence of acute graft-versus-host disease. Blood 1984,63:1416-1423.

35. Anderson KC, Ritz J, Takvorian T, Coral F, Daley H, Gorgone BC, Freedman AS, Canellos GP, Schlossman SF, Nadler LM: Hematologic engraftment and immune reconstitution posttransplantation with anti-B1 purged autologous bone marrow. Blood 1987;69:597-604.

36. Ault KA, Antin JH, Ginsburg D, Orkin SH, Rappeport JM, Keohan ML, Martin P, Smith BR: The phenotype of recovering lymphoid cell populations following marrow transplantation. J Exp Med 1985;161:1483-1502.

37; Smith BR, Rappeport JM, Burakoff SJ, Ault KA: Clinical correlates of unusual circulating lymphocytes appearing post marrow transplantation. In *Progress in Bone Marrow Transplantion*, edited by Gale RP, Champlin R. Alan R Liss, Inc., New York, 1987; pp. 659-663.

38. Ginsburg D, Antin JH, Smith BR, Orkin SH, Rappeport JM: Origin of cell populations after bone marrow transplantation. Analysis using DNA sequence polymorphisms. J Clin Invest 1985;75:596-603.

39. Lopez CD, Sorell M, Kirkpatrick D, O'Reilly RJ, Change C: Association between pre-transplant natural kill and graft-versus-host disease after stem cell transplantation. Lancet 1979,2:1103-1106.

40. Livnat S, Seigneuret M, Storb R, Prentice RL: Analysis of cytotoxic effector cell function in patients with leukemia or aplastic anemia before and after marrow transplantation. J Immun 1980;124:481-490.

41. Charley M, Mikhael A, Bennett M, Gilliam JM, Sortheimer RD: Prevention of lethal minor-determinate graft-versus-host disease in mice by the in vivo administration of anti-asial GM. J Immunol 1983;131:2101-2103.

42. Velardi A, Terenzi A, Cucciaioni S, Millo R, Grossi CE, Grignani F, Martelli MF: Imbalances within the peripheral blood T-helper (CD4+) and T-suppressor (CD8+) cell populations in the reconstitution phase after human bone marrow transplantation. Blood 1988,71:1196-1200.

43. Hess AH, Horwitz L, Beschorner WE, Santos GW: Development of graft-vs.-host disease-like syndrome in cyclosporine-treated rats after syngeneic bone marrow transplantation. J Exp Med 1985;161:718-730.

44. Glazier A, Tutschka PJ, Farmer ER, Santos GW: Graft-versus-host disease in cyclosporin A treated rats after syngeneic and autologous bone marrow reconstitution. J Exp Med 1983;158:1-8.

45. Beschorner WE, Hess AD, Shinn CA, Santos GW: Transfer of cyclosporine-associated syngeneic graft-versus-host disease by thymocytes. Transplantation 1988;45: 209-215.

46. Trainin M, Small M, Globerson A: Immunocompetence of spleen cells from neonatally thymectomized mice conferred in vitro by a syngeneic thymus extract. J Exp Med 1969;130:765-775.

47. Jenkins MK, Schwartz RH, Pardoll DM: Effects of cyclosporine A on T cell development and clonal deletion. Science 1988;241:1655-1658.

25

Viral Infections and Graft-vs.-Host Disease

Olle Ringdén
Huddinge Hospital
Huddinge, Sweden

I. INTRODUCTION

Acute GVHD is a major problem in clinical bone marrow transplantation (BMT), and even with genotypic identity of donor and patient for the human major histocomptibility antigens, life-threatening GVHD may occur. The frequency of GVHD is also highly dependent on the method of prophylaxis. Thus, in experimental animals and in man, T-cell depletion may completely abrogate acute GVHD (1-3). Pharmacologic immunosuppression, using methotrexate, cyclosporine, prednisolone, and anti-thymocyte globulin or combinations thereof, has been reported to result in an incidence of moderate to severe acute GVHD between 10 and 70% (4-8). Acute GVHD is a complex disease. Its mechanism is not completely understood, but it is generally accepted that cytotoxic donor T cells are mainly responsible for this disorder (Chapter 2). Zinkernagel and Doherty found that T cells react with virus-infected histocompatible cells as if they were allogeneic (9). In clinical BMT there are several recent reports demonstrating an association between herpesviruses in recipient or donor (or both) and GVHD, suggesting that viral antigens may mimic minor histocompatibility antigens and trigger immune reactions which may induce acute or chronic GVHD.

Due to immunoincompetence, viral infections, especially by herpesviruses and other opportunistic infections, are common causes of morbidity and mortality in BMT recipients of allogeneic as well as syngeneic and autologous marrow. The most important factor influencing cellular immune recovery after BMT is time (10-12). However, acute GVHD and its treatment with immunosuppressive drugs further impair immune function and increase the risk for infections (12-14). Chronic GVHD is associated with a prolonged immune deficiency (15-16; for review see Chapter 36) and infections, especially by gram-positive bacteria and varicella-zoster virus (VZV) (17-18). In leukemic patients acute and chronic GVHD have antileukemic effects and reduce the risk of relapse (19-10; for review see Chapter 39). Preliminary data also indicate that CMV may be associated with a reduced risk of recurrent leukemia after BMT. The various associations between viruses and GVHD will be discussed in this chapter.

II. ROLE OF VIRAL INFECTIONS IN THE DEVELOPMENT OF ACUTE GVHD

Overall, infections play an important role for the subsequent development of GVHD, a fact known from extensive experiments in animals. For instance, in mice treated with antibiotics, the severity of GVHD was decreased as compared to untreated animals (21). A germ-free environment reduced the severity of or prevented GVHD. C3H/He mice irradiated with 1000 rads and given allogeneic bone marrow in a germ-free environment had a 98% survival rate 120 days after transplantation, while conventionally treated mice all died (22). Moreover, in xenogeneic chimeras the germ-free state allowed for prolonged survival time, but mortality from GVHD was not prevented. In line with these experiments Heit and co-workers found that animals treated with antibiotics and allogeneic bone marrow had a superior survival compared to controls not treated with antibiotics, though both groups developed histologic signs and symptoms of GVHD (23). In man, a study from Seattle showed a beneficial effect of laminar air flow treatment on the severity of acute GVHD in BMT patients with severe aplastic anemia (24). The patients treated in laminar air flow rooms had significantly less acute GVHD ($p = 0.02$), which also affected patient survival rates: actuarial survival at 800 days was 87% compared to 69% for those treated in conventional rooms ($p = 0.03$). These studies suggest a role of bacterial infections in the development and severity of acute GVHD in experimental animals and in man.

More recently, some clinical studies in BMT recipients also indicated a role for viruses in the subsequent development of acute GVHD. The interactions between humoral and cellular immunity to herpes simplex viruses (HSV) in bone marrow donors, the occurrence of active HSV infections, and the development of moderate to severe acute GVHD were studied in recipients of marrow from HLA-identical siblings by Gratama and co-workers (25). The study included 70 BMT recipients with a median age of 25 years. The presence of IgG anti-HSV antibodies in marrow donors was associated with a high incidence of acute GVHD. Among recipients with HSV seropositive donors, 72% (38/53) developed grade II-IV acute GVHD compared to 13% (2/15) among patients with HSV seronegative donors ($p = 0.0004$). The cellular immunity to HSV was studied in vitro by evaluating the degree of lymphocyte proliferative responses to stimulation with fibroblasts infected with HSV type I. Seventy percent of recipients of marrow from donors with a positive cellular test developed moderate to severe acute GVHD as compared to 40% among recipients of marrow from donors with a negative test ($p = 0.03$). Donor CMV seropositivity further increased the risk of acute GVHD due to donor HSV antibodies. Thus, 85% of the recipients of marrow from donors who were both HSV and CMV seropositive developed moderate to severe acute GVHD as compared to 50% of recipients with marrow from HSV and CMV seronegative donors ($p = 0.0008$). Logistic regression analysis revealed that HSV seropositive donors ($p = 0.0006$), sex mismatch between recipient and donor ($p = 0.0008$), and a CMV seropositive donor ($p = 0.05$) were all independent risk factors for acute GVHD. Gratama and co-workers suggested the following hypothesis (25). Activation of memory T cells by HSV associated antigens may lead to the release of gamma-interferon (26). This may result in an increased expression of class I and class II HLA antigens on endothelial cells and fibroblasts. The presence of increased amounts of class I and II HLA antigens is important for the presentation and induction of an immune response to non-HLA antigens and the subsequent development of acute GVHD. However, one problem is that the anatomic location of GVHD in skin, gut, liver, and lymphoid tissue does not coincide with the location of HSV infection such as lips and oropharynx. Therefore, the possible effect of HSV immunity and infection on acute GVHD may be indirect. In line with this there are data that suggest that HSV can interface with cell surface antigens and alter the immune reactivity. The addition of HSV antigens to mixed lymphocyte cultures (MLC) of HLA-identical MLC mutually non-reactive and HSV seronegative siblings induced a strong proliferative response (27).

A subsequent study from Leiden including 126 HLA-identical marrow transplant recipients studied the role of recipient and donor pretransplant immunity against the four most common herpesviruses, donor and recipient age, sex and sex matching, the type of gastrointestinal decontamination, the type of GVHD prophylaxis, and the diagnostic in-dictions for BMT in relation to development of acute GVHD (28). If both donor and re-cipient were HSV seronegative, grades II-IV acute GVHD occurred in 18% of patients as compared to 56% when both were seropositive (p = 0.0001). A similar pattern was seen for varicella-zoster virus (VZV) serology (15% vs. 45% (p = 0.01)). If both recipient and donor were negative for CMV, 26% developed acute GVHD as compared to 69% when both were seropositive (p = 0.01). GVHD was less common in EBV-seronegative recipi-ents (8% vs. 51%; p = 0.0002). The incidence of GVHD also rose with recipient age, sex mismatch and selective compared to total gastrointestinal decontamination. Logistic regression procedures were used to control for confounding factors. The following fac-tors were found to be associated with grades II-IV acute GVHD (negative vs. positive for odds ratio): positive recipient EBV serology (odds ratio 10.1, p = 0.005), positive donor HSV serology (odds ratio 0.1, p = 0.003), selective vs. total gut decontamination (odds ratio 0.1, p = 0.004), and high donor age (odds ratio 3.7, p = 0.02). Sex mismatch (p = 0.054) and recipient age (p = 0.08) did not reach statistical significance. Due to these findings Gratama and co-workers speculated that EBV nonimmune donor cells may become infected and induce a polyclonal T-cell activation as seen in primary EBV infections. They suggested that this polyclonal T-cell activation contributed to the de-velopment of acute GVHD. If in contrast EBV immune cells were transferred with the marrow, these would rapidly kill the EBV-infected cells and prevent polyclonal T-cell activation and the risk of GVHD.

Inspired by the reports of Gratama and co-workers, we retrospectively analyzed herpesvirus serology in recipients and donors and acute GVHD in 111 consecutive HLA-identical bone marrow recipients at Huddinge Hospital (29). Age among the recipients ranged from 1 to 55 years, with a median of 17 years. As prophylaxis for GVHD, 65 pa-tients received methotrexate and 46 patients received cyclosporine (30). Acute GVHD grade I was treated with 2 mg/kg/day of prednisolone. IgG antibodies to CMV, HSV, and VZV were measured by enzyme-linked immunosorbent assay (ELISA) (31). For EBV, indirect immunofluorescence was used to measure virus capsid antigen IgG (32). HSV infection was defined as clinical signs of infection and a positive culture from local sites. Logistic regression analysis showed that a positve serology for HSV in the donors (odds ratio 3.12; p = 0.0176), a positive serology for CMV in the recipients (odds ratio 4.01; p = 0.013), and a low marrow cell dose (odds ratio 1.89; p = 0.05) were signifi-cantly associated with grade II-IV acute GVHD. Donor or recipient age, donor and re-cipient sex, donor CMV and recipient HSV immunity, EBV and VZV immunity in donor and recipient and splenectomy were not significantly associated with acute GVHD. The

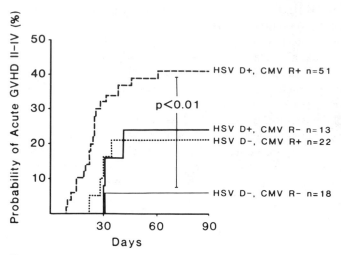

Figure 1 Probability and time to grade II active GVHD in patients were donor (D) was either immune (+) or nonimmune (−) to herpes simplex virus (HSV). Recipient (R) immunity to cytomegalovirus (CMV) is also considered. (Source: Ref. 29.)

cumulative incidence of grades II-IV acute GVHD in patients with an HSV seropositive donor was 37% as compared to 13% when the donor was HSV seronegative (p = 0.02). Patients with or without HSV infection had a similar incidence of moderate to severe acute GVHD (27% vs. 29%, respectively). In a multivariate analysis CMV seropositive recipients had an increased risk of GVHD (odds ratio 3.3; p = 0.049), and recipients with HSV seropositive donors had a marginal association (odds ratio 2.5; p = 0.067). None of the other analyzed factors were significantly associated with acute GVHD. If the recipient was CMV seropositive and the donor was HSV seropositive, 41% (20/51) of the patients developed moderate to severe acute GVHD as compared to only 6% (1/18) if both were seronegative (Fig. 1, p < 0.01). If the donor was HSV seropositive and the recipient CMV seronegative, 23% developed grades II-IV acute GVHD, and if the donor was HSV seronegative and the recipient was CMV seropositive, 21% developed acute GVHD. A positive serology for 1-2 herpesviruses among recipients or donors resulted in a 12% incidence of moderate to severe acute GVHD, whereas a positive serology for 3-4 herpes viruses in recipient or donor resulted in an incidence of 32% and 37% of acute GVHD, respectively (p = 0.05). In agreement with the findings of Gratama et al. (25,28), we found that positive donor immunity to HSV showed an association with grades II-IV acute GVHD. However, we could not confirm the role of EBV immunity. In contrast, our data indicated that CMV immunity in the recipients played a role. Taken together, the data suggest that HSV immune T cells in the graft could initiate a GVH reaction. HSV reactivation occurs early after transplantation before acute GVHD develops. Our study did not find any correlation between recipient HSV infection and acute GVHD, but Gratama et al. found a trend for more GVHD in recipients with HSV infection (25). In agreement with this, a study in pediatric marrow transplant recipients reported that HSV infection tended to be more common in patients with GVHD than in those without GVHD (30% vs. 15%, n.s.) (33). As mentioned above, HSV antigens can also induce blast transformation in MLC between otherwise MLC-nonreactive nonimmune siblings (27). Therefore, it is possible that latent HSV in donor or recipient cells have initiated acute

GVHD. In our material CMV seropositivity in the recipient was the strongest factor associated with grades II-IV acute GVHD (29). Latent CMV can be widely spread in various tissues in the body, and it is possible that CMV antigens could act as targets in the effector phase of acute GVHD.

Syngeneic transplant recipients can also develop signs of acute GVHD (34). In a study of nine patients undergoing syngeneic BMT, seven presented with symptoms resembling acute GVHD grades I-III (35). In at least three of these cases demonstration of CMV and HSV reactivation or seroconversion of an active hepatitis B infection prior to the occurrence of the GVHD-like organ manifestations suggested viral triggering or promotion of the disease.

There seems to be conflicting data regarding a correlation between CMV infection and acute GVHD (36-39). Among other risk factors found to be associated with acute GVHD are high recipient and donor age, sex mismatch, previous sensitization by pregnancy in female donors or transfusions, and splenectomy (40-46). The increasing incidence of acute GVHD dependent on increasing age of recipients and donors may be due to the fact that older people have become immune to more infectious agents. Thus, with increasing age more recipients and donors are immune against HSV, EBV, CMV, and VZV. In the study by Gratama et al. higher donor age, sex mismatch, and gut decontamination were independently associated with acute GVHD apart fro m the role of herpesviruses (28). In the study from Huddinge Hospital none of these factors were significantly associated with acute GVHD (29).

De Gast and co-workers suggested that four phases occurred in the development of acute GVHD (47). The first phase comprises infection and immunity before transplantation, including latent virus infections, protozoa, and colonization with bacteria and fungi in the recipient, and the generation of sensitized T cells in the donor. In the second phase cytoreduction therapy-induced immune deficiency and mucosal damage in the patient lead to reactivation of latent virus and invasion of bacteria and fungi. The sensitized donor marrow T cells are reactivated by these microbial agents resulting in gamma-interferon production (26). Gamma-interferon increases expression of HLA class I antigens and also induces expression of HLA class II antigens on endothelial cells and fibroblasts (48-49). However, a trial of patients transplanted for acute lymphoblastic leukemia in remission and randomized to receive or not to receive human leukocyte interferon every 3 days, beginning after marrow engraftment and continued to day 80 after transplantation, did not show any difference in the probability or severity of GVHD (50). Therefore, the role of interferon for the induction of GVHD may have been overemphasized. Next, epithelial cells, targets of acute GVHD are able to present antigen to T cells and cause sensitization (51-52). In the effector phase of GVHD, donor T cells attack recipient cells expressing HLA class I antigens.

To conclude, herpesvirus infections and immunity in marrow recipients and donors have to be considered among other risk factors associated with acute GVHD in recipients of HLA-identical bone marrow.

III. ACUTE GVHD AND THE DEVELOPMENT OF CMV INFECTIONS AND CMV INTERSTITIAL PNEUMONITIS

The incidence of CMV infection after BMT ranges from 50 to 90% (36,53-55). Around one third of the patients acquire asymptomatic disease, whereas latent CMV infections are reactivated without symptoms in the remaining patients. Symptoms of CMV infections include, fever, nausea, vomiting, esophagitis, gastrointestinal symptoms, arthralgias, and, more rarely in BMT patients, chorioretinitis and encephalitis. The most serious complication of CMV is pneumonitis, which occurs between 10 and 30% of allogeneic BMT recipients (36,56-58). The fatality rate of CMV interstitial pneumonitis is 80-90% (58-61). The strongest risk factor for the subsequent development of a CMV infection is a positive recipient CMV serology prior to transplantation (36-37,54-55). These studies suggest that CMV infection often occurs through reactivation of latent virus in CMV seropositive recipients. Some studies have also shown a correlation between granulocyte transfusions and CMV infection (36,62-63), presumably because CMV can be transferred via transfused blood products.

As indicated above, some investigators have found a correlation between CMV infection and acute GVHD (36-37). In a recent analysis from our hospital, however, acute GVHD was not associated with symptomatic CMV infection after BMT (39). A study in children demonstrated that CMV tended to be more common in patients with GVHD (33%) than in those without GVHD (11%) (33). In the same study adenoviruses were not notably more common in patients with GVHD (20%) as compared to patients without GVHD (17%). The cause of CMV infections in some patients with acute GVHD is most probably immunosuppression caused by this disease and its treatment with immunosuppressive drugs (10-12). CMV infection by itself also causes immunosuppression. This was shown by a faster recovery of lymphocyte mitogenic responses in BMT recipients who did not have CMV infection after marrow transplantation than in patients with CMV infection who did not experience GVHD (64). Impaired immune function may be the reason why patients undergoing CMV infection have superimposed an increased incidence of bacterial and fungal infections after allogeneic BMT (14). Even allogeneic effects not manifest as GVHD may have an effect on herpesvirus reactivation. In BMT recipients who were seropositive for various herpesviruses there was a significantly higher incidence of reactivation in patients undergoing allogeneic BMT as compared to autologous BMT (65). This was found for HSV (p = 0.007), CMV (p = 0.02), and VZV (p = 0.02). After autologous BMT, the restoration of cellular immunity to the three viruses occurred at a faster rate than after allogeneic BMT. The enhanced cellular immunity to the three viruses may have contributed to the low incidence of active infections with those viruses after autologous BMT. There was also a tendency for acute and chronic GVHD to decrease the immune responses to the three herpesviruses. Furthermore, cytotoxicity against CMV-infected targets by blood lymphocytes from patients with acute GVHD was reduced 20-40 days after transplant as compared to responses seen in patients without GVHD (p = 0.04) (66). Survival from CMV infection is superior in patients who had greater than or equal to 15% lysis of CMV infected targets during the first 20-60 days after BMT (p = 0.04). The study suggested that natural cytotoxicity of CMV targets is of importance for the acquisition and outcome of CMV infection after BMT.

The most feared complication of CMV infection is interstitial pneumonitis, and several clinical observations clearly indicate a correlation between GVHD and CMV interstitial pneumonitis. For instance, CMV interstitial pneumonitis is rare in syngeneic BMT recipients. In a report from Seattle none of 100 syngeneic BMT recipients developed CMV interstitial pneumonitis compared to 19% among 353 HLA-identical siblings (67). True idiopathic pneumonitis seems to be as common after syngeneic as after allogeneic BMT. There was a clear relationship between total lung irradiation dose and the incidence of lung complications after BMT (68). CMV interstitial pneumonitis is also rarely reported in autologous marrow transplant recipients (69). Several clinical reports have shown an association between acute GVHD and CMV interstitial pneumonitis (36,39,57-58,60). In a prospective study of 80 BMT recipients GVHD was significantly associated with an increase in both the incidence and severity of interstitial pneumonitis (p < 0.01) (58). Among the recipients who had no clinical manifestations of GVHD, the incidence of interstitial pneumonitis was 40% with a mortality rate of 52% for those affected. In contrast, among the 28 patients with GVHD of any degree, the incidence was 79% and the mortality rate 77%. In a more recent retrospective analysis from Seattle among 952 patients receiving allogeneic BMT, 35% developed interstitial pneumonia within 100 days of transplant (70). Development of CMV or idiopathic interstitial pneumonia was infrequent in patients with aplastic anemia treated with cyclophosphamide only in contrast to leukemic patients pretreated with total body irradiation. In that study total body irradiation, increasing patient age, pretransplant seropositivity for CMV antibody, and the development of GVHD all increased the risk of CMV pneumonia. This is in accordance with the analysis by Meyers et al. where factors which increased the incidence of CMV pneumonitis and CMV infection included the Caucasian race, GVHD grade II or greater, age above 12 years, lung irradiation greater than 600 rads, preceding recipient CMV seropositivity, granulocyte transfusions, and the extent of recipient/donor HLA matching (60). Pneumonitis was twice as common after BMT for acute leukemia as after aplastic anemia (p < 0.0005). In a French study of 130 consecutive BMT patients the overall mortality due to pneumonia was 20%. GVHD clearly increased the incidence of infectious pneumonia and the mortality (71).

According to our experience at Huddinge Hospital, the following factors were associated with CMV interstitial pneumonitis in bivariate analysis: acute GVHD grades II-IV (p = 0.009), donor age above 17 years (p = 0.02), and a positive recipient CMV serology (p = 0.014) (39). In multivariate analysis only grades II-IV acute GVHD was significantly associated with CMV interstitial pneumonitis (p = 0.01). In our experience among 197 consecutive HLA-identical siblings undergoing allogeneic BMT between 1975 and May 1988, the cumulative incidence of CMV interstitial pneumonitis was 26% in patients with moderate to severe acute GVHD compared to 11% in patients with no or mild acute GVHD (p = 0.01, Fig. 2). Thus, in clinical BMT several studies show an association between allogeneic BMT and especially acute GVHD, and the subsequent development of CMV interstitial pneumonia. This is supported by experimental data in mice presented by Grundy and co-workers (72).

Mice given a high dose of spleen cell challenge but not infected with CMV developed acute GVHD measured as an increased spleen/body weight ratio. After infection with murine CMV and challenge with extremely low doses of parenteral spleen cells, GVHD was augmented. Mice receiving murine CMV and GVHD challenge died, with interstitial pneumonitis being the most prominent pathological lesion. These experimental data demonstrate that CMV infections play a primary role in both provoking or accentuating acute GVHD and in the development of CMV interstitial pneumonitis. It was also shown that murine CMV infection can, after an early phase of immunosuppression, modulate the host immune response to enhance responsiveness to allogeneic and hapten-modified syngeneic histocompatibility antigens (73). Recently Grundy and co-workers postulated that CMV interstitial pneumonitis in transplant recipients may be an immunopathologic condition (74). Their hypothesis is that limited CMV replication in the lungs leads to the display of a virus-coded protein which is recognized by host T cells, and the pneumonitis is due to an uncontrolled accumulation and recruitment of such cells in the

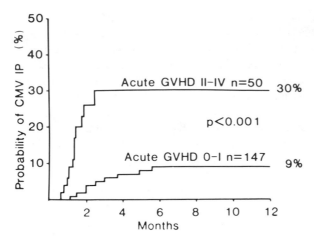

Figure 2 Probability and time to cytomegalovirus interstitial pneumonitis (CMV-IP) in 197 out of 210 consecutive bone marrow recipeints who engrafted and were evaluable for acute GVHD. The patients underwent bone marrow transplantation from 1975 to June 1988 at Huddinge Hospital. Analysis was performed on August 10, 1988. Patients with moderate to severe acute GVHD had an increased probability of CMV-IP compared to those with mild or no acute GVHD (log-rank analysis).

lungs. They suggested that evidence from studies in man and in murine models of CMV showed that virus replication in the lung is unrelated to the development of pathologic effects. Furthermore, the host immune response is required for the induction of pneumonitis. Using DNA probes, viral DNA was measured by dot-blot hybridization, and this correlated with infectious CMV in a study by Zaia (75). However, neither CMV DNA nor CMV viral titers correlated with time from the onset of pneumonia to death. It was, therefore, suggested that CMV pneumonitis was caused by immunologic events induced after CMV infection. Such events were CMV alterations in recipient cell surfaces inducing donor alloreactivity to minor histocompatibility differences leading to subsequent pneumonitis.

In conclusion, clinical studies and experimental data demonstrate a relationship between GVHD and CMV interstitial pneumonitis.

IV. IMMUNITY AND CMV PNEUMONITIS

Deficient recipient CMV immunity seems to play a role in the development of CMV pneumonitis. Neiman et al. (58) reported that a failure to respond serologically to CMV infection markedly increases the hazard of dying of interstitial pneumonia. All 13 patients with CMV-associated pneumonia who failed to seroconvert died, whereas the mortality rate was 3/7 among those who did respond serologically. This finding was also confirmed in a more recent analysis from Seattle (36). In this study it was found that patients who seroconverted had a risk of dying from CMV pneumonitis of 29% as compared to 7% among patients who did not seroconvert ($p < 0.02$). In accordance with these findings we found that patients with CMV interstitial pneumonitis, and who all died, had significantly lower CMV IgG titers than patients with other symptomatic CMV infections who survived (55). An indication that deficient T-cell immunity plays a role in the subsequent development of CMV pneumonitis is that treatment with antithymo-cyte globulin was reported to be correlated with CMV pneumonitis (36,57). In a more recent study the use of antithymocyte globulin for the treatment of acute GVHD was associated with a high incidence of CMV pneumonia only among CMV seropositive, but not seronegative patients (36). Treatment with antithymocyte globulin not only elimi-nates GVHD-reactive T cells but also T cells immune to CMV, thereby paving the way for serious CMV infections (76). It was also shown that allogeneic BMT recipients with fatal CMV infections had depressed natural killer cells and antibody dependent cytotoxic activities before and during CMV infection as compared to patients who survived (77).

Whether donor immunity is of importance for the prevention of CMV pneumoni-tis is controversial. Antitetanus toxin titers after BMT were highest if both donor and recipient were immunized shortly prior to transplantation (78). If neither donor nor recipient was immunized to tetanus toxin prior to transplantation the antibody titer was low, and if either donor or recipient alone was immunized the antibody titer re-sponse was intermediate. We have also reported that virus-specific antibodies disap-peared more frequently during the first year after BMT in seropositive patients who had seronegative donors than in patients who had seropositive donors (79). These studies indicate transfer of immunocompetent cells from the donor. In accordance with this, it was noted that among CMV seropositive recipients of T-cell-depleted marrow, those with a CMV seropositive donor had a decreased incidence of CMV pneumonitis (4/27) as compared to recipients with CMV seronegative donors (8/13) ($p < 0.001$) (80). The mortality by CMV pneumonitis was 1/27 and 6/13 in the two groups, respectively, a dif-ference which was significant in multivariate analysis ($p = 0.01$). The data from Grob et al. (80) could not be confirmed by us (81). Thus, among 170 consecutive allogeneic BMT recipients, those with a CMV seropositive donor had, instead, an increased risk of developing CMV pneumonitis (16/95) as compared with a seronegative donor (3/75) ($p = 0.01$). If only CMV seropositive recipients were included in the analysis, the dif-ference was not statistically significant ($p = 0.2$). According to a previous report from Grob and co-workers at the Royal Free Hospital, T-cell-depleted marrow recipients receiving a higher dose of total body irradiation had an increased risk of CMV pneumo-nitis (82). Even if the role of donor CMV serology was significant in multivariate analy-sis, irradiation dose may have contributed to the high incidence of CMV interstitial pneu-monitis in their report. In comparison the incidence of CMV pneumonitis was 12/40 (30%) among the CMV seropositive patients from Royal Free Hospital, compared to 17/112 (15%) at Huddinge Hospital, a difference which was statistically significant ($p = 0.05$). The lower incidence at our institution may be due to the use of lung shielding. Our patients received a total dose toward the lungs of 900 rads at a dose rate of 4 rads/min (83). In contrast to the data from the Royal Free Hospital, most of our patients received unmanipulated marrow. However, two of our patients who developed CMV interstitial pneumonitis received T-cell-depleted marrow and both had CMV seropositive donors. In two other studies, a lower frequency of CMV interstitial pneumonitis was also found in recipients of marrow from CMV seronegative donors (57,84). This may be partly due to primary CMV infections in CMV seronegative recipients with seropositive donors. However, preliminary data from Seattle indicate that among CMV seropositive recipients of T-cell-depleted marrow, those with a CMV seropositive donor tended to have a lower incidence of CMV pneumonitis (Meyers, personal communication). Fur-thermore, a study using T-cell depletion with CAMPATH-1 also showed a lower incidence of CMV pneumonitis in recipients of marrow from CMV seropositive donors (85). Therefore, it may be possible that donor CMV immunity is more important in recipients of T-cell-depleted marrow than in recipients of nonmanipulated marrow as suggested by Brenner et al. (86). More data are needed to elucidate the role of donor immunity in the prevention of recipient CMV pneumonitis. However, recipient immunity to CMV posttransplantation seems important to prevent later CMV pneumonitis.

V. VIRAL INFECTIONS AND RISK FACTORS FOR CHRONIC GVHD

The major risk factor for the development of chronic GVHD is previous acute GVHD (87-89). In a bivariate analysis Lönnqvist and co-workers from our group found that CMV infection was associated with or preceded chronic GVHD (90). Thus, chronic GVHD was seen in 20/36 (56%) of the patients who had previously experienced a symptomatic or an asymptomatic CMV infection as compared to only 2/17 patients (12%) without signs of active CMV infection (p < 0.01). The CMV infections preceded the development of chronic GVHD by a median of 128 days (range 33-322 days). In a subsequent multivariate analysis of factors associated with chronic GVHD performed in 75 consecutive allogeneic BMT recipients at our center a preceding CMV infection did not reach statistical significance (p = 0.07) (88). In the bivariate analysis, patients with a preceding CMV infection had a cumulative incidence of chronic GVHD of 65% as compared to 17% in those without CMV infection (p = 0.003). In the multivariate analysis, donor age >17 years (p = 0.003), donor buffy-coat treatment (p = 0.003) and preceding grades II-IV acute GVHD (p = 0.047) were significantly associated with chronic GVHD. This partly supports the results of an analysis of chronic GVHD in patients with severe aplastic anemia by Storb and co-workers where preceding acute GVHD, high recipient age, and treatment with unirradiated donor buffy coat cells predisposed to chronic GVHD (87). In our study among patients with an otherwise low occurrence rate of chronic GVHD, such as recipients under the age of 17 years or in recipients with donor below 17 years of age and in patients with grade 0-I acute GVHD, those with CMV infection had a significantly increased risk of chronic GVHD (p < 0.01) (88). Experimental data in mice also show that CMV infection enhances host reactivity to foreign antigens by T-cell cytotoxicity and host reactivity to self-antigens by auto-antibody production (72-73). However, the suggestive correlation found by us between CMV infection and chronic GVHD was not confirmed by others (36-37). In the study from Seattle including 545 BMT patients, patients with or without CMV infection had the same incidence of chronic GVHD (36). However, in the study from Seattle only 36% of the patients were diagnosed to have a CMV infection as compared to 59% of our patients. Outpatients were followed much more frequently, and we used an ELISA technique for serologic diagnosis, whereas Seattle used a complement fixation test which may be less sensitive. These differences may partly explain the discrepant findings. In the study by Miller et al. chronic GVHD was diagnosed in 24% of CMV uninfected patients and in 41% of CMV-infected patients (p = 0.13) (37). An analysis from the International Bone Marrow Transplant registry found a correlation between CMV infection and chronic GVHD in bivariate analysis, but this correlation was not significant in multivariate analysis, confirming our findings of Huddinge Hospital (Atkinson et al., in preparation).

Jacobsen and co-workers analyzed donor and recipient immunity to CMV and recipient CMV infection and their role for the subsequent development of chronic GVHD (91). They found that donor immunity to CMV was important for the development of chronic GVHD, but not CMV infection in the recipient. Thus, among patients with a posttransplant CMV infection, 7/12 with a CMV seropositive donor developed chronic GVHD as compared to 3/22 patients with a CMV seronegative donor (p < 0.05). A subsequent multivariate analysis by the Nordic Bone Marrow Transplantation Group demonstrated that high donor age (p = 0.01), female donor above 20 years to male recipient (p = 0.003), preceding acute GVHD grades II-IV (p = 0.04), and a CMV seropositive donor (p = 0.002) were associated with chronic GVHD (92). Since donor age was correlated to seropositive CMV immune status, donor age was excluded in the analysis where a CMV seropositive donor was a significant factor. Recently Bostrom et al. from Huddinge Hospital analyzed the role of immunity in recipients and donors against the four most common herpesviruses for the development of chronic GVHD in 150 consecutive HLA-identical marrow recipients (93). Bivariate Cox's regression analysis showed that seropositivity for CMV in patients (p = 0.04) and donors (p = 0.0005), donor seropositivity for HSV (p = 0.04), donor age (p = 0.01), and grades II-IV acute GVHD (p = 0.001) were associated with an increased incidence of chronic GVHD. In multivariate analysis, previous grade II-IV acute GVHD (p = 0.0001) and a positive donor CMV serology (p < 0.01) were statistically significant associated with chronic GVHD. High donor age did not reach statistical significance in this multivariate analysis (p = 0.09). If the patients had previous grades II-IV acute GVHD, and the donor was seropositive for CMV, the probability of developing chronic GVHD was above 80% (Table 1). In patients who developed grades 0-I acute GVHD and the donors were CMV seronegative, the incidence of chronic GVHD was only 13%. If only one of these factors were positive (either acute GVHD occurred or the donor was CMV seropositive), approximately half of the patients developed chronic GVHD. When the recipient or the donor were immune to three or four herpesviruses before marrow transplantation compared to zero to two herpesviruses, there was an increased risk for chronic GVHD (p = 0.025 and 0.0008, respectively).

Also, viruses outside the herpes group may play a role in GVHD. Thus, a measles exanthema was reported to initiate chronic GVHD, and the skin involved was limited to the area of viral eruption (94).

In addition to acute GVHD, donor immunity to CMV seems to play a role in the subsequent development of chronic GVHD in the recipient. I, therefore, would like to speculate about a possible mechanism behind this finding. Recently it was reported that proteins from human CMV bound to B_2 microglobulin, a protein that is part of the class I major histocompatibility complex antigens (95,96). Furthermore, DNA sequence analysis demonstrated that CMV encodes a molecule similar to the class I antigens (97). It may be possible that CMV immune donor cells cross-react with beta-2-microglobulin

Table 1 Probability of Chronic GVHD One Year After Bone Marrow Transplantation in HLA-Matched Siblings in Relation to Acute GVHD and Donor CMV Immunity

Grades II-IV acute GVHD	Donor CMV immunity	Number of patients	Chronic GVHD (%)
+	+	15	82%
+	−	11	50%
−	+	56	46%
−	−	50	13%

Source: Ref. 93.

and the class I HLA antigens and, subsequently, trigger an allogeneic immune reaction that may lead to chronic GVHD. Thus, latent CMV or a previous CMV infection in the recipient may not always be needed to trigger the CMV immune donor cells. Although latent CMV in the recipient or CMV infection were not statistically significantly associated with chronic GVHD in the multivariate analysis, these factors may in any case play a role for the subsequent development of chronic GVHD. Factors such as recipient CMV serology, CMV infection, acute GVHD, and chronic GVHD are all closely interrelated. Since acute GVHD is a major factor predisposing to chronic GVHD this may mask a role of recipient CMV serology and CMV infection for the subsequent development of chronic GVHD. It is, therefore, also possible that CMV immune donor cells are triggered by recipient CMV antigens, which in turn may lead to chronic GVHD.

In addition to acute GVHD, a positive donor CMV immunity seems to increase the risk of developing chronic GVHD.

VI. PRELIMINARY INDICATIONS THAT CYTOMEGALOVIRUS MAY INDUCE ANTILEUKEMIC ACTIVITY AFTER MARROW TRANSPLANTATION

In 72 consecutive marrow transplant recipients with hematologic malignancies at Huddinge Hospital, all relapses occurred in patients with acute leukemia below 18 years of age transplanted in second of later remission, or with more than 10% blasts in the marrow before BMT (98). The probability of relapse was increased in patients without CMV infection (p = 0.001) and in patients without chronic GVHD (p = 0.049). When leukemic patients below 18 years of age with a high risk of relapse were analyzed separately, 8/11 of patients without CMV infection relapsed compared to none of 13 with CMV infection (p = 0.006). In an analysis by the Nordic Bone Marrow Transplant Group, none of 12 AML patients with CMV seropositive donors had posttransplantation relapse in contrast to 7/10 AML patients with CMV seronegative donors (p = 0.0005) (99). This effect was independent of disease status, donor and recipient age, recipient pretransplant CMV immunity, or posttransplant CMV infection. The effect was not mediated through an increased occurrence of acute or chronic GVHD, and no such effect was observed in patients with acute lymphoblastic leukemia. In a subsequent analysis by the Nordic Bone Marrow Transplantation Group of 163 patients with acute myeloid leukemia, acute lymphoblastic leukemia, or malignant lymphoma, the following factors were found to increase the risk of relapse in multivariate analysis: marrow transplantation during relapse (p = 0.006), marrow transplantation later than in first remission (p < 0.0001), a CMV seronegative donor (p = 0.0002), donor age above 20 years (p = 0.005), and absence of chronic GVHD (p = 0.0009) (92). In this analysis CMV infection did not decrease the risk of relapse. However, in a recent analysis from Huddinge Hospital including 127 patients with leukemia, donor CMV immune status was not correlated with the incidence of relapse (100). In these patients those grafted in first remission of acute leukemia or in first chronic phase of chronic myeloid leukemia had a 5-year probability of relapse of 8% as compared to 50% in patients grafted in second or later remission or in early relapse (p = 0.0001). In addition, patients with leukemia with asymptomatic CMV infection had a significantly lower incidence of relapse than patients with symptomatic CMV infection or with no CMV infection (Fig. 3). By multivariate analysis a decreased risk of relapse was seen in patients in first remission or first chronic

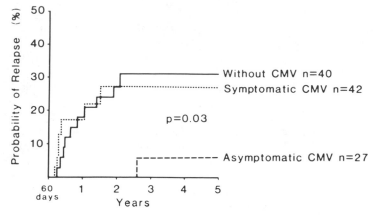

Figure 3 Probability and time to relapse (from day 60 after BMT) in patients undergoing marrow transplantation for acute leukemia in remission or early relapse (less than 25% blasts in marrow). Only patients surviving at least 60 days were included in the analysis to avoid the bias by selecting patients who lived long enough to develop CMV infection. The log-rank test was used for statistical analysis, taking censored data into account. CMV infection was diagnosed by virus isolation from blood, bone marrow, or urine, appearance of specific IgM titers > 100, specific IgG titers, seroconversion > 100 and/or a 5-fold ELISA CMV IgG rise. (Source: Ref. 100.)

phase ($p = 0.002$), while asymptomatic CMV infection did not reach statistical significance ($p = 0.09$).

These studies suggest an antileukemia effect by either CMV immune donor cells, overall CMV infection or asymptomatic CMV infection. In this context I would like to speculate that viral infections could activate natural killer cells which may be involved in this suggested antileukemia effect. Natural killer cells are capable of killing syngeneic tumor transplants (101). Patients with asymptomatic disease may have an immune system that is competent to depress symptomatic CMV disease and may also activate natural killer cells which are competent to kill leukemic cells. In patients with symptomatic CMV infection this antileukemic activity may be depressed. It is also possible that interferon which is released during CMV infection may have an anti-leukemic effect. Thus, a randomized trial in patients with acute lymphoblastic leukemia showed that patients treated with interferon had a probability of relapse of 0.36, which was significantly lower ($p = 0.04$) than in untreated controls where the relapse rate was 0.74 (50). In this study treatment with interferon did not affect the incidence of CMV infection or the probability or severity of GVHD.

The decreased incidence of relapse associated with CMV infection or donor CMV immunity needs to be further explored by other centers and also in larger patient series.

ACKNOWLEDGMENTS

OR was supported by research grants from Barncancerfonden, the Swedish Cancer Society (770-B88-01XA), The Swedish Medical Research Council (16X-05971), Jennyfonden and the Karolinska Institute.

REFERENCES

1. Dicke KA, Tridente G, van Bekkum DW: The selective elimination of immunologically competent cells from bone marrow and lymphocytic cell mixtures. III. In vitro test for detection of immunocompetent cells in fractionated mouse spleen cells suspension and primate bone marrow suspensions. Transplantation 1969;8:422-434.
2. Korngold R, Sprent J: T cell subsets and graft-versus-host disease. Transplantation 1987;44:335-339.
3. Prentice HG, Blacklock HAA, Janossy G, Gilmore MJML, Prince-Jones L, Tidman N, Trejdosiewicz LK, Skeggs DBL, Panjwani O, Ball S, Graphakos S, Pattersson J, Ivory K, Hoffbrand AV: Depletion of T lymphocytes in donor marrow prevents significant graft versus host disease in matched allogeneic leukaemic marrow transplant recipients. Lancet 1984;1:472-475.
4. Thomas ED, Storb R, Clift RA, Fefer A, Jonson FL, Neiman PE, Lerner KG, Glucksberg H, Buckner SD: Bone-marrow transplantation. N Engl J Med 1975;292:832-843, 895-902.
5. Weiden PL, Doney K, Storb R, Thomas ED: Anti-human thymocyte globulin (ATG) for prophylaxis and treatment of graft-versus-host disease in recipients of allogeneic marrow grafts. Transplant Proc 1978;10:213-216.
6. Storb R, Deeg HJ, Whitehead J, Appelbaum F, Beatty P, Bensinger W, Buckner CD, Clift R, Doney K, Farewell V, Hansen J, Hill R, Lum L, Martin P, McGuffin R, Sanders J, Stewart P, Sullivan K, Witherspoon R, Yee GY, Thomas ED: Methotrexate and cyclosporine compared with cyclosporine alone for prophylaxis of acute graft versus host disease after marrow transplantation for leukemia. N Engl J Med 1986; 314:729-735.
7. Ringdén O, Persson U, Johansson SGO, Gahrton G, Groth CG, Lundgren G, Lönnqvist B: Early diagnosis and treatment of acute human graft-versus-host disease. Transplant Proc 1983;15:1490-1494.
8. Ramsay NKC, Kersey JH, Robison LL, McGlave PB, Woods WG, Krivit W, Kim TH, Goldman AI, Nesbit ME Jr: A randomized study of the prevention of acute graft-versus-host disease. N Engl J Med 1982;306:392-397.
9. Zinkernagel RM, Doherty PC: Restriction of in vitro T cell-mediated cytotoxicity in lymphocytic choriomeningitis within a syngeneic or semi-allogeneic system. Nature 1974;248:701-712.
10. Witherspoon RP, Storb R, Ochs HD, Flournoy N, Kopecky KJ, Sullivan KM, Deeg HJ, Sosa R, Noel DR, Atkinson K, Thomas ED: Recovery of antibody production in human allogeneic marrow graft recipients: Influence of time posttransplantation, the presence or absence of chronic graft-versus-host disease, and antithymocyte globulin treatment. Blood 1981;58:360-368.
11. Witherspoon RP, Matthews D, Storb R, Atkinson K, Cheever M, Deeg HJ, Doney K, Kalbfleisch J, Noel D, Prentice R, Sullivan KM, Thomas ED: Recovery of in vivo cellular immunity after human marrow grafting. Influence of time postgrafting and acute graft-versus-host disease. Transplant 1984;37:145-150.
12. Paulin T, Ringdén O, Nilsson B: Immunological recovery after bone marrow transplantation. Role of age, graft-versus-host disease, prednisolone treatment and infections. Bone Marrow Transplantation 1987;1:317-328.
13. Gale RP, Opelz G, Mickey MR, Graze PR, Saxon A: for the UCLS Bone Marrow Transplant Team: Immunodeficiency following allogeneic bone marrow transplantation. Transplant Proc 1978;10:223-227.
14. Paulin T, Ringdén O, Nilsson B, Lönnqvist B, Gahrton G: Variables predicting bacterial infections after allogeneic marrow engraftment. Transplantation 1987;43:393-398.

15. Noel DR, Witherspoon RP, Storb R, Atkinson K, Doney K, Mickelson EM, Ochs HD, Warren RP, Weiden PL, Thomas ED: Does graft-versus-host disease influence the tempo of immunologic recovery after allogeneic human marrow transplantation? An observation of 56 long-term survivors. Blood 1978;51:1087-1104.

16. Ringdén O, Witherspoon R, Storb R, Ekelund E, Thomas ED: B cell function in human marrow transplant recipients assessed by direct and indirect hemolysis in gel assays. J Immunol 1979;123:2729-2734.

17. Atkinson K, Storb R, Prentice RL, Weiden PL, Witherspoon RP, Sullivan K, Noel D, Thomas ED: Analysis of late infections in 89 long-term survivors of bone marrow transplantation. Blood 1979;53:720-731.

18. Atkinson K, Farewell V, Storb R, Tsoi M-S, Sullivan KM, Witherspoon RP, Fefer A, Clift R, Goodell B, Thomas ED: Analysis of late infections after human bone marrow transplantation: Role of genotypic nonidentity between marrow donor and recipient and of nonspecific suppressor cells in patients with chronic graft-versus-host disease. Blood 1982;60:714-720.

19. Weiden PL, Flournoy N, Thomas ED, Prentice R, Fefer A, Buckner CD, Storb R: Antileukemic effect of graft-versus-host disease in marrow transplantation. N Engl J Med 1979;300:1068-1073.

20. Weiden PL, Sullivan KM, Flournoy N, Storb R, Thomas ED: and the Seattle Marrow Transplant Team: Antileukemic effect of chronic graft-versus-host disease. Contribution to improved survival after allogeneic marrow transplantation. N Engl J Med 1981;304:1529-1533.

21. van Bekkum DW, Vos O: Treatment of secondary disease in radiation chimeras. Int J Radiat Biol 1961;3:173-181.

22. Jones JM, Wilson R, Bealmear PM: Mortality and gross pathology of secondary disease in germfree mouse radiation chimeras. Radiat Res 1971;45:577-588.

23. Heit H, Wilson R. Fliedner TM, Kohne E: Mortality of secondary disease in antibiotic-treated mouse radiation chimers. In *Germfree Research*, edited by Heneghan IJ. Academic Press, New York, 1973; pp. 477-483.

24. Storb R, Prentice RL, Buckner CD, et al.: Graft-versus-host disease and survival with aplastic anemia treated by marrow grafts from HLA-identical siblings. Beneficial effect of a protective environment. N Engl J Med 1983;308:302-307.

25. Gratama JW, Sinnige LGF, Weijers TF, Zwaan FE, van Heugten JG, Stijnen T, D'Amaro J, The TH, Hekker AC, de Gast GC: Marrow donor immunity to herpes simplex virus: association with acute graft-versus-host disease. Exp Hematol 1987; 15:735-740.

26. Trinchieri G, Perussia B: Immune interferon: a pleiotropic lymphokine with multiple effects. Immunol Today 1985;6:131-136.

27. Singal DP, Rawls WE: Effects of herpes simplex virus antigens on human mixed lymphocyte culture. Transplantation 1980;29:500-502.

28. Gratama JW, Zwaan FE, Stijnen T, Weijers TF, Weiland HT, D'Amaro J, Hekker AC, The TH, de Gast GC, Vossen JMJJ: Herpes-virus immunity and acute graft-versus-host disease. Lancet 1987;1:471-474.

29. Boström L, Ringdén O, Sundberg B, Linde A, Tollemar J, Nilsson B: Pretransplant herpes virus serology and acute graft-versus-host disease. Transplantation 1988;46: 548-552.

30. Ringdén O, Bäckman L, Lönnqvist B, Heimdahl A, Lindholm A, Bolme P, Gahrton G: A randomized trial comparing the use of cyclosporin and methotrexate for graft-versus-host disease prophylaxis in bone marrow transplant recipients with haematologic malignancies. Bone Marrow Transplant 1986;1:41-51.

31. Sundqvist V-A, Wahren B: An interchangeable ELISA for cytomegalovirus antigen and antibody. J Virol Methods 1981;2:301-312.

32. Linde A, Andersson J, Lundgren G, Wahren B: Subclass reactivity to Epstein-Barr virus capsid antigen in primary and reactivated EBV infections. J Med Virol 1987; 21:109-121.
33. Wasserman R, August CS, Plotkin SA: Viral infections in pediatric bone marrow transplant patients. Pediatr Infect Dis J 1988;7:109-115.
34. Rappeport J, Mihm M, Reinherz E, Lopansri S, Parkman R: Acute graft-versus-host disease in recipients of bone marrow transplants from identical twin donors. Lancet 1979;2:717-720.
35. Einsele H, Ehninger G, Schneider EM, Krüger GFR, Vallbracht A, Dopfer R, Schmidt H, Waller HD, Müller CA: High frequency of graft-versus-host-like syndromes following syngeneic bone marrow transplantation. Transplantation 1988;45:579-585.
36. Meyers JD, Flournoy N, Thomas ED: Risk factors for cytomegalovirus infection after human marrow transplantation. J Infect Dis 1986;153:478-488.
37. Miller W, Flynn P, McCullough J, Balfour HH Jr, Goldman A, Haake R, McGlave P, Ramsay N, Kersey J: Cytomegalovirus infection after bone marrow transplantation: An association with acute graft-v-host disease. Blood 1986;67:1162-1167.
38. Gratama JW, Fibbe WE, Naipal AMIH, Slats J, Stijnen T, D'Amaro J, Bolhuis RLH, The TH, Janssen J: Cytomegalovirus immunity and T lymphocytes in bone marrow donors and acute graft-versus-host disease. Bone Marrow Transplant 1986;1: 141-146.
39. Paulin T, Ringdén O, Sundberg B, Lönnqvist B, Tollemar J: Symptomatic cytomegalovirus infection after bone marrow transplantation. Importance of high marrow cell dose. Bone Marrow Transplant 1988;3(Suppl 1):251-252.
40. Storb R, Prentice RL, Thomas ED: Treatment of aplastic anemia by marrow transplantation from HLA identical siblings: prognostic factors associated with graft versus host disease and survival. J Clin Invest 1977;59:625-632.
41. Baughan ASJ, Worsley AM, McCarthy DM, Hows JM, Catovsky D, Gordon-Smith EC, Galton DAG, Goldman JM: Haematological reconstitution and severity of graft-versus-host disease after bone marrow transplantation for chronic granulocytic leukaemia: the influence of previous splenectomy. Br J Haematol 1984;56:445-454.
42. Bross DS, Tutschka PJ, Farmer ER, Beschorner WE, Braine HG, Mellits ED, Bias WB, Santos GW: Predictive factors for acute graft-versus-host disease in patients transplanted with HLA-identical bone marrow. Blood 1984;63:1265-1270.
43. Ringdén O, Nilsson B: Death by graft-versus-host disease is associated with HLA mismatch, high recipient age, low marrow cell dose and splenectomy. Transplantation 1985;40:39-44.
44. Atkinson K, Farrell C, Chapman G, Downs K, Penny R, Biggs J: Female marrow donors increase the risk of acute graft-versus-host disease: effect of donor age and parity and analysis of cell subpopulations in the donor marrow inoculum. Br J Haematol 1986;63:231-239.
45. Gale RP, Bortin MM, van Bekkum DM, Biggs JC, Dicke KA, Gluckman E, Good RA, Hoffmann RG, Kay HEM, Kersey JH, Marmont A, Masaoka T, Rimm AA, van Rood JJ, Zwaan FE: Risk-factors for acute graft-versus-host disease. Br J Hematol 1987; 67:397-406.
46. Michallet M, Corront B, Bosson JL, Reiffers J, Marit G, Maraninchi D, Gaspart MH: Risk factors for GVHD: study of 157 patients from Bordeaux, Grenoble, Marseille. Bone Marrow Transplant 1988;3(Suppl 1):226.
47. de Gast GC, Gratama JW, Ringdén O, Gluckman E: The multifactorial etiology of graft-versus-host disease. Immunology Today 1987;8:209-212.
48. Pober JS, Collins T, Gimbrone MA Jr, Cotran RS, Gitlin JD, Fiers W, Clayberger C, Krensky AM, Burakoff SJ, Reiss CS: Lymphocytes recognize human vascular endo-

thelial and dermal fibroblast Ia antigens induced by recombinant immune interferon. Nature 1983;305:726-729.

49. Collins T, Korman AJ, Wake CT, Boss JM, Kappes DJ, Fiers W, Ault KA, Gimbrone MA Jr, Strominger JL, Pober JS: Immune interferon activates multiple class II major histocompatibility complex genes and the associated invariant chain gene in human endothelial cells and dermal fibroblasts. Proc Natl Acad Sci USA 1984;81:4917-4921.

50. Meyers JD, Flournoy N, Sanders JE, McGiffin RW, Newton BA, Fisher LD, Lum LG, Appelbaum FR, Doney K, Sullivan KM, Storb R, Buckner CD, Thomas ED: Prophylactic use of human leukocyte interferon after allogeneic marrow transplantation. Ann Int Med 1987;107:809-816.

51. Lampert IA, Suitters AJ, Chisholm PM: Expression of Ia antigen on epidermal keratinocytes in graft-versus-host disease. Nature 1981;293:149-150.

52. Mason DW, Dallman M, Barclay AN: Graft-versus-host disease induces expression of Ia antigen in rat epidermal cells and gut epithelium. Nature 1981;293:150-151.

53. Würsch AM, Gratama JW, Middledorp JM, Nissen C, Gratwohl A, Speck B, Jansen J, D'Amaro J, The TH, de Gast GC: The effect of cytomegalovirus infection on T lymphocytes after allogeneic marrow grafting. Clin Exp Immunol 1985;62:278-287.

54. Gratama JW, Middeldorp JM, Sinnige LGF, van der Meer JWM, D'Amaro J, Jansen J, Zwaan FE, Brand A, de Gast GC, The TH: Cytomegalovirus immunity in allogeneic marrow grafting. Transplantation 1985;40:510-514.

55. Paulin T, Ringdén O, Lönnqvist B, Wahren B, Nilsson B: The importance of pre bone marrow transplantation serology in determining subsequent cytomegalovirus infection. An analysis of risk factors. Scand J Infect Dis 1986;18:199-209.

56. Neiman P, Wasserman PB, Wentworth BB, Kao, GF, Lerner KG, Storb R, Buckner CD, Clift RA, Fefer A, Fass L, Glucksberg H, Thomas ED: Interstitial pneumonia and cytomegalovirus infection as complications of human marrow transplantation. Transplantation 1973;15:478-485.

57. Meyers JD, Spencer HC Jr, Watts JC, Gregg MB, Stewart JA, Troupin RH, Thomas ED: Cytomegalovirus pneumonia after human marrow transplantation. Ann Int Med 1975;82:181-188.

58. Neiman PE, Reeves W, Ray G, Flournoy N, Lerner KG, Sale GE, Thomas ED: A prospective analysis of interstitial pneumonia and opportunistic viral infection among recipients of allogeneic marrow graft. J Infect Dis 1977;136:754-767.

59. Bortin MM, Kay HEM, Gale RP, Rimm AA: Factors associated with interstitial pneumonitis after bone-marrow transplantation for acute leukaemia. Lancet 1982; 1:437-439.

60. Meyers JD, Flournoy N, Thomas ED: Nonbacterial pneumonia after allogeneic marrow transplantation: A review of ten years' experience. Rev Infect Dis 1982; 4:1119-1132.

61. Weiner RS, Bortin MM, Gale RP, Gluckman E, Kay HEM, Kolb H-J, Hartz AJ, Rimm AA: Interstitial pneumonitis after bone marrow transplantation. Assessment of risk factors. Ann Int Med 1986;104:168-175.

62. Winston DJ, Ho WG, Howell CL, Miller MJ, Mickey R, Martin WJ, Lin CH, Gale RP: Cytomegalovirus infections associated with leukocyte transfusions. Ann Inter Med 1980;93:671-675.

63. Hersman K, Meyers JD, Thomas ED, Buckner CD, Clift R: The effect of granulocyte transfusions on the incidence of cytomegalovirus infection after allogeneic marrow transplantation. Ann Intern Med 1982;96:149-152.

64. Paulin T, Ringdén O, Lönnqvist B: Faster immunological recovery after bone marrow transplantation in patients without cytomegalovirus infection. Transplantation 1985;39:377-384.

65. Gratama JW, Verdonck LF, van der Linden JA, van Heugten JG, Kreeft HA, D'Amaro J, Zwaan FE, de Gast GC: Cellular immunity to vaccinations and herpesvirus infections after bone marrow transplantation. Transplantation 1986;41:719-724.

66. Bowden RA, Day LM, Amos DE, Meyers JD: Natural cytotoxic activity against cytomegalovirus-infected target cells following marrow transplantation. Transplantation 1987;44:504-508.

67. Appelbaum FR, Meyers JD, Fefer A, Flournoy N, Cheever MA, Greenberg PD, Hackman R, Thomas ED: Nonbacterial nonfungal pneumonia following marrow transplantation in 100 identical twins. Transplantation 1982;33:265-268.

68. Barrett A, Depledge MH, Powles RL: Interstitial pneumonitis following bone marrow transplantation after low dose rate total body irradiation. Int J Rad Oncol Biol Phys 1983;9:1029-1033.

69. Pecego R, Hill R, Appelbaum FR, Amos D, Buckner CD, Fefer A, Thomas ED: Interstitial pneumonitis following autologous bone marrow transplantation. Transplantation 1986;42:515-517.

70. Sullivan KM, Meyers JD, Flournoy N, Storb R, Thomas ED: Early and late interstitial pneumonia following human bone marrow transplantation. Int J Cell Cloning 1986;4(Suppl 1):107-121.

71. Cordonnier C, Bernaudin JF, Bierling P, Huet Y, Vernant JP: Pulmonary complications occurring after allogeneic bone marrow transplantation. A study of 130 consecutive transplanted patients. Cancer 1986;58:1047-1054.

72. Grundy JE, Shanley JD, Schearer GM: Augmentation of graft-versus-host reaction by cytomegalovirus infection resulting in interstitial pneumonitis. Transplantation 1985;39:548-553.

73. Grundy JE, Shearer GM: The effect of cytomegalovirus infection on the host response to foreign and hapten-modified self histocompatibility antigens. Transplantation 1984;37:484-490.

74. Grundy JE, Shanley JD, Griffiths PD: Is cytomegalovirus interstitial pneumonitis in transplant recipients an immunopathological condition? Lancet 1987;2:996-999.

75. Zaia JA: The biology of human cytomegalovirus infection after bone marrow transplantation. Int J Cell Cloning 1986;4(Suppl 1):135-154.

76. Ljungman P, Lönnqvist B, Gahrton G, Ringdén O, Wahren B: CMV specific lymphocyte proliferation and in vitro CMV IgG production for diagnosis of CMV infections after bone marrow transplantation. Blood 1986;68:108-112.

77. Quinnan GV Jr, Kirmani N, Rook AH, Manischewitz JF, Jackson L, Moreschi G, Santos GW, Saral R, Burnes WH: Cytotoxic cells in cytomegalovirus infection. HLA-restricted T-lymphocyte and non-T-lymphocyte cytotoxic responses correlate with recovery from cytomegalovirus infection in bone-marrow-transplant recipients. N Engl J Med 1982;307:6-13.

78. Wimperis JZ, Brenner MK, Prentice HG, Reittie JE, Karayiannis P, Griffiths PD, Hoffbrand AV: Transfer of a functioning humoral immune system in transplantation of T-lymphocyte-depleted bone marrow. Lancet 1986;1:339-343.

79. Wahren B, Gahrton G, Linde A. Ljungman P, Lönnqvist B, Ringdén O, Sundqvist VA: Transfer and persistence of viral antibody producing cells in bone marrow transplantation. J Infect Dis 1984;150:358-365.

80. Grob JP, Grundy JE, Prentice HG, Griffiths PD, Hoffbrand AV, Hughes MD, Tate T, Wimperis JZ, Brenner MK: Immune donors can protect marrow-transplant recipients from severe cytomegalovirus infections. Lancet 1987;1:774-776.

81. Ringdén O, Lönnqvist B, Sundberg B: Cytomegalovirus immune bone-marrow donors and interstitial pneumonitis. Lancet 1987;2:105-106.

82. Grob J-P, Grundy JE, Prentice HG, Griffiths PD, Brenner MK, Milburn HJ, duBois R, Skeggs D, Hoffbrand AV: Interstitial pneumonitis in recipients of HLA-matched T-depleted BMT: apparent effect of received lung TBI dose. Bone Marrow Transplant 1986;1(Suppl 1):49.

83. Ringdén O, Baryd I, Johansson B, Gahrton G, Groth CG, Lundgren G, Lönnqvist B: Increased mortality by septicemia, interstitial pneumonitis and pulmonary fibrosis among bone marrow transplant recipients receiving an increased mean dose rate of total irradiation. Acta Radiol Oncol 1983;22:423-428.

84. Mudde GC, de Gast GC, Verdonck LF, van den Linden J, van Heugten H, de Graan-Hentzen YCE: Recovery from CMV infection/reactivation after T cell depleted BMT is dependent on T cell immunity and neutralizing antibodies. Bone Marrow Transplant 1987;2(Suppl 1):295.

85. Engelhard D, Or R, Naparstek E, Aker M, Breuer R, Ravid Z, Morag A, Sarov I, Slavin S: Cytomegalovirus infection and disease after T-cell depleted allogeneic bone marrow transplantation for malignant hematological diseases. Transplant Proc 1989;21:3101-3102.

86. Brenner MK, Griffiths PD, Prentice HG: Cytomegalovirus pneumonitis after allogeneic marrow transplantation. Lancet 1987;2:286-287.

87. Storb R, Prentice RL, Sullivan KM, Shulman HM, Deeg HJ, Doney KC, Buckner CD, Clift RA, Witherspoon RP, Appelbaum FA, Sanders JE, Stewart PS, Thomas ED: Predictive factors in chronic graft-versus-host disease in patients with aplastic anemia treated by marrrow transplantation from HLA-identical siblings. Ann Int Med 1983;98:461-466.

88. Ringdén O, Paulin T, Lönnqvist B, Nilsson B: An analysis of factors predisposing for chronic graft-versus-host disease. Exp Hematol 1985;13:1062-1067.

89. Horowitz MM, for the Writing Committee, Atkinson K, van Bekkum DW, Bortin MM, Gluckman E, Gale RP, Good RA, Jacobsen N, Kolb H-J, Rimm AA, Ringdén O, Rozman C, Zwaan FE: Risk factors for chronic graft-versus-host disease: a preliminary report from the International Bone Marrow Transplant Registry. Bone Marrow Transplant 1988;3(Suppl 1):215.

90. Lönnqvist B, Ringdén O, Wahren B, Gahrton G, Lundgren G: Cytomegalovirus infection associated with and preceding chronic graft-versus-host disease. Transplantation 1984;38:465-468.

91. Jacobsen N, Andersen HK, Skinhöj P, Ryder LP, Platz P, Jerne D, Faber V: for the Copenhage Bone Marrow Transplantation Group: Correlation between donor cytomegalovirus immunity and chronic graft-versus-host disease after allogeneic bone marrow transplantation. Scand J Haematol 1986;36:499-506.

92. Jacobsen N, Badsberg JH, Lönnqvist B, Ringdén O, Volin L, Ruutu T, Rajantie J, Siimes MA, Nikoskelainen J, Toivanen A, Andersen HK, Keiding N, Gahrton G: for the Nordic Bone Marrow Transplatation Group: Predictive factors for chronic graft-versus-host disease and leukemic relapse after allogeneic bone marrow transplantation. In *Recent Advances and Future Directions in Bone Marrow Transplantation*, edited by Baum SJ, Santos GW, Takaku F. Springer-Verlag, 1988.

93. Boström L, Ringdén O, Sundberg B, Linde A, Ljungman P, Nilsson B: Pretransplant herpes virus serology and chronic graft-versus-host disease. Bone Marrow Transplant 1989;4:547-552.

94. Fenyk JR Jr, Smith CM, Warkentin PI, Krivit W, Goltz RW, Neely JE, Nesbit ME, Ramsay NKC, Coccia PF, Kersey JH: Sclerodermatous graft-v-host disease limited to an area of measles exanthem. Lancet 1978;1:472-473.

95. McKeating JA, Griffiths PD, Grundy JE: Cytomegalovirus in urine specimens has host B_2 microglobulin bound to the viral envelope: a mechanism of evading the host immune response. J Gen Virol 1978;68:785-792.

96. Grundy JE, McKeating JA, Ward PJ, Sanderson AR, Griffiths PD: B_2 microglobulin enhances the infectivity of cytomegalovirus and when bound to the virus enables class I HLA molecules to be used as a virus receptor. J Gen Virol 1987;68:793-803.

97. Beck S, Barrell BG: Human cytomegalovirus encodes a glycoprotein homologous to MHC class-I antigens. Nature 1988;331:269-272.

98. Lönnqvist B, Ringdén O, Ljungman P, Wahren B, Gahrton G: Reduced risk of recurrent leukemia in bone marrow transplant recipients after cytomegalovirus infection. Br J Haematol 1986;63:671-679.

99. Jacobsen N, Lönnqvist B, Ringdén O, Rajantie J, Siimes M, Volin L, Ruutu T, Nikoskelainen J, Ryder L, Andersen HK, Keiding N, Gahrton G: For the Nordic BMT Group: Graft-versus-leukaemia activity associated with cytomegalovirus seropositive bone marrow donors but separated from graft-versus-host disease in allograft recipients with AML. Eur J Hematol 1987;38:350-355.

100. Ringdén O, Sundberg B, Lönnqvist B, Tollemar J, Gahrton G, Nilsson B: Allogeneic bone marrow transplantation for leukemia: factors of importance for long-term survival and relapse. Bone Marrow Transplant 1988;3:281-290.

101. Ojo E: Positive correlation between the levels of natural killer cells and the in vivo resistance to syngeneic tumor transplants as influenced by various routes of administration of corynebacterium parvum bacterium. Cell Immunol 1979;45:182-187.

26

Treatment of Acute Graft-vs.-Host Disease

P. Jean Henslee-Downey
University of Kentucky Medical Center
Lexington, Kentucky

I. INTRODUCTION

The theoretical constructs regarding the pathophysiology of acute Graft-vs.-Host Disease (GVHD) are considered in depth in Chapters 1 and 16 of this book. Briefly, both animal models and human transplant experience have supported the concept that alloreactive lymphocytes are mediators of tissue destruction and severe immune dysregulation, which comprise the major effects of GVHD. Since the development of acute GVHD significantly contributes to mortality following allogeneic marrow grafting (1), various techniques have been devised to abrogate or ameliorate this immunologic reaction and are explored in depth in other sections of this volume. Despite techniques to either remove GVHD-producing lymphocytes or suppress their function, the incidence of GVHD has still been reported to occur in 20-55% of histocompatible and over 80% of histoincompatible allogeneic recipients (2-4). Therefore, investigators have explored methods to reverse and control the manifestations of established GVHD. Most therapies have been directed at the regulation or inactivation of T-lymphocyte function.

The severity of acute GVHD can be graded according to established methods which indicate the extent of organ involvement, primarily involving skin, gastrointestinal tract, and liver (5). This staging system can be used as a tool to assess the effectiveness of treatment. The treatment of acute GVHD tends to be successful in mild to moderate disease (grade I or II), whereas the treatment of severe disease (grades III and IV) is often unsuccessful in large part due to intervening fatal infections. In addition to specific therapy directed toward immunologic control of acute GVHD, the management of patients must include supportive care measures designed for both protection from and treatment of life-threatening infections, as well as the prevention of acute GVHD recurrence or progression to chronic GVHD. Meticulous and repeated evaluations are mandated for the successful long-term follow-up of these patients. Furthermore, the ultimate goal for the successful management of acute GVHD must enhance the process of competent im-

munoreconstitution and development of tolerance without disturbing freedom from relapse of an underlying malignancy.

II. THERAPEUTIC AGENTS

A. Corticosteroids

Corticosteroids have a catabolic effect on lymphoid cells suppressing their function or
rendering them inactive. With high doses of glucocorticoids, lymphoid cells may actually
be destroyed. Early case reports indicated that steroid preparations could be beneficial
in reversing a GVHD reaction (6-8). Bacigalupo and colleagues reported a series of 19
patients with acute GVHD who received bolus 6-Methylprednisolone at doses of 20 mg/kg/
day i.v. for the first 3 days, 10 mg/kg/day i.v. for the following 4 days, and gradually
tapered to a maintenance dose of 1 mg/kg/day i.v. thereafter (9). Among 16 recipients
of HLA-identical marrow, 43% demonstrated a complete response and an additional 37%
obtained a partial response. No responses were observed in the three patients who received HLA-nonidentical marrow. Side effects were felt to be minimal, consisting primarily of hyperglycemia and gastritis, which could be managed with conventional treatment. Patients with minimal disease were most likely to become complete responders.
Relapse in GVHD activity did occur in some patients after tapering of the corticosteroid
dose.

   Encouraging results were also obtained by the University of Minnesota Transplant
Team, where patients with mild to moderate GVHD were treated with systemic prednisone, 60 mg/m^2/day for 3 weeks and tapered over 4 to 5 months, resulting in a probability of survival comparable to that of patients who never developed GVHD (10). However, patients with severe (grades III and IV) GVHD who were treated with high-dose
methylprednisolone at 60 mg/kg/day for 5 days followed by gradual taper had poor survival and the majority of patients died with opportunistic infections. In this study, the
authors observed that patients treated with steroids for acute GVHD had a relatively low
incidence of severe chronic GVHD.

   Better responses in patients with advanced stages of severe acute GVHD were obtained by Kanojia and colleagues, following administration of a 10-day course of high-
dose methylprednisolone starting at a dose of 500 mg/m^2/ every 6 hours for 2 days and
reduced 50% after each 8 doses (11). Eighteen treatments were given to 14 patients resulting in complete responses in 3 and partial responses in 15. There were 5 long-term
survivors and all developed chronic GVHD. Most deaths were attributed to opportunistic
infection or intersitital pneumonitis. A similar regimen was administered to haploidentical marrow recipients at the University of Kentucky, and while complete responses
could be obtained in patients with early manifestations of skin or gastrointestinal GVHD,
all patients developed recurrent GVHD after reduction in the steroid dose (unpublished data). Other case reports have also confirmed the ability to reverse acute GVHD
with the administration of high-dose methylprednisolone (12,13). The response to
systemic prednisone therapy may be enhanced in patients who develop GVHD while
receiving cyclosporine as compared to methotrexate prophylaxis (14).

   Although the observed response rates vary from study to study, and although doses
from 1 to 60 mg/kg/day have been used, many investigators now employ steroids as standard therapy for acute GVHD. As will be discussed later, regimens with a higher probability of responses have been described. It appears, therefore, that the widepread use of

steroids is due to the extensive experience and the ease of administration rather than scientific reasons.

The untoward effects associated with the administration of corticosteroids are varied and often enhanced with long-term administration. Increased appetite, hypertension, fluid retention, hyperglycemia, glycosuria, gastritis or gastric ulceration, mood changes, weight gain, and development of cushingoid changes frequently occur. Patients receiving corticosteroids over long periods of time also remain at significant risk for opportunistic infections, muscle wasting, weakness, and bony lesions including osteoporosis, aseptic necrosis, and possible growth retardation.

B. Antithymocyte Globulin

Antithymocyte globulin (ATG) has been produced in rabbits, goats, and horses following the inoculation of thoracic duct or peripheral blood lymphocytes to produce a high antihuman lymphocytotoxicity titer. Antibodies can be purifed from serum to form a product which can be safely adminstered to human patients with the purpose of specific T-lymphocyte suppression although the net effect may be nonspecific immunosuppression. After initial experiments in dogs demonstrating activity of anti-dog lymphocyte serum (ALS) in established GVHD, anti-human ATG has been applied to several aspects of marrow transplantation including prevention of rejection and prophylaxis and treatment of GVHD (14-20). Storb and colleagues used both rabbit and goat preparations to treat 19 patients with established GVHD and observed complete responses in 12 and partial responses in the remaining 7 patients (15). Five patients were surviving at the time of reporting, 3 of whom showed no recurrence of GVHD and 2 developed chronic GVHD. The majority of deaths was due to infectious complications, particularly the development of interstitial pneumonitis.

In a later report, Weiden extended this investigation by the Seattle Transplant Team to 60 patients with GVHD treated with ATG noting improvement in 36, no change in 12, and progression in 12 patients (16). This report also included 15 patients who were randomized, 9 to receive and 6 not to receive ATG. In this group of patients ATG had no beneficial effect and, furthermore, more infections were noted in the study group, although the difference was not statistically significant. A subsequent randomized trial including 37 patients compared ATG, given every other day over 6 days, and prednisolone, 2 mg/kg daily for 10 days (17). The overall response rate was higher in the steroid group although not significantly so. Furthermore, responses occurred in all organ systems in the steroid group, whereas patients in the ATG group experienced only few and incomplete responses in the gastrointestinal tract and liver.

Subsequently, Deeg and colleagues conducted a trial comparing the efficacy of ATG in combination with cyclosporine with or without the addition of methylprednisolone to further evaluate the usefulness of combination regimens in the treatment of acute GVHD (18). Among 48 patients, 29 received ATG, 15 mg/kg i.v. on days +1, +3, and +5 of treatment, and cyclosporine was started on day +3 at a dose of 1.5 mg/kg i.v. twice daily. Nineteen patients received the same regimen of ATG and cyclosporine combined with methylprednisolone, 2 mg/kg/day starting on day +1 of treatment with tapering of the dose beginning on day +14. On day +14 approximately 50% of patients demonstrated responses with a somewhat higher response rate observed in patients receiving ATG and cyclosporine only. Of concern, survival was diminished in patients on triple immunosuppressives apparently due to an increase in the frequency of complications, in particular infections. The authors cautioned that the addition of methylprednisolone to ATG and cyclosporine may lead to excessive immunosuppression without apparent benefit in GVHD control. Most patients escaping fatal infections subsequently developed chronic GVHD. These and other reports demonstrate therefore that ATG is an effective agent for the control of acute GVHD (19,20). Further trials will be required to optimize the use of this drug in the management of acute GVHD.

Untoward effects which have been associated with the administration of ATG include hemolytic anemia, thrombocytopenia, neutropenia, fever, chills, polyarthritis, myalgias, nausea and vomiting, and urticaria. Sedatives, antipyretics, and antihistamines may ameliorate some of the symptoms which appear to be related to a serum sickness reaction. Using a product from a different species may be tolerated in patients with severe reactions.

C. Cyclosporine

Cyclosporine is a fungal metabolite shown to have potent immunosuppressive properties resulting in improved survival of solid organ grafts, as well as reduction in GVHD when used prophylactically following allogeneic marrow grafting. The mechanism of action is not completely defined, although there appears to be a preferential effect on T helper lymphocytes favoring the development of suppressor cells, thereby exerting a more specific immunosuppressive effect. Cyclosporine is the first immunosuppressive agent with some selectivity for T lymphocytes. Through the inhibition of the release of various lymphokines, activation and proliferation of T-lymphocyte clones appear to be blocked (21,22).

Initial preclinical and clinical evaluations examining the use of cyclosporine for treatment of established GVHD, however, were not encouraging (23,24). Powles and colleagues administered cyclosporine intramuscularly or orally in escalating doses to five allogeneic recipients with acute GVHD obtaining prompt responses in the skin (24). However, four patients went on to develop hepatic failure, and other complications including renal dysfunction, felt to be a drug-related toxic effect. The dose of cyclosporine given to these patients was much higher (25 mg/kg/day) than in general usage today.

Subsequently, the Seattle Transplant Team reported responses in a pilot trial with cyclosporine which prompted their instigation of a randomized comparison between cyclosporine and prednisolone for the management of severe (grade II or greater) acute GVHD (25). Methylprednisolone was given at doses of 2 mg/kg daily for 14 days and tapered gradually thereafter, dependent upon clinical course. Cyclosporine was administered to the first 9 patients as a loading dose of 12.5 mg/kg i.v., followed by oral administration at a dose of 6.25 mg/kg twice daily. The subsequent 28 patients were given an intravenous product at a dose of 1.5-2.5 mg/kg twice daily. Reduction in GVHD, particularly when skin was the target organ, was obtained in 26 of 39 patients receiving methylprednisolone and 28 of 38 patients receiving cyclosporine. The response to cyclosporine was not clearly dose related. The development of chronic GVHD occurred with similar frequency in both groups, however, slightly fewer patients receiving cyclosporine required secondary therapy. No difference in the survival projections for the two groups was demonstrated.

A most concerning untoward effect of cyclosporine is the development of renal dysfunction. This effect appears to be dose related and with dose adjustments in response to serum creatinine levels, renal manifestations are usually reversible. However, patients have occasionally required hemodialysis. Associated electrolyte abnormalities include hypomagnesimia and either hypokalemia or hyperkalemia. Other generalized side effects have included hypertension, hirsutism, anorexia, nausea, malaise, peripheral extremity pain and burning, tremor, and, in several cases, seizures have occurred. Hepatic dysfunction has been noted with high serum levels. Complications may be worsened when cyclosporine is given in combination with other immunosuppressive drugs. A high incidence of hypertension has been observed in patients receiving both cyclosporine and steroids and can become uncontrollable unless the drug is discontinued (26). The administration of cyclosporine has also been associated with the development of hemolytic anemia and lymphoproliferative disorders (27,28).

D. Monoclonal Antibodies

Conceptually, the use of monoclonal antibodies raised to specific antigens expressed on lymphocyte subsets felt to be cellular effectors in the GVHD process has been attractive and sought after by many investigators. Utilizing cell hybridization techniques, monoclonal antibodies to specific membrane determinants can be reliably produced. Increasing experience with such biologic agents has allowed even the production of antibodies with predesigned specificities.

An early clinical trial in renal allograft patients demonstrated the efficacy of monoclonal antibody immunotherapy. Cosimi and colleagues treated eight patients given renal transplants from cadaver donors with OKT3 (CD3) monoclonal antibody at the time of diagnosis of acute rejection (29). All patients showed a complete loss of OKT3 reactive cells from the peripheral circulation, which coincided with a return to normal serum creatinine levels and apparent reversal of the rejection process. Thereafter, Gratama reported early experience with this same antibody given to eight allogeneic marrow recipients with grade II and IV acute GVHD (30). Circulating CD3 positive T cells virtually disappeared within one hour following administration of antibody. However, by the second week of treatment, lymphocytes with T-cell markers suggesting modulation of the CD3 antigen reemerged in small numbers. Six of the eight patients showed beneficial clinical responses, which were most dramatic in patients with minimal acute GVHD.

Subsequently, Gluckman and colleagues studied 10 patients given OKT3 antibody for grade III to IV acute GVHD resistant to treatment by cyclosporine and methylprednisolone (31). OKT3 antibody was given at a dose of 5 mg/day for 15 consecutive days. Response to therapy was seen within one to four days of beginning treatment, resulting in complete responses in five, partial responses in four, and no response in one patient. Recurrence of acute GVHD occurred both during and after cessation of therapy, and all surviving patients developed limited chronic GVHD. One patient developed a monoclonal B-cell lymphoma. The investigators speculated that the selective activity of monoclonal antibodies on T cells might allow for B-cell activation and clonal expansion by Epstein-Barr virus (EBV) infected cells.

A similar observation was made by Martin and colleagues in the analysis of a dose escalation trial utilizing an IgG 2a anti-CD3 monoclonal antibody for the treatment of acute GVHD (32). An improvement in skin disease was reliably achieved at doses of 0.1 mg/kg/day. Higher doses were required to achieve responses in the gastrointestinal tract or liver. Four of 24 patients developed EBV associated lymphoproliferative disorders within 7 to 18 days of starting antibody therapy. The occurrence of this complication markedly exceeded the incidence in patients not given anti-CD3 monoclonal antibody. Two additional patients with severe steroid-resistant acute GVHD were treated by the same investigator with an IgM anti-CD3 monoclonal antibody, 64.1, and both developed fatal EBV-associated lymphoproliferative disorders (33). Both patients received daily drug doses up to 20 mg/day for greater than 2 weeks leading to dramatic responses in GVHD. However, the resultant severe immunodysregulation may have permitted uncontrolled expansion of EBV-infected B cells suggesting the need to limit both the dose and duration of therapy when potent T-lymphocyte activating and lytic agents are administered.

Reinherz and colleagues used a T-lymphocyte-specific monoclonal antibody, T12, administered intravenously for the treatment of acute GVHD which developed despite ex vivo purging of the marrow graft with the same monoclonal antibody preparation (34). Complete reversal of GVHD manifestations was obtained in this sequential fashion.

A phase I clinical trial was instituted by Remlinger and colleagues to evaluate the feasibility and toxicity associated with administrating murine monoclonal antibodies to patients with established acute GVHD (35). Four different IgG 2a antibodies designated 9.6, 35.1, 10.2, and 12.1 were administered to 15 patients for a total of 151 infusions ranging in doses from 1 to 20 mg given daily. No severe toxicities were encountered, and 6 of 10 patients receiving intermittent to high doses (5-20 mg) had evidence of at least partial improvement in GVHD in at least one involved organ system. The unanswered questions emerging from these studies require definition of whether specific functional alterations of lymphocytes can be caused by binding antibody to cell surface receptors or whether disruption or lysis of cellular effectors must be mediated (36). Furthermore, the effectiveness of an infused foreign protein may be diminished over time due to its antigenic potential which may elicit a neutralizing antibody response.

Postulating that the use of a nonmitogenic monoclonal antibody of the IgG isotype would reduce the likelihood of uncontrolled T-cell proliferation, Beelen and colleagues investigated the effect of administering a 5-day course of an anti-T-cell receptor antibody designated DMA031 (37). When given to two recipients of haploidentical marrow grafts, complete resolution of GVHD manifestations was obtained. Neither of these patients went on to develop chronic GVHD although they may have been protected from this event by the ongoing administration of cyclosporine.

The fate and impact of circulating T-lymphocyte specific monoclonal antibodies is not well defined. With the intent of ensuring destruction of the target cell, monoclonal antibody conjugates have been produced for both ex vivo and in vivo reduction of mature lymphocytes (38,39). A phase I-II trial to evaluate the toxicity and efficacy of a 14-day course of an IgG, ricin-A-chain conjugated monoclonal antibody, XomaZyme®-H65, has recently been completed (Byers et al., unpublished data). This immunotoxin targeted to and internalized by mature T lymphocytes has the potential advantage of achieving cell death due to ribosomal inhibition by the ricin-A-chain toxin. In this study 34 patients with steroid refractory, moderate to severe, acute GVHD were treated at a dose ranging between 0.05 mg/kg to 0.33 mg/kg daily for up to 14 days. Of 32 evaluable patients, 72% responded in at least one organ system and an additional 16% had stable disease. The development of a lymphoproliferative disorder was not observed in this series of patients. To date all clinical trials utilizing monoclonal antibody preparations have been applied primarily to patients with advanced stages of acute GVHD which produces a state of profound immunodeficiency contributing further to a high incidence of infectious complications. Therefore, the benefit of using this highly specific control of immune function may be better understood when applied to patients earlier in the disease process when a greater survival probability can be captured. Successful control of acute GVHD has not been shown to protect patients from the development of chronic GVHD.

The untoward effects of administering murine monoclonal antibodies has consisted primarily of febrile reactions. This response seems to improve with ongoing therapy and can be ameloriated with the administration of antipyretics or antihistamines. Although fluctuations in white count and platelet count have been described, an adverse effect on marrow production has not conclusively been demonstrated. An association with the development of B-cell lymphoproliferative disorders has been described with monoclonal antibodies directed at the CD3 receptor. The potential side effects associated with the administration of a monoclonal antibody ricin-A-chain conjugate (XomaZyme®-H65) has been recently examined. Transient and reversible flu-like symptoms, including fever, tremors, lethargy, anorexia, myalgias, and arthralgias, are often encountered. However, these symptoms are rarely observed in patients receiving XomaZyme®-H65 as GVHD prophylaxis early in their posttransplant course (unpublished data). Hypoalbuminemia of unknown etiology has been seen in approximately 1/3 of patients without clinical significance when promptly corrected with replacement therapy. Renal insufficiency has occasionally been noted, particularly in patients with a preexisting renal dysfunction.

E. Other Immunosuppressive Agents

Cytotoxic drugs including cyclophosphamide, methotrexate, 6-mercaptopurine, and mechlorethamine have been tested in animal models for control of established acute GVHD (40). Of these, cyclophosphamide could prevent GVHD mortality; however, treated animals remained immunologically depressed and low grade GVHD persisted. These agents have been extremely disappointing when applied to established GVHD in man. There is no clinical evidence to support the inclusion of these agents in therapeutic regimens for the management of acute GVHD. Vogelsang and colleagues have recently examined an immunosuppressive drug, Thalidomide, known best for its sedative and teratogenetic effects (41,42). In a mismatched animal model this drug has been shown to be effective for both prophylaxis and treatment of acute GVHD. Thalidomide is particularly attractive due to the lack of untoward effects, limited primarily to mild sedation and neuropathies.

III. SUPPORTIVE CARE

Patients with acute GVHD with profound immune dysregulation and deficiency remain at great risk for fatal overwhelming infectious diseases. The ease by which exposure and entry of organisms can occur is enhanced by breakdown in skin and mucosal protective barriers, as well as the administration of drugs which further cripple and interfere with immune defense mechanisms. Every effort must be made to provide the patients with a constant environment which will limit or prevent exposure to infectious organisms with particular attention to the avoidance of fungal, viral, or parasitic microbial agents. It is advisable to nurse patients in isolation rooms with special air handling devices adequate to remove fungal spores and maintain a positive pressure with constant flow away from the patient's surroundings. The skin must be cleansed frequently, and close observation and attention paid to any desquamated areas where infection can breed. Broad spectrum antibacterial and antifungal preparations should be applied liberally. When severe grade IV skin lesions develop, management techniques are similar to the care of severe burn victims.

Along the entire gastrointestinal tract, particularly when severe damage of the mucosal barrier has occurred, there is opportunity for entry of infecting organisms. The oral cavity must be cleansed frequently and treated with antibacterial and antifungal preparations. When and if grossly bloody diarrhea ensues, the patient's diet should be limited to sterilized fluids and advanced gradually to include low bacterial foods when healing is evident. Nonabsorbable antibiotics for gut decontamination may be helpful. Treatment of suspected or proven gastrointestinal infections, such as Clostridium difficile or Cryptosporidium should be instituted empirically. Stools should be repeatedly cultured and when diarrhea is unrelenting, biopsy of mucosal surfaces may aid in the identification of secondary infections, which often include viral agents such as cytomegalovirus, adenovirus, and rotavirus. Identification of the virus may facilitate obtaining experimental antiviral therapy.

It is advisable to administer prophylactic antimicrobials shown to decrease the incidence of opportunistic infection including pneumocystis carinii, herpes simplex and zoster, cytomegalovirus, and streptococcus pneumonia. These drugs include penicillin preparations, trimethoprim sulfamethoxazole, Acyclovir and Ganciclovir, and immunoglobulin preparations. Whenever the patient's clinical course suggests acute infection, broad-spectrum antibacterial, antifungal, and antiviral therapy should be instituted. Frequent culture surveillance and screening chest radiographs may aid in the early detection of infectious processes, thereby becoming more amenable to management.

Since many patients undergoing aggressive treatment for severe acute GVHD require extensive transfusion support with both packed red blood cells and platelets, every effort should be made to avoid exposure to infectious agents or alloreactive lymphocytes capable of initiating a new GVHD reaction. Guidelines for the preparation of blood products should include the use of serologically screened products which are concentrated or washed to remove leukocytes or administered through leukopoor filters. All products must be irradiated to destroy any alloreactive lymphocytes capable of producing a GVHD reaction.

Careful attention must be applied to the maintenance of fluid and electrolyte balance. Hyperalimentation may be required to meet protein and caloric needs, particularly in patients with severe gastrointestinal involvement. Prompt response to early signs and symptoms of developing organ complications is essential. Patients must be evaluated daily or more frequently as indicated during the acute stages of GVHD.

IV. CONCLUSIONS

The focus of this chapter has been to review clinical investigations in the treatment of acute GVHD. In the field of marrow transplantation, a much larger effort has been applied to the development of techniques for successful prophylaxis of GVHD. This approach has certainly been warranted as the long-term survival achieved in patients developing moderate to severe GVHD has generally been less than 30% of patients regardless of therapy used. It is clear that complete response rates which can favor survival are obtained in patients when treated with early manifestations of GVHD. Therefore, when GVHD prophylaxis fails, there should be no hesitation in applying effective therapeutic agents during the early development of acute GVHD. The experience to date does not suggest that broad combination therapy will be more effective, and in fact, it may be detrimental by increasing complication rates.

ACKNOWLEDGMENTS

The author's investigations have been supported in part by the Xoma Corporation, Berkeley, California. I would like to express my appreciation to Paula Hollingsworth and Jennifer C. Nix for their assistance with the preparation of this manuscript.

REFERENCES

1. Storb R, Prentice RL, Buckner CD, Clift RA, Appelbaum F, Deeg HJ, Doney K, Hansen JA, Mason M, Sanders JE, Singer J, Sullivan KM, Witherspoon RP, Thomas ED: Graft-versus-host disease and survival in patients with aplastic anemia treated by marrow grafts from HLA-identical siblings. N Engl J Med 1983;308:302-306.

2. Deeg HJ, Storb R: Acute and chronic graft-versus-host disease: Clinical manifestations, prophylaxis, and treatment. J Nat Clin Investig 1986;76:1325-1328.

3. Gale RP. Graft-versus-host disease. Immunol Rev 1985;88:193-214.

4. Henslee PJ, Thompson JS, Romond EH, Doukas MA, Metcalfe M, Marshall ME, Macdonald JS: T cell depletion of HLA and haploidentical marrow reduces graft-versus-host disease but it may impair a graft-versus-leukemia effect. Transpl Proc 1987, XIX:2701-2706.

5. Glucksberg H, Storb R, Fefer, A, Buckner CD, Neiman PE, Clift RA, Lerner KG, Thomas ED: Clinical manifestations of graft-versus-host disease in human recipients of marrow from HLA matched sibling donors. Transplantation 1974;18:295-304.

6. O'Reilly R, Dupont B, Pahwa S, Grimes E, Smithwich M, Pahwa R, Schwartz S, Hansen JA, Siegal FP, Sorell M, Svejgaard A, Jersild C, Thomsen M, Platz P, L'Esperance P, Good RA: Reconstitution in severe combined immunodeficiency by transplantation of marrow from an unrelated donor. N Engl J Med 1977;297:1311-1318.

7. Marmont AM, Damasio EE, Bacigalupo A, Giordano D, Rossi E, Realli G, Gay A, Dagna-Bricarell F, Brema F, Carella A, Santini G: A to O bone marrow transplantation in severe aplastic anemia: Dynamics of blood group conversion and demonstration of early dyserythropoiesis in the engrafted marrow. Br J Haemat 1977; 36:511-518.

8. Groth CG, Gahrton G, Lundgren G, Moller E, Pihlstedt P, Ringden O, Sundelin P: Successful treatment with prednisone of graft-versus-host disease in an allogeneic bone marrow transplant recipient. Scand J Haemat 1979;22:333-338.

9. Bacigalupo A, vanLint MT, Frassoni F, Podesta M, Veneziano G, Avanzi G, Vitale V, Marmont AM: High dose bolus methylprednisolone for the treatment of acute graft-versus-host disease. Blut 1983;46:125-132.

10. Neudorf S, Filipovich A, Ramsay N, Kersey J: Prevention and treatment of acute graft-versus-host disease. Seminars in Hemat 1984;21:91-100.

11. Kanojia, MD, Anagnostou AA, Zander AR, Vellekoor L, Spitzer G, Verma DS, Jagannath S, Dicke KA: High dose methylprednisolone treatment for acute graft-versus-host disease after bone marrow transplantation in adults. Transplantation 1984;37:246-249.

12. Hall RR, Anagnostou A, Kanojia M, Zander A. Pneumatosis intestinalis associated with graft-versus-host disease of the intestinal tract. Transpl Proc 1984;XVI:1666-1668.

13. Kendra J, Barrett AJ, Lucas C, Joshi R, Joss V, Desai M, Halil O, Rogers TR, Hobbs JR, Hugh-Jones K: Response of graft-versus-host disease to high doses of methylprednisolone. Clin Lab Haemat 1981;3:19-26.

14. Deeg HJ, Storb R, Thomas ED, Flournoy N, Kennedy MS, Banaji M, Appelbaum FR, Bensinger WI, Buckner CD, Clift RA, Doney K, Fefer A, McGuffin R, Sanders JE, Singer J, Stewart P, Sullivan KM, Witherspoon RP: Cyclosporine as prophylaxis for graft-versus-host disease: A randomized study in patients undergoing marrow transplantation for acute nonlymphoblastic leukemia. Blood 1985;65:1325-1334.

15. Storb R, Kolb HJ, Graham TC, Kolb H, Weiden PL, Thomas ED: Treatment of established graft-versus-host disease in dogs by antithymocyte serum or prednisone. Blood 1973;42:601.

16. Storb R, Gluckman E, Thomas ED, Buckner CD, Clift RA, Fefer A, Glucksberg H, Graham TC, Johnson FL, Lerner KG, Neiman PE, Ochs H: Treatment of established human graft-versus-host disease by antithymocyte globulin. Blood 1974; 44:57-75.

17. Weiden PL, Doney K, Storb R, Thomas ED: Anti-human thymocyte globulin for prophylaxis and treatment of graft-versus-host disease in recipients of allogeneic marrow grafts. Transplan Proc 1978;X:213-216.

18. Doney KC, Weiden PL, Storb R, Thomas ED: Treatment of graft-versus-host disease in human allogeneic marrow graft recipients: A randomized trial comparing antithymocyte globulin and corticosteroids. Am J Hemat 1981;11:1-8.

19. Deeg HJ, Loughran TP Jr, Storb R, Kennedy MS, Sullivan KM, Doney K, Appelbaum FR, Thomas ED: Treatment of human acute graft-versus-host disease with antithymocyte globulin and cyclosporine with or without methylprednisolone. Transplantation 1985,40:162-166.

20. Sullivan KM, Deeg HJ, Sanders J, Klosterman A, Amos D, Shulman H, Sale G, Martin P, Witherspoon R, Appelbaum F, Doney K, Stewart P, Meyers J, McDonald GB, Weiden P, Fefer A, Buckner CD, Storb R, Thomas ED: Hyperacute graft-versus-host disease in patients not given immunosuppression after allogeneic marrow transplantation. Blood 1986;67:1172-1175.

21. Storb R, Thomas ED: Graft-versus-host disease in dog and man: The Seattle experience. Immunol Rev 1985;88:215-238.

22. Bunjes D, Hardt C, Deusch K: Studies on the mechanism of action of cyclosporine A in the murine and human T cell, respectively in vitro. In *Cyclosporine A*, edited by White DJG. Elsevier, Amsterdam, New York, Oxford; 1982, p. 261.

23. Borel JF, Feurer C, Magnee C: Effects of the new lymphocytic peptide cyclosporine A in animals. Immunology 1900;32:1017.

24. Markwick JR, Hobbs JR, Chambers JD, Pegrum GD: Timing of cyclosporine-A therapy for abrogation of HVG and GVH responses in rats. Lancet 1979;II:1037-1039.

25. Powles RL, Clink H, Sloane J, Barrett AJ, Kay HEM, McElwain TJ: Cyclosporine-A for the treatment of graft-versus-host disease in man. Lancet 1978;II:1327-1331.

26. Kennedy MS, Deeg HJ, Storb R, Doney K, Sullivan KM, Witherspoon RP, Appelbaum FR, Stewart P, Sanders J, Buckner CD, Martin P, Weiden P, Thomas ED: Treatment of acute graft-versus-host disease after allogeneic marrow transplantation. Amer J Med 1985;78:978-983.

27. Loughran RP Jr, Deeg HJ, Dahlberg S, Kennedy MS, Storb R, Thomas ED: Incidence of hypertension after marrow transplantation among 112 patients randomized to either cyclosporine or methotrexate as graft-versus-host disease prophylaxis. Br J Haematol 1985,59:547-553.

28. Hows J, Beddow K, Gordon-Smith E, Branch DR, Spruce W, Sniecinski I, Krance RA, Petz LD: Donor-derived red blood cell antibodies and immune hemolysis after allogeneic bone marrow transplantation. Blood 1986;67:177-181.

29. Starzl TE, Porter KA, Iwatsuki S, Rosenthal JT, Shaw BW Jr, Atchison RW, Nalesnik MA, Ho M, Griffith BP, Hakala TR, Hardesty RL, Jaffe R, Bahnson HT: Re-

versibility of lymphomas and lymphoprolifcrative lesions developing under cyclosporin-steroid therapy. Lancet 1984,II:583-587.

30. Cosimi AB, Burton RC, Colvin RB, Goldstein G, Delmonico RL, LaQuaglia MP, Tolkoff-Rubin N, Rubin RH, Herrin JT, Russell PS: Treatment of acute renal allograft rejection with OKT3 monoclonal antibody. Transplantation 1981;32: 535-539.

31. Gratama JW, Jansen J, Lopovich RA, Tanke HJ, Goldstein G, Zwaan FE: Treatment of acute graft-versus-host disease with monoclonal antibody OKT3. Transplantation 1984;38:469-474.

32. Gluckman E, Devergie A, Varin F, Rabian C, D'Agay MF, Benbunan M: Treatment of steroid resistant severe acute graft-versus-host disease with a monoclonal PAN T OKT3 antibody. Exp Hemat 1984;12:66-67.

33. Martin PJ, Hansen JA, Anasetti C, Zutter M, Durnam D, Storb R, Thomas ED: Treatment of acute graft-versus-host disease with anti-CD3 monoclonal antibodies. Am J Kidney Dis 1988;XI:149-152.

34. Martin PJ, Shulman HM, Schubach WH, Hansen JA, Fefer A, Miller G, Thomas ED: Fatal Epstein-Barr-virus-associated proliferation of donor B cells after treatment of acute graft-versus-host disease with a murine anti-T-cell antibody. Ann Intern Med 1984;101:310-315.

35. Reinherz EL, Geha R, Rappeport JM, Wilson M, Penta AC, Hussey RE, Fitzgerald KA, Daley JF, Levine H, Rosen FS, Schlossman SF: Reconstitution after transplantation with T-lymphocyte-depleted HLA haplotype-mismatched bone marrow for severe combined immunodeficiency. Proc Natl Acad 1982;79:6047-6051.

36. Remlinger K, Martin PJ, Hansen JA, Doney KC, Smith A, Deeg HJ, Sullivan K, Storb R, Thomas ED: Murine monoclonal antibodies for treatment of steroid-resistant acute graft-versus-host disease. Hum Immun 1984;9:21-35.

37. Martin PJ, Remlinger K, Hansen JA, Storb R, Thomas ED, and Members of the Seattle Marrow Transplant Team: Murine monoclonal anti-T cell antibodies for treatment of refractory acute graft-versus-host disease. Transplan Proc 1984; XVI:1494-1495.

38. Beelen DW, Graeven U, Schulz G, Grosse-Wilde H, Doxiadis I, Schaefer UW, Quabeck K, Sayer H, Schmidt CG: Treatment of acute graft-versus-host disease after HLA-partially matched marrow transplantation with a monoclonal antibody (BMA031) against the T cell receptor. Onkologie 1988;11:56-58.

39. Filipovich AH, Vallera DA, Youle RJ, Haake R, Blazar BR, Arthur D, Neville D, Ramsay NK, McGlave P, Kersey JH: Graft-versus-host disease prevention in allogeneic bone marrow transplantation from histocompatible siblings. Transplantation 1987;44:62-69.

40. Kernan NA, Byers V, Scannon PJ, Mischak RP, Brochstein J, Flomenberg N, Dupont B, O'Reilly RJ: Treatment of steroid-resistant acute graft-versus-host disease by in vivo administration of an anti-T-cell ricin-A-chain immunotoxin. JAMA 1988,259:3154-3157.

41. Owens AH, Santos GW: The effect of cytotoxic drugs on graft-versus-host disease in mice. Transplantation 1971;11:378-382.

42. Vogelsang GB, Taylor S, Gordon G, Hess AD: Thalidomide, a potent agent for the treatment of graft-versus-host disease. Transplan Proc 1986;XVIII:904-906.

43. Vogelsang GB, Hess AD, Santos GW: Acute graft-versus-host disease: Clinical characteristics in the cyclosporine era. Medicine 1988;67:163-174.

27

Pharmacologic Monitoring of Immunosuppressive Therapy

Gary C. Yee
University of Florida
Gainesville, Florida

I. INTRODUCTION

As reviewed elsewhere in this volume, the rationale for the administration of immunosuppressive drugs to prevent GVHD is based on numerous studies in rodents and dogs which demonstrate that immunosuppressive drugs could reduce the severity and mortality from GVHD. Although the effectiveness of GVHD prophylaxis has never been established in a randomized, placebo-controlled clinical study, most (1,2) but not all (3) studies have shown that the incidence of grades II-IV acute GVHD is increased when no GVHD prophylaxis is given. Therefore, most patients receive at least one immunosuppressive drug as GVHD prophylaxis. The effectiveness of different immunosuppressive drug regimens used as GVHD prophylaxis is reviewed elsewhere in this volume.

In this chapter, we will review the clinical pharmacology of immunosuppressive drugs used in the prevention and treatment of GVHD. Although the pharmacology of each drug will be discussed individually, it is important to note that many centers are now giving combinations of drugs as GVHD prophylaxis. Therefore, drug-drug interactions can occur, which can result in changes in either immunosuppressive activity or organ toxicity. Finally, it is important to note that, with the exception of cyclosporine, few pharmacologic studies of these drugs have been conducted in marrow transplant recipients. Many of the principles discussed below are therefore based on studies in other patient populations and may not entirely apply to the marrow transplant setting.

II. CYCLOSPORINE

Cyclosporine is a neutral, hydrophobic cyclic peptide of 11 amino acids, one of which is a novel amino acid (4). Although the drug has been used to prevent or treat acute GVHD for more than 10 years, its precise role in GVHD prophylaxis regimens is not clear. It is clear, however, that cyclosporine is as effective as methotrexate (5) and that cyclosporine combined with either methotrexate or prednisone prevents acute GVHD in more than 50% of recipients of HLA-identical marrow grafts (6-8). The drug is also as effective as methylprednisolone in the treatment of established acute GVHD (9).

A. Pharmacokinetics

1. Absorption

As in other transplant patients, oral cyclosporine is usually diluted in milk or juice prior to administration to marrow transplant recipients. After oral administration, about one-third (range 20-60%) of the dose reaches the systemic circulation (10). Peak concentrations are usually reached 3-5 hr after oral dosing (11). At steady state, peak serum concentrations of 800-900 ng/ml (as measured by radioimmunoassay (RIA)) are achieved after oral doses of 6.25 mg/kg given every 12 hr (11,12).

Several factors can influence oral cyclosporine absorption in marrow transplant recipients. In patients with transplant-related gut dysfunction, oral cyclosporine absorption can be impaired. Mean peak serum concentrations are reduced from about 900 ng/ml in patients with no gastrointestinal disease to 350 and 125 ng/ml (RIA) in patients with chemoradiation-induced enteritis and acute GVHD of the gastrointestinal tract, respectively (12).

2. Distribution

Cyclosporine is highly tissue-bound in humans, as evidenced by a mean steady-state volume of distribution of 5-35 L/kg based on serum concentrations (13,14), and 4-13 L/kg based on whole blood concentrations (15). Measurement of tissue cyclosporine concentration from marrow transplant recipients who were autopsied also shows that cyclosporine is widely distributed and that the drug can be measured for at least 2 weeks after cyclosporine therapy is discontinued (16).

In human blood at 37°C, cyclosporine partitions equally between red blood cells and plasma (17). In plasma, cyclosporine is highly bound to lipoproteins, which comprise 10-15% of all plasma proteins (18,19). Although the effect of diseases or other drugs on cyclosporine binding to lipoproteins in vivo is not known, an association between high serum cyclosporine concentrations and hypertriglyceridemia (20) or hypercholesteremia (21) has been observed. As discussed later, this association between cyclosporine and lipoproteins can influence the risk of serious toxicity.

The steady-state volume of distribution based on serum cyclosporine concentration varies according to patient age (Fig. 1) (14). Patients less than 10 years old have the highest volume of distribution, while those older than 40 years have the lowest volume of distribution. Patients 11-20, 21-30, and 31-40 years old have intermediate volume of distribution values. The physiologic basis for the age-dependent differences are not known, but may be related to age-related changes in binding of cyclosporine to lipoproteins. In contrast to most plasma proteins, lipoprotein concentrations gradually increase with age (22). Increases in lipoprotein concentrations would result in a corresponding decrease in the fraction unbound in plasma (i.e., free fraction). For drugs with a large volume of distribution (>100L), such as cyclosporine, a decrease in free fraction would result in a lower volume of distribution. This model is supported by studies in rabbits showing that decreases in free fraction are associated with a decrease in volume of distribution (23). Since cyclosporine is a highly lipophilic drug, we have also studied the effect of obesity on cyclosporine distribution in man (15,24). There was no significant effect of obesity on cyclosporine volume of distribution, which suggests that cyclospo-

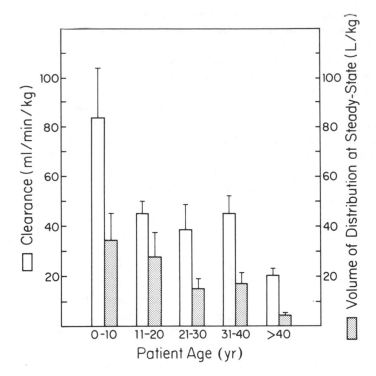

Figure 1 Effect of age on cyclosporine clearance and volume of distribution. Bar heights and error bars represent mean values and SEM, respectively. (Source: Ref. 14.)

rine distribution is limited primarily to lean body mass. These results indicate that obese patients do not require a higher loading dose than nonobese patients.

3. Metabolism

Cyclosporine is extensively metabolized, with subsequent biliary and, to a lesser extent, urinary elimination. At least nine cyclosporine metabolites have been isolated and identified from bile, feces, and urine from animals and urine from humans (25). None of the metabolites identified thus far are conjugated. Some of these metabolites can be measured from human blood or plasma samples; blood concentrations of the major metabolite (no. 17) can exceed those of parent drug (26,27). In marrow transplant recipients, trough blood concentrations of cyclosporine metabolite no. 17 are about 80% that of parent drug concentrations (26). At least some of the metabolites have been shown to possess immunosuppressive activity (27,28). There is also indirect evidence that some of the cyclosporine metabolites may be nephrotoxic (29).

The liver is probably the major site of cyclosporine metabolism, as evidenced by metabolism in in vitro liver microsomal systems and numerous drug interactions between cyclosporine and microsomal enzyme inducers or inhibitors (25). Total plasma (or serum) clearance ranges from 13 to 80 ml/min/kg, depending on patient age (14). Corresponding values for blood cyclosporine clearance range from 7 to 13 ml/min/kg, which classifies cyclosporine as a low-to-intermediate clearance drug (15).

Hepatic dysfunction occurs in many marrow transplant recipients during the postgrafting period. The etiology is often unclear but the most common causes are venocclusive disease and acute GVHD (30). Although hepatic dysfunction has been shown to delay clearance of cyclosporine or cyclosporine metabolites (11), additional studies show that standard biochemical tests of liver function—bilirubin, SGOT, and alkaline phosphatase— are not accurate indicators of the ability of the liver to metabolize cyclosporine.

Cyclosporine clearance based on serum cyclosporine concentrations is age-related; infants and young children less than 10 years old have a more rapid clearance than older patients (Fig. 1) (14). Conversely, patients older than 40 years have a lower clearance than those 11-40 years old. Similar age-related differences are observed with cyclosporine clearance values based on whole blood concentrations, but the differences between age groups are less apparent (15). The physiologic basis for the age-related changes in plasma cyclosporine clearance is not known but may also be related to the gradual increase in lipoprotein concentration with increasing age. Since cyclosporine is a low-to-intermediate clearance drug, decreases in free fraction would theoretically reduce hepatic clearance (31). This theoretical model is supported by studies in rabbits showing that a decrease in free fraction results in a decrease in cyclosporine clearance (23).

Other studies in humans indicate that changes in the erythrocyte mass, as measured by hematocrit, can influence blood cyclosporine clearance (15). Patients with higher hematocrit values had lower blood cyclosporine clearance values. Although the precise mechanism of this phenomenon is not known, it is possible that the effect of hematocrit on blood cyclosporine clearance is related to changes in the fraction of cyclosporine bound to erythrocytes. Since marrow transplant recipients usually are anemic during the early posttransplant period, differences in hematocrit may explain in part the higher blood cyclosporine clearance values reported in this patient population compared with renal transplant recipients.

Obesity does not appear to influence cyclosporine clearance (15,24), which is consistent with the observation that obesity has little if any effect on the clearance of drugs that are metabolized via oxidative pathways. Thus, if cyclosporine is dosed according to actual body weight, obese patients will tend to have higher steady-state concentrations than nonobese patients, which may increase their risk of renal dysfunction. These data also suggest that if one wishes to achieve and maintain steady-state cyclosporine concentrations in an obese patient that are comparable to those found in nonobese patients, then maintenance doses should probably be given on the basis of ideal body weight rather than actual body weight.

Many drugs have been reported to increase or decrease cyclosporine concentration; a partial list of these drug-drug interactions is shown in Table 1 (32-35). Although it is often stated that these interactions are related to inhibition or induction of microsomal enzyme activity, very little is actually known concerning the underlying mechanism. For example, a recent study of the erythromycin-cyclosporine interaction indicates that the primary effect of erythromycin is to alter cyclosporine absorption after oral administration (36), with little or no effect on cyclosporine clearance, as previously stated by other investigators (37,38).

4. Excretion

A relatively minor amount of unchanged cyclosporine, comprising less than 1% of an administered dose, is excreted renally (39). In marrow transplant recipients, mean renal cyclosporine clearance is 25.5 ml/min, which is less than 10% of total systemic clearance (40). As with hepatic clearance, renal cyclosporine clearance is also age-related. Urinary cyclosporine concentrations are frequently over 1000 ng/ml, which are several-fold higher

Table 1 Selected List of Drugs Reported to Have a Pharmacokinetic Interaction with Cyclosporine

Drugs that may increase cyclosporine concentration:
  Erythromycin
  Verapamil
  Nicardipine
  Diltiazem
  Steroids
  Ketoconazole
  Metoclopramide

Drugs that may decrease cyclosporine concentration:
  Phenytoin
  Rifampin
  Phenobarbital
  Carbamazepine

Source: Refs. 32-35.

than systemic (blood or serum/plasma) concentrations associated with toxicity. It is not known if high urinary cyclosporine (or cyclosporine metabolite) concentrations contribute to renal dysfunction.

B. Adverse Effects

1. Renal Dysfunction

The dose-limiting toxicity of cyclosporine is nephrotoxicity. Three major syndromes have been described in transplant patients (41-43). The first and most common syndrome is transient acute renal failure, manifested by increases in serum creatinine that occur after several days or weeks of daily cyclosporine therapy (Fig. 2). The incidence of this syndrome is high. In one study, about 85% of marrow transplant recipients developed acute renal dysfunction, defined as an increase in serum creatinine to twice the baseline value (44). Although the major risk factor for acute renal dysfunction is cyclosporine therapy, about 50% of patients who received single-agent methotrexate as GVHD prophylaxis also developed renal dysfunction. In both methotrexate- and cyclosporine-treated patients, mean weekly serum creatinine increased during the first few weeks posttransplant. However, the rate of increase and the peak serum creatinine were greater in cyclosporine-treated patients. Among patients treated with cyclosporine, peak serum creatinine was reached during the fourth week posttransplant and gradually decreased thereafter (Fig. 3). Other risk factors for acute renal dysfunction include baseline serum creatinine, concurrent amphotericin or aminoglycoside therapy, sepsis, hepatic venocclusive disease, or elevated cyclosporine concentration (discussed below) (29,45-47). Age or the type of underlying hematologic disease did not appear to influence the risk of renal dysfunction (29). Concurrent high-dose intravenous acyclovir therapy has also been associated with a higher risk of cyclosporine-induced acute renal dysfunction (48).

Increases in serum creatinine are usually rapidly reversible after cyclosporine doses are temporarily held or reduced. The pathophysiology of transient acute renal failure is not clear, but the reduction of glomerular filtration rate appears to be caused by cyclo-

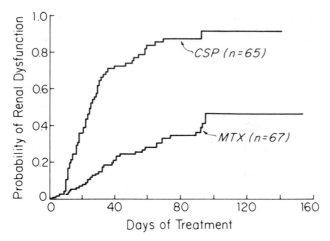

Figure 2 Probability of developing renal dysfunction in patients receiving cyclosporine (CSP) or methotrexate (MTX). (Source: Ref. 44.)

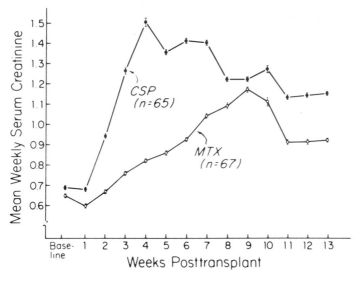

Figure 3 Mean (± SEM) weekly serum creatinine (mg/dl) in patients receiving cyclosporine (CSP) or methotrexate (MTX). (Source: Ref. 44.)

sporine-induced renal vasoconstriction, which results in increased renal vascular resistance and reduced renal perfusion rate (49,50).

The second syndrome is a more severe form of acute renal failure, which lasts for more than one week. The incidence of this syndrome in marrow transplant recipients is not known, but several centers have observed that about 10% of marrow transplant recipients treated with cyclosporine require hemodialysis during the first few weeks posttransplant. Although histopathologic data or results of detailed renal function tests are not available, it is likely that many of these patients have this more severe form of acute renal failure. Protracted acute renal failure can be associated with the development of thrombosis of glomerular arterioles or diffuse, interstitial fibrosis (51). The pathophysiology of this syndrome is probably related to protracted renal vasoconstriction, which may prevent the increase in renal blood flow that has been shown to be necessary to recover from postischemic renal injury. Alternatively, cyclosporine may exacerbate intravascular thrombus formation or may serve as a stimulus to interstitial cell proliferation. Recovery of renal function after protracted acute renal failure is usually not complete, even when cyclosporine is withdrawn.

The third and most serious syndrome is chronic nephropathy, which has been reported to occur in cardiac transplant patients receiving continuous cyclosporine for more than one year (52). Since most marrow transplant recipients receive cyclosporine for no more than 6 months, this syndrome is probably rare. In one series, patients who had their cyclosporine therapy tapered and discontinued by day 180 had a mean serum creatinine at one year that was not significantly different from that in patients treated with methotrexate alone (53). Mean serum creatinine at one year was also not significantly different from pretransplant values. Furthermore, none of the cyclosporine-treated patients had an abnormally elevated serum creatinine. Daily cyclosporine therapy for more than 6 months appears to increase the risk of chronic nephropathy. For example, only patients who received more than 6 months of cyclosporine therapy because of chronic GVHD had evidence of chronic nephrotoxicity at one year, defined as an increase in serum creatinine to more than twice the pretransplant value (53). These results are similar to those reported by Gratwohl and colleagues, who routinely administer daily cyclosporine for one year as acute GVHD prophylaxis (54). In their study, mean serum creatinines at one year were higher than pretransplant values.

More specific tests of glomerular filtration or renal biopsies have not been performed in marrow transplant recipients. In cardiac transplant recipients, chronic nephropathy is associated with a reaction in the number of functional nephrons with an attendant loss of glomerular filtration surface area. Because these changes may be accompanied by a rise in tubular creatinine secretion, only modest changes in serum creatinine may be observed.

2. Hypertension

The incidence of cyclosporine-induced hypertension in marrow transplant recipients is high, occurring in about 60% of patients (55). The mechanism of hypertension is not clear (56), but in some patients it is related to hypomagnesemia caused by renal magnesium wasting (57). Studies in renal transplant recipients indicate that cyclosporine-treated patients have sodium retention and presumably a volume-dependent hypertension (58). Plasma renin was normal in cyclosporine-treated patients, which explains why patients in that study had minimal blood pressure responses to captopril. The major risk factor is concurrent use of glucocorticoids (55). In another study, the duration of infusion influenced the risk of hypertension (59). Patients who received intravenous cyclosporine as a 12-18-hour infusion had a higher incidence of hypertension than those who received cyclosporine as a short one-hour infusion. It should be noted, however, that a higher percentage of patients given cyclosporine as a 12-18-hour infusion received glucocorticoids than those given cyclosporine as a one-hour infusion. Other factors such as age, sex, underlying disease, cyclosporine concentration, and renal function do not appear to be significantly associated with cyclosporine-induced hypertension (55).

3. Neurotoxicity

Central nervous system abnormalities that have been associated with cyclosporine use in children and adults undergoing marrow transplantation include seizures, cerebellar ataxia, tremor, depression, aphasia, drowsiness, confusion, quadriparesis, amnesia, transverse myelitis, and paraparesis (60-63). Seizures generally occur within the first few weeks of cyclosporine therapy while other subacute episodes such as cerebellar ataxia, tremor, and depression tended to occur after prolonged cyclosporine therapy (61). In liver transplant patients, cortical blindness and abnormalities of the white matter on cerebral computerized tomography and magnetic resonance scans were also observed and progressed to coma in two patients (64). Cyclosporine-induced neurotoxicity has been associated with hypomagnesemia in marrow transplant recipients (61) and with hypocholesterolemia in liver transplant recipients (64). The mechanism for the association between low serum cholesterol and cyclosporine-induced central nervous system toxicity is not known. Since cyclosporine is primarily bound to lipoproteins, low serum cholesterol may allow greater amounts of "free" or unbound cyclosporine to pass through the blood-brain barrier. Other risk factors that have been reported include concurrent use of high-dose steroids, conditioning regimens that include total body irradiation, intrathecal methotrexate, and elevated cyclosporine concentrations (60,62).

4. Hepatotoxicity

Cyclosporine-induced hepatotoxicity has been reported in marrow transplant recipients but is not a major cause of hepatic dysfunction during the first few weeks posttransplant (30). It is of interest that the combination of cyclosporine and methotrexate is associated with more frequent and more severe increases in serum bilirubin than the use of cyclosporine alone (6). Similarly, the concurrent use of cyclophosphamide and cyclosporine has been associated with an increased risk of hepatic venocclusive disease (65).

5. Other Toxicities

The time to discontinuation of red blood cell transfusions or the number of red blood cell transfusions required has been reported to be increased in cyclosporine-treated patients (66-68). The mechanism for this observation is not known but cyclosporine has been shown to interfere with the function of an accessory cell of erythropoiesis (69).

C. Monitoring Blood/Plasma Concentrations

Because cyclosporine concentrations during the first few weeks posttransplant vary considerably between patients receiving identical mg per kg doses due to interpatient variability in pharmacokinetics (44), it has been recommended that cyclosporine concentration be monitored to ensure adequate immunosuppression and avoid unnecessary toxicity. However, before monitoring of cyclosporine concentration can be applied, the "target" or "therapeutic" concentration range for cyclosporine must be known. This target concentration range must be established with studies of the relationship between drug concentration and therapeutic effect or toxicity.

Since only a few pharmacodynamic studies of cyclosporine have been reported, many of the "therapeutic" concentration ranges for cyclosporine that are used clinically have been based on anecdotal cases or small numbers of patients (32). None of the published studies have included concurrent measurements of cyclosporine concentration in different biologic fluids (whole blood versus plasma/serum) or analyzed by different assay methods (radioimmunoassay versus high-performance liquid chromatography). Therefore, the most appropriate biologic fluid or assay method—as measured by the clinical response or toxicity—to use for monitoring cyclosporine concentration is not known.

Theoretical considerations can be used to support the use of one biologic fluid or one assay method over another (70-72). For example, proponents of the use of whole blood argue that because of the temperature-dependent binding of cyclosporine to red blood cells or plasma proteins and because other factors (e.g., hematocrit, lipoproteins, etc.) can affect the distribution of cyclosporine between blood and plasma or serum, whole blood is preferable to plasma or serum. Alternatively, proponents of plasma or serum argue that because of the extensive binding of cyclosporine to body tissues, plasma or serum concentration represents a more accurate index of cyclosporine concentration at the site of action. These investigators also point out that most of the published pharmacodynamic studies have used plasma or serum cyclosporine data. Similarly, proponents of the use of high-performance liquid chromatographic methods argue that because cyclosporine concentrations measured by radioimmunoassay are variably higher than concentrations measured by high-performance liquid chromatography and because other factors (e.g., degree of hepatic function) can influence the ratio between radioimmunoassay and high-performance liquid chromatography measurements, high-performance liquid chromatographic methods are preferable to nonspecific radioimmunoassay methods. Proponents of radioimmunoassay argue that some cyclosporine metabolites are immunosuppressive or nephrotoxic and that for most patients, the ratio between radioimmunoassay and high-performance liquid chromatographic measurements does not significantly change.

1. Immunosuppression

Several in vitro (73) and in vivo (74) studies have shown that the immunosuppressive effects of cyclosporine are reversible and require a minimum concentration of drug in the supernatant or blood. Theoretically, a minimum effective (i.e., immunosuppressive) cyclosporine concentration must be maintained to prevent acute GVHD in most patients. This minimum level will be different for different patients depending on other factors that influence the risk of acute GVHD such as patient age, the concurrent use of other immunosuppressive agents, and the degree of immunologic incompatibility between donor and recipient (HLA-identical vs. HLA-nonidentical). For example, the minimum effective cyclosporine concentration in a 15-year-old recipient of an HLA-identical marrow graft is probably lower than that in a 45-year-old recipient of an HLA-nonidentical marrow graft. Further, since many marrow transplant recipients receive cyclosporine combined with other immunosuppressive agents, systemic concentrations of each individual drug will influence the overall effectiveness of the regimen.

Although many marrow transplant teams routinely monitor cyclosporine concentrations, most studies have failed to find a significant correlation between cyclosporine levels and the risk of developing acute GVHD (32). In one study by Gluckman and colleagues, patients who developed acute GVHD had a significantly lower mean plasma level

(84 ng/ml (RIA)) than those who did not develop acute GVHD (211 ng/ml) (75). In another study, Santos and colleagues observed that cyclosporine concentration during the first week posttransplant correlated with the incidence of acute GVHD (7). However, none of these studies used multivariate statistical methods that adjusted for the potential influence of other factors on the risk of acute GVHD.

We studied 179 marrow transplant recipients who received cyclosporine as acute GVHD prophylaxis to determine the relationship between serum cyclosporine concentration and risk of acute GVHD (76). Trough serum cyclosporine concentrations were measured by RIA. The relationship between patient characteristics and risk of acute GVHD was analyzed with a multivariate relative risk regression model; weekly trough cyclosporine concentration was modeled as a time-dependent covariate. Sixty-six patients (37%) developed grades II-IV acute GVHD 7 to 66 (median 13) days posttransplant. The mortality rate in patients who developed grades II-IV acute GVHD was 1.95 times higher than in those who did not develop acute GVHD. Trough cyclosporine concentration significantly influenced the risk of developing acute GVHD during the next week (Fig. 4). Patients who developed acute GVHD had a lower average cyclosporine concentration during the previous week than those who did not develop acute GVHD. The relative risk was 0.7 for every 100 ng/ml increase in cyclosporine concentration and was 1.0, 0.60, and 0.20 for cyclosporine concentrations of <100, 100-199, and ⩾200 ng/ml, respectively (Table 2). Patient age, GVHD prophylaxis regimen, and year of transplant also significantly influenced the risk of acute GVHD.

These data indicate that serum cyclosporine concentration influences the level of in vivo immunosuppression and that low cyclosporine concentration can be a cause for treatment failure. These results also illustrate the complexities associated with the use of

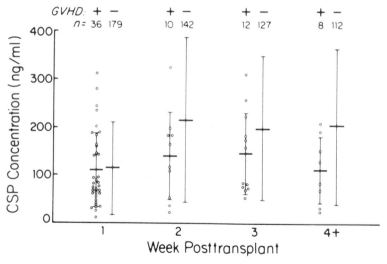

Figure 4 Mean (± SD) trough cyclosporine (CSP) concentrations, according to the number of weeks posttransplant, in patients who developed acute GVHD during the next week (+) and in those who were at risk for GVHD at the start of the week (−). Each circle represents the average cyclosporine concentration in one patient who developed acute GVHD during the next week. (Source: Ref. 76.)

Table 2 Multivariate Relative Risk Regression Model of the Association Between Patient Characteristics or Cyclosporine Concentration and Risk of Acute GVHD

Covariate	Relative risk	p value
GVHD prophylaxis regimen		
Cyclosporine	1.00	<0.01
Cyclosporine and methotrexate	0.37	
Patient Age (yr)		
<20	1.00	0.05
20-29	1.70	
30-39	2.26	
≥40	3.71	
Year of Transplantation		
1983 or earlier	1.00	0.02
After 1983	1.75	
Cyclosporine Concentration		
Continuous	0.70[a]	<0.01
<100 ng/ml	1.00	<0.01
100-199 ng/ml	0.60	
≥200 ng/ml	0.20	

[a]Risk shown is estimated for every increase in cyclosporine concentration of 100 ng/ml.

Source: Modified from Ref. 76.

a therapeutic concentration range. For example, a relatively low cyclosporine concentration may be acceptable for patients who are at relatively low risk of developing acute GVHD (i.e., children). Conversely, even high cyclosporine concentrations may not be adequate for patients who are at high risk for developing acute GVHD; combinations of immunosuppressive agents should be considered in these patients. Examples of high-risk groups include patients older than 40 years and recipients of HLA-nonidentical marrow grafts (77).

2. Renal Dysfunction

In our studies, we have defined renal dysfunction as a doubling of baseline serum creatinine, which is associated with a significant reduction in glomerular filtration rate (29,44, 46). Using this relatively severe definition of renal dysfunction, 85-90% of patients receiving cyclosporine as GVHD prophylaxis developed renal dysfunction (Fig. 2). Serum cyclosporine concentrations, as measured by RIA, correlated with the risk of developing renal dysfunction in marrow transplant recipients (Fig. 5A). The median days of onset of renal dysfunction were 46, 29, and 20 in patients with mean trough concentrations of <150, 150-250, and >250 ng/ml, respectively (46). Eight of nine patients who did not develop renal dysfunction had a mean trough cyclosporine concentration of <150 ng/ml. However, even in the group with the lowest mean trough cyclosporine concentration, 73% developed renal dysfunction.

Since the radioimmunoassay measures both cyclosporine and cyclosporine metabolites, these data are difficult to interpret because the relative role of parent drug and

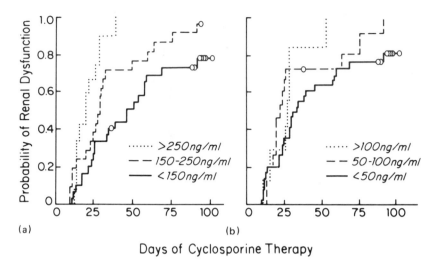

(a)   (b)

Days of Cyclosporine Therapy

Figure 5 Probability of developing renal dysfunction in patients with different mean trough cyclosporine concentrations, as measured by (a) radioimmunoassay or (b) high-performance liquid chromatography. Circles represent patients who did not develop renal dysfunction. (Source: Ref. 29.)

cross-reactive metabolites in the development of renal dysfunction cannot be determined. If some of these metabolites accumulate in patients with early clinically undetectable renal dysfunction, they may be important in the development of renal dysfunction. We indirectly addressed this question by remeasuring cyclosporine concentrations in serum samples from the original 63 patients by high-performance liquid chromatography (29). Cyclosporine concentrations measured by high-performance liquid chromatography were about one-third as high as values measured by radioimmunoassay. Contrary to our results with cyclosporine concentrations measured by radioimmunoassay, cyclosporine concentrations measured by high-performance liquid chromatography did not significantly correlate with renal dysfunction (Fig. 5B) (Table 3), which suggests that cyclosporine metabolites play a role in the development of renal dysfunction. These results

Table 3 Multivariate Relative Risk Regression Model of the Association Between Patient Characteristics or Cyclosporine Concentration and Risk of Acute Renal Dysfunction

Covariate	Relative risk	p value
Baseline serum creatinine (mg/dl)	0.1	0.01
Cyclosporine Concentration (RIA)		
<150 ng/ml	1.00	<0.001
150–250 ng/ml	1.90	
>250 ng/ml	4.30	
Cyclosporine Concentration (HPLC)	–	0.34

Abbreviations: RIA = radioimmunoassay, HPLC = high-performance liquid chromatography.
Source: Modifed from Ref. 29.

also suggest that monitoring of serum cyclosporine concentrations by high-performance liquid chromatography provides no clinical advantage to monitoring serum cyclosporine concentrations by radioimmunoassay. It is not known if whole blood cyclosporine concentrations measured by radioimmunoassay or high-performance liquid chromatography would also correlate with renal dysfunction.

3. Clinical Guidelines

Indications for monitoring cyclosporine concentrations are listed in Table 4. In general, trough or predose cyclosporine concentrations should be monitored at least twice weekly in marrow transplant recipients. "Peak" cyclosporine concentrations are more difficult to interpret because of the marked effect of the time of sampling on the measured concentration. For example, after intravenous administration, a difference of 30 minutes can result in a 50% or more difference in "peak" cyclosporine concentration. After oral administration, however, small differences in time do not markedly influence cyclosporine concentration. Similarly, a difference of 1-2 hours usually does not change the trough concentration by more than 10-20%. A cyclosporine concentration 4 hours after oral administration can sometimes be helpful if a clinician suspects that poor oral cyclosporine absorption is the cause for low cyclosporine concentrations. The therapeutic or toxicologic importance of high "peak" cyclosporine concentration is probably small. In one comparison of two intravenous cyclosporine infusion schedules, the incidence of acute GVHD and renal dysfunction was similar regardless of whether patients received cyclosporine as a one-hour infusion or a 12-18 hour infusion (59).

Most pharmacodynamic studies in marrow transplant recipients are based on serum or blood cyclosporine concentration measured by the polyclonal radioimmunoassay developed by Sandoz (78). However, this assay is no longer available and has been replaced by two monoclonal radioimmunoassays (79,80). One of the monoclonal radioimmunoassays is specific for parent drug while the other assay measures parent drug and cross-reactive metabolites. It should also be noted that another radioimmunoassay kit which uses an iodinated labeled tracer is commercially available (81). A polyclonal fluorescence polarization immunoassay has recently been introduced for clinical use (82,83). The major advantages of that assay are improved precision, rapid turnaround time, and simpler technical operation. Many high-performance liquid chromatography procedures have also been developed to measure cyclosporine concentration (70). Two studies have attempted to compare the correlation between cyclosporine concentration measured by several different assays and the occurrence of GVHD (or graft rejection) or renal dysfunction (84,85). Although no definitive conclusions can be drawn from these preliminary studies, these types of studies are needed to determine the preferred biologic fluid or assay method for measurement of cyclosporine concentration. The available assays and

Table 4 Indications for Monitoring Cyclosporine Concentration

Maintain adequate immunosuppression and reduce serious toxicity
Document adequate oral absorption
Aid in diagnosis of suspected cyclosporine-associated renal dysfunction
Onset of possible acute GVHD
Change in route of administration (i.e., intravenous to oral or vice versa)
Change in hepatic or renal function
Concurrent therapy with potentially interacting drug

Table 5 Assays Available for Measurement of Cyclosporine Concentration and Approximate Therapeutic Ranges

Assay	Biologic fluid	Therapeutic range (ng/ml)
Radioimmunoassay (polyclonal)[a]	Serum/Plasma	100-250
	Whole blood	200-800
Radioimmunoassay (monoclonal)[b]	Serum/Plasma	50-125
	Whole blood	150-400
Fluorescence polarization	Serum/Plasma	150-400
immunoassay (polyclonal)	Whole blood	200-800
High-performance liquid chromatography	Whole blood	150-400

[a]No longer available.

[b]Refers to monoclonal radioimmunoassay specific for parent drug.

their approximate therapeutic ranges as of December 1988 are listed in Table 5. It is important to note that these ranges are not based on pharmacodynamic studies in large numbers of patients but on clinical experience.

III. METHOTREXATE

Methotrexate is a folic acid antagonist with immunosuppressive and antineoplastic activity (86,87). The immunosuppressive activity of methotrexate is directly related to its cytotoxic activity. As discussed elsewhere, the use of methotrexate as GVHD prophylaxis is based on murine and canine studies that demonstrate its effectiveness in MHC-identical and -nonidentical marrow transplantation (Chapter 16).

A. Pharmacokinetics

The oral absorption of methotrexate after marrow transplantation has not been studied. In cancer patients, oral methotrexate absorption is erratic and incomplete (88-91). Methotrexate is therefore not usually given by the oral route in marrow transplant recipients. Peak concentrations are usually achieved 2 hours after oral administration but can vary from 1 to 5 hours (90). The average oral bioavailability is about 40% (range 6-95%).

   After intravenous administration, the steady-state volume of distribution for methotrexate is about 40-80% of body weight (91-93). The drug is about 50% bound to plasma proteins, primarily albumin (88,92,94). Methotrexate can accumulate in extravascular compartments or "third spaces," such as pleural or peritoneal effusions (94,95). The latter is of clinical importance because many patients develop ascites associated with hepatic venocclusive disease during the first few weeks posttransplant. Methotrexate that accumulates into these extravascular compartments, including the cerebrospinal fluid space, is slowly released into the systemic circulation and can result in excessive toxicity (96). In patients with leukemia, the gradual release of methotrexate from the extravascular compartments is the reason that intravenous methotrexate is not given along with intrathecal methotrexate. It is assumed (but has never been proven) that an adequate amount of methotrexate is released from the cerebrospinal fluid space to cause systemic immunosuppression. For example, when single-agent methotrexate is given as GVHD prophylaxis, during the weeks that intrathecal methotrexate is administered, intravenous drug is not given (66-68).

The plasma half-life after low-dose methotrexate administration is 2-3 hours (88-93). In one study, a terminal half-life of 27 hours was observed (93). However, since radiolabeled methotrexate was used in that study, the long half-life may represent elimination of a less active methotrexate metabolite and not parent drug. The major route of elimination for methotrexate is renal excretion (88,92,93). Renal methotrexate clearance involves glomerular filtration, tubular secretion, and tubular reabsorption. The renal excretion of methotrexate has not been studied after low (<25 mg/m^2) intravenous doses or in marrow transplant recipients. Excessive methotrexate-related toxicity has been observed in marrow transplant recipients with impaired renal function; in some instances the drug may have been responsible for poor engraftment or graft failure posttransplant. Thus, methotrexate concentrations should be monitored in patients with impaired renal function or fluid accumulation in "third spaces" and leucovorin should be administered if needed.

A relatively minor excretory pathway for methotrexate is biliary secretion, with enterohepatic recycling (88,97). In a patient given intramuscular methotrexate, severe vomiting and diarrhea has been reported to increase plasma clearance of the drug, probably via reduced enterohepatic recycling and increased fecal excretion (98). It is therefore possible that severe vomiting or diarrhea posttransplant may have similarly increased nonrenal elimination of methotrexate.

B. Adverse Effects

1. Mucositis

In marrow transplant recipients conditioned with cyclophosphamide and total body irradiation, randomized comparisons show that the incidence of mucositis is higher in methotrexate-treated patients than in those treated with cyclosporine alone (66–68). In another study of patients who also received cyclophosphamide and total body irradiation, 15 of 43 patients (35%) randomized to receive low-dose intravenous methotrexate on days 1, 3, 6, and 11 in combination with cyclosporine developed severe mucositis compared with only 4 of 50 patients (8%) who received cyclosporine alone (6).

2. Myelosuppression

The time to engraftment and recovery of granulocytes and platelets has been reported to be delayed by about one week in patients treated with methotrexate compared to those treated with cyclosporine alone in some (66,68) but not all studies (67). The addition of four doses of methotrexate on days 1, 3, 6, and 11 to cyclosporine has been found to delay engraftment in patients with leukemia prepared with cyclophosphamide and total body irradiation (67). Collectively, these studies suggest that methotrexate interferes not only with T lymphocytes, but also with hematopoietic precursor cells.

3. Hepatotoxicity

Although prolonged low-dose methotrexate regimens used in the treatment of various autoimmune diseases have been associated with hepatotoxicity (86,87), methotrexate-induced hepatic dysfunction is infrequent in marrow transplant recipients (30). However, the incidence of hyperbilirubinemia during the first 2 weeks posttransplant is higher in patients treated with a combination of methotrexate and cyclosporine than in patients given either single-agent cyclosporine (6) or methotrexate (99). The mechanism for this apparent additive or synergistic effect on the liver is not known.

4. *Pulmonary Toxicity*

Interstitial pneumonitis has rarely been associated with methotrexate, particularly when given in low doses for prolonged periods. In the marrow transplant setting, it is not clear whether methotrexate as compared to cyclosporine increases the risk of interstitial pneumonitis. In a report by the International Bone Marrow Transplant Registry, the risk of interstitial pneumonitis was increased 2.3 times in patients receiving methotrexate as GVHD prophylaxis (100). In another uncontrolled study, marrow transplant recipients who received methotrexate GVHD prophylaxis had a higher risk of interstitial pneumonitis (15/34) than those not receiving any GVHD prophylaxis (3/21) (3). In randomized comparisons of cyclosporine versus methotrexate, methotrexate-treated patients had a slightly higher incidence of interstitial pneumonitis during the first year posttransplant compared with cyclosporine-treated patients (30% versus 22%) (5). This difference, however, was not statisically significant.

C. Monitoring Plasma/Serum Concentrations

Because of the low doses used in marrow transplantation, methotrexate concentrations probably do not have to be monitored after every dose. They should, however, be monitored in patients who are likely to have high methotrexate concentrations, such as those with renal dysfunction, moderate-to-severe hepatic dysfunction, or accumulation of fluid into "third spaces." Blood samples should be drawn about 24 hours after the intravenous or intrathecal dose and methotrexate concentration should be measured with an assay method with a limit of sensitivity of at least 0.01 μM. Figure 6 shows a nomogram

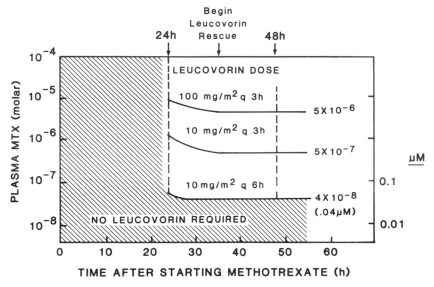

Figure 6 Nomogram for methotrexate concentrations after low-dose intravenous or intrathecal administration in marrow transplant recipients.

that was developed by Dr. Archie Bleyer and has been used by the Seattle marrow transplant team as a guide for "acceptable" methotrexate levels.

IV. GLUCOCORTICOIDS

Glucocorticoids remain important immunosuppressive agents in the prevention and treatment of acute GVHD. Although glucocorticoids are often included in acute GVHD prophylaxis regimens, they have never been shown in a randomized study to be necessary or beneficial (Chapter 20). In the treatment of acute GVHD, however several randomized studies have demonstrated their efficacy compared with antithymocyte globulin (101) or cyclosporine (91) (Chapter 26). Since the most commonly used preparations are prednisone orally and methylprednisolone intravenously, these preparation will be discussed in detail.

A. Pharmacokinetics

After oral administration, about 80% of prednisone is absorbed and converted in vivo to prednisolone, the active metabolite (102-104). Peak concentrations of the drug are usually achieved 1-3 hours after oral administration. The rate and extent of absorption is variable and can be influenced by the specific commercial preparation of prednisone. In solid organ transplant recipients, rejection episodes have been observed shortly after the patients changed to different generic brands of oral prednisone (103). The cause of poor bioavailability with some brands of oral prednisone has been shown to be related to slow dissolution rates.

Because of poor water solubility, methylprednisolone is adminstered intravenously as an ester, such as the sodium succinate ester. The succinate ester of methylprednisolone is converted in vivo to methylprednisolone by esterases in the blood and liver. The inactive sodium succinate ester of methylprednisolone should, therefore, be considered as a pro-drug for the active form, methylprednisolone. After intravenous administration of radiolabeled drug, 75% of the total radioactivity was recovered in urine in 96 hours and 9% was recovered in feces (105). Recent studies show that about 10% of the drug is excreted unchanged in the urine as the succinate ester, which indicates incomplete conversion of the pro-drug (106). After high-dose administration (10 mg/kg), the terminal half-life for conversion of the methylprednisolone succinate ester to active drug is about 30 minutes.

After conversion to methylprednisolone, the drug is extensively metabolized, with only about 5% of the drug excreted unchanged in the urine (106,107). Total plasma clearance of methylprednisolone appears to be nonlinear, averaging about 340 ml/min after an 80 mg dose and 277 ml/min after a 10 mg/kg dose in adults (106). The mechanism for the apparent nonlinear elimination is not known but may be related to saturation of metabolizing enzymes. The average plasma half-life for methylprednisolone is about 2.7 hours after low-dose administration and 3.6 hours after high-dose administration (106). The volume of distribution for methylprednisolone has been reported to be 80-90 liters in two studies (106,108) and 50 liters in a third study (109); these values do not appear to be dose-dependent.

All glucocorticoids are variably bound to transcortin and albumin (102-104). The affinity of methylprednisolone for these proteins relative to other glucocorticoids is not known. The binding of prednisolone to plasma proteins has been reported to be markedly concentration-dependent (110), but it is not known if methylprednisolone exhibits similar binding characteristics.

B. Adverse Effects

When given as GVHD disease prophylaxis or treatment, glucocorticoids are usually given for relatively short periods at high dosages. The risk of toxicities associated with long-term chronic use are therefore small.

1. Hypertension

When given as single agent therapy for established acute GVHD, glucocorticoids occasionally cause hypertension. When combined with cyclosporine, however, glucocorticoids have been associated with an increased risk of hypertension (7,8,55). In one study, 37 of 54 patients randomized to receive cyclosporine and prednisone as GVHD prophylaxis developed hypertension, defined as a blood pressure greater than 140/90 mm Hg (8). For comparison, only 8 of 53 patients randomized to received methotrexate and prednisone developed hypertension.

2. Other Toxicities

Other adverse effects that have been reported after "standard" dosages of glucocorticoids (1-2 mg/kg methylprednisolone or equivalent) include abdominal pain (101), gastrointestinal bleeding (101), and pancreatitis (9). After high-dose ($>$5 mg/kg) therapy, the major adverse effects include gastrointestinal bleeding and transient hyperglycemia (111, 112). Aseptic necrosis and acute psychotic reactions have also been observed.

V. ANTITHYMOCYTE GLOBULIN

Antithymocyte globulin is a solution of immunoglobulin G prepared from plasma or serum of healthy animals hyperimmunized with human thymus lymphocytes. The current animal source for most preparations is the horse.

A. Pharmacokinetics

The pharmacokinetics of antithymocyte globulin have not been well characterized in man. After intravenous infusion of 10 mg/kg daily for 5 days, mean equine IgG concentration was 727 μg/ml (113). The plasma half-life of equine IgG is about 6 days. About 1% of the dose is eliminated in the urine, primarily as unchanged equine IgG (113). The disposition of equine IgG in man is not known, but it is believed to be catabolized and extensively bound to most body tissues.

B. Adverse Effects

1. Infusion-Related Toxicities

The most common toxicities of antihymocyte globulin are those related to administration of an animal protein. Despite prior skin testing in every patient, most patients develop fever and chills after every infusion. Pretreatment with sedatives, antihistamines, and antipyretics can reduce the severity of symptoms but does not prevent their occurrence. In patients with extreme hyperpyrexia, 25-50 mg of intravenous hydrocortisone may be helpful (101). Since febrile reactions also occur in patients receiving prednisone as GVHD prophylaxis, higher dosages of glucocorticoids probably offer no additional benefit (114). The severity of these reactions tends to decrease after the first few infusions (115). The mechanism of these febrile reactions is not known but may be related to release of endogenous leukocyte pyrogens. Occasionally patients develop a serum sickness syndrome.

2. Myelosuppression

The incidence and severity of myelosuppression appears to vary depending on the specific preparation of antithymocyte globulin. Although lymphocytopenia occurs in most patients receiving subcutaneous or intramuscular rabbit or goat antithymocyte globulin (116), leukopenia and thrombocytopenia are uncommon toxicities of equine antithymocyte globulin. Two randomized studies have shown that the addition of antithymocyte globulin does not delay engraftment after marrow grafting (114,115). One study, however, reported that additional platelet support was required during the period of antithymocyte globulin therapy (114). Furthermore, other studies have noted marked leukopenia and thrombocytopenia temporally related to antithymocyte therapy, which required discontinuation of therapy in some patients (101,115).

3. Infection

Two randomized studies have shown that the incidence or severity of bacterial, fungal, and nonpulmonary viral infections does not appear to be increased in patients receiving antithymocyte globulin as GVHD prophylaxis (115) or treatment (101). In a retrospective analysis of 545 marrow transplant recipients, however, the use of antithymocyte globulin for treatment of established acute GVHD was associated with a 1.9 times greater risk of cytomegaloviral pneumonia in seropositive patients (117). This association was not observed in other subgroups of patients, such as those receiving prophylactic antithymocyte globulin or those who were seronegative for cytomegalovirus. Similar associations between antithymocyte globulin use and an increased risk of cytomegalovirus infection have been observed in renal transplant recipients (118,119). It is not clear whether this increased risk of cytomegalovirus infection is related to a specific effect of antithymocyte globulin or merely to a greater degree of generalized immunosuppression.

VI. CONCLUSIONS

Potent immunosuppressive drugs are usually given after allogeneic marrow transplantation as prophylaxis or treatment of GVHD. Many of the drugs have potentially serious toxicities and narrow therapeutic indexes. With the exception of cyclosporine, the pharmacology of drugs used in marrow transplantation have not been well characterized. Most drug regimens have been designed empirically, and additional studies are needed to determine the optimal dosage schedules. Finally, further studies in man are needed to determine if monitoring of blood or plasma concentrations of these drugs can maximize the immunosuppressive activity and reduce the risk of serious toxicity.

REFERENCES

1. Sullivan KM, Deeg HJ, Sanders J, Klosterman A, Amos D, Shulman H, Sale G, Martin P, Witherspoon R, Appelbaum F, Doney K, Stewart P, Meyers J, McDonald GB, Weiden P, Fefer A, Buckner CD, Storb R, Thomas ED: Hyperacute graft-versus-host disease in patients not given immunosuppression after allogeneic marrow transplantation. Blood 1986;67:1172-1175.

2. Gale RP, Bortin MM, van Bekkum DW, Biggs JC, Dicke KA, Gluckman E, Good RA, Hoffmann RG, Day HEM, Kersey JH, Marmont A, Masaoka T, Rimm AA, van Rood JJ, Zwann FE: Risk factors for acute graft-versus-host disease. Br J Haematol 1987; 67:397-406.

3. Lazarus HM, Coccia PF, Herzig RH, Graham-Pole J, Gross S, Strandjord S, Gordon E, Cheung NKV, Warkentin PI, Spitzer TR, Warm SE: Incidence of acute graft-versus-host disease with and without methotrexate prophylaxis in allogeneic bone marrow transplant patients. Blood 1984;64:214-220.

4. Wegner R: Synthesis of cyclosporine and analogues: structure, activity, relationships of new cyclosporine derivatives. Transplant Proc 1983;15(Suppl 1):2230-2241.

5. Storb R, Deeg HJ, Fisher L, Appelbaum F, Buckner CD, Bensinger W, Clift R, Doney K, Irle C, McGuffin R, Martin P, Sanders J, Schoch G, Singer J, Stewart P, Sullivan K, Witherspoon R, Thomas ED: Cyclosporine versus methotrexate for graft-versus-host disease prevention in patients given marrow grafts for leukemia: long-term follow-up of three controlled trials. Blood 1988;71:293-298.

6. Storb R, Deeg HJ, Whitehead J, Appelbaum F, Beatty P, Bensinger W, Buckner CD, Clift R, Doney K, Farewell V, Hansen J, Hill R, Lum L, Martin P, McGuffin R, Sanders J, Stewart P, Sullivan K, Witherspoon R, Yee G, Thomas ED: Methotrexate and cyclosporine compared with cyclosporine alone for prophylaxis of acute graft-versus-host disease after marrow transplantation for leukemia. N Engl J Med 1986;314:729-735.

7. Santos GW, Tutschka PJ, Brookmeyer R, Saral R, Beschorner WE, Bias WB, Braine HG, Burns WH, Farmer ER, Hess AD, Kaizer H, Mellits D, Sensenbrenner LL, Stuart R, Yeager AM: Cyclosporine plus methylprednisolone versus cyclophosphamide plus methylprednisolone as prophylaxis for graft-versus-host disease: a randomized double-blind study in patients undergoing allogeneic marrow transplantation. Clin Transplant 1987;1:21-28.

8. Forman SJ, Blume KG, Krance RA, Miner PJ, Metter GE, Hill LR, O'Donnell MR, Nademanee AP, Snyder DS: A prospective randomized study of acute graft-versus-host disease in 107 patients with leukemia: methotrexate/prednisone versus cyclosporine A/prednisone. Transplant Proc 1987;19:2605-2607.

9. Kennedy MS, Deeg HJ, Storb R, Doney K, Sullivan KM, Witherspoon RP, Appelbaum FR, Stewart P, Sanders J, Buckner CD, Martin P, Weiden P, Thomas ED: Treatment of acute graft-versus-host disease after allogeneic marrow transplantation: randomized study comparing corticosteroids and cyclosporine. Amer J Med 1985;78:978-983.

10. Wood AJ, Maurer G, Niederberger W, Beveridge T: Cyclosporine: pharmacokinetics, metabolism, and drug interactions. Transplant Proc 1983;15(Suppl 1):2409-2412.

11. Yee GC, Kennedy MS, Storb R, Thomas ED: Effect of hepatic dysfunction on oral cyclosporine pharmacokinetics in marrow transplant patients. Blood 1984;64:1277-1279.

12. Atkinson K, Biggs JC, Britton K, Short R, Mrongovius R, Concannon A, Dodds A: Oral administration of cyclosporine A for recipients of allogeneic marrow transplant: implications of clinical gut dysfunction. Br J Haematol 1984;56:223-231.

13. Yee GC, Kennedy MS, Storb R, Thomas ED: Pharmacokinetics of intravenous cyclosporine in bone marrow transplant patients: comparison of two assay methods. Transplantation 1984;38:511-513.

14. Yee GC, Lennon TP, Gmur DJ, Kennedy MS, Deeg HJ: Age-dependent cyclosporine pharmacokinetics in marrow transplant recipients. Clin Pharmacol Ther 1986; 40:438-443.

15. Yee GC, McGuire TR, Gmur DJ, Lennon TP, Deeg HJ: Blood cyclosporine pharma-

cokinetics in patients undergoing marrow transplantation: influence of age, obesity, and hematocrit. Transplantation 1988;46:399-402.

16. Atkinson K, Boland J, Britton J, Biggs J: Blood and tissue distribution of cyclosporine in humans and mice. Transplant Proc 1983;15(Suppl 1):2430-2433.
17. Gurecki J, Warty V, Sanghvi A: The transport of cyclosporine in association with plasma lipoproteins in heart and liver transplant patients. Transplant Proc 1985; 17:1997-2002.
18. Lemaire M, Tillement JP: Role of lipoproteins and erythrocytes in the in vitro binding and distribution of cyclosporin A in the blood. J Pharm Pharmacol 1982;34:715-718.
19. Mraz W, Zink RA, Graf A, Preis D, Illner WD, Land W, Siebert W, Zottlein H: Distribution and transfer of cyclosporine among the various human lipoprotein classes. Transplant Proc 1983;15:2462-2429.
20. Nemunaitis J, Deeg HJ, Yee GC: High cyclosporin levels after bone marrow transplantation associated with hypertriglyceridemia. Lancet 1986; ii:744-745.
21. Lindholm A, Henricsson S, Gang P: The free fraction of cyclosporine in plasma : clinical findings with a new method. Transplant Proc 1988;20(Suppl 2):377-381.
22. Schaefer EJ, Levy RI: Pathogenesis and management of lipoprotein disorders. N Engl J Med 1985;312:1300-1310.
23. Awni WM, Sawchuk R: The pharmacokinetics of cyclosporine. II. Blood-plasma distribution and binding studies. Drug Metab Dispos 1985;13:133-138.
24. Yee GC, Lennon TP, Gmur DJ, Cheney CL, Deeg HJ: Effect of obesity on cyclosporine disposition. Transplantation 1988;45:649-651.
25. Maurer G: Metabolism of cyclosporine. Transplant Proc 1985;17(Suppl 1):19-26.
26. Yee GC, Gmur DJ, Meier P: Measurement of blood cyclosporine metabolite concentrations with a new column-switching high-performance liquid chromatographic assay. Transplant Proc 1988;20(Suppl 2):585-590.
27. Rosano TG, Freed BM, Cerilli J, Lempert N: Immunosuppressive metabolites of cyclosporine in the blood of renal allograft recipients. Transplantation 1986;42: 262-267.
28. Freed BM, Rosano TG, Lempert N: In vitro immunosuppressive properties of cyclosporine metabolites. Transplantation 1987;43:123-127.
29. Yee GC, Kennedy MS, Gmur DJ, Self SG, Deeg HJ: Monitoring cyclosporin concentrations in marrow transplant recipients: comparison of two assay methods. Bone Marrow Transplantation 1987;1:289-295.
30. Shulman HM, McDonald GB: In *The Pathology of Bone Marrow Transplantation*, Ch. 7., edited by Sale GE, Shulman HM. Masson, New York, 1984; pp. 104-135.
31. Gibaldi M, Koup JR: Pharmacokinetic concepts—drug binding, apparent volume of distribution and clearance. Eur J Clin Pharmacol 1981;20:299-305.
32. Yee GC, Kennedy MS: Cyclosporine. In *Applied Pharmacokinetics: Principles of Therapeutic Drug Monitoring*, edited by Evans WE, Schentag JJ, Jusko WJ. Applied Therapeutics, Spokane WA, 1986, pp. 826-851.
33. Scott JP, Higenbottam TW: Adverse reactions and interactions of cyclosporin. Med Toxicol 1988;3:107-127.
34. Wadhwa NK, Schroeder TJ, Pesce AJ, Myre SA, Clardy CW, First MR: Cyclosporine drug interactions: a review. Ther Drug Monitor 1987;9:399-406.
35. Cockburn I: Cyclosporine A: a clinical evaluation of drug interactions. Transplant Proc 1986;18(Suppl 5):50-55.
36. Gupta SK, Bakran A, Johnson RWG, Rowland M: Erythromycin enhances the absorption of cyclosporin. Br J Clin Pharmacol 1988;25:401-402.
37. Jensen CWB, Flechner SM, Van Buren CT, Frazier OH, Cooley DA, Lorber MI, Kahan BD: Exacerbation of cyclosporine toxicity by concomitant administration of erythromycin. Transplantation 1987;43:263-270.

38. Martell R, Heinrichs D, Stiller CR, Jenner M, Keown PA, Dupre J: The effects of erythromycin in patients receiving cyclosporine. Annal Intern Med 1986;104:660-661.
39. Beveridge T, Gratwohl A, Michot F, Niederberger W, Nuesch E, Nussbaumer K, Schaub P, Speck B: Cyclosporin A: pharmacokinetics after a single dose in man and serum levels after multiple dosing in recipients of allogeneic bone-marrow grafts. Curr Ther Res 1981;30:5-18.
40. Yee GC, Mills G, Schaffer RS, Lennon TP, Kennedy MS, Deeg HJ: Renal cyclosporine clearance in marrow transplant recipients: age-related variation. J Clin Pharmacol 1986;26:658-661.
41. Bennett WM, Pulliam JP: Cyclosporine nephrotoxicity. Annal Intern Med 1983;99: 851-854.
42. Humes HD, Jackson NM, O'Connor RP, Hunt DA, White MD: Pathogenetic mechanisms of nephrotoxicity: insights into cyclosporine nephrotoxicity. Transplant Proc 1985;17(Suppl 1):51-62.
43. Myers BD: Cyclosporine nephrotoxicity. Kid International 1986;30:964-974.
44. Yee GC, Kennedy MS, Deeg HJ, Leonard TM, Thomas ED, Storb R: Cyclosporine-associated renal dysfunction in marrow transplant recipients. Transplant Proc 1985;17:196-201.
45. Kennedy MS, Deeg HJ, Siegel M, Crowley JJ, Storb R, Thomas ED: Acute renal toxicity with combined use of amphotericin B and cyclosporine after marrow transplantation. Transplantation 1983;35:211-215.
46. Kennedy MS, Yee GC, McGuire TR, Leonard TM, Crowley JJ, Deeg HJ: Correlation of serum cyclosporine concentration with renal dysfunction in marrow transplant recipients. Transplantation 1985;40:249-253.
47. Hows JM, Chipping PM, Fairhead S, Smith J, Baughan A, Gordon-Smith EC: Nephrotoxicity in bone marrow transplant recipients treated with cyclosporin A. Br J Haematol 1983;54:69-78.
48. Shepp DH, Dandiker PS, Meyers JD: Treatment of varicella-zoster virus infections in severely immunocompromised patients: a randomized comparison of acyclovir and vidarabine. N Engl J Med 1986;314:208.
49. English J, Evan A, Houghton DC, Bennett WM: Cyclosporine-induced renal dysfunction in the rat: evidence for arteriolar vasoconstriction with preservation of tubular function. Transplantation 1987;44:135-141.
50. Murray BM, Paller MS, Ferris TF: Effect of cyclosporine administration on renal hemodynamics in conscious rats. Kid Intern 1985;28:767-774.
51. Shulman H, Striker G, Deeg HJ, Kennedy M, Storb R, Thomas ED: Nephrotoxicity of cyclosporin A after allogeneic marrow transplantation. N Engl J Med 1981;305: 1392-1395.
52. Myers BD, Ross J, Newton L, Luetscher J, Perlroth M: Cyclosporine-associated chronic nephropathy. N Engl J Med 1984;311:699-705.
53. Yee GC, McGuire TR, St. Pierre BA, Self SG, Zager RA, Sullivan KM, Deeg HJ: Minimal risk of chronic renal dysfunction in marrow transplant recipients treated with cyclosporine for 6 months. Bone Marrow Transplant 1989;4:691-694.
54. Gratwohl A, Lori A, Osterwalder B, Nissen C, Speck B: Low incidence of nephrotoxicity in long-term recipients of cyclosporine following bone marrow transplantation. Transplant Proc 1986;18:1434-1436.
55. Loughran TP, Deeg HJ, Dahlberg S, Kennedy MS, Storb R, Thomas ED: Incidence of hypertension after marrow transplantation among 112 patients randomized to either cyclosporine or methotrexate as graft-versus-host disease prophylaxis. Br J Haematol 1985;59:547-553.
56. Bennett WM, Porter GA: Cyclosporine-associated hypertension. Am J Med 1988; 85:131-132.

57. June CH, Thompson CB, Kennedy MS, Loughran TP, Deeg HJ: Correlation of hypomagnesemia with the onset of cyclosporine-associated hypertension in marrow transplant patients. Transplantation 1986;41:47-51.
58. Curtis JJ, Luke RG, Jones P, Diethelm AG: Hypertension in cyclosporine-treated renal transplant recipients is sodium dependent. Am J Med 1988;85:134-138.
59. Tallman MS, Nemunaitis JJ, McGuire TR, Yee GC, Hughes TE, Almgren JD, Appelbaum FR, Higano CS, McGuffin RW, Singer JW, Thomas ED: Comparison of two intravenous cyclosporine infusion schedules in marrow transplant recipients. Transplantation 1988;45:810-813.
60. Atkinson K, Biggs J, Darveniza P, Boland J, Concannon A, Dodds A: Cyclosporine-associated central nervous system toxicity after allogeneic bone marrow transplantation. Transplantation 1984;38:34-37.
61. Thompson CB, June CH, Sullivan KM, Thomas ED: Association between cyclosporin neurotoxicity and hypomagnesaemia. Lancet 1984; ii:1116-1120.
62. Labar B, Bogdanic V, Plavsic F, Francetic I, Dobric I, Kastelan A, Grgicevic D, Vrtar M, Grgic-Markulin L, Balabanic-Kamauf B, Boban D, Kerhin-Brkljacic V, Boranic M: Cyclosporin neurotoxicity in patients treated with allogeneic bone marrow transplantation. Biomed Pharmacother 1986;40:148-150.
63. Barrett AJ, Kendry JR, Lucas CF, Joss DV, Joshi R, Pendharker P, Hugh-Jones K: Cyclosporin A as prophylaxis against graft-versus-host disease in 36 patients. Br Med J 1982;285:162-166.
64. De Groen PC, Aksamit AJ, Rakela J, Forbes GS, Krom RAF: Central nervous system toxicity after liver transplantation: the role of cyclosporine and cholesterol. N Engl J Med 1987;317:861-866.
65. Deeg HJ, Shulman HM, Schmidt E, Yee GC, Thomas ED, Storb R: Marrow graft rejection and veno-occlusive disease of the liver in patients with aplastic anemia conditioned with cyclophosphamide and cyclosporine. Transplantation 1986;42:497-502.
66. Deeg HJ, Storb R, Thomas ED, Flournoy N, Kennedy MS, Banaji M, Appelbaum FR, Bensinger WI, Buckner CD, Clift RA, Doney K, Fefer A, McGuffin R, Sanders JE, Singer J, Stewart P, Sullivan KM, Witherspoon RP: Cyclosporine as prophylaxis for graft-versus-host disease: a randomized study in patients undergoing marrow transplantation for acute nonlymphoblastic leukemia. Blood 1985;65:1325-1334.
67. Storb R, Deeg HJ, Thomas ED, Appelbaum FR, Buckner CD, Clift RA, Doney KC, Flournoy N, Kennedy MS, Loughran TP, McGuffin RW, Sale GE, Sanders JE, Singer JW, Stewart PS, Sullivan KM, Witherspoon RP: Marrow transplantation for chronic myelocytic leukemia: a controlled trial of cyclosporine versus methotrexate for prophylaxis of graft-versus-host disease. Blood 1985;66:698-702.
68. Irle C, Deeg HJ, Buckner CD, Kennedy M, Clift R, Storb R, Appelbaum FR, Beatty P, Bensinger W, Doney K, Cheever M, Fefer A, Greenberg P, Hill R, Martin P, McGuffin R, Sanders J, Stewart P, Sullivan K, Witherspoon R, Thomas ED: Marrow transplantation for leukemia following fractionated total body irradiation. A comparative trial of methotrexate and cyclosporine. Leuk Res 1985;9:1255-1261.
69. Lennon TP, Yee GC, Kennedy MS, Torok-Storb B, Burstein SA, Deeg HJ: Monitoring of cyclosporine therapy with in vitro biological assays. Transplantation 1987; 44:799-804.
70. National Academy of Clinical Biochemistry/American Association for Clinical Chemistry Task Force on Cyclosporine Monitoring: Critical issues in cyclosporine monitoring: report of the task force on cyclosporine monitoring. Clin Chem 1987;33: 1269-1288.
71. Burckhart GJ, Canafax DC, Yee GC: Monitoring cyclosporine concentration. Drug Intell Clin Pharm 1986;20:649-652.

72. Shaw LM: Cyclosporine Monitoring. Clin Chem 1989;35:5-6.
73. Hess AD, Colombani PM: Cyclosporine mechanism of action: in-vitro studies. Prog Allergy 1986;38:198-221.
74. Keown PA, Stiller CR, Ulan RA, Sinclair NR, Wall WJ, Carruthers G, Howson W: Immunological and pharmacological monitoring in the clinical use of cyclosporin A. Lancet 1981;i:686-689.
75. Gluckman E, Lokiec F, Devergie A: Pharmacokinetic monitoring of cyclosporine in allogeneic bone marrow transplants. Transplant Proc 1984;17:500-501.
76. Yee GC, Self SG, McGuire TR, Carlin J, Sanders JE, Deeg HJ: Serum cyclosporine concentration and risk of acute graft-versus-host disease after allogeneic marrow transplantation. N Engl J Med 1988;319:65-70.
77. Beatty PG, Clift RA, Mickelson EM, Nisperos BB, Flournoy N, Martin PJ, Sanders JE, Stewart P, Buckner CD, Storb R, Thomas ED, Hansen JA: Marrow transplantation from related donors other than HLA-identical siblings. N Engl J Med 1985;313: 765-771.
78. Donatsch P, Abisch E, Homberger M, Traber R, Trapp M, Voges R: A radioimmunoassay to measure cyclosporin A in plasma and serum samples. J Immunoassay 1981; 2:19-32.
79. Wong PY, Mee AV, Taylor G, Uchimaru D, Sun C, Alspector F: Comparison of two radioimmunoassay kits for the determination of cyclosporine concentrations in transplantation. Transplant Proc 1988;20(Suppl 2):348-353.
80. Marsden JT, Johnston A, Holt DW: Monoclonal antibodies for the radioimmunoassay of cyclosporine. Transplant Proc 1988;20(Suppl 2):319-322.
81. Schran HF, Rosano TG, Hassell AE, Pell MA: Determination of cyclosporrine concentrations with monoclonal antibodies. Clin Chem 1987;33:2225-2229.
82. Sanghvi A, Divan W, Seltman H, Starzl T: Abbott's fluorescence polarization immunoassay for cyclosporine and metabolites compared with the Sandox "Sandimmune" RIA. Clin Chem 1988;34:1904-1906.
83. Schroeder TJ, Pesce AJ, Hassan FM, Wermeling JR, Warner A, Schlueter KT, First MR: Comparison of Abbott TDx fluorescence polarization immunoassay, Sandoz immunoassay, and high-performance liquid chromatography methods for the assay of serum cyclosporine. Transplant Proc 1988;20(Suppl 2):345-347.
84. Rosano TG, Pell MA, Freed BM, Dybas MT, Lempert N: Cyclosporine and metabolites in blood from renal allograft recipients with nephrotoxicity, rejection, or good renal function: comparative high-performance liquid chromatography and monoclonal raadioimmunoassay studies. Transplant Proc 1988;20(Suppl 2):330-338.
85. McGuire TR, Yee GC, Carlin J: unpublished data.
86. Weinstein GD: Methotrexate. Annal Intern Med 1977;86:199-204.
87. Willkens RF, Watson MA: Methotrexate: a perspective of its use in the treatment of rheumatic diseases. J Lab Clin Med 1982;100:314-321.
88. Evans WE, Crom WR, Yalowich JC: Methotrexate. In *Applied Pharmacokinetics: Principles of Therapeutic Drug Monitoring*, edited by Evans WE, Schentag JJ, Jusko WJ. Applied Therapeutics, Spokane, WA, 1986.
89. Pinkerton CR, Welshman SG, Kelly JG, Shanks RG, Bridges JM: Pharmacokinetics of low-dose methotrexate in children receiving maintenance therapy for acute lymphoblastic leukemia. Cancer Chemother Pharmacol 1982;10:36-39.
90. Balis FM, Savitch JL, Bleyer WA: Pharmacokinetics of oral methotrexate in children. Cancer Res 1983;43:2342-2345.
91. Campbell MA, Perrier DG, Dorr RT, Alberts DS, Finley PR: Methotrexate: bioavailability and pharmacokinetics. Cancer Treat Rep 1985;69:833-838.

92. Henderson ES, Adamson RH, Oliverio VT: The metabolic fate of tritiated methotrexate. II. Absorption and excretion in man. Cancer Res 1965;25:1018-1024.

93. Huffman DH, Wan SH, Azarnoff DL, Hoogstraten B: Pharmacokinetics of methotrexate. Clin Pharmacol Ther 1973;14:572-579.

94. Evans WE, Pratt CB: Effect of pleural effusion on high-dose methotrexate kinetics. Clin Pharmacol Ther 1978;23:68-72.

95. Wan SH, Huffman DH, Azarnoff DL, Stephens R, Hoogstraten B: Effect of route of administration and effusions on methotrexate pharmacokinetics. Cancer Res 1974;34:3487-3491.

96. Jacobs SA, Bleyer WA, Chabner BA, Johns DG: Altered plasma pharmacokinetics of methotrexate administered intrathecally. Lancet 1975; i:465-466.

97. Strum WB, Liem HH: Hepatic uptake, intracellular protein binding, and biliary excretion of amethopterin. Biochem Pharmacol 1977;26:1235-1240.

98. Van Den Berg HW, Murphy RF, Kennedy DG: Rapid plasma clearance and reduced rate and extent of urinary elimination of parenterally administered methotrexate as a result of severe vomiting and diarrhea. Cancer Chemother Pharmacol 1980;4:47-48.

99. Storb R, Deeg HJ, Farewell V, Doney K, Appelbaum F, Beatty P, Bensinger W, Buckner CD, Clift R, Hansen J, Hill R, Longton G, Lum L, Martin P, McGuffin R, Sanders J, Singer J, Stewart P, Sullivan K, Witherspoon R, Thomas ED: Marrow transplantation for severe aplastic anemia: methotrexate alone compared with a combination of methotrexate and cyclosporine for prevention of acute graft-versus-host disease. Blood 1986;68:119-125.

100. Weiner RS, Bortin MM, Gale RP, Gluckman E, Kay HEM, Kolb HJ, Hartz AJ, Rimm AA: Interstitial pneumonitis after bone marrow transplantation: assessment of risk factors. Annal Intern Med 1986;104:168-175.

101. Doney KC, Weiden PL, Storb R, Thomas ED: Treatment of graft-versus-host disease in human allogeneic marrow graft recipients: a randomized trial comparing antithymocyte globulin and corticosteroids. Amer J Hematol 1981;11:1-8.

102. Pickup ME: Clinical pharmacokinetics of prednisone and prednisolone. Clin Pharmacokin 1979;4:111-128.

103. Gambertoglio JG, Amend WJC, Benet LZ: Pharmacokinetics and bioavailability of prednisone and prednisolone in healthy volunteers and patients: a review. J Pharmacokin Biopharm 1980;8:1-52.

104. Jusko WJ, Rose JQ: Monitoring prednisone and prednisolone. Ther Drug Monitor 1980;2:169-176.

105. Shaunwhite WR, Sandberg AA: Disposition of radioactive 17α-hydroxy-progesterone, 6α-methyl-17α-acetoxyprogesterone and 6α-methylprednisolone in human subjects. J Clin Endocrinol Metab 1971;21:753-764.

106. Derendorf H, Mollmann H, Rohdewald P, Rehder J, Schmidt EW: Kinetics of methylprednisolone and its hemisuccinate ester. Clin Pharmacol Ther 1985;37:502-507.

107. Antal EJ, Wright CE, Gillespie WR, Albert KS: Influence of route of administration on the pharmacokinetics of methylprednisolone. J Pharmacokin Biopharm 1983;11:561-576.

108. Mollmann H, Rohdewald P, Barth J, Mollmann C, Verho M, Derendorf H: Comparative pharmacokinetics of methylprednisolone phosphate and hemisuccinate in high doses. Pharmaceu Res 1988;5:509-513.

109. Narang PK, Wilder R, Chatterji DC, Yeager RL, Gallelli JF: Systemic bioavailability and pharmacokinetics of methylprednisolone in patients with rheumatoid arthritis following "high-dose" pulse administration. Biopharm Drug Dispos 1983; 4:233-248.

110. Rose JQ, Yurchak AM, Jusko WJ: Dose dependent pharmacokinetics of predni-
     sone and prednisolone in man. J Pharmacokin Biopharm 1981;9:389-417.
111. Bacigalupo A, van Lint MT, Frassoni F, Pedesta M, Veneziano G, Avanzi G, Vitale
     V, Marmont AM: High dose bolus methylprednisolone for the treatment of acute
     graft-versus-host disease. Blut 1983;46:125-132.
112. Kanojia MD, Anagnostou A, Zander AR, Vellekoop L, Spitzer G, Verma DS,
     Jagannath S, Dicke KA: High-dose methylprednisolone treatment for acute graft-
     versus-host disease after bone marrow transplantation in adults. Transplantation
     1984;37:246-249.
113. The Upjohn Company: Drug reference: Atgam®, Kalamazoo, MI, 1981.
114. Ramsay NKC, Kersey JH, Robison LL, McGlave PB, Woods WG, Krivit W, Kim TH,
     Goldman AI, Nesbit ME: A randomized study of the prevention of acute graft-
     versus-host disease. N Engl J Med 1982;306:392-397.
115. Weiden PL, Doney K, Storb R, Thomas ED: Antihuman thymocyte globulin for
     prophylaxis of graft-versus-host disease. Transplantation 1979;27:227-230.
116. Storb R, Gluckman E, Thomas ED, Buckner CD, Clift RA, Fefer A, Glucksberg
     H, Graham TC, Johnson FL, Lerner KG, Neiman PE, Ochs H: Treatment of es-
     tablished human graft-versus-host disease by antithymocyte globulin. Blood 1974;
     44:57-75.
117. Meyers JD, Flournoy N, Thomas ED: Risk factors for cytomegalovirus infection
     with human marrow transplantation. J Infect Dis 1986;153:478-488.
118. Pass RF, Whitley RJ, Diethelm AG et al.: Cytomegalovirus infection in patients
     with renal transplants: potentiation by antithymocyte globulin and an incom-
     patible graft. J Infect Dis 1980;142:9-17.
119. Rubin RH, Cosimi AB, Hirsch MS, et al.: Effects of antithymocyte globulin on
     cytomegalovirus infection in renal transplant recipients. Transplantation 1981;
     31:143-145.

28

Infections in Patients with Graft-vs.-Host Disease

Raleigh A. Bowden
Fred Hutchinson Cancer Research Center
University of Washington
Seattle, Washington

I. INTRODUCTION

Infections remain a major cause of morbidity and mortality after allogeneic marrow transplantation (1). One of the major risk factors for the development of infection is the presence of Graft-vs.-Host Disease (GVHD) (2). The risk of particular infections with respect to GVHD is thought to be related not only to the immunosuppressive nature of GVHD but to the additional immunosuppression associated with the treatment required for this disease. Patients with GVHD usually do not die of target organ failure but rather of the complications of associated infections.

Bacterial, viral, and fungal infections occur in a very predictable manner during the months that follow marrow transplant (see Table 1). The factors in host defense which influence these patterns presumably include a balance between the recovery of normal granulocyte and lymphocyte function and the ongoing immunosuppressive influence of GVHD, the treatments used to prevent or control it, or both.

This chapter will focus on the types of infections seen and the factors associated with increased infectious risk in acute GVHD following marrow transplant. Specific attention will include comparisons between infections in patients with and without GVHD. The relationship between specific modalities used to prevent or treat GVHD and specific types of infections will also be discussed. The primary emphasis will be on bacterial, fungal, and parasitic infections during acute GVHD, although a brief summary of viral infections and infections associated with chronic GVHD is included. The reader should refer to other chapters in this volume for more details in these later specific areas. Finally, an approach to prevention and treatment of infections in patients with GVHD will also be discussed.

Table 1 The Relationship Between Types of Infections, GVHD, and Time After Marrow Transplant

	Months after transplant						
	1	2	3	4	5	6-12	12-18

————Acute GVHD———   ———Chronic GVHD———————————————————————>

Bacteria
————Gram-negative enteric organisms————————————————————————————>
                                        ————encapsulated organisms————————————>
————Coagulase-positive————
    staphlococcus
————Coagulase-negative—————————
    staphlococcus

Fungi
————Candida———————— ——————————————————————————————————————>
————————Aspergillus—————————>

Viruses
————HSV————————————VZV————————VZV————————————————————————>
—————————CMV————————————————————>
————EBV?————————
————Adenovirus————

Parasites
————Toxoplasmosis————————
————Pneumocystis ———————————————————>

Abbreviations: GVHD = Graft-vs.-Host Disease. HSV = herpes simplex virus. CMV = cytomegalovirus. EBV = Epstein-Barr virus. The solid line (——) signifies the time period during which the majority of infections are observed, and the broken line (— — —) signnifies the time when infection occurs less frequently.

II. INFECTIONS IN PATIENTS WITH ACUTE GVHD

A. Bacterial and Fungal Infections

The risk of bacterial infections after transplant is highest immediately following transplant during the period of neutropenia. The neutropenic period generally lasts for 3-4 weeks following marrow infusion until the absolute neutrophil count is $\geq 500/mm^3$. When patients develop infections with bacteria during this early period, it is usually with gram-negative enteric organisms, gram-positive mouth flora or with either gram-positive or gram-negative organisms colonizing the skin. The major risk factors contributing to the increase in these infections include not only neutropenia but the breakdown of integumentary barriers, specifically the gastrointestinal tract, from the conditioning regimens used for transplant, and the skin from either side effects of conditioning or from the intravascular catheters placed to assist in supportive care.

The spectrum of bacterial pathogens has changed following marrow transplantation since the early 1970s. Previously, gram-negative organisms including the enterobacteriaceae and pseudomonas accounted for 71% of bacteremias observed (1). More recently, gram-positive organisms, including both coagulase-positive and -negative staphylococci have accounted for 61% of bloodborne infections after marrow transplant (1). However, the proportion of gram-negative infections may be proportionally higher in patients with acute GVHD compared to those without acute GVHD because active gastrointestinal tract GVHD may continue to provide a source of entry for these organisms. The increase in the proportion of coagulase-negative staphylococci is thought to be the result of more aggressive use of antimicrobial agents which has reduced the proportion of gram-negative organisms, leading to an increase in the proportion of catheter-associated gram-positive organisms. Fortunately, despite its frequency, coagulase-negative staphylococcus is a relatively nonvirulent organism and is not a major cause of life-threatening infection, although shock and hypotension have been observed in association with this infection.

Fungal infections are also common during this period. Colonization of the gastro-intestinal tract is seen frequently, and the risk of invasive bloodstream and systemic organ involvement increases with the duration of neutropenia and the use of broad spectrum antibiotics. Candida species are the most common cause of fungal infection. In our institution, *C. albicans* accounts for approximately half and *C. tropicalis* for one quarter of infections with other species making up the remainder.

The median time of onset of GVHD occurs during the first month after transplant, and because of this, differences in the types of severity of bacterial infections during the first month in patients with and without acute GVHD may not be apparent. However, the risk of bacterial and fungal infections may be prolonged in patients with acute GVHD for several reasons. First, the presence of skin or gastrointestinal disease may result in the breakdown of barriers of host defense against the normal bacterial organisms that inhabit the skin and gastrointestinal tract. Patients with severe GVHD of the skin may have infection problems similar to burn patients with sepsis originating from normal skin flora or from colonization with hospital-acquired gram-negative organisms. Patients with severe gastrointestinal disease have persistent portals of entry for intestinal organisms and may be at particular risk for polymicrobial sepsis.

Second, GVHD may have an effect on the function of neutrophils even after the neutrophils return in adequate numbers to protect against infection. Neutrophils appear to be important for the prevention and elimination of both bacterial and fungal infections. Clark et al. found decreased chemotactic activity, more pronounced in patients with acute GVHD or in patients who had received goat or rabbit antithymocyte globulin (ATG) (3). Sosa found a similar association with GVHD but not with horse ATG (4).

Third, because of the persistent fever often associated with acute GVHD, patients with GVHD frequently remain on broad spectrum antibiotics for prolonged periods of time. This may increase the risk of bacterial infection by interfering with the balance of normal flora in the gastrointestinal tract or by resulting in an increase in the frequency of antibiotic resistant organisms.

Patients with acute GVHD may be at particular risk for invasive fungal infection for several additional reasons. First, as with bacterial infections, involvement of the gastro-intestinal tract with GVHD provides a portal of entry for colonizing organisms, and the prolonged use of antibiotics results in the potential for fungal overgrowth in the gastro-intestinal tract and genital area. Second, in addition to the importance of granulocytes as a mechanism of host defense against fungal infection, cell-mediated immune responses may also be important against invasive fungal infection, although the specific contribution has not been defined. These responses may be persistently abnormal in patients with GVHD. An increase in fungal infections has been observed in patients receiving T-cell-depleted marrow (5). One might suspect that other forms of T-cell immunosuppressive therapy such as the use of antithymocyte globulin, for example, are associated with an increase in fungal infections, but these studies have not been performed.

And finally, an increase in bacterial or fungal infections may also be in part due to the immunosuppressive effects of other infections. For example, it is not uncommon to see an increase in bacterial or fungal infections in patients with cytomegalovirus infection, an infection closely associated with GVHD (see below) (2,6).

While recovery of neutrophils is clearly important to reducing the incidence of bacterial infection during the early posttransplant period, an adequate number of neutrophils alone are not enough to ensure protection. Unless acute GVHD is brought under control, the abnormalities in the skin and gastrointestinal tract barriers continue as a risk for bacterial as well as fungal infection.

B. Prevention and Treatment of Bacterial and Fungal Infection During the Period of Acute GVHD

The mainstay of prevention of the morbidity and mortality of bacterial infection after transplant has been the early institution of empiric systemic antibiotics when fever develops. Patients with acute GVHD may be particular management problems since they often have persistent fever without a clear source. In general, the best approach in these patients is to initiate treatment with empiric broad spectrum antibiotics with activity against gram-negative enteric organisms during febrile periods and continue treatment until engraftment occurs. Once patients are able to maintain an absolute neutrophil count above $500/mm^3$, they should be cultured carefully when fever occurs and placed on an empiric antibiotic regimen only until all cultures prove negative (usually 48 to 72 hours). Other causes of fever, such as recrudescence of GVHD or viral infections, should also be investigated.

The use of a total protective environment including a laminar air flow room, oral nonabsorbable antibiotics, sterile food, and skin decontamination have also been shown to reduce the incidence of bacterial infection (7). There is evidence that the prevention of bacterial infections may also have an effect on the development of GVHD. Studies in mice have suggested that decontamination in the early posttransplant period may delay the onset of acute GVHD (8). The mechanisms for this phenomenon are unknown, but gram-negative bacteria seem to play an important role. After human marrow transplantation, a delay in acute GVHD in patients with aplastic anemia managed in a protected environment has been reported (9). This topic is discussed in more detail elsewhere in this volume. The cost of such an approach is high and may not be justified in all cases until the effect on long-term survival has been established. The use of nonabsorbable antibiotics outside the protected environment is of unknown benefit.

Other forms of antibacterial prophylaxis have been or are currently being evaluated. The use of prophylactic granulocytes has given conflicting results in the past (10,11) and is not used routinely in most centers. Weekly intravenous globulin during the first several months after transplant has been used in some centers to prevent a variety of infections, and results have varied (12). In an analysis of the incidence of bacterial infections occurring in conjunction with the administration of CMV immunoglobulin for the prevention of CMV infection, septicemia was 2.1 times more likely to develop in patients not receiving CMV immunoglobulin compared to patients receiving no prophylaxis following engraftment (p = 0.039) (13). A similar controlled trial at UCLA showed that standard intravenous immunoglobulin had no effect on the development of bacterial, fungal, or viral infections (14). The role of oral immunoglobulin given as daily prophylaxis during the first month after transplant to prevent infections has been considered (15), but its efficacy has not been established.

Amphotericin B remains the treatment of choice for suspected or proven fungal infection and is often used empirically for patients with fever which is unresponsive to broad spectrum antibiotics. The mortality from fungemia with tissue involvement in our center is particularly high. When tissue involvement occurs, it involves multiple organs in over half of patients with a mortality rate of greater than 90%. Oral nonabsorbable antifungal agents such as nystatin or chlotrimazole are used as prophylaxis in most centers during the preengraftment period without specific data about their efficacy.

C. Viral Infections During Acute GVHD

Herpesvirus infections, including herpes simplex virus (HSV), cytomegalovirus (CMV), and varicella-zoster virus (VZV), continue to be the most common causes of viral infections after marrow transplant despite recent advances in antiviral therapy (1). Because the reconstitution of normal lymphocyte function is critical to both the prevention of reactivation of the herpesviruses as well as to the recovery from infection, it would appear likely that GVHD would have a major impact on the incidence and severity of these infections.

1. Herpes Simplex Virus (HSV) Infection

HSV infection develops primarily from reactivation of latent virus in patients who are seropositive for HSV at the time of transplant (16). HSV infection occurs early after transplant with a median time of onset of 9 days in patients not receiving prophylactic acyclovir and 78 days in patients routinely receiving prophylaxis from the time of conditioning until day 30 after transplant. Prior to the use of acyclovir, HSV infection generally occurred before the onset of GVHD and because the incidence of HSV infection has been reduced from 68% to 20% with the routine use of acyclovir prophylaxis, the effect of GVHD on this infection is difficult to determine. However, because cell-mediated immunity appears to be critical to the control of herpesvirus infections after marrow transplant, it is likely that patients with GVHD are at higher risk of having ongoing problems with recurrent HSV infection than are patients without GVHD.

2. Cytomegalovirus (CMV) Infection

CMV infection remains the major cause of infectious morbidity and mortality during the first 100 days after allogeneic transplant. The median time of onset of infection is 7-9 weeks after transplant, with an 80% infection rate in patients who are CMV seropositive (17). The risk of CMV infection in patients who are seronegative has been dramatically reduced by the use of CMV seronegative blood products in patients with CMV seronegative donors but remains a significant problem in those with CMV seropositive marrow donors (18).

Approximately 30% of patients who become infected with CMV during the first 100 days after transplant will develop invasive CMV disease, usually CMV enteritis or pneumonia. Of those who develop pneumonia, the survival rate has improved substantially with treatment using ganciclovir in combination with CMV immunoglobulin (19), although the fatality rate remains at approximately 50% (31).

There is a clear association with the development of acute GVHD and the risk for CMV pneumonia (1,2,6). There has been ongoing debate as to whether CMV infection precedes and, therefore, increases the risk for GVHD or whether patients who develop GVHD are subsequently at risk for infection with CMV. An association between CMV and GVHD has also been implicated in graft rejection. An association of CMV infection and subsequent chronic GVHD has been described (20). More recently, Meyers et al. demonstrated in a study of more than 500 patients undergoing allogeneic transplant that the occurrence of acute GVHD significantly increases the risk of CMV infection and the risk of CMV pneumonia (5). In contrast, CMV did not increase the risk of either acute or chronic GVHD.

3. Other Viral Infections

Little is known about the incidence and severity of Epstein-Barr virus (EBV) infection after marrow transplant. This is due in part to the difficulty in culturing this virus and interpretation of serological changes with respect to EBV after transplant (21). Oro-pharyngeal shedding and seroconversion have been documented to occur in marrow transplant patients, but these patients usually do not have specific symptoms referrable to EBV infection (21,22). EBV has been associated with the lymphoproliferative dis-orders seen during the first 3 months after transplant (23-25). The true incidence is unknown but proably is less than 1% in patients undergoing allogeneic marrow trans-plantation (24). As with the other herpesviruses, the only clear risk factors for the development of EBV lymphoproliferative disorder have been occurrence of acute GVHD (24,25), treatment with anti-T-cell monoclonal antibodies (23,24), and T-cell depletion (24).

Adenovirus infection occurs in approximately 5% of patients undergoing marrow transplantation (26). As many as one fifth of patients will develop invasive tissue infec-tion of lung, liver, or kidney with a high mortality rate. The only risk factor which has been identified for the development of adenovirus after marrow transplant has been the presence of moderate-to-severe GVHD.

D. Prevention and Treatment of Viral Infections in Patients with Acute GVHD

The major effort in prevention and treatment strategies against viral infections during the first 3 months after transplant have been directed at HSV and CMV infections. It is quite clear that acyclovir given intravenously twice a day (27) or orally (28) from the time of conditioning until day 30 after transplant can effectively prevent HSV infection in more than 90% of patients. Although reactivation often occurs after discontinuing prophy-laxis, it is often not necessary to treat patients with systemic acyclovir, thus allowing expo-sure to viral antigens important for immunologic reconstitution required to prevent sub-sequent reactivations.

Prevention of CMV infection has been more difficult, especially in patients who are CMV seropositive or who are seronegative with a seropositive marrow donor at the time of transplant. For patients who are CMV seronegative with a seronegative marrow donor, the use of CMV seronegative blood products can effectively prevent CMV infection in more than 95% of patients (29). The use of CMV hyperimmune globulin in seronegative patients with seronegative or seropositive marrow donors remains contoversial. While earlier studies showed complete protection against acquisition of primary CMV infection (30), subsequent studies have shown a protective benefit in reducing the incidence of pneumonia but not CMV infection itself (14,29).

Ganciclovir (DHPG) has demonstrated antiviral activity against CMV in vitro and has been shown to successfully treat CMV retinitis in patients with acquired immuno-deficiency syndrome. It is not know whether ganciclovir can be safely used to prevent CMV infection early after transplant, in part because its major side effect is marrow toxicity. Ganciclovir when used in combination with CMV immunoglobulin to treat CMV pneumonia has recently been shown to improve survival from 15% (17) to 52% (19).

III. INFECTIONS IN PATIENTS WITH CHRONIC GVHD

A. Bacterial and Fungal Infections in Patients with Chronic GVHD

Although bacterial infections in most patients occur during the early posttransplant period, patients with chronic GVHD continue to have problems with bacterial infections. In fact, bacterial infections are a major cause of late infectious deaths in patients with chronic GVHD.

Patients with chronic GVHD have persistent problems with host defense barriers due to mucosal atrophy and decreased lubrication of mucosal surfaces (sicca syndrome) as well as decreased or absent secretory IgA, decreased opsonizing antibody, and functional neutrophil defects (31). The most common cause of all bacterial infections is encapsulated bacteria, particularly with respect to infection of the sinuses and respiratory tract. The most common organisms are *Streptococcus pneumoniae* and *Haemophilus influenzae*, related presumably to the inability of B cells of patients with chronic GVHD to produce opsonizing antibody. Infections with *Staphylococcus aureus* are also seen in this setting.

The major bacterial infectious complications seen in patients with chronic GVHD are infections of the upper and lower respiratory tracts, skin infections, and septicemia (32). Sinusitis, otitis media, and bacterial pharyngitis are the most common sites of bacterial infection. Except for sinusitis, the organisms may be difficult to identify but often include gram-negative organisms as well as staphylococcus and pneumococcus. Pneumonia and bronchitis are also common and are seen with equal frequency. The most common causes are either *S. pneumoniae* or *S. aureus*. It remains unclear whether pulmonary complications are a cause or effect of the chronic obstructive and restrictive lung disease seen in some patients with chronic GVHD. Septicemia also remains a serious, though less frequent cause of infection in patients with chronic GVHD. Purulent conjunctivitis and cystitis are also seen with increased frequency in patients with chronic GVHD.

Fungal infections, the most common of which include the Candida species, are also increased in patients with chronic GVHD (33). These infections are generally localized to oral mucosal surfaces and rarely disseminate. Aspergillus and nocardia can also be seen in this setting. Treatment of chronic GVHD with azathioprine and corticosteroids likely contributes to the ongoing risk of fungal infection.

B. Viral Infections During Chronic GVHD

Patients with chronic GVHD have an increase in nonspecific suppressor cell activity which has been shown to suppress antigen-specific transformation responses (33) and may be related to the increase in both viral and fungal infections seen in patients with chronic GVHD. Humoral responses may also be delayed in patients with chronic GVHD (34).

Infection with varicella-zoster virus (VZV) is the most frequent viral infection during the period of chronic GVHD, with a median time of onset of 5 months (35). During the first year after transplant, the overall incidence of VZV infection is 30%, with 45% of patients with chronic GVHD experiencing this infection. In a review of 231 patients by Locksley et al., 80% of cases occurred within the first 9 months after transplant, during which time the risk of disseminated infection was 45% (35). Death, seen in patients who developed disseminated infection, also occurred only during the first 9 months after transplant, with a mortality rate of 5-10% before effective antiviral therapy became available. Significant risk factors for the development of VZV infection included allogeneic transplantation, acute GVHD, and chronic GVHD in patients surviving ≥90 days after transplant. Acute GVHD was also associated with the risk for disseminated VZV infection or death. The use of antithymocyte globulin as treatment for acute GVHD was also associated with a risk of subsequent VZV infection in patients surviving ≥90 days after transplant.

A distinct syndrome of fever, severe abdominal pain, nausea, and vomiting preceding the development of skin lesions was observed in 18 patients in this review, including 13 patients with GVHD (35). All but two of the patients were receiving prednisone as immunosuppressive therapy for GVHD. Ten patients developed herpes zoster in dermatomes T6-T12, and three of these subsequently developed disseminated infection. Eight patients developed a disseminated rash without dermatomal localization. Six patients died. Five of these patients underwent autopsy, which showed extensive visceral involvement in all cases.

In an analysis of infections in 89 aplastic anemia patients occurring more than 6 months after transplant, chronic GVHD associated with the presence of nonspecific suppressor cells was also found to predispose to late VZV infection but not to late non-VZV infections (32). The factor predisposing most strongly to VZV infection was genotypic nonidentity between marrow donor and recipient.

Although the most common viral infection after the first 100 days is VZV infection, patients with active chronic GVHD continue to be at risk for other herpesvirus infections, the most problematic of which is CMV pneumonia. In general, other viral infections, with the exception of CMV pneumonia, are not life threatening.

C. Prevention of Infection in Patients with Chronic GVHD

Treatment of infection in patients with chronic GVHD is guided by the organism identified. Infectious prophylaxis has been focused, for the most part, on the prevention of recurrent bacterial infections and *Pneumocystis carinii*. Prophylaxis with daily cotrimoxazole for the duration of treatment for GVHD has been successful in reducing bacterial infections from 66% among patients not taking prophylaxis to 47% in patients receiving prophylaxis when evaluated 5 years after diagnosis of GVHD ($p < 0.0001$) (36). Oral penicillin has been used as an alternative in patients who are allergic to sulfa drugs. Prevention of pneumococcal infection by immunization is difficult because of poor antibody response to this immunogen.

Patients with chronic GVHD often have subnormal levels of circulating immunoglobulin which may predispose them to recurrent sinopulmonary infections. In our center, such patients are currently being given monthly or bimonthly replacement with intravenous immunoglobulin at a dose of 100-500 mg/kg until they can maintain normal levels of IgG and IgA. The use of monthly adjuvant immunoglobulin replacement in patients with chronic GVHD is currently being evaluated to determine if this approach can reduce the infection and pulmonary complications in all patients with chronic GVHD during the first year after transplant.

Since VZV is the most common potentially life-threatening viral infection seen after the first 100 days after transplant, efforts have been made to prevent VZV infection with the use of acyclovir. In a placebo-controlled trial reported by Lundgren et al., 400 mg given orally three times a day for 6 months resulted in a significant reduction in both VZV and HSV infections in the treatment group (37). The success in preventing infection in patients with chronic GVHD obviously depends on successful treatment of their underlying GVHD.

IV. OTHER OPPORTUNISTIC INFECTIONS IN PATIENTS WITH ACUTE AND CHRONIC GVHD

A. *Pneumocystis carinii*

Pneumocystis carinii infection has been seen with decreasing frequency since the routine use of the prophylactic cotrimoxazole before and after transplant (1). When pneumocystis does occur, it is usually seen in patients who have a history of sulfa allergy or, because of poor engraftment status, have not received prophylaxis. The effect of GVHD on the incidence of pneumocystis infection has not been studied.

B. *Toxoplasma gondii*

The incidence of toxoplasma infection following marrow transplant has been difficult to determine because it is difficult to diagnose. However, its occurrence appears to be relatively infrequent. In a review by Shepp et al., only 10 cases among more than 2000 transplants were identified, all diagnosed by post-mortem tissue samples (38). A majority of the patients had acute GVHD. An additional report described three marrow transplant patients with disseminated toxoplasmosis who all had severe GVHD (39). Because cell-mediated immune responses are critical for the control of this infection, and patients with GVHD have abnormal cell-mediated immune responses, it is perhaps surprising that toxoplasmosis is not seen more often. It has been suggested that prophylaxis with trimethoprim-sulfamethoxazole against *Pneumocystis carinii* may have some effect in suppressing the reactivation of toxoplasmosis as well (39).

V. THE EFFECT OF GVHD PROPHYLAXIS OR TREATMENT ON THE RISK OF INFECTION

Strategies used to prevent or treat GVHD may increase the risk of infection by interfering with aspects of host defense important for protection by a variety of mechanisms. Unfortunately, very few studies have specifically addressed the relationship between infection and specific GVHD treatment or prevention modalities (see Table 2). In addition it may technically be very difficult to separate the effects of GVHD from the effects of regimens used to treat it.

Because cell-mediated immune responses are important for host defense against both viruses and fungi, drugs such as methotrexate which interfere with DNA synthesis and suppress the normal T-cell function necessary to control GVHD, increase the risk of these infections. In addition, methotrexate also interferes with production of normal bone marrow precursors resulting in delayed engraftment and can delay normal tissue repair resulting in increased or prolonged mucositis. Both of these factors add to the increased risk of infection during the early posttransplant period (40).

Table 2 The Relationship Between Specific Modalities Used to Prevent or Treat Acute GVHD and Specific Infectious Risks and Mechanisms

GVHD prophylaxis or treatment	Infection with an increased risk (reference)	Mechanism (reference)
Methotrexate	Bacterial HSV	Delayed engraftment (40) Increased mucositis (40) Local trauma
Antithymocyte globulin	Viral (CMV) Fungal	Decreased cell-mediated immunity Decreased chemotaxis of neutrophils (3)
Corticosteroids	Bacterial Fungal	Decreased neutrophil function (8) Decreased cell-mediated immunity
Intravenous anti-T-cell monoclonal antibodies	EBV lymphoproliferative disorder (24,25)	Decreased cell-mediated immunity
T-cell depletion	No increased risk (12,13) Fungal (5) EBV lymphoproliferative disorder (25)	Decreased cell-mediated immunity

Corticosteroids, while used to suppress cell-mediated immune responses which mediate GVHD, may also interfere with cell-mediated immune responses required to contain viral or fungal infections. In addition, their antiinflammatory activity may interfere with neutrophil chemotaxis and degranulation. Other modalities such as the use of anti-T-cell monoclonal antibodies, cyclosporine, or antithymocyte globulin are aimed at limiting the T-cell response which mediates GVHD. Therefore, infections which require cell-mediated immune responses for their control, and specifically viral and fungal infections, may be increased, although controlled data are not available.

It is often difficult to separate the effects of GVHD prophylaxis or treatment from the effects of GVHD itself. For example, in a study comparing methotrexate alone with cyclosporine plus methotrexate for the prevention of GVHD in patients with aplastic anemia, there was a higher number of non-CMV infection-related deaths in patients with GVHD receiving methotrexate alone than in patients receiving combined prophylaxis (41). Eight of nine deaths in this study were directly attributable to interstitial pneumonias or bacterial or fungal infections. Because the incidence of GVHD was higher in the methotrexate only arm, it is possible that the increase in infectious deaths was closely related to the presence of active GVHD. Similar results were observed in the cyclosporine only arm when methotrexate plus cyclosporine was compared to cyclosporine alone in patients undergoing allogeneic transplant for hematologic malignancies (42).

The increasing use of T-cell depletion of marrow as a means of GVHD prophylaxis has the theoretical potential to affect the incidence of infection, particularly infections requiring intact T-cell-mediated responses such as viral, fungal, or protozoan infections in several ways. First, the effect of T-cell depletion on reducing the risk of acute GVHD could possibly lower the incidence of herpesvirus infections by eliminating the immunologic abnormalities associated with this disease and its treatment. Or alternatively, T-cell depletion of marrow may remove the necessary cells important for the reconstitution of herpesvirus immunity after marrow transplant. Although one report found an increased risk of systemic fungal infection in patients receiving T-cell-depleted marrows (5), others have found no difference in the incidence of infection, including viral infections (43,44). It is possible that the reduction in the incidence of GVHD offsets the possible immunodeficiency that results from the depletion of lymphocytes that may be important for host defense against infectious pathogens.

VI. CONCLUSIONS

Infections of all types remain a serious problem after marrow transplant, with an increased risk for many types of infections in patients with acute GVHD. Infection remains a leading cause of death in patients with active GVHD, and this risk continues in patients with chronic GVHD. The risk of bacterial infections in patients with GVHD is increased due to the combined effects of breakdown of mechanical barriers, problems with granulocyte function, and the prolonged usage of antibiotics compared to patients without GVHD. Viral and fungal pathogens remain a particular challenge in patients with GVHD. Host defense against these organisms requires intact cell-mediated immune responses which continue to be abnormal in patients with GVHD either because of GVHD itself or because of the agents used to prevent or treat GVHD.

The long-term success of marrow grafting depends on the successful eradication and control of the closely associated problems of GVHD and infection. Although it is likely that the reduction or elimination of GVHD will lead to a reduction in infection, the treatment or prophylaxis aimed at its elimination may increase the risk of bacterial or fungal infections by disruption of mucosal barriers (e.g., methotrexate) or by altering the number or function of T cells required to maintain adequate host defense required for protection against viral and fungal pathogens (e.g., antithymocyte globulin, T-cell depletion of marrow, methotrexate, cyclosporine). The result may be that factors which increase the risk of infection are balanced by factors associated with a decrease in the incidence of GVHD. Alternatively, attempts at infection prevention may reduce both the risk of infection and the risk of GVHD (e.g., the association of the use of protective isolation or immunoglobulin and the decreased incidence of GVHD), resulting in a decrease in the morbidity and mortality from infection in patients with GVHD after marrow transplant.

REFERENCES

1. Bowden RA, Meyers JD: Infectious complications following marrow transplantation. In *Plasma Therapy and Transfusion Technology*, Vol. 6, No. 2, 1985; pp. 285-302.
2. Paulin T, Ringdén O, Nilsson B, Lönnqvist B, Gahrton G. Variables predicting bacterial and fungal infections after allogeneic marrow engraftment. Transplantation 1987;43:393-398.
3. Clark RA, Johnson FL, Klebanoff SJ, Thomas ED: Defective neutrophil chemotaxis in bone marrow transplant patients. J Clin Invest 1976;58:22-31.
4. Sosa R, Weiden PL, Storb R, Syrotuck J, Thomas ED: Granulocyte function in human allogeneic marrow graft recipients. Exp Hematol 1980;8:1183-1189.
5. Pirsch JD, Maki DG: Infectious complications in adults with bone marrow transplantation and T-cell depletion of donor marrow. Increased susceptibility to fungal infections. Ann Intern Med 1986;104:619-631.

6. Meyers JD, Flournoy N, Thomas ED: Risk factors for cytomegalovirus infection after human marrow transplantation. J Infect Dis 1986;153:478-488.
7. Buckner CD, Clift RA, Sanders JE, Meyers JD, Counts GW, Farewell VT, Thomas ED: Protective environment for marrow transplant recipients. A prospective study. Ann Intern Med 1978;89:893-901.
8. Watson JG: Problems of infection after bone marrow transplantation. J Clin Pathol 1983;36:683-692.
9. Storb R, Prentice RL, Thomas ED: Marrow transplantation for treatment of aplastic anemia. An analysis of factors associated with graft rejection. N Engl J Med 1977; 296:61-66.
10. Clift RA, Sanders JE, Thomas ED, Williams B, Buckner CD: Granulocyte transfusions for the prevention of infection in patients receiving bone-marrow transplants. N Engl J Med 1978;298:1052-1057.
11. Winston DJ, Ho GW, Young LS, Gale RP: Prophylactic granulocyte transfusions during human bone marrow transplantation. Am J Med 1980;68:893-897.
12. Sullivan KM: Immunoglobulin therapy in bone marrow transplantation. Am J Med 1987;83:34-45.
13. Petersen FB, Bowden RA, Thornquist M, Meyers JD, Buckner CD, Counts GW, Nelson MT, Newton BA, Sullivan KM, McIver J, Thomas ED: The effect of prophylactic intravenous immune globulin on the incidence of septicemia in marrow transplant recipients. Bone Marrow Transplantation 1987;2:141-148.
14. Winston DJ, Ho WG, Lin C-H, Budinger MD, Champlin RE, Gale RP: Intravenous immunoglobulin for modification of cytomegalovirus infections associated with bone marrow transplantation. Am J Med 1984,76:128-133.
15. Tutschka PJ: Diminishing morbidity and mortality of bone marrow transplantation. Vox Sang 1986;51:87-94.
16. Wade JC, Newton B, Flournoy N, Meyers JD: Oral acyclovir for prevention of herpes simplex virus reactivation after marrow transplantation. Ann Intern Med 1984,100:823-828.
17. Meyers JD: Infection in recipients of marrow transplants, in *Current Clinical Topics in Infectious Diseases*, edited by Remington JS, Swartz MN. McGraw-Hill, New York, 1985, pp. 261-292.
18. Bowden RA, Sayers M, Gleaves CA, Banaji M, Newton BA, Meyers JD: Cytomegalovirus-seronegative blood components for the prevention of primary cytomegalovirus infection after marrow transplantation: Consideration for blood banks. Transfusion 1987,27:478-481.
19. Reed EC, Bowden RA, Dandliker PS, Lilleby KE, Meyers JD: Treatment of cytomegalovirus pneumonia in marrow transplant patients with ganciclovir and intravenous cytomegalovirus immunoglobulin. Ann Intern Med 1988;109:783-788.
20. Lönnqvist B, Ringdén O, Wahren B, Gahrton G, Lundgren G: Cytomegalovirus infection associated with and preceding chronic graft-versus-host disease. Transplantation 1984,38:465-468.
21. Lange B, Henle W, Meyers JD, Yang LC, August C, Koch P, Arbeter A, Henle G: Epstein-Barr virus-related serology in marrow transplant recipients. Int J Cancer 1980;26:151-157.
22. Ambinder RE: The use of viral probes in bone marrow transplant patients. Leukemia 1987;1:263a (abstr).
23. Martin PJ, Shulman HM, Schubach WH, Hansen JA, Fefer A, Miller G, Thomas ED; Fatal Epstein-Barr-virus-associated proliferation of donor B cells after treatment of acute graft-versus-host disease with a murine anti-T-cell antibody. Ann Intern Med 1984;101:310-315.

24. Zutter MM, Martin PJ, Sale GE, Shulman HM, Fisher L, Thomas ED, Durnam DM: Epstein-Barr virus lymphoproliferation after bone marrow transplantation. Blood 1988;72:520-529.

25. Shapiro RS, McClain K, Frizzera G, Gajl-Peczalska KJ, Kersey JH, Blazar BR, Arthur DC, Patton DF, Greenberg JS, Burke B, Ramsay NKC, McGlave P, Filipovich AH. Epstein-Barr virus associated B cell lymphoproliferative disorders following bone marrow transplantion. Blood 1988;71:1234-1243.

26. Shields AF, Hackman RC, Fife KH, Corey L, Meyers JD: Adenovirus infections in patients undergoing bone-marrow transplantation. N Engl J Med 1985;312:529-533.

27. Saral R, Burns WH, Laskin OC, Santos GW, Lietman PS. Acyclovir prophylaxis of herpes-simplex-virus infections. A randomized, double-blind, controlled trial in bone-marrow-transplant recipients. N Engl J Med 1981;305:63-67.

28. Wade JC, Newton B, Glournoy N, Meyers JD: Oral acyclovir for prevention of herpes simplex virus reactivation after marrow transplant. Ann Intern Med 1984; 100:823-828.

29. Bowden RA, Sayers M, Flournoy N, Newton B, Banaji M, Thomas ED, Meyers JD: Cytomegalovirus immune globulin and seronegative blood products to prevent primary cytomegalovirus infection after marrow transplantation. N Engl J Med 1986; 314:1006-1010.

30. O'Reilly RJ, Reich L, Gold J, Kirkpatrick D, Dinsmore R, Kapoor N, Condie R: A randomized trial of intravenous hyperimmune gobulin for the prevention of cytomegalovirus (CMV) infections following marrow transplantation: Preliminary results. Transplant Proc 1983,15:1405-1411.

31. Sullivan KM, Deeg HJ, Sanders JE, Shulman HE, Witherspoon RP, Doney K, Appelbaum FR, Schubert MM, Stewart P, Springmeyer S, McDonald GB, Storb R, Thomas ED: Late complications after marrow transplantation. Semin Hematol 1984;21: 53-63.

32. Atkinson K, Farewell V, Storb R, Tsoi M-S, Sullivan KM, Witherspoon RP, Fefer A, Clift R, Goodell B, Thomas ED: Analysis of late infections after human bone marrow transplantation: Role of genotypic nonidentity between marrow donor and recipient and of nonspecific suppressor cells in patients with chronic graft-versus-host disease. Blood 1982,60:714-720.

33. Reinherz EL, Parkman R, Rappeport J, Rosen FS, Schlossman SF: Aberrations of suppressor T cells in human graft-versus-host disease. N Engl J Med 1979;300: 1061-1067.

34. Witherspoon RP, Storb R, Ochs HD, Flournoy N, Kopecky KJ, Sullivan KM, Deeg HJ, Sosa R, Noel DR, Atkinson K, Thomas ED: Recovery of antibody production in human allogeneic marrow graft recipients: Influence of time posttransplantation, the presence or absence of chronic graft-versus-host disease, and antithymocyte globulin treatment. Blood 1981;58:360-368.

35. Locksley RM, Flournoy N, Sullivan KM, Meyers JD: Infection with varicella-zoster virus after marrow transplantation. J Infect Dis 1985;152:1172-1181.

36. Sullivan KM, Dahlberg S, Storb R, Meyers JD, Witherspoon RP: Infection acquisition and prophylaxis in chronic graft-versus-host disease (GVHD). Blood 1983; 62:230a (Abstract).

37. Lundgren G, Wilczek HK, Lonnqvist B, Lindholm A, Wahren B, Ringdén O: Acyclovir prophylaxis in bone marrow transplant recipients. Scan J Infect Dis 1985; Suppl;1-8.

38. Shepp DH, Hackman RC, Conley FK, Anderson JB, Meyers JD: Toxoplasma gondii reactivation identified by detection of parasitemia in tissue culture. Ann Intern Med 1985,103:218-221.

39. Hirsch R, Burke BA, Kersey JH: Toxoplasmosis in bone marrow transplant recipients. J Pediatr 1984;105,426-428.

40. Atkinson K, Biggs JC, Ting A, Concannon AJ, Dodds AJ, Pun A: Cyclosporine A is associated with faster engraftment and less mucositis than methotrexate after allogeneic bone marrow transplantation. Br J Haematol 1983;53:265-270.

41. Storb R, Deeg HJ, Farewell V, Doney K, Appelbaum F, Beatty P, Bensinger W, Buckner CD, Clift R, Hansen J, Hill R, Longton G, Lum L, Martin P, McGuffin R, Sanders J, Singer J, Stewart P, Sullivan K, Witherspoon R, Thomas ED: Marrow transplantation for severe aplastic anemia: Methotrexate alone compared with a combination of methotrexate and cyclosporine for prevention of acute graft-versus-host disease. Blood 1986;68:119-125.

42. Storb R, Deeg HJ, Whitehead J, Appelbaum F, Beatty P, Bensinger W, Buckner CD, Clift R, Doney K, Farewell V, Hansen J, Hill R, Lum L, Martin P, McGuffin R, Sanders J, Stewart P, Sullivan KM, Witherspoon R, Yee G, Thomas ED: Methotrexate and cyclosporine compared with cyclosporine alone for prophylaxis of acute graft versus host disease after marrow transplantation for leukemia. N Engl J Med 1986,314:729-735.

43. Martin PJ, Hansen JA, Buckner CD, Sanders JE, Deeg HJ, Stewart P, Appelbaum FR, Clift R, Fefer A, Witherspoon RP, Kennedy MS, Sullivan KM, Flournoy N, Storb R, Thomas ED: Effects of in vitro depletion of T cells in HLA—identical allogeneic marrow grafts. Blood 1985;66:664-672.

44. Mitsuyasu RT, Champlin RE, Gale RP, Ho WG, Lenarsky C, Winston D, Selch M, Elashoff R, Giorgi JV, Wells J, Terasaki P, Billing R, Feig S: Treatment of donor bone marrow with monoclonal anti-T-cell antibody and complement for the prevention of graft-versus-host disease. A prospective, randomized, double blind trial. Ann Intern Med 1986;105:20-26.

29

Transfusion-Induced Graft-vs.-Host Disease

Thomas R. Spitzer
Vincent T. Lombardi Cancer Research Center
Georgetown University Hospital
Washington, D.C.

I. INTRODUCTION

Graft-vs.-Host Disease (GVHD) following transfusion of whole blood or blood components is an uncommon yet increasingly recognized complication in immunocompromised individuals (1-5). First described as a possible complication of blood transfusion by Hathaway et al. in 1965 (6), transfusion-induced GVHD has subsequently been described with increasing frequency as potent immunosuppressive therapies became more widely used. Because of uncertainties regarding definition of patients at risk, recommendations for prevention have remained controversial (1-5,7-10). The purpose of this chapter will be to describe the incidence, postulated pathogenesis, and the clinical situations in which the risk is thought to be increased, and strategies for the prevention in patients at highest risk.

II. INCIDENCE

Given the likelihood of mistaken diagnoses and varied reporting practices, the true incidence of transfusion-induced GVHD is unknown. Von Fliedner et al. estimated a 0.1-1.0% incidence in patients with hematologic and lymphoproliferative malignancies at Roswell Park Memorial Institute based on 12 suspected (one confirmed) cases of transfusion-induced GVHD over 10 years (1). Two series of intensively treated cancer patients suggest a higher incidence, however. Stutzman et al. reported two cases of fatal GVHD following unirradiated blood product transfusion in 105 intensively treated patients with Hodgkin's disease (11). Murphy et al. observed four cases of fatal transfusion-induced GVHD out of 47 patients with grade IV neuroblastoma (12). The incidence of GVHD following granulocyte transfusions from patients with chronic myelogenous leukemia

(CML) has also been addressed (13,14). Bussel reported six cases of probable GVHD in 1332 transfusions (13). Nonfatal GVHD was described to occur in 20% of neutropenic patients treated with CML leukocytes by Schwarzenberg et al. (14). GVHD, following transfusion of CML leukocytes has been shown to be considerably more common (although less severe) than when normal donor blood products are used (1). The overall incidence of transfusion-induced GVHD has likely been underestimated given the multiple reports of "probable" GVHD that are clinically mild and nonfatal.

III. PATHOGENESIS

Similar to the postulated mechanism for GVHD following bone marrow transplantation, transfusion-induced GVHD results from infusion of allogeneic immunocompetent T lymphocytes disparate for major or minor histocompatibility antigens into an immuno-compromised host (1-5). The minimum degree of host immune deficiency necessary for transfusion-induced GVHD in unknown, but significant impairment of cell-mediated immunity is thought to be a prerequisite. Disorders characterized by inadequate antibody production (e.g., common variable hypogammaglobulinemia) or neutrophil dysfunction alone (e.g., chronic granulomatous disease) have not been associated with transfusion-induced GVHD (5). Most transfusion-induced GVHD has occurred in individuals with severely impaired cellular immunity such as that seen in congenital T-cell immune deficiency syndromes (e.g., severe combined immune deficiency syndrome or Wiskott-Aldrich syndrome) or advanced lymphoproliferative malignancies (1,2,5).

One disorder characterized by severely dysfunctional cellular immunity, the acquired immunodeficiency syndrome (AIDS), has not been reported to be associated with transfusion-induced GVHD (5). Such an observation might result from failure of reporting, misdiagnosis (given overlapping clinical features such as rash and diarrhea), or widespread use of irradiated blood products. Lack of GVHD in six patients with AIDS treated with monthly infusions of unirradiated haplotype identical lymphocytes (4-8.5 $\times$ 10^9 lymphocytes/infusion) suggests the possibility that patients with AIDS are less susceptible to the risk of transfusion-induced GVHD than patients with other disorders of cellular immunity, however (15). The role of partially HLA-matched blood products versus preservation of immune responsiveness preventing GVHD in this phenomenon is unclear. Several conditions in which transfusion-induced GVHD has been reported (infancy, pregnancy, aplastic anemia, post-cardiac surgery) are not generally associated with impaired cellular immunity. In these instances subtle immune defects combined with infusion of large numbers of genetically disparate immunocompetent lymphocytes likely led to a full-blown GVHD syndrome. Presently, any patient with a disorder characterized by clinically overt T-cell dysfunction is believed to be susceptible to acquiring transfusion-induced GVHD and should be considered for prophylactic measures.

The minimal inoculum of transfused lymphocytes necessary to induce GVHD is also uncertain. Plavljanic et al. used a murine model to show that GVHD is observed after transfusing as few as 2×10^6 allogeneic lymphocytes. Lethally irradiated F_1 hybrid mice receiving 2-4 $\times$ 10^6 allogeneic lymphocytes died after 8-9 days from a graft-vs.-host-like illness while those receiving 10^7 lymphocytes died within 6 days from a similar illness (16). On the other hand, van Bekkum et al. demonstrated that a minimum

Table 1 Blood Products and Associated Risk of GVHD

Blood product	Estimated number of viable lymphocytes	GVHD risk	Reference
Fresh frozen plasma	None	None	5
Cryoprecipitate	None	None	5
Frozen red blood cells	3.0×10^7/unit[a]	Unknown	85,86
Fresh plasma	8×10^4/kg	Low (limited to CIS[b])	18
Platelets—single donor	4.0×10^7/unit	Intermediate	5
—apheresis donor	3.0×10^8/unit	Intermediate	5
Whole blood	1×10^9/unit	Intermediate	24
Packed red blood cells	5.0×10^8/unit	Intermediate	5
Washed red blood cells	2.5×10^8/unit	Intermediate	5
Leukocytes (normal donor)	$5\text{-}10 \times 10^9$/unit	High	5
Leukocytes (CML donor)	$12\text{-}120 \times 10^9$/unit	High[c]	2

[a]Assuming 6% viable mononuclear cells following deglycerolization and washing.

[b]Congenital immune deficiency syndrome.

[c]Increased compared to normal donor leukocytes.

of 10^7 lymphocytes per kg recipient weight was necessary to induce GVHD in lethally irradiated mice (17). Hematologically normal newborn and adult hybrid F_1 mice required 2×10^8/kg and 10^9/kg lymph node cells, respectively, to cause a graft-versus-host reaction (GVHR).

Most transfusion-induced GVHD in man has occurred following infusion of greater than 10^7 lymphocytes/kg recipient weight (1,2,5). Reports of GVHD following plasma infusion (estimated lymphocyte dose of 8×10^4/kg in one instance (18)) have underscored the importance of the degree of underlying immune deficiency in addition to the number of infused lymphocytes. Blood products most commonly implicated in the pathogenesis of GVHD along with the calculated number of lymphocytes per product are listed in Table 1. With the exception of an increased risk of GVHD following infusion of granulocytes from patients with chronic myelogenous leukemia (1), no relationship between number of transfused lymphocytes and incidence or severity of GVHD has been established.

Finally, the degree of genetic disparity probably influences the incidence (and severity) of transfusion-induced GVHD. Given the lack of attempt to provide HLA-matched or partially matched products in most instances, multiple HLA-A,B, and DR antigen mismatched donor lymphocytes were likely transfused. DR antigen identity between donor lymphocytes and the host has been observed in two instances of transfusion-induced GVHD leading the authors to conclude that engraftment may be facilitated by HLA compatibility (19,20). Other cases of transfusion-induced GVHD confirmed by HLA typing have not been associated with HLA antigen identity (21). In any event, HLA-antigen disparity probably contributes to the fulminant course and high mortality rate observed in transfusion-induced GVHD. In the worst case scenario, it is not difficult to envision fatal GVHD occurring in a relatively immunocompetent individual if the genetic disparity and infused lymphocyte dose are sufficient.

IV. CLINICAL FEATURES

Transfusion-induced GVHD is characterized by abrupt onset (median 8 (range 3-30) days) following transfusion, severe multiorgan system involvement including bone marrow hypoplasia or aplasia with peripheral pancytopenia, and usually fatal outcome (1-5). Compared to GVHD following bone marrow transplantation, transfusion-induced GVHD occurs earlier and is more likely to have a fulminant course. Bone marrow hypoplasia/ aplasia is also not a feature regularly observed in GVHD following transplantation.

Presenting features of transfusion-induced GVHD include fever and severe skin involvement (maculopapular rash progressing to erythroderma and exfoliation) in most cases. Fever may precede skin manifestations but more commonly occurs concomitant with or after skin changes are observed (1). Intestinal involvement with moderate to severe diarrhea and hepatic involvement with hyperbilirubinemia are common but not universal features.

Pathological features of transfusion-induced GVHD are typical of those seen following bone marrow transplantation with the exception of almost uniform hypoplasia or aplasia of the bone marrow. Thymic dysplasia with severe epithelial injury (including loss of Hassall's corpuscles), similar to the pathological changes observed in severe combined immune deficiency, has been described in neonates affected with transfusion-induced GVHD (22).

Documentation of transfusion-induced GVHD requires identification of donor lymphocytes (by HLA typing or karyotype analysis) or, in the case of transfused CML leukocytes, presence of the Philadelphia chromosome. Only 15 of the reported 78 cases (19%) of transfusion-induced GVHD have fulfilled these criteria. Diagnosis of GVHD in all other cases was established by typical clinical and histopathological features.

V. DISEASE ASSOCIATIONS

Transfusion-induced GVHD has been described in association with numerous malignant and nonmalignant immune deficiency disorders. To date, 78 cases have been reported either as individual case reports or as part of retrospective series evaluating the incidence of transfusion-induced GVHD. Disease categories and associated clinical findings are listed in Table 2. For purpose of discussion, diseases have been divided into those associated with uncertain immunologic abnormalities, and malignant and nonmalignant diseases, congenital and acquired, associated with impaired cell-mediated immunity.

A. Uncertain Immunologic Abnormalities

1. Neonates

Seven cases of GVHD have been reported in infants following exchange transfusion (22-26). Four of the infants also received intrauterine transfusions for hemolytic disease of the newborn. Six of the infants were born prematurely (28-36 weeks of gestation). Given the likelihood that the capacity of rejecting allogeneic cells is developed by midgestation (22), establishment of GVHD in otherwise immunologically intact infants is thought to be dependent on the induction of tolerance, either through previous maternal or intrauterine transfusion (22). Persistence of circulating allogeneic lymphocytes (maternal or from transfused random blood) in some children without GVHD indicates that a spectrum of induced tolerance and chimerism likely exists following neonatal transfusions (27,28).

2. Post-Cardiac Surgery

Recently, several Japanese investigators have described a syndrome entitled "postoperative erythroderma" following open heart surgery (29,30). An additional case was reported by Aoki et al. in a 66-year-old man following massive transfusion for aortic aneurysm repair (31). The syndrome is characterized by fever, rash (erythroderma), abnormal liver function tests, diarrhea, and marrow hypoplasia or aplasia beginning approximately 10 days postoperatively. The incidence, which has been estimated at 1 in every 300-400 cases of heart surgery, has been uniformly fatal (30). Pathological changes of GVHD have not been well documented. Two cases in which peripheral blood lymphocytes were obtained for HLA typing were associated with circulating lymphocytes likely derived from donor transfusions. The authors speculated that the common practice of using fresh blood for transfusion in Japan may increase the risk of transfusion-induced GVHD, particularly in relatively immunocompetent individuals (30).

GVHD has not been described following open heart surgery in the United States (1). A mononucleosis-like syndrome due in most cases to cytomegalovirus with overlapping clinical features (e.g., rash, liver function abnormalities) is not uncommonly seen following open-heart surgery and emphasizes the importance of careful documentation of GVHD (32,33).

3. Aplastic Anemia

Fatal transfusion-induced GVHD was described in a 12-year-old female with aplastic anemia secondary to hepatitis who received unirradiated CML leukocyte transfusions (34). GVHD was documented by clinical course, pathological findings, and the occurrence of myeloid engraftment. Defective cell-mediated immunity is generally not a feature of aplastic anemia and immunosuppressive therapy was not given to the patient. A baseline (pretransfusion) absolute lymphocyte count of 200/μl was consistent with the presence of at least a quantitative abnormality of cellular immunity.

4. Pregnancy

Sheehan et al. reported the occurrence of fatal GVHD in a previously healthy 22-year-old female given two units of packed red blood cells immediately following induced delivery for mild preeclampsia (35). Although lymphoid engraftment was not documented, clinical findings (erythroderma, hepatopathy) and autopsy findings were typical of GVHD. Impaired cellular immunity is not an expected feature of pregnancy (36), and no precipitating immunologic disturbance was apparent in this patient.

B. Impaired Cell-Mediated Immunity: Nonmalignant Disorders

Seventeen cases of transfusion-induced GVHD in children with severe combined immune deficiency disease (SCID) or Wiskott-Aldrich syndrome have been reported (6,18, 37-49). The only two cases of transfusion-induced GVHD due to fresh plasma infusion have been seen in this population emphasizing the importance of the severity of the underlying disorder of cell-mediated immunity in the pathogenesis of transfusion-induced GVHD (18,41). In the case described by Seemayer and Bolande, a premature infant developed fatal GVHD following an exchange transfusion for neonatal jaundice (22). A normal thymic shadow was observed on chest X-ray prior to transfusion. Pathological features at post-mortem included severe injury to thymic epithelium. The authors speculated that this acquired form of thymic dysplasia was similar to that seen in SCID and that some cases of SCID or other T-cell dysfunction syndrome of childhood may result from intrauterine transplacental maternal or blood transfusion-induced GVHD (22).

Table 2 Transfusion-Induced GVHD: Patient Characteristics

Immunologic disorder disease	Number of reported cases	Type of transfused blood product	Outcome	Comments	References
I. Uncertain immunologic abnormality					
A. Neonates (prematurity, HDN)	7	ET(1) ET+IUT(5)	7D		22-26
B. Post-open heart surgery	2	WB(2)	2D	Fresh whole blood	29,30
C. Post-aortic aneurysm surgery	1	WB (1)	1D		31
D. Aplastic anemia	1	CML–L(1)	1D		34
E. Pregnancy	1	PRBC(1)	1D	Pre-tx lymphopenia	35
II. Impaired cellular immunity					
A. Congenital immunodeficiency Syndrome					
1. SCID	15	P(1) PRBC(3) WB(4) BC(4) WB+PRBC(1) UK(2)	1A,14D	P only in survivor, survivor 2/chronic GVHD: one patient also received fetal liver and thymus.	6,18,37-41,43,45-49 42,44
2. Wiskott-Aldrich	2	P(1) PRBC(1)	2D		

B. Malignancy

1. Lymphoproliferative					
a. Hodkin's disease	12	WB(1) PRBC(3) PLT(2) PRBC+PLT(1) ND–L(3) CML–L(2)	1A,11D	CML–L in survivor	1,11,19, 50–54
b. Non-Hodgkin's lymphoma	7	PRBC(1) WB+PRBC+PLI(1) ND–L(3) CML–L(1) BC(1)	7D		20,50,57–61
2. Acute leukemia					
a. ANLL	12	WB+PLT(1) WB+BC(1) BC(1) W–RBC+PLT(2) ND–L(4) ND–L+PLT(1) CML–L(2)	4A,8D		34,50,63–67 70,72,73
b. ALL	9	WB(1) ND–L(3) CML–L(5)	7A,2D		68,71
3. CLL	1	CML–L(1)	1A	CML–L in 5 of 7 survivors; 1 survivor w/chronic GVHD	64
4. Solid tumors					
a. Neuroblastoma	6	PRBC(2) UK(4)	6D		12,78,79
b. Glioblastoma	1	BC(1)	1D		53
c. Rhabdomyosarcoma	1	PRBC(1)	1D		21

Abbreviations: HDN = Hemolytic Disease of the Newborn; SCID - severe combined immune deficiency syndrome; CML = chronic myelogenous leukemia, ET = exchange transfusion, IUT = intrauterine transfusion, WB = whole blood; PRBC = packed red blood cells; BC = buffy coat; CML–L: CML leukocytes, ND–L: normal donor leukocytes, P: plasma, PLT: plateletes, UK = unknown; Tx: transfusion; CLL: chronic lymphocytic leukemia; ANLL: acute nonlymphocytic leukemia, ALL. acute lymphoblastic leukemia; A. alive, D = dead.

C. Impaired Cell-Mediated Immunity: Maliganant Disorders

1. Lymphoproliferative Malignancies

The majority of patients with transfusion-induced GVHD and underlying malignancy were receiving intensive chemo- or chemoradiotherapy for advanced Hodgkin's disease (1,11,19,50-54). Characteristics of the 12 reported cases of Hodgkin's disease in association with transfusion-induced GVHD include young age (median 24 years) advanced (stages IIB, III, or IV) but potentially curable disease and fatal outcome in 11 of the cases (1,11,19,50-54). An underlying defect in cellular immunity (which may persist following successful therapy) in addition to the immunosuppressive effects of chemoradiotherapy may render patients with Hodgkin's disease more susceptible to transfusion-induced GVHD than patients with other advanced malignancies (55,56).

Seven cases of fatal transfusion-induced GVHD have been reported in patients with non-Hodgkin's lymphoma (20,50,57-61). One patient had previously received a cadaveric renal transplant and was receiving combination chemotherapy for a posttransplant immunoblastic sarcoma at the time of development of GVHD (60). Given the variable clinical presentations and histologic subtypes in this group, conclusions regarding risk factors for GVHD are difficult to establish. As expected, all patients had intermediate to high grade histologies (NCI Working Classification) (62), advanced stage disease, and had recently received intensive chemotherapy.

2. Acute Leukemia

Despite the need for intensive transfusional support during induction and consolidation therapy, obligatory period of marrow aplasia, and lack of widespread use of irradiated blood products, transfusion-induced GVHD in patients with acute leukemia has been a relatively rarely reported event (34,50,63-73). Some patients, moreover, have shown transient evidence of myeloid engraftment when CML leukocytes were used followed by "rejection" of the graft 2-3 weeks later (when endogenous marrow recovery occurred) (34). Lack of significant impairment of T-cell immunity in many cases of acute leukemia probably accounts for the rarity of reported transfusion-induced GVHD (74,75).

3. Chronic Lymphocytic Leukemia

Clinical GVHD developed in a 54-year-old female with chronic lymphocytic leukemia following infusion of CML leukocytes (64). Although primarily a B-cell neoplasm, T-cell dysfunction is a common accompaniment of advanced stage disease (76).

4. Solid Tumors

Thoracic Duct Lymphocyte Infusion Experience

Transfusion-induced GVHD is a rare occurrence in patients with solid tumors given preservation of cell-mediated immunity in most instances (1). Yonemoto et al. transfused large numbers ($20-71 \times 10^9$) of allogeneic thoracic duct lymphocytes into six patients with advanced solid tumors in an effort to evaluate antitumor efficacy (77). Two patients demonstrated transient evidence of mild GVHD (rash, fever), demonstrating possible induction of GVHD if sufficient numbers of genetically disparate donor lymphocytes are transfused. On the other hand, given the large number of transfused allogeneic lymphocytes, the six patients demonstrated remarkably little GVHD-related morbidity.

Neuroblastoma

To date, most reported cases of transfusion-induced GVHD in solid tumor patients have involved patients with metastatic neuroblastoma. In addition to the estimated 8.5% incidence (4 of 47) of transfusion-induced GVHD following use of unirradiated blood products in patients with neuroblastoma undergoing intensive chemotherapy (12), two case reports have been published (78,79). Factors implicated in the pathogenesis of transfusion-induced GVHD in neuroblastoma include young age (median 2 years) and the known impairment of cellular immunity that accompanies stage IV neuroblastoma (80).

Glioblastoma Multiforme

Schmidmeier et al. described a case of fatal transfusion-induced GVHD occurring in a 59-year-old woman with glioblastoma multiforme (53). The patient had previously received cranial irradiation and combination chemotherapy and was severely neutropenic when she received buffy coat infusions (with an estimated mononuclear cell infusion number of $5\text{-}7.5 \times 10^7$/kg body weight). A diagnosis of GVHD was established by typical clinical (fever, rash, diarrhea, hyperbilirubinemia) and pathologic findings.

Rhabdomyosarcoma

Fatal posttransfusion GVHD developed in a 9-year-old female who was receiving combination chemotherapy for advanced rhabdomyosarcoma (21). Clinically, GVHD was suspected by the presence of a typical skin rash and progressive pancytopenia. HLA typing of circulating lymphocytes and skin fibroblasts confirmed the presence of an allogeneic lymphoid graft.

VI. TREATMENT

The outcome was fatal in 64 of 78 (82%) of the reported cases of transfusion-induced GVHD. No therapy including high-dose corticosteroids has clearly had an impact on the natural history of the disease. Surviving cases have been characterized by relatively mild disease manifestations, spontaneously reversible tissue injury, and in some cases, at least partial resolution of the underlying immune deficit (e.g., successful remission induction in acute leukemia). Supportive care (antibiotics, transfusional support, etc.) is essential during periods of peripheral cytopenia. Bone marrow transplantation from a mismatched sibling donor was attempted in one patient with marrow aplasia but early posttransplant death occurred due to overwhelming candidal sepsis (H. J. Deeg, personal communication).

VII. PROGNOSIS

Small numbers of patients in each disease category make statistically meaningful conclusions difficult. Nonetheless, several probable prognostic associations have emerged from examination of the data and are summarized in Table 3. Use of leukocytes obtained from patients with chronic myelogenous leukemia results in a higher incidence of GVHD (perhaps due to a significantly higher number of lymphocytes infused) but a significantly lower mortality than transfusion of non-CML blood products. GVHD mortality rates following non-CML donor blood products and CML leukocytes are 92% (61 of 66 patients) and 25% (3 of 12 patients) ($p < 0.01$), respectively. Use of leukocyte transfusions for therapy of neutropenia-related infections has declined recently, however, and given the lack of proven superiority, CML leukocytes are rarely used.

Table 3 Prognostic Factors for Outcome of Transfusion-Induced GVHD

Factor	Better prognosis	Poor prognosis
Transfusion product	CML leukocytes	Normal donor leukocytes
Disease	Acute leukemia	Congenital immune-deficiency syndrome
		Malignant lymphoma
Age	Adult	Infant (less than 1 year)

Age is potentially an independent prognostic factor particularly if the mortality in infancy (including premature infants, HDN, and congenital immune deficiency syndromes) is compared to the mortality of older children and adults. All 21 infants under one year of age with transfusion-induced GVHD have died compared to 43 of 57 (75%) older individuals with transfusion-induced GVHD ($p < 0.05$). Excess mortality is more likely due to poorly tolerated GVHD-related complications (e.g., exfoliative dermatitis, overwhelming diarrhea) than the underlying immune deficiency since several infants had no apparent immunologic deficit other than their age.

Disease status may also influence outcome of transfusion-induced GVHD. Mortality of transfusion-induced GVHD in nonleukemic conditions is 95% (54 of 57 patients), which is significantly greater than the 48% (10 of 21 patients) mortality rate for patients with acute leukemia ($p < 0.01$). However 10 of 14 (71%) patients with acute leukemia who developed GVHD from blood products other than CML leukocytes died, which is not significantly different from the overall mortality of transfusion-induced GVHD. Eighteen of 19 (95%) patients with malignant lymphoma and 16 of 17 (94%) patients with congenital immune deficiency syndromes have died constituting the disease groups with the largest numbers of reported deaths. Although outcome of GVHD has not been clearly shown to correlate with diagnosis (independent of transfusion source), relatively immunocompetent individuals frequently appear to have a milder course (as evidenced by the "rejection" of transfused myeloid cells when patients with acute leukemia achieve remission) (34).

VIII. PREVENTION OF TRANSFUSION-INDUCED GVHD

Removal of immunocompetent lymphocytes from transfused blood products by either physicochemical methods or irradiation-induced functional inhibition has been proposed as a method of preventing transfusion-induced GVHD (1-5,10). Given the ease of irradiating blood products and lack of data regarding efficacy of physicochemical methods of lymphocyte removal, efforts have been largely directed towards establishing optimal methods of blood cell irradiation. Lack of irradiation facilities in some blood banks, however, necessitates a discussion of both methods.

A. Physicochemical Methods

Since transfusion-induced GVHD has been observed in severely immunocompromised patients receiving fresh plasma only, "safe" numbers of residual lymphocytes (i.e., minimum number sufficient to cause GVHD) following leukocyte separation procedures are unknown. Fresh whole blood contains large numbers (1×10^9 lymphocytes/unit) of immunocompetent lymphocytes. Storage in ACD (acid-citrate-dextrose) anticoagulant for 2-3 weeks causes minimal change in in vitro lymphocyte function (81). Washed red cells and leukocyte-poor red cells prepared by centrifugation contain at least 2.5 × 10^8 leukocytes/unit postprocessing, a number in the range generally agreed to cause transfusion-induced GVHD in immunocompromised humans (82). Even use of cotton filtration to remove leukocytes has been shown to result in 4.0 × 10^7 residual leukocytes (3.2 × 10^7 lymphocytes/unit postprocessing) (83). Use of frozen deglycerolized red cells has also been suggested as a means of preventing transfusion-induced GVHD. Small numbers (6% of the original leukocytes or approximately 3.0 × 10^7 total lymphocytes) of viable mononuclear cells demonstrating normal mitogenesis and blast transformation have been shown to be present following deglycerolization and washing, raising questions about the prophylactic potential of frozen cells (84,85). Use of fresh frozen plasma and cryoprecipitate is believed to be without risk of transfusing viable lymphocytes since cryoprotective agents are not used in the freezing process (5).

B. Blood Product Irradiation

Irradiation of blood products, usually from a cesium-137 source, is a well-accepted method of inhibiting lymphocyte proliferation and eliminating GVHD potential (1-5, 7,8,10). Controversy continues, however, regarding optimal irradiation dose (both in terms of effective inhibition of lymphocyte reactivity and lack of significant injury to other blood elements) (2,3,5,10). Mixed lymphocyte culture techniques have shown that 500 rads is sufficient to completely inhibit host lymphocyte proliferative response to allogeneic cells (86). Suppression of mitogen-induced blast transformation requires higher irradiation doses, however. Blast transformation is reduced by 70-90% following treatment with 1500-1600 rads (87,88), 97-98.5% by 5000 rads (86,88), and 100% by 7500 rads (88). B lymphocytes have been shown to be more sensitive to irradiation than T cells and T suppressor cells more sensitive than T helper cells (89). Antigen-specific suppressor cells are particularly sensitive to irradiation with complete functional ablation following 400 rads (89).

Extent of injury to other blood elements following irradiation is also an important factor in determining optimal irradiation doses. Neutrophil function (i.e., chemotaxis, bactericidal activity, endotoxin-stimulated nitroblue tetrazolium reduction) is not significantly affected by irradiation doses less than 500 rads (86,90,91). Remarkable resistance to radiation is exemplified by preservation of normal neutrophil bactericidal activity and 60% of phagocytic activity after 40,000 and 100,000 rads, respectively (86,90). Expected posttransfusion platelet count was found to be reduced by 33% following exposure to 5000 rads by Button et al. (88). In vivo platelet survial (measured by ^{51}Cr-labeling studies) was not altered following radiation doses of 5000 to 7500 rads, however (88,92). Platelet function studies following platelet irradiation (5000 rads) have included diminished neutralization of aspirin effect on the template bleeding time and impaired collagen (although not epinephreine or ADP) induced in vitro aggregation (93).

Despite ample data concerning effects of irradiation on cellular blood elements, debate persists regarding optimal irradiation doses to prevent transfusion-induced GVHD. Incomplete inhibition of mitogen-induced lymphocyte blast transformation occurs after exposure to 1500 rads (87,88); no cases of transfusion-induced GVHD have been reported following use of blood products treated with 1500 rads, however (5). Recommendations for an effective irradiation dose have, therefore, ranged from 1500 rads (presumed adequate lymphocyte functional inhibition and clinical experience) to 5000 rads (near complete inhibition of lymphocyte blastogenesis but lack of sufficient data regarding safety to other blood elements above that dose). A compromise recommendation which allows for adequate margin of error and which has been adopted by many centers is to irradiate all appropriate blood products with 2500-3500 rads (2,3).

IX. BLOOD PRODUCT IRRADIATION FOR GVHD PROPHYLAXIS: RECOMMENDATIONS

Controlled studies evaluating the efficacy of blood product irradiation have not been performed. Recommendations are therefore made on the basis of (1) low risk (no known toxicity from administration of irradiated blood products), (2) significant prevalence of transfusion-induced GVHD in certain immune deficiency states, (3) high fatality rate of transfusion-induced GVHD, and (4) clinical (and supporting laboratory) evidence for a GVHD protective effect of blood product irradiation. Arguments concerning cost of a cesium irradiator ($40,000-$60,000) and labor of irradiating blood products cannot be ignored by but are probably inconsequential relative to the physcal and emotional demands of treating an iatrogenic fatal illness in otherwise potentially curable individuals.

Accordingly, irradiation of blood products (fresh frozen plasma and cryoprecipitate excluded) using a cesium-137 or other appropriate irradiation source to deliver 2500-3500 rads is recommended for the following high-risk disorders:

1. Intrauterine and exchange transfusions for premature infants or hemolytic disease of the newborn.
2. Congenital immune deficiency syndromes characterized by impairment of cellular immunity (e.g., SCID, Wiskott-Aldrich syndrome).
3. Patients undergoing syngeneic, allogeneic, or autologous bone marrow transplantation.
4. Hodgkin's disease: Given the underlying dysfunctional cellular immunity, all patients with active disease should receive irradiated blood products.
5. Non-Hodgkin's lymphoma: All patients with intermediate to high grade histologies or any patient undergoing therapy.
6. Acute leukemia: Despite the relatively low risk, the intensive transfusional support required during therapy necessitates use of irradiated blood products.
7. Acquired immunodeficiency syndrome: No cases of transfusion-induced GVHD have been reported, but the underlying defect in cellular immunity is sufficiently severe to recommend use of irradiated blood products.
8. Metastatic neuroblastoma: A high incidence of transfusion-induced GVHD relative to other solid tumors has been reported.
9. Miscellaneous: Other disorders (e.g., advanced solid tumors, aplastic anemia) in which defective cellular immunity is suspected.

X. SUMMARY AND CONCLUSIONS

Transfusion-induced GVHD is an infrequently reported but increasingly recognized complication of blood transfusion in immunocompromised individuals. Factors influencing the development of GVHD include nature (and degree) of impairment of cellular immunity, number of infused immunocompetent T lymphocytes, and possibly degree of genetic disparity between donor and host. Clinical features are similar to those of GVHD following bone marrow transplantation but include severe bone marrow involvement in most cases and more fulminant clinical course (and higher mortality). No effective therapy is known for transfusion-induced GVHD. Since transfusion-induced GVHD can be prevented by irradiating blood products with 2500-3500 rads, patients at high risk (by virtue of impaired cellular immunity and/or clinical experience) should receive irradiated blood products only.

ACKNOWLEDGMENT

Supported in part by grants CA14626 awarded by the National Institutes of Health, Bethesda, MD.

REFERENCES

1. Von-Fliedner V, Higby DJ, Kim U: Graft-versus-host reaction following blood transfusion. Am J Med 1982;72:951-961.
2. Brubaker DB: Human posttransfusion graft-versus-host disease. Vox Sang 1983; 45:401-420.
3. Pflieger H: Graft-versus-host disease following blood transfusions. Blut 1983;46: 61-66.
4. Fagiolo E, D'Addasio AM: Post-transfusion graft-versus-host disease (GVHD): immunopathology and prevention. Haematologica 1985;70:62-74.
5. Leitman SF, Holland PV: Irradiation of blood products: indications and guidelines. Transfusion 1985;25:293-300.
6. Hathaway WE, Githens JA, Blackburn JR, Fulginiti V, Kempe CH: Aplastic anemia, histiocytosis, and erythroderma in immunologically deficient children. N Engl J Med 1965;273:953-958.
7. Perkins HA: Granulocyte concentrates: should they be routinely irradiated? Prog Clin Biol Res 1981;65:49-57.
8. Weiden P: Graft-vs-host disease following blood transfusions (editorial). Arch Intern Med 1984;144:1557-1558.
9. Lind SE: Has the case for irradiating blood products been made? (editorial). Am J Med 1985;78:543-544.
10. Pritchard SL, Rogers PC: Rationale and recommendations for the irradiation of blood products. CRC Crit Rev Onc/Hematol 1987;7:115-124.
11. Stutzman L, Nisce L, Friedman M: Increased toxicity of total nodal irradiation (TNI) following combination chemotherapy (abstract). Proc Am Soc Clin Oncol 1977,18:388.
12. Murphy ML, Helson L: Chemotherapy of metastic neuroblastoma stage IV (abstract). Proc Am Soc Clin Oncol 1977;18:388.
13. Bussel A, Benbunan M, Weil M, Reviron J, Jacquillot C, Boiron M, Bernard J: White blood cell transfusions in leukemic patients with severe infections. Recent Results Cancer Res 1974;49:40-47.
14. Schwarzenberg L, Mathe G, Amiel JL, Cattan A, Schneider M, Schlumberger JR: Study of factors determining the usefulness and complications of leukocyte transfusions. Am J Med 1967;43:206-213.
15. Hauptman SP, Batuman O, Friedman L, Balaban D, Allen-Hagen B, Ifft N, Shapiro SS: Amelioration of immunologic deficits and clinical manifestations of the acquired immunodeficiency syndrome (AIDS) by allogeneic lymphocyte transfusions (abstract). Blood 1985;66 (suppl 1):113a.
16. Plavljanic D, Hrsak M, Vitale B: Acute graft-versus-host reaction in mice. 5. Cell interaction. Period Biol 1977;79:129-140.
17. Van Bekkum DW: Transfusion or transplantation? Isr J Med Sci 1965;1:879-882.

18. Rubenstein A, Radl J, Cottier H, Rossi E, Gugler E: Unusual combined immuno-deficiency syndrome exhibiting kappa-IgD paraproteinemia, residual gut-immunity and graft-vs-host reaction after plasma infusion. Acta Pediatr Scand 1973;62:365–372.

19. Dinsmore RE, Straus DJ, Pollack MS, Woodruff JM, Garrett TJ, Young CW, Clarkson BD, Dupont B: Fatal graft-versus-host disease following blood transfusion in Hodgkin's disease documented by HLA typing. Blood 1980;55:831–833.

20. Weiden PL, Zuckerman N, Hansen JA, Sale GE, Remlinger K, Beck TM, Buckner CD: Fatal graft-versus-host disease in a patient with lymphoblastic leukemia following normal granulocyte transfusions. Blood 1981;57:328-332.

21. Labotka RJ, Rodvany R: Graft-versus-host disease in rhabdomyosarcoma following transfusion with non-irradiated blood products. Med Pediatr Oncol 1985;13:101-104.

22. Seemayer TA, Bolande RP: Thymic involution mimicking thymic dysplasia. Arch Pathol Lab Med 1980;104:141-144.

23. Naiman JL, Punnett HH, Lischner HW, Destine MI, Arey JB: Possible graft-versus-host reaction after intrauterine transfusion for Rh erythroblastosis fetalis. N Engl J Med 1969;281:697-701.

24. Parkman R, Mosier D, Umansky I, Cochran W, Carpenter C, Rosen FS: Graft-versus-host disease after intra-uterine and exchange transfusions for hemolytic disease of the newborn. N Engl J Med 1974;290:359-363.

25. Bohm N, Kleine W, Enzel U: Graft-versus-host disease in two newborns after repeated blood transfusions because of Rhesus incompatibility. Beitr Path Vol 1977; 160:381-400.

26. Hathaway WE, Brangle RS, Nelson TL, Roeckel IE: Aplastic anemia and alymophocytosis in an infant with hypogammaglobulinemia: graft-versus-host reaction? J Pediatr 1966;69:713-722.

27. Cohen F, Zuelzer WW, Kadowski J, Thompson R, Kennedy D: Temporary persistence of replicating donor cells after intra-uterine transfusion (abstract). J Pediatr 1965,67:937-938.

28. Hutchinson DL, Turner JH, Schlesinger ER: Persistence of donor cells in neonates after fetal and exchange transfusion. Am J Obstet Gynecol 1971;109:281-284.

29. Ino T, Matsuura A, Takahashi R, et al.: GVHD like syndrome following transfusion at the time of surgery. Geka 1986;48:706-712.

30. Sakakibara T, Juji T: Post-transfusion graft-versus-host disease after open heart surgery (letter). Lancet 1986;ii:1099.

31. Aoki Y, Nakamura H, Sakakibara Y: Probable graft-versus-host reaction following massive blood transfusion in an aged patient with postoperative aortic aneurysm: a case report. Nippon Naika Gakkai Zasshi 1984;73:99-106.

32. Wheeler ED, Turner JD, Scannell JG: Fevery, splenomegaly and atypical lymphocytes: syndrome observed after cardiac surgery utilizing pump oxygenator. N Engl J Med 1962;266:454-456.

33. Caul EO, Clarke SKR, Mott MG, Perham TGM, Wilson RSE: Cytomegalovirus infections after open heart surgery: a prospective study. Lancet 1971;i:777-781.

34. Lowenthal RM, Grossman L, Goldman JM, Storring RA, Buskard NA, Park DS, Murphy BC, Spiers ASD, Gattan DAG: Granulocyte transfusions in treatment of infections in patients with acute leukemia and aplastic anemia. Lancet 1975;i:353-358.

35. Sheehan T, McLaren KM, Brettle R, Parker AC: Transfusion-induced graft-versus-host disease in pregnancy. Clin Lab Hemat 1987;9:205-207.

36. Faulk WP, McIntrye JA: Trophoblast survival. Transplantation 1981;32:1-5.

37. Fulginiti VA, Pearlman DS, Reiquam CW, Claman HN, Hathaway WE, Blackburn WJ,

Githens JH, Kempe CH: Dissociation of delayed-hypersensitivity and antibody-synthesizing capacities in man. Lancet 1966;ii:5-8.

38. Hathaway WE, Fulginiti VA, Pierce CW, Githens JH, Pearlman DS, Muschenheim F, Kempe CH: Graft-versus-host reaction following a single blood transfuion. JAMA 1967;201:1015-1020.

39. Shapiro M: Familial autohemolytic anemia and runting syndrome with Rho-D specific autoantibody. Transfusion 1967;7:281-296.

40. Hong R, Cooper MD, Allan MJG, Kay HEM, Meuwissen H, Good RA: Immunological restitution in lymphopenic immunological deficiency syndrome. Lancet 1968; i:503-506.

41. Jacobs JC, Blanc WA, Capor A, Heird WC, McGilvray E, Miller OJ, Morse JH, Rossen RD, Schullinger JN, Walzer RA: Complement deficiency and chromosomal breaks in a case of Swiss-type agammaglobulinemia. Lancet 1968;i:499-503.

42. Douglas SD, Fudenberg HH: Graft-versus-host reaction in Wiskott-Aldrich syndrome: antemortem diagnosis of human GVH in an immunologic deficiency disease. Vox Sang 1969;16:172-178.

43. Gatti RA, Platt N, Pomerance HH, Hong R, Langer LO, Kay HEM, Good RA: Hereditary lymphopenic agammaglobulinemia associated with a distinctive form of short-limbed dwarfism and ectodermal dysplasia. J Pediatr 1969;75:675-684.

44. Robertson NRC, Berry CL, Macaulay JC, Soothill JF: Partial immuno-deficiency and graft-versus-host disease. Arch Dis Child 1971;46:571-574.

45. Soriano R, South MA, Montgomery J, Salmon S: Attempted immunologic reconstitution of a child with severe combined immune deficiency using the "suicide" radioactive thymidine technique. Clin Res 1972;20:102.

46. Park BH, Good RA, Gate J, Burke B: Fatal graft-versus-host reaction following transfusion of allogeneic blood and plasma in infants with combined immunodeficiency disease. Transplant Proc 1974;6:385-387.

47. Niethammer D, Goldman SF, Flad HD, Meigel W, Tollner U, Pohlandt F, Heymer B, Kleihauer E: Graft-versus-host reaction after blood transfusion in a patient with cellular immunodeficiency: the role of histocompatibility testing. Eur J Pediatr 1979;132:43-48.

48. Brubaker DB: Fatal graft-versus-host disease occurring after transfusion with unirradiated normal donor red cells in an immunodeficient neonate. Plasma Ther Transfus Techol 1984;5:117.

49. Billard V, Taboureau O, Lambilliotte A, Delattre A, Genet B: Reaction du greffon contre l'hote apres transfusion materno-foetale. Pediatrie 1986;41:657-663.

50. Mathe G, Schwarzenberg L, deVries MJ, Amiel JL, Cattan A, Schneider M, Binet JL, Tubiana JL, Lalanne M, Schwarzman V, Nordman R: Les divers aspects du syndrome secondaire compliquent les transfusions allogeniques de moelle osseuse ou de leukocytes chez des sujets d'hemopathies malignes. Eur J Cancer 1965;1:75-113.

51. Groff P, Torhorst J, Speck B, Nissen C, Weber W, Cornu P, Rossier J, Biland L: Die Graft-versus-Host Krankheit, eine wenig bekannte Komplikation der Bluttransfusion. Schweiz Med Wschr 1976;106:634-636.

52. Schaerer R, Schaerer L, Sotto JJ, et al.: La reaction du greffon contre l'hote (GVHD) comme complication letale des transfusions de sang us cours de la maladie de Hodgkin: a propos de deux observations (abstract). Premier Congress Francais d'Hematologie. Vittel, 1975.

53. Schmidmeier W, Feil W, Gebhard W, Grisold W, Gschnait F, Hinterberger W, Hocker P, Jellinger K, Krepier R, Machacek E: Fatal graft-versus-host reaction following granulocyte transfusions. Blut 1982;45:115-119.

54. Burns LJ, Westberg MN, Burns CP, Klassen LW, Goeken NE, Ray TL, Macfarlane DE: Acute graft-versus-host disease resulting from normal donor blood transfusions. Acta Haematol 1984;71:270-276.

55. Fisher RI, DeVita VT, Bostick F, Vanhaelen C, Howser DM, Hubbard SM, Young RC. Persistent immunologic abnormalities in long-term survivors of advanced Hodgkin's disease. Ann Intern Med 1980;92:595-599.

56. Twomey JJ, Rice L: Impact of Hodgkin's disease upon the immune system. Semin Oncol 1980,7:114-125.

57. DeDobbeleer GD, Ledoux-Corbusier MH, Achten GA: Graft-versus-host reaction. An ultrastructural study. Arch Dermatol 1975;8:1597-1602.

58. Betzhold J, Hong R: Fatal graft-versus-host disease after a small leukocyte transfusion in a patient with lymphoma and varicella. Pediatrics 1978;62:63-66.

59. Saab GA, Kurban AA, Mutasimi DF: Graft-versus-host disease in lymphoblastic lymphoma following blood transfuions. MEJ Anesth 1983;7:221-225.

60. Tolbert B, Kaufman CE, Burgdorf W, Brubaker DB: Graft-versus-host reaction from leukocyte transfusions: a case of irreversible bone marrow failure. J Am Acad Derm 1983;9:416-419.

61. Gossi U, Bucher U, Brundel RG: Acute Graft-versus-Host-Krankheit nach einer einzigen Erythrozytentransfusion. Schweiz Med Wschr 1985;115:34-40.

62. National Cancer Institute-sponsored study of classification of non-Hodgkin's lymphoma. Summary and description of a working formulation for clinical usage. Cancer 1982;49:2112-2135.

63. Schwarzenberg L, Mathe G, deGrouchy J, DeNava C, DeVries MJ, Amiel JL, Cattan A, Schneider M, Schlumberger JR: White blood cell transfusions. Isr J Med Sci 1965;1:923-926.

64. Mathe G, Amiel JL, Schwarzenberg L: Leukocyte transfusions. In *Bone Marrow Transplantation and Leucocyte Transfusion*, edited by Kugelmass. CC Thomas, Springfield, IL, 1971; pp. 104-130.

65. Szaly F, Buki B, Kalonics I, Keleman I: Graft-versus-host reaction (GVHD). Post-transfusion GVHR in an adult, diagnosed during life. Orv Hetil 1972;113:1275-1280.

66. Ford JM, Cullen MH, Lucey JJ, Tobias JS, Lister TA: Fatal graft-versus-host disease following transfusion of granulocytes from normal donors. Lancet 1976;ii:1167-1169.

67. Rosen RC, Huestis DW, Corrigan JJ: Acute leukemia and granulocyte transfusion of cells obtained from normal donors. J Pediatr 1978;93:268-270.

68. Salfner B, Borberg H, Kruger C, Schumacher K, Siebel E: Graft-versus-host Reaktion nach Granulozyten-transfusion von einem Normaspender. Blut 1978;36:27-34.

69. Cohen D, Weinstein H, Mohm M, Yankee R: Non-fatal graft-versus-host disease occurring after transfusion with leukocytes and platelets obtained from normal donors. Blood 1979;53:1053-1057.

70. Lowenthal RM, Menon C, Challis DR: Graft-versus-host disease in consecutive patients with acute myeloid leukemia treated with blood cells from normal donors. Aust NZJ Med 1981;11:179-183.

71. Siimes MA, Koskimies S: Chronic graft-versus-host disease after blood transfusions confirmed by incompatible HLA antigens in bone marrow (letter). Lancet 1982;i:42-43.

72. Schmitz N, Kayser W, Gassman W, Huhn A, Kruger G, Sachs V, Loffler H: Two cases of graft-versus-host disease following transfusion of non-irradiated blood products. Blut 1982;44:83-88.

73. Nikoskelainen J, Soderstrom KO, Rajamaki A, Meurman L, Korvenranta H, Kalliomaki JL, Toivanen A: Graft-versus-host reaction in 3 adult leukemia patients after transfusion of blood cell products. Scand J Haematol 1983;31:403-409.

74. Hersh EM, Whitecar JP, McCredie KB, Bodey GP, Freireich EJ: Chemotherapy, immune-competence, immunosuppression and prognosis in acute leukemia. N Engl J Med 1971,285:1211-1216.

75. Char DH, Lepourhiet A, Leventhal BF, Herberman RB: Cutaneous delayed hypersensitivity responses to tumor associated with other antigens in acute leukemia. Int J Cancer 1973,12:409-419.

76. Kay NE, Burton J, Allen JL, Eagon C, Perri R: Immunoregulatory cells in B-chronic lymphocytic leukemia. In *Chronic Lymphocytic Leukemia: Recent Progress and Future Direction*, edited by Gale RP, Rai KR. Alan R. Liss, Inc., New York, 1987; pp. 103-113.

77. Yonemoto RH, Terasaki PI: Cancer immunotherapy with HLA-compatible thoracic duct lymphocyte transplantation: a preliminary report. Cancer 1972;30:1438-1443.

78. Woods WG, Lubin BH: Fatal graft-versus-host disease following a blood transfusion in a child with neuroblastoma. Pediatrics 1981;67:217-221.

79. Kennedy JS, Ricketts RR: Fatal graft-versus-host disease in a child with neuroblastoma following a blood transfusion. J Pediatr Surg 1986;21:1108-1109.

80. Rosanda C, DeBernardo B, Pasino M, Bisogni C, Maggio A, Haupt R, Tonini GP, Ponzoni M: Immune evaluation of 50 children with neuroblastoma at onset. Med Pediatr Oncol 1982;10:321-330.

81. McCullough J, Benson SJ, Yunis EJ, Quie PG: Effect of blood bank storage on leukocyte function. Lancet 1969;ii:1333-1337.

82. Buchholz DH, Charette JR, Bove JR: Preparation of leukocyte-poor red blood cells using the IBM 2991 blood cell processor. Transfusion 1978;18:653-661.

83. Swensen S, Gilcher RO: Evaluation of cotton wool filter for preparation of leukocyte poor blood (abstract). South Central Association of Blood Banks, 1981.

84. Crowley JP, Skrabut EM, Valeri CR: Immunocompetent lymphocytes in previously frozen washed red cells. Vox Sang 1974;26:513-517.

85. Crowley JP, Wade PH, Wish C, Valeri CR: The purification of red cells for transfusion by freeze-preservation and washing. V. Red cell recovery and residual leukocytes after freeze-preservation with high concentrations of glycerol and washing in various systems. Transfusion 1977;17:1-7.

86. Valerius NH, Johansen KS, Nielsen OS, Platz P, Rosenkvist J, Sorensen H: Effect of in vitro x-irradiation on lymphocyte and granulocyte function. Scand J Hematol 1981,27:9-18.

87. Rotstein S, Baral E, Blomgren H, Johansson B: The effect of in vitro irradiation on mitogenic responsiveness of peripheral blood lymphocytes from untreated patients with Hodgkin's disease and non-Hodgkin's lymphoma. Cancer 1982;50:900-903.

88. Button LN, DeWolf WC, Newburger PE, Jacobson MS, Kevy SV: The effects of irradiation on blood components. Transfusion 1981;21:419-426.

89. Doria G, Agarossi G, Adorini L: Selective effects of ionizing radiation on immunoregulatory cells. Immunol Rev 1982;65:23-54.

90. Holley TR, Van Epps DE, Harvey RL, Anderson RE, Williams RC: Effects of high doses of radiation on human neutrophil chemotaxis, phagocytosis, and morphology. Am J Pathol 1974;75:61-68.

91. Patrone F, Dallegri F, Brema F, Sacchetti C: Effects of irradiation and storage on granulocytes harvested by continuous-flow centrifugation. Exp Hematol 1979;7:131-136.

92. Greenberg ML, Chanana AD, Cronkite EP, Schiffer LM, Stryckmans PA: Extracorporeal irradiation of blood in man: radiation resistance of circulating platelets. Radiat Res 1968;35:147-154.

93. Zuck TF, Brown GL, Buck LL: Effects of in vitro irradiation on platelet function and lymphocyte viability (abstract). Transfusion 1973;13:344a.

30

Graft Failure Following Transplantation of T-Cell-Depleted Marrow

Nancy A. Kernan
Memorial Sloan-Kettering Cancer Center
New York, New York

I. INTRODUCTION

Graft failure in recipients of unmodified bone marrow transplants from an HLA-identical sibling has been almost exclusively limited to patients affected by aplastic anemia with a history of repeated transfusions (1-3). Among patients with leukemia who have received total body irradiation in addition to cyclophosphamide, the incidence of graft failure following unmodified marrow transplants is less than 1% (4). In contrast, with similar immunosuppressive regimens the reported incidence of graft failure among recipients of T-cell-depleted HLA-identical transplants ranges from 10 to 30% independent of the method of T-cell depletion (5-10). For patients transplanted with T-cell-depleted marrow from HLA-nonidentical donors, the incidence of graft failure has been as high as 50-75% depending upon the degree of MHC disparity between the donor and recipient (11,12). These results are in sharp contrast to those seen in leukemic recipients of unmodified HLA-nonidentical marrow in which failure to achieve sustained marrow engraftment occurs in 5% of recipients (4,13).

An increase in the incidence of graft failure or rejection following transplants of T-cell-depleted marrow or fetal liver cells is not unique to man. It has been observed in murine, canine, and primate models (14-20) where it has been possible to differentiate between two immune mediated etiologies of graft failure: graft rejection secondary to prior sensitization and graft failure due to genetic resistance in a nonsensitized animal. The earliest studies demonstrated that lymphocytes in the fetal thymus promoted engraftment of T-cell-deficient fetal liver hematopoietic cells without contributing additional hematopoietic progenitor cells (21,22). Subsequent studies of transplants of T-cell-depleted marrow enriched with thymocytes (23) or spleen cells (24) derived from the donor have suggested that donor T cells promote, but are not mandatory for engraftment of hematopoietic progenitors in an allogeneic host. Although T lymphocytes elaborate several cytokines that may promote hematopoietic progenitor growth, deficiencies of such stimulatory factors do not adequately explain the increased need for T cells for engraftment in allogeneic as opposed to syngeneic hosts. The need for donor T lymphocytes to ensure engraftment in allogeneic hosts suggests that graft failure may be secondary to recognition and suppression of donor marrow by host immune cells.

II. ANIMAL MODELS

A. Presensitized Recipients

Resistance to hematopoietic grafts contributing to graft failure has been most extensively characterized in murine and canine models, in which at least two immune-mediated mechanisms have been distinguished. One reflects an unprimed (hybrid) host resistance to engraftment and the other an apparent rejection secondary to prior sensitization to donor antigens; lethally irradiated dogs or mice, previously sensitized to MHC-matched or mismatched allogeneic donors through infusions of whole blood or marrow cells, reject marrow grafts by what is presumed to be a classic immune response (18,19,25,26). In the mouse, Cantor has demonstrated that cytotoxic T cells generated in vitro in response to major or minor alloantigens are capable of suppressing hematopoietic cell growth in vivo (27). Additionally, the distinct contribution of T cells to rejection of bone marrow allografts has been directly demonstrated by Dennert et al. (18). In a mouse strain not exhibiting genetically determined hybrid resistance, cytotoxic T cells generated following presensitization to allogeneic, H-2-incompatible donor tumor cells could, upon passive transfer to secondary unsensitized syngeneic lethally irradiated recipients, precipitate rejection of a marrow graft from the sensitizing donor strain.

B. Unprimed Recipients

Resistance has been described in certain genetic strains of mice, by which unsensitized, lethally irradiated recipients are able to reject marrow from either H-2-nonidentical (allogeneic) or H-2-compatible (F_1 rejection of parental strain marrow) donors (15,16,28). This form of resistance is T-cell-independent, in that it is observed in both nude (athymic) and neonatally thymectomized mice (15-17). It is selectively directed against hematopoietic cells homozygously expressing certain non-H-2 antigens which are noncodominantly expressed, termed Hh antigens (16). In the canine model a similar form of resistance has been described but believed to be controlled through MHC-associated genes which are codominantly expressed (19,29,30). In both species this form of resistance appears to be mediated by effector cells with the genetic and cytotoxic characteristics of natural killer (NK) cells (17,31).

Although there is strong evidence in murine and canine models and substantial human data suggesting a primary role of NK cells in resistance to T-cell-depleted haploidentical (parental) marrow engraftment in patients with severe combined immunodeficiency (32), a role for NK cells in rejection of hematopoietic grafts by immunologically competent individuals has not been demonstrated. In fact, in a series of durably engrafted leukemic recipients of marrow depleted of T cells by soybean agglutinin and E-rosettes (SBA⁻E⁻), NK cells of donor origin appeared in the early phase of hematopoietic reconstitution posttransplant (33). In recipients of SBA⁻E⁻ marrow these cells do not have marrow suppressive activity against hematopoietic precursors (34). Since NK cells have been reported to secrete several lymphokines including interleukin-2, interleukin-1, and interferons as well as cytokines with colony stimulating activity

(35,36), the engrafted donor NK cells may actually play an important role post transplant in the regulation and differentiation of hematopoiesis.

III. CLINICAL TRANSPLANTATION

A. Evaluation of the Marrow Graft

All clinical studies involving the use of T-cell depletion have been complicated by an increased incidence of graft failure. Bone marrow manipulations associated with the different techniques utilized for T-cell depletion could be responsible for graft failure through a number of different mechanisms, including loss of stem cells, elimination of lymphoid and nonlymphoid cells with accessory functions for hematopoietic development, and removal of T cells capable of down-regulating residual host effectors responsible for graft rejection. Even though it is possible that all these mechanisms contribute to some extent to graft failure, there is considerable experimental and clinical evidence suggesting that it is unlikely that stem cell damage represents the predominant cause of graft failure. In animal models treated, syngeneic or autologous marrow transplants rarely fail. In clinical trials of T-cell-depleted marrow transplants there are no reports that demonstrate a significant correlation between the risk of graft failure and the number of nucleated cells or committed hematopoietic progenitors (CFU-GM). Furthermore, in two recently reported studies, T-cell depletion of *autologous* marrow was not associated with graft failure after transplantation, whereas there was a 15% and 27% incidence of graft failure among recipients of allogeneic marrow treated by the same methods (5,37).

Although stem cell damage does not appear to be the predominant cause of graft failure and most patients with graft failure show an initial engraftment with donor cells, there are reports of patients with primary graft failure (9,38,39). Whether this pattern of primary graft failure reflects stem cell damage, a defective microenvironment or residual host immunocompetence is unclear. Patients with primary graft failure have engrafted following additional immunosuppression and transplantation of unmodified same donor marrow. This would suggest that residual host resistance and not a defective marrow microenvironment was the predominant cause of marrow failure even in the setting of primary graft failure.

There is evidence that host marrow fibroblasts can be infected with virus in patients with active viral infection (40). Theoretically, at least, such an infection could actively interfere with the production of lymphokines necessary for hematopoietic growth.

B. HLA-Nonidentical T-Cell-Depleted Transplants

Analysis of the clinical and laboratory factors associated with graft failure indicate that the biology of graft failure may differ between recipients of HLA-nonidentical and HLA-identical transplants. Following an HLA-nonidentical T-cell-depleted transplant the course of hematopoietic recovery and subsequent rejection is very similar in all reported series (11,12,41,42). Bone marrow and peripheral blood studies reveal myeloid cells of donor origin between day 7 and 12. At 11-25 days posttransplant, patients develop an abrupt and absolute neutropenia accompanied by a lymphocytosis that lasts for 2-4 days. At the time of lymphocytosis, only cells of host origin can be detected in the peripheral blood and bone marrow by HLA serotyping, karyotype analysis, or both. By phenotypic analysis the circulating host cells are $CD3^+$ T cells predominantly of the $CD8^+$ lymphoid subset (42). These lymphocytes proliferate in response to and are cytotoxic toward donor peripheral blood targets. Sondel et al. have shown that peripheral blood mononuclear cells obtained from a recipient of an HLA-D mismatched marrow demonstrated a selective proliferative response against donor cells in a mixed lymphocyte culture reaction with a kinetic pattern suggesting a secondary response seen in in vitro primed lymphocyte testing (41). In another series of patients who rejected HLA-nonidentical grafts depleted of T cells with soybean agglutinin and sheep erythrocytes (SBA⁻E⁻), a correlation between the degree of HLA allodisparity unique to the bone marrow donor and the incidence of graft rejection was observed (11). The host T lymphocytes isolated from these recipients at the time of graft failure demonstrated cell mediated toxicity against donor target cells but not against host targets or the natural killer cell target, K562 (42). This pattern of reactivity suggested an active rejection process in a host sensitized to donor HLA antigens. And, in fact, it was possible to demonstrate that PBMC from a patient exhibited allospecific cytotoxic reactivity directed against a single class I (B7) MHC disparity unique to the donor. In a subsequent study, not only did a patient's PBMC exhibit allospecific (B46) cytotoxicity, but the cytotoxic activities of the PBMC and an interleukin-2 expanded T-cell line derived from the patient's PBMC at the time of graft failure were blocked by prior incubation of the target cells with an anti HLA-B locus monoclonal antibody (Kernan, N. A., and Keever, C. A., unpublished observations). Consistent with these findings the circulating T cells were CD8⁺ Leu7⁻ by surface phenotype analysis (Kernan, N. A. and Small T. N., unpublished observations). To date, cytotoxic responses directed against class II antigens unique to the donor have not been reported. In our series, an interleukin-2 expanded CD3⁺ CD4⁺ T-cell line lysed DR1 (donor)-bearing targets, but a sufficient number of PBMC from the patient were not available for direct cytotoxic assays.

C. HLA-Identical T-Cell-Depleted Transplants

1. Clinical Analyses

Prior to the introduction of T-cell-depletion techniques, graft failure following an HLA-identical sibling transplant was almost exclusively limited to patients with aplastic anemia (1-3). Although the effector cells mediating rejection of unmodified marrow grafts in these patients have not been fully characterized, they are presumed to be alloimmune T cells, since such rejections occur infrequently among untransfused individuals. In rare instances patients with aplastic anemia who have experienced graft failure or rejection have on occasion been found to have circulating lymphocytes capable of generating mixed lymphocyte reactions or cytotoxic reactions to donor antigens at the time of graft failure (43,44).

Graft failure has been a relatively frequent occurrence in virtually every study in which marrow transplants depleted of T lymphocytes have been used for prevention of GVHD. This has been a consistent observation independent of the method employed for depletion. Analyses of clinical and laboratory parameters that may affect the incidence of graft failure following a T-cell-depleted transplant have suggested five factors, listed in Table 1. Three reports have demonstrated an inverse relationship between the risk of graft failure and the amount of total body irradiation (37,38,45). However, the addition of total lymphoid irradiation to standard doses of total body irradiation has not affected the incidence of engraftment in all series (46). In contrast to the clear effect of increased doses of total body irradiation on engraftment, retrospective analyses of other character-

Table 1 Factors Associated with Graft Failure (HLA Identical)

Total dose of TBI
Underlying diagnosis
Sex of the donor
Donor/Recipient sex match
Age of the patient

istics have shown conflicting results. One study showed an increase in graft failure in patients with actue leukemia as compared to patients with chronic myelogenous leukemia (CML) (37). However, in a series of 115 leukemic recipients of T-cell-depleted (SBA⁻E⁻) HLA-identical marrow, the underlying diagnosis did not influence the rate of engraftment (39). This same study demonstrated a markedly increased risk of graft failure in patients with male donors that was even more significant among female recipients of male donor grafts (39). That this finding has not been confirmed in other studies may reflect small sample sizes, heterogeneous patient populations, or possibly the additional posttransplant immunosuppression used in other studies.

Few studies of T-cell depletion have included patients under the age of 15 years. In one series (SBA⁻E⁻), in which there were 17 evaluable patients under the age of 15, no patient rejected his/her graft. In this entire series (115 patients) the presence of specific HLA antigens, an intact spleen or antidonor leukocyte antibodies in the recipient did not constitute a significant risk factor for graft failure. Thus, graft failures occurred in patients without antidonor leukocyte antibodies and in patients who had had a splenectomy prior to transplantation. Since prior sensitization to donor HLA antigens has been associated with graft rejection among transfused patients with aplastic anemia, patients who suffered graft failure have been examined for exposure to sensitizing antigen (transfusion and pregnancy). In two studies no association was found between pretransplant transfusion history and graft failure following T-cell-depleted marrow transplantation (37,39). In both studies graft failures occurred in untransfused males.

In summary, the reported studies indicate that increasing doses of total body irradiation decrease the incidence of graft failure and that if pretransplant sensitization to alloantigens affects engraftment it is not the only cause of graft failure, as even untransfused males have failed to engraft following a T-cell-depleted marrow transplant. Since it is unlikely that the causes of graft failure are different for each series of patients, it is unclear why there are contradictory results with respect to underlying diagnosis and sex of the donor. Perhaps varied prior chemotherapy and posttransplant immunosuppression account for these observed discrepancies.

2. Laboratory Analyses

In an effort to understand the biology of marrow graft failure, several investigators have attempted to identify and characterize peripheral blood mononuclear cells found circulating either in patients with durable engraftment or in patients at the time of graft failure. Several patterns of graft failure have been observed: failure of initial engraftment, prompt early engraftment followed by the development of pancytopenia and marrow aplasia, development of early myeloid activity followed by an abrupt lymphocytosis identical to the pattern observed in patients who have rejected HLA-nonidentical T-cell-depleted transplants, and late graft failure associated with or without cytogenetic evidence of leukemic relapse.

In several studies natural killer (NK) cells were found to be the first lymphoid population to recover posttransplant as measured by both phenotypic and functional analyses (33,47). The cytolytic activity of these cells toward K562 was either normal or high. Although NK cells are known to inhibit hematopoiesis (48,49), the circulating cells in patients with durable engraftment following a T-cell-depleted marrow transplant have not been found to be marrow suppressive (34,39).

In marked contrast to patients with durable engraftment, lymphoid cells circulating in patients with graft failure following an HLA-identical T-cell-depleted transplant have lacked NK surface markers and function (39). Surface phenotype analysis has revealed $CD3^+$, $CD8^+$, $Leu7^+$, $HLA-DR^+$ T cells that do not express the CD25-associated IL-2 receptor (39,50). Although these cells were not lytic toward donor peripheral blood targets in chromium release assays, a role for these cells in the pathogenesis of graft failure has been suggested by their inhibitory activity against donor marrow colony forming units in in vitro assays (39,51).

In normal subjects the lymphoid subset of $CD3^+$, $CD8^+$, $Leu7^+$, $HLA-DR^+$ T cells has been described in adult bone marrow and less often in the peripheral blood (52). Vinci et al. have recently demonstrated that this subset of marrow T cells was able to inhibit in vitro hematopoiesis (53). Furthermore, the suppression was genetically restricted by the HLA DR locus. Other investigators have reported similar HLA DR restricted inhibitory effects on hematopoiesis by HLA DR positive T cells in both normal subjects (54) and patients with lymphoproliferative syndromes (55).

In the setting of marrow transplantation, Vinci et al. (56,57) have examined circulating monocytes, lymphocytes, and peripheral blood CFU-C and BFU-E in patients undergoing unmodified allogeneic bone marrow transplantation with apparent full donor engraftment. A subset of lymphocytes characterized by the presence of mature T-cell antigens, CD3, CD8, CD2 as well as Leu 7 and HLA DR suppressed peripheral blood CFU-C and BFU-E derived from the donor and family members sharing one HLA DR determinant with the donor and recipient (56). Interestingly, whereas the HLA DR restricted hematopoietic suppressive T cells described by Torok-Storb and Hansen (54) affected both haploidentical DR phenotypes, only one haplotype seemed to be involved in the genetic restriction described following marrow transplantation.

All genetic studies of the origin of hematopoietic and lymphoid cells in patients following a T-cell-depleted marrow have demonstrated a higher incidence of mixed chimerism in both cell populations as compared to that seen in recipients of unmodified marrow grafts (37,58-61). In our series the cytogenetic results of marrow metaphases in the early posttransplant period in patients who ultimately suffered graft failure or who were experiencing graft failure were no different from those observed in patients who experienced durable engraftment. However, interleukin 2 expanded T cells derived from peripheral blood mononuclear cells at the time of graft failure were 100% host origin in 12 of 14 cases (Kernan, N. A., unpublished observations). The high incidence of mixed chimerism observed in patients following a T-cell-depleted transplant as compared to recipients of unmodified marrow grafts suggests that host hematopoietic and lymphoid cells are targets for and are eliminated by donor T cells. The data from Vinci et al. indicate (1) $CD3^+$, $CD8^+$, $Leu7^+$ T cells suppress hematopoiesis in normal subjects and (2) following an unmodified marrow graft this same subset recovers early and demonstrates marrow inhibitory activity in an HLA DR restricted manner. In two studies of patients with graft failure, this same T-cell subset has been shown to demonstrate donor specific marrow suppression (39,51) and in one of these studies the cells have been shown to be of host origin (39). Thus, in the setting of full engraftment following an allogeneic transplant the subset may reflect recapitulation of normal ontogeny. However, should this host lymphoid subset persist following total body irradiation and chemotherapy and maintain its inhibitory capacity, it may completely suppress donor marrow growth in vivo. Whether these cells initiate marrow graft failure by a direct lytic or suppressive action on hematopoietic progenitors or by suppression of the growth or other donor cells (e.g., natural killer cells) or by the secretion of lymphokines remains to be determined.

3. Identificaton of the Target Antigen

In recipients of HLA-nonidentical grafts the target antigen appears to be in disparate HLA locus unique to the donor. The isolated effector cells are capable of both lysing B lymphoblastoid cell lines and suppressing CFU-GM progenitor cell growth of targets sharing the donor sensitizing HLA antigen (39). What the target cell or antigen is in the setting of HLA identity is entirely unclear. Clearly, in vitro studies indicate that the target structure is present in cells giving rise to CFU-GM. If graft failure is GVHD in reverse as has been suggested by some (62), then a system of minor antigens which can be recognized following an HLA-restricted interaction between host cells and their targets may play an important role in graft failure. In the setting of GVHD, sex-linked or Y-encoded minor antigens have been described as target antigens which can be recognized in association with HLA-A2 and B7 (63). The association of male donor-derived grafts with graft failure following transplantation with a T-cell-depleted marrow suggests that the H-Y antigen may well be a significant target antigen for effector cells involved in marrow graft failure.

IV. CONCLUSION

Despite increased incidences of graft failure in all clinical series and leukemic relapses in some series, T-cell depletion of donor marrow has proven to be the most successful approach to the prevention of both acute and chronic GVHD, certainly between HLA-identical pairs and most significantly between HLA-nonidentical pairs. However, for clinical trials of T-cell depletion to continue, successful approaches to overcome these new obstacles must be developed. The use of more intensive pre- or posttransplant immunosuppression and methods for less complete removal of T cells are presently under active investigation as approaches for preventing both graft failure and leukemic relapse. More intensive immunosuppression can increase the incidence of engraftment, however, at the cost of increased toxicity to the patient (12). The identification of residual host T lymphocytes (cytotoxic $CD8^+$, $Leu7^-$, $CD25^-$ cells in recipients of HLA-nonidentical transplants and suppressive $CD8^+$, $Leu7^+$ DR^+ $CD25^-$ cells in recipients of HLA-identical transplants) suggests that specific anti-pan-T-cell or anti-$CD8^+$ T-cell reagents might prevent the emergence of host effector cells capable of suppressing donor hematopoiesis. Clinical trials that are evaluating the potential of antithymocyte globulin preparations and anti-T-cell ricin A chain immunotoxins to decrease host resistance to engraftment are presently in progress.

Alternatively, the introduction of specific lymphokines, hematopoietic growth factors, or both into posttransplant regimens may provide sufficient stimuli for the growth of donor-derived marrow. In the setting of autologous marrow transplantation, leukocyte recovery has been accelerated by both recombinant human GM-CSF and G-CSF administered in vivo in the posttransplant period (64). Murine studies by Blazer et al. have suggested, however, that certain cytokines may actually increase the incidence of mixed chimerism following a T-cell-depleted marrow transplant (65) and thus, theoretically, could increase the incidence of graft failure.

It may be that durable engraftment of T-cell-depleted HLA-identical and HLA-non-identical transplants will be achieved by combining antihost specific reagents with hematopoietic cell growth promoting factors. Exploration of phase III studies combining two such reagents await the completion of phase I and II studies with each antilymphoid reagent and each cytokine used alone.

ACKNOWLEDGMENTS

The author's investigation was supported by Grants CA22507, CA23766, and CA08748 awarded by the National Cancer Institute, Department of Health and Human Services. I thank Carolynn Barnes for assistance in preparation of the manuscript.

REFERENCES

1. Storb R, Prentice RL, Thomas ED, Appelbaum FR, Deeg HJ, Doney K, Fefer A, Goodell BW, Mickelson E, Stewart P, Sullivan KM, Witherspoon RP: Factors associated with graft rejection after HLA-identical marrow transplantation for aplastic anemia. Br J Hematol 1983;55:573-585.
2. Champlin RE, Feig SA, Ho WG, Gale RP: Graft failure following bone marrow transplantation: its biology and treatment. Exp Hematol 1984;12:728.
3. Deeg HJ, Self S, Storb R, Doney K, Appelbaum FR, Witherspoon RP, Sullivan KM, Sheehan K, Sanders J, Mickelson E, Thomas ED: Decreased incidence of marrow graft rejection in patients with severe aplastic anemia: changing impact of risk factors. Blood 1986;68:1363-1368.
4. Beatty PG, Clift RA, Mickeson EM, Nisperos BB, Flournoy N, Martin PJ, Sanders JE, Stewart P, Buckner CD, Storb R, Thomas ED, Hansen JA: Marrow transplantation from related donors other than HLA-identical siblings. N Engl J Med 1985; 313:765-771.
5. Hale G, Cobbold S, Waldmann H: For CAMPATH-1 Users, T cell depletion with CAMPATH-1 in allogeneic bone marrow transplantation. Transplantation 1988; 45:753-759.
6. Patterson J, Prentice HG, Brenner MK, Gilmore M, Janossy G, Ivory K, Skeggs D, Morgan H, Lord J, Blacklock HA, Hoffbrand AV, Apperley JF, Goldman JM, Burnett A, Gribben J, Alcorn M, Pearson C, McVickers I, Hann IM, Reid C, Wardel D, Gravett PJ, Bacigalupo A, Robertson AG: Graft rejection following HLA matched T-lymphocyte depleted bone marrow transplantation. Br J Haematol 1986;63:221-230.
7. Mitsuyasu RT, Champlin RE, Gale RP, Ho WG, Lenarsky C, Winston D, Selch M, Elashoff R, Giorgi JV, Wells J, Terasaki P, Billing R, Feig S: Treatment of donor bone marrow with monoclonal anti-T cell antibody and complement for the prevention of graft versus host disease. Ann Intern Med 1986;105:20-26.
8. Filipovich AH, Vallera DA, Youle RJ, Haake R, Blazer BR, Arthur D, Neville D, Ramsay NK, McGlave P, Kersey JH: Graft versus host disease prevention in allogeneic bone marrow transplantation from histocompatible siblings. Transplantation 1987;44:62-69.
9. Martin PJ, Hansen JA, Buckner CD, Sanders JE, Deeg HJ, Stewart P, Appelbaum FR, Clift R, Fefer A, Witherspoon RP, Kennedy MS, Sullivan KM, Flournoy N, Storb R, Thomas ED: Effects of in vitro depletion of T cells in HLA-identical allogeneic marrow grafts. Blood 1985;66:664-672.

10. O'Reilly RJ, Collins NH, Brochstein J, Kernan NA, Keever C, Castro-Malaspina H, Flomenberg N, Laver J, Gulati S, Burns J, Emanuel D, Bordignon C, Small T, Hornick D, Kushner B, Shank B: Soybean lectin agglutination and E rosette depletion for removal of T cells from HLA identical marrow grafts: results in 60 consecutive patients transplanted for hematopoietic malignancy. In *Minimal Residual Disease in Acute Leukemia*, Edited by Hagenbeck A, Löwenberg B. Martinus Nijhoff, Dordrecht, The Netherlands 1986; pp. 337-433.

11. O'Reilly RJ, Collins NH, Kernan NA, Brochstein J, Dinsmore R, Kirkpatrick D, Siena S, Keever C, Jordan B, Shank B, Wolf L, Dupont B, Reisner Y. Transplantation of marrow depleted of T cells by soybean lectin agglutination and E rosette depletion: major histocompatibility complex-related graft resistance in leukemic transplant recipients. Transplant Proc 1985;17:455-459.

12. Bozdech MJ, Sondel PM, Trigg ME, Longo W, Kohler PC, Flynn B, Billing R, Anderson SA, Hank JA, Hong R: Transplantation of HLA-haploidentical T-cell depleted marrow for leukemia: addition of cytosine arabinoside to the pretransplant conditioning prevents rejection. Exp Hematol 1985;13:1201-1210.

13. Powles RL, Morgenstern GR, Kay HEM, McElwain TJ, Clink HA, Dady PJ, Barrett A, Jameson B, Depledge MH, Watson JG, Sloane J, Leigh M, Lumley H, Hedley D, Lawler SD, Filshie J, Robinson B: Mismatched family donors for bone-marrow transplantation as treatment for acute leukemia. Lancet 1983;1:612-615.

14. Uphoff D: Preclusion of secondary phase of irradiation syndrome by inoculation of fetal hematopoietic tissue following lethal total body x-irradiation. J Natl Cancer Inst 1958;20:625.

15. Cudkowicz G, Bennett M: Peculiar immunobiology of bone marrow allografts. I. Graft rejection by irradiated responder mice. J Exp Med 1971;134:83-102.

16. Cudkowicz G, Bennett M: Peculiar immunobiology of bone marrow allografts. II. Rejection of parental grafts by resistance F_1 hybrid mice. J Exp Med 1971;134:1513-1529.

17. Kiessling R, Hochman PS, Haller O, Shearer GM, Wigzell H, Cudkowicz G: Evidence for a similar or common mechanism for natural killer activity and resistance to hemopoietic grafts. Eur J Immunol 1977;7:655-663.

18. Dennert G, Anderson CG, Warner J: T killer cells play a role in allogeneic bone marrow graft rejection but not in hybrid resistance. J Immunol 1985;135:3729-3734.

19. Storb R, Deeg HJ: Failure of allogeneic canine marrow grafts after total body irradiation: Allogeneic "resistance" versus transfusion-induced sensitization. Transplantation 1986;42:571-580.

20. Wagamaker G, Vriesendorp HM, van Bekkum DW: Successful bone marrow transplantation across major histocompatibility barriers in rhesus monkeys. Transplant Proc 1981;13:875-880.

21. Bortin MM, Saltzstein EC: Graft versus host inhibition: fetal liver and thymus cells minimize secondary disease. Science 1969;164:316-318.

22. Lowenberg B: Radiological Institute of the Organization for Health Research TNO. Rijswijk 56, The Netherlands, 1975.

23. Deeg HJ, Storb R, Weiden PL, Shulman HM, Graham TC, Torok-Storb BJ, Thomas ED: Abrogation of resistance to and enhancement of HLA-nonidentical unrelated marrow grafts in lethally irradiated dogs by thoracic duct lymphocytes. Blood 1979;53:552-557.

24. Vallera DA, Soderling C, Carlson GJ, Kersey JH: Bone marrow transplantation across major histocompatibility barriers in mice II: T cell requirement for engraftment in total lymphoid irradiaton-conditioned recipients. Transplantation 1982;33:243-248.

25. Storb R, Epstein RB, Rudolph RH, Thomas ED: The effect of prior transfusion on

marrow grafts between histocompatible canine siblings. J Immunol 1970;105:627-633.

26. Storb R, Rudolph RH, Graham TC, Thomas ED: The influence of transfusions from unrelated donors upon marrow grafts between histocompatible canine siblings. J Immunol 1971,107:409-413.

27. Cantor H: Control of allograft response and GVH disease. In *Natural Resistance Systems Against Foreign Cells, Tumors and Microbes*, edited by Cudkowicz G, Landy M, Shearer GM, Academic Press, New York 1978; p. 252.

28. Bonmassar E, Campanile F, Houchens D, Crino L, Goldwin A: Impaired growth of a radiation induced lymphoma in intact or lethally irradiated allogeneic athymic (nude) mice. Transplantation 1975;20:343-346.

29. Storb R, Weiden PL, Graham TC, Thomas ED: Failure of engraftment and graft versus host disease after canine marrow transplantation: two phenomena linked to but not exclusively determined by known antigens of the major histocompatibility complex. Transplant Proc 1978;10:113-118.

30. Deeg HJ, Storb R, Raff RF, Weiden PL, DeRose S, Thomas ED: Marrow grafts between phenotypically HLA-identical and haploidentical unrelated dogs: additional antigens controlling engraftment are not detected by cell-mediated lympholysis. Transplantation 1982;33:17-21.

31. Raff RF, Deeg HJ, Loughran TP, Graham TC, Aprile JA, Sale GE, Storb R. Characterization of host cells involved in resistance to marrow grafts in dogs transplanted from unrelated HLA-nonidentical donors. Blood 1986;68:861-868.

32. Friedrich W, Goldmann SF, Ebell W, Blutters-Sawatzki R, Gaedicke G, Raghavachar A, Peter HH, Belohradsky B, Kreth W, Kubanek B, Kleihauer E: Severe combined immunodeficiency: treatment by bone marrow transplantation in 15 infants using HLA-haploidentical donors. Eur J Pediatr 1985;144:125-130.

33. Keever CA, Welte K, Small T, Levick J, Sullivan M, Hauch M, Evans RL, O'Reilly RJ: Interleukin 2-activated killer cells in patients following transplants of soybean lectin separated and E rosette depleted bone marrow. Blood 1987;70:1893-1903.

34. Bordignon C, Kernan NA, Keever CA, Cartagena T, Benazzi E, Burns J, Flomenberg N, Dupont B, O'Reilly RJ: Graft failures following SBA⁻E⁻ T cell depleted marrow transplants for leukemia: in vitro correlates, in *T Cell Depletion in Allogeneic Bone Marrow Transplantation*, edited by Martelli MF, Grignani F, Reisner Y. Ares-Serono Symposia, Rome, Italy 1988; pp. 57-60.

35. Kasahara T, Djeu JY, Dougherty SF, Oppenheim JJ: Capacity of human large granular lymphocytes (LGL) to produce multiple lymphokines: interleukin 2, interferon, and colony stimulating factor. J Immunol 1983;131:2379-2385.

36. Djeu JY: Release of cytokines by large granular lymphocytes, In *Natural Immunity, Cancer and Biological Response Modification*, edited by Lotova E, Herberman RB. Karger, Basel, 1986; pp. 50-55.

37. Martin PJ, Hansen JA, Torok-Storb B, Durnam D, Przepioka D, O'Quigley J, Sanders J, Sullivan KM, Witherspoon RP, Deeg HJ, Appelbaum FR, Stewart P, Weiden P, Doney K, Buckner CD, Clift R, Storb R, Thomas ED: Graft failure in patients receiving T cell depleted HLA-identical allogeneic marrow transplants. Bone Marrow Transplantation 1988;3:445-456.

38. Patterson J, Prentice HG, Brenner MK, Gilmore M, Janossy G, Ivory K, Skeggs D, Morgan H, Lord J, Blacklock HA, Hoffbrand AV, Apperley JF, Goldman JM, Burnett A, Gribben J, Alcorn M, Pearson C, McVickers I, Hann AM, Reid C, Wardle D, Gravett PJ, Bacigalupo A, Robertson AG: Graft rejection following HLA matched T lymphocyte depleted bone marrow transplantation. Br J Haemat 1986;63:221-230.

39. Kernan NA, Bordignon C, Keever CA, Cunningham I, Castro-Malaspina H, Collins NH, Small TN, Brochstein J, Emanuel D, Laver J, Shank B, Burns J, Flomenberg N,

Gulatin S, Dupont B, O'Reilly RJ: Graft failure after T cell depleted marrow transplants for leukemia: clinical and in vitro characteristics. Transplant Proc 1987;19: 29-32.

40. Torok-Storb B, Simmons P, Przepioka D: Impairment of hemopoiesis in human allografts. Transplant Proc 1987,19:33-37.

41. Sondel PM, Hank JA, Trigg ME ME, Kohler PC, Finlay JL, Blank J, Meisner L, Borcherding W, Hong R, Steeves R, Billing R, Flynn B, Bozdech MJ: Transplantation of HLA-haploidentical T-cell depleted marrow for leukemia: Autologous marrow recovery with specific immune sensitization to donor antigens. Exp Hematol 1986;14:278-286.

42. Kernan NA, Flomenberg N, Dupont B, O'Reilly RJ: Graft rejection in recipients of T-cell depleted HLA-nonidentical marrow transplants for leukemia. Transplantation 1987;43:482-487.

43. Tsoi MS, Warren RP, Storb R, Witherspoon RP, Mickelson E, Giblett ER, Schanfield MS, Weiden P, Thomas ED: Autologous marrow recovery and sensitization to non-HLA antigens after HLA-identical marrow transplantation for aplastic anemia. Exp Hematol 1983;11:73-81.

44. Goulmy E, Termijtelen A, Bradley BA, van Rood JJ: Y-antigen killing by T cells of women is restricted by HLA. Nature 1977;266:544-545.

45. Guyotat D, Dutou L, Erhsam A, Campos L, Archimbaud E, Fiere D: Graft rejection after T cell-depleted marrow transplantation: Role of fractonated irradiation. Br J Haematol 1987;65:499-507.

46. Ganem G, Kuentz M, Beaujean F, Lebourgeois J, Vinci G, Cordonnier C, Vernant JP: Additional total-lymphoid irradiation in preventing graft failure of T-cell depleted bone marrow transplantation from HLA-identical siblings. Transplantation 1987; 45:244-248.

47. Brenner MK, Reittie JE, Grob J-P, Wimperis JZ, Stephens S, Patterson J, Hoftbrand AV, Prentice HG: The contribution of large granular lymphocytes to B cell activation and differentiation after T-cell-depleted allogeneic bone marrow transplantation. Transplantation 1986,42:257-261.

48. Mangan KF, Hartnett ME, Matis SA, Winkelstein A, Abo T: Natural killer cells suppress human erythroid stem cell proliferation in vitro. Blood 1984;63:260-269.

49. Degliantoni G, Perussia B, Mangoli L, Trinchieri G: Inhibition of bone marrow colony formation by human natural killer cells and by natural killer cell-derived colony inhibiting activity. J Exp Med 1985;161:1152-1168.

50. Sandell L, Johnson G, Przepiorka D, Torok-Storb B: Phenotype and function of T cells associated with marrow graft failure and rejection, In *T-Cell Depletion in Allogeneic Bone Marrow Transplantation*, edited by Martelli MF, Grignani F, Reisner Y. Ares-Serono Symposia, Rome, Italy, 1988; pp. 49-56.

51. Bunjes D, Heit W, Arnold R, Schmeiser X, Wiesneth M, Carbonell F, Porzsolt F, Raghavachar A, Heimpel H: Evidence of the involvement of host derived OKT8-positive T cells in the rejection of T-depleted, HLA-identical bone marrow grafts. Transplantation 1987;43:501-505.

52. Abo T, Miller CA, Gartland L, Balch CM: Differentiation stages of human natural killer cells in lymphoid tissues from fetal to adult life. J Exp Med 1983;157:273-284.

53. Vinci G, Vernant JP, Nakazawa M, Zohair M, Katz A, Henri A, Rochant H, Breton-Gorius J, Vainchenkes W: In vitro inhibition of normal human hematopoiesis by marrow CD3+, CD8+, HLA-DR+, HNK+ lymphocytes. Blood 1988;72:1616-1621.

54. Torok-Storb B, Hansen JA: Modulation of in vitro BFU-E growth by normal Ia-positive T cells is restricted by HLA-DR. Nature 1982;298:473-474.

55. Lipton JM, Nadler LM, Canellos GP, Kudisch M, Reiss CS, Nathan DG: Evidence for genetic restriction in the suppression of erythropoiesis by a unique subset of T lymphocytes in man. J Clin Invest 1983,72:694-706.

56. Vinci G, Vernant JP, Cordonnier C, Bracq C, Rochant H, Breton-Gorius J, Vain-chenker W: HLA-DR restriction in suppression of hematopoiesis by T cells from allogeneic bone marrow transplants. J Immunol 1986;136:3225-3230.

57. Vinci G, Vernant JP, Cordonnier C, Henri A, Breton-Gorius J, Rochant H, Vain-chenker W: In vitro inhibition of hematopoiesis by HNK1, DR-positive T cells and monocytes after allogeneic bone marrow transplantation. Exp Hematol 1987;15:54-64.

58. Bretagne S, Vidaud M, Kuentz M, Cordonnier C, Henni T, Vinci G, Goossens M, Vernant JP: Mixed blood chimerism in T cell-depleted bone marrow transplant recipients: Evaluation using DNA polymorphisms. Blood 1987;70:1692-1695.

59. Lawler SD, Harris H, Millar J, Barrett A, Powles RL: Cytogenetic follow-up studies of recipients of T cell depleted allogeneic bone marrow. Br J Haematol 1987;65:143-150.

60. Bertheas MF, Maraninchi D, Lafage M, Fraisse J, Blaise D, Stoppa AM, Michel G, Brizard CP, Gaspard MH, Novakovitch G, Mannoni P, Viens P, Carcassonne Y: Partial chimerism after T-cell depleted allogeneic bone marrow transplantation in leukemic HLA-matched patients: A cytogenetic documentation. Blood 1988;72:89-93.

61. Schouten HC, Sizoo W, van't Veer MB, Hagenbeek A, Lowenberg B: Incomplete chimerism in erythroid, myeloid and B lymphocyte lineage after T cell-depleted allogeneic bone marrow transplantation. Bone Marrow Transplantation 1988;3:407-412.

62. Gale RP, Reisner Y: Graft rejection and graft-versus-host disease: mirror images. Lancet 1986;1:1468-1470.

63. Goulmy E, Gratama JW, Blokland E, Zwaan FE, van Rood JJ: A minor transplantation antigen detected by MHC-restricted cytotoxic T lymphocytes during graft-versus-host disease. Nature 1983;302:159-161.

64. Peters WP, Kurtzburg J, Atwater S, Borowitz M, Gilbert L, Rao M, Currie M, Shogan J, Jones RB, Shpall EJ, Souzer L: Comparative effects of rHuG-CSF and rHuGM-CSF on hematopoietic reconstitution and granulocyte function following high dose chemotherapy and autologous bone marrow transplantation (BMT). Blood 1988;72:(Suppl 1).432.

65. Blazar BR, Widmer MB, Soderling C, Gillis S, Vallera DA: Enhanced survival but reduced engraftment in murine recipients of recombinant granulocyte/macrophage colony-stimulating factor following transplantation of T-cell depleted histoincompatible bone marrow. Blood 1988;72:1148-1154.

31

Clinical Spectrum of Human Chronic Graft-vs.-Host Disease

Kerry Atkinson
St. Vincent's Hospital
Sydney, New South Wales, Australia

I. INTRODUCTION

The first cases of human chronic GVHD were reported in the mid-1970s as recipients of HLA-identical sibling marrow allografts began to become long-term survivors. Since this was a new disease in the 1970s, early patients were often diagnosed late in their course when disabling complications had already set in. Manifestations in these patients included severe skin and subcutaneous fibrosis with contractures, severe wasting, and frequent infections, the latter often being the ultimate cause of death. Early attempts at treatment of this late advanced disease, often with single agents, were ineffective. However, increased physician awareness of the disease, with subsequent early monitoring posttransplant, has resulted in earlier diagnosis and instititution of treatment (Chapter 38). Additionally, the development of effective therapy (Chapter 38) has enabled the majority of patients diagnosed early to be treated satisfactorily, with very few subsequently developing severe life-threatening complications or complications that impair the quality of life. Therefore, the possibility of chronic GVHD should not be regarded as an argument against allogeneic transplantation for otherwise fatal diseases. Furthermore, the disease has been shown to contribute positively to increased survival in patients at high risk of leukemic relapse due to an associated graft-vs.-leukemia effect (Chapter 39).

The incidence of chronic GVHD is between 25 and 50% in different reported series. In 2534 patients given HLA-identical sibling marrow transplants for hematological malignancy or severe aplastic anemia and reported to the International Bone Marrow Transplant Registry between January 1982 and June 1987, the actuarial probability of developing chronic GVHD by 3 years posttransplant was 46% (1).

The common target organs involved in chronic GVHD are the skin, liver, eyes, and mouth (2-4). Less commonly, the esophagus, small intestine, lung, vagina, muscles, and tendons are involved. Isolated cases of renal and brain involvement have also been reported. The systemic and widespread nature of the disease, as well as the clinical manifestations of the individual target organs, have produced analogies between chronic GVHD and the connective tissue disorders such as progressive systemic sclerosis, systemic lupus erythematosus, Sjögren's syndrome, eosinophilic fasciitis, and rheumatoid arthritis. These similarities have been further emphasized by the finding of circulating autoantibodies in patients with chronic GVHD. The immune system is also a target organ, and this is manifested clinically by the susceptibility to infectious complications, both bacterial and viral, in these patients (5-8).

By convention, GVHD occurring 100 days or later after marrow transplantation has been designated chronic. Clearly, however, the two syndromes of acute and chronic GVHD differ not only by their timing posttransplant and in their clinical manifestations, but also in their responsiveness to treatment and their prognosis. While acute GVHD is primarily an alloreactive disorder (Chapter 16), there is evidence both in the clinic and in the laboratory of an autoreactive component in chronic GVHD. Clearly, the pathogenetic mechanisms involved have no respect for the time-frame definitions used by the clinician, and lesions clinically typical of chronic GVHD can occur in individual patients much earlier than 100 days posttransplant (9).

II. INCIDENCE OF CHRONIC GVHD

In most reported series of patients given HLA-identical sibling marrow grafts, the incidence of chronic GVHD is between 25 and 50%. The largest series is that from the International Bone Marrow Transplant Registry (IBMTR) in which 2534 patients given HLA-identical sibling marrow transplants were included. The incidence of chronic GVHD in this population was 39%, while the actuarial probability of developing chronic GVHD at 3 years posttransplant was 46% (1).

A number of factors are known to predispose to the development of chronic GVHD, and the prevalence of these factors in a given series will influence the incidence of chronic GVHD. These factors include the incidence and severity of preceding acute GVHD, recipient age, and the type of GVHD prophylaxis used posttransplant. Thus, older recipients have a higher incidence of chronic GVHD than younger recipients, while T-cell-depleted marrow transplants are associated with a lower incidence of chronic GVHD than T-cell-replete transplants (1). In a study in which the recipients were children (median age 10 years) who were given the conventional long methotrexate immunosuppressive prophylactic regime, the incidence of chronic GVHD was 11% (10). Likewise, in another study in which the median age was 16 but in which posttransplant immunosuppression was not utilized, the incidence was 18% (11). Conversely, analyses in which the recipients were older (median ages 47 and 55 years) the incidence of chronic GVHD was 70% and 60%, respectively (12).

As noted above, chronic GVHD has been defined as GVHD present 100 days or later posttransplant. In practice, the typical clinical lesions of chronic GVHD (for example the lichen planus-like lesions seen in the mouth) can be seen as early as 40 days posttransplant (9). Seldom, however, does chronic GVHD develop later than 400 days posttransplant (Fig. 1).

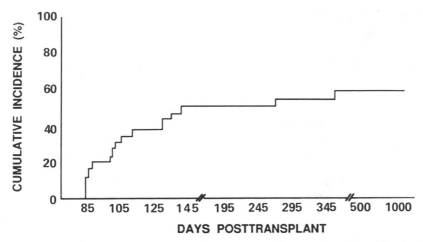

Figure 1 Incidence and time of onset of chronic GVHD after HLA-identical sibling marrow transplantation for acute leukemia. Recipients (n = 76) were prepared for transplantation with cyclophosphamide 120 mg/kg and fractionated total body irradiation 12 Gy. Unmanipulated marrow was used and immunoprophylaxis for GVHD was with cyclosporine or methotrexate (K. Atkinson, unpublished data).

III. CLASSIFICATION OF CHRONIC GVHD

A. Type of Onset

Most commonly chronic GVHD will become clinically manifest sometime after the clinical manifestations of acute GVHD have resolved—the so-called "quiescent" mode of development of chronic GVHD. Alternatively, acute GVHD will clinically merge slowly into chronic GVHD—the so-called "progressive" mode of development of chronic GVHD. In a third (and rarer) pattern, chronic GVHD will develop without any preceding clinically recognizable syndrome of acute GVHD—the so-called "de novo" pattern of development of chronic GVHD.

B. Extent of Disease

Early in the recognition of this disease a limited form was differentiated from an extensive form (2). The limited form was defined as localized skin involvement with or without hepatic dysfunction. Extensive chronic GVHD was defined as either generalized skin involvement, or as localized skin involvement with or without hepatic dysfunction, but with liver histology showing chronic aggressive hepatitis, bridging necrosis or cirrhosis, or eye involvement, or oral involvement or involvement of any other target organ (Table 1). While localized skin involvement alone is relatively rare, an asymptomatic and isolated elevation of the serum alkaline phosphatase concentration due to chronic GVHD is not uncommon. The usefulness of this demarcation of the disease into limited and extensive forms has been validated by the response to a questionnaire sent to transplant centers by the IBMTR (9).

While involvement with chronic GVHD may also be subjectively divided into mild, moderate, or severe by individual physicians, objective criteria for such definitions are lacking. The Karnofsky performance score, however, has proven to be a useful and ob-

Table 1 Clinical Grading of Chronic GVHD

Limited chronic GVHD
    Either or both:
        1. Localized skin involvement
        2. Hepatic dysfunction
Extensive chronic GVHD
    Either:
        1. Generalized skin involvement; or
        2. Localized skin involvement with or without hepatic dysfunction, plus:
            a. Liver histology showing chronic aggressive hepatitis, bridging necrosis or cirrhosis; or
            b. Involvement of eye:Schirmer's test with less than 5 mm wetting; or
            c. Involvement of minor salivary glands or oral mucosa demonstrated on lip biopsy; or
            d. Involvement of any other target organ

Source: Adapted from Ref. 2.

Table 2 The Karnofsky Performance Score

Able to carry on normal activity; no special care is needed.	100%	Normal; no complaints; no evidence of disease.
	90%	Able to carry on normal activity.
	80%	Normal activity with effort.
Unable to work; able to live at home, care for most personal needs; a varying amount of assistance is needed.	70%	Cares for self; unable to carry on normal activity or to do active work.
	60%	Requires occasional assistance but is able to care for most needs.
	50%	Requires considerable assistance and frequent medical care.
Unable to care for self; requires equivalent of institutional or hosptial care; disease may be progressing rapidly.	40%	Disabled; requires special care and asistance.
	30%	Severely disabled; hospitalization indicated, although death not iminent.
	20%	Very sick; hospitalization necessary.
	10%	Moribund; fatal process progressing rapidly.
	0%	Dead.

jective means of defining the extent and severity of this disease and is currently widely utilized for this purpose (Table 2).

IV. CLINICAL MANIFESTATIONS

A. Skin

The skin is the most common organ involved in chronic GVHD (Fig. 2). The clinical manifestations include dyspigmentation (hyper- and hypopigmentation), lichenoid papules (often purplish with white striae criss-crossing their surface), and areas of local erythema (13). Areas of hyperpigmentation can be the sole clinical manifestation but may be cosmetically important, particularly if on the face. Lichenoid papules can occur anywhere including the palms, soles, and genitals. A typical mottled appearance of the skin is produced when alternating hyperpigmentation and hypopigmentation develop. The tempo of development of these changes is variable, but sometimes they can develop remarkably quickly, particularly if prophylactic immunosuppression is being tapered or ceased. Photoactivation of chronic GVHD by sunlight has been reported but is now virtually eliminated with advice on sun exposure and the routine use of strong UV-blocking creams.

The more serious manifestation of dermal and subcutaneous fibrosis can also develop rapidly and in a widespread manner. All areas of the skin can become involved. Less commonly the localized form of subcutaneous fibrosis occurs (localized morphoea). Hair loss (scarring alopecia) is a consequence of this subcutaneous fibrosis and conversely, as the fibrosis resolves, hair regrowth is an excellent early sign of skin improvement. Without treatment, the generalized form of fibrosis will result in hidebound skin and joint contractures. Interestingly, when the fibrosis is localized it may resolve spontaneously without treatment, or it may wax and wane in different areas over a period of several years. Rarely, a blistering (bullous) eruption can occur on top of skin involved by the scleroderma-like syndrome (14), and vascular tumours have also been reported (15).

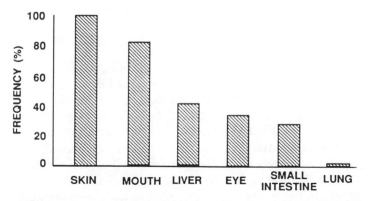

Figure 2 Frequency of organ involvement in chronic GVHD. The data are derived from the same population as in Figure 1.

Table 3 Liver Function Test Profiles in Various Complications Causing Jaundice After Bone Marrow Transplantation

Diagnosis	Elevation of serum values		
	Bilirubin	Transaminase	Alkaline Phosphatase
Hepatic GVHD	++	+	+++
Hepatic VOD	++	+	+++
CSP hepatotoxicity	+	±	±
Acute viral hepatitis	+ to ++	+++	+
Hemolysis	± (unconjugated)	−	−

Abbreviations: GVHD = Graft-vs.-Host Disease; VOD = veno-occlusive disease; CSP = cyclosporine.

B. Liver

Liver involvement occurs in approximately 80% of patients with chronic GVHD. It can range in severity from a completely asymptomatic elevation of the serum alkaline phosphatase concentration, which may resolve spontaneously without treatment, to marked cholestatic jaundice. As with acute hepatic GVHD the serum alkaline phosphatase concentration is markedly increased (median six times normal) (2) while the alanine transaminase concentration, although increased, does not reach levels seen in acute viral hepatitis. The primary differential diagnosis in marrow transplant recipients late posttransplant includes other causes of obstructive jaundice, including that due to sludge or cotrimoxazole or to a phenothiazine. Differentiation from other causes of jaundice in the marrow transplant recipient is usually relatively easily made on the basis of the liver function test profile (Table 3) (16). Differentiation from the cholestatic phase of a viral hepatitis is important in view of the low but definite incidence of progression of non-A non-B hepatitis to cirrhosis and its possible prevention with the use of α-interferon. Liver biopsy can be useful in this regard with atypia, inflammation, and a generalized decrease in the number of small bile ducts being a sensitive, but not specific, indicator of involvement by GVHD (17). Endothelialitis of portal or central hepatic veins has been suggested as a more predictive change for GVHD (18).

   Interestingly, and encouragingly, progression of chronic hepatic GVHD to either hepatic failure (17) or cirrhosis and portal hypertension (19) are reported but rare.

C. Mouth

Mouth involvement occurs in 80% of patients with chronic GVHD. Characteristic clinical changes include the development of white, lichen planus-like striae and plaques, ulceration, atrophy, patchy erythema, and dryness (20). The lichenoid changes can occur on the buccal mucosa, tongue, and gums, as can the ulceration. Mouth ulcers can be painful and prevent adequate nutrition. The lichenoid changes can usually be differentiated from candida of the mouth relatively easily. Atrophy of the gums together with poor oral hygiene (consequent to oral pain) can predispose rapidly to severe dental damage. In addition to this mucosal damage, involvement of the minor salivary glands and ducts by chronic GVHD leads to dryness of the mouth. However, since one study has suggested that reduction of salivary flow rate is related to the use of total body irradiation in the pretransplant preparative regime (21), some caution should be exercised in initiating treatment when dryness of the mouth is the only clinical manifestation. In this situation, lip biopsy is a helpful diagnostic test as obliterative sialadenitis correlates strongly with the oral sicca syndrome of chronic GVHD (22). Unchecked, oral chronic GVHD can progress to give a firm leathery appearance to the buccal mucosa and a reduced ability to open the mouth.

Salivary gland involvement in chronic GVHD is associated with decreased or absent levels of salivary IgA and inorganic phosphate, decreased salivary flow rates and increased concentrations of salivary sodium, albumin, and IgG (23). This secretory IgA deficiency may contribute to the frequent sino-bronchial infections observed in patients with chronic GVHD (see below).

D. Eye

Ocular involvement occurs in 80% of patient with chronic GVHD (24-26). The commonest symptom is dryness of the eyes, and all patients should be monitored with a Schirmer's test at 3 months and then annually posttransplant for detection of lacrimal gland involvement. The keratoconjuctivitis sicca thus produced by lacrimal gland damage can progress to cause small pits on the surface of the conjunctivae with eventual conjunctival ulceration and scarring.

Occasionally acute uveitis occurs. Additionally, skin involvement of the eyelid sometimes progresses to thickening and stiffening of the lids resulting in lagophthalmos and ectropion, which only compounds the effects of the kerato-conjunctivitis sicca. The long-term use of corticosteroids for the treatment of chronic GVHD predisposes to cataract formation, which may require glasses or lens replacement.

E. Sinuses

Sinusitis is common in patients with chronic GVHD and results from a combination of a mucosal sicca syndrome involving the sinuses, together with the well-known predisposition of these patients to gram-positive bacterial infections, particularly with pneumococcus (5,7). Besides immunosuppressive therapy for the underlying GVHD, antibiotic therapy is required for acute exacerbations, and surgical drainage is necessary for the management of recurrent episodes.

F. Lung

1. Acute Infections

The broncho-pulmonary system is the commonest site for the acute infections to which patients with chronic GVHD are susceptible (5,6). When late infectious complications were analyzed in 89 recipients of HLA-identical sibling marrow transplants, 45 of 152 infectious episodes occurred in the lungs. In 20 of these the infection was a bacterial pneumonia, in 20 an acute bronchitis, and in 5 an interstitial pneumonia. Cotrimoxazole has been shown to decrease the incidence of both interstitial pneumonitis and bacterial infections in patients with chronic GVHD.

2. Large Airways Involvement

This is a relatively rare occurrence and is characterized by cough with bronchorrhoea (27).

3. Small Airways Involvement

Again rare, but of ominous significance, is the recognition over the last 4-5 years of an obliterative bronchiolitis syndrome in 5-10% of recipients of HLA-identical sibling transplants (28-34). This syndrome is characterized by nonreversible bronchospasm, cough, dyspnea, and pneumothoraces. The forced expiratory volume in one second is markedly decreased, and lung biopsy shows obliterative bronchiolitis. This syndrome only occurs in patients with chronic GVHD, although the activity of the GVHD in other organs may be minimal. It responds poorly to both bronchodilators and immune suppression and is not infrequently fatal. Risk factors for the development of this syndrome, besides the presence of chronic GVHD, include increased age, a lower FEV 1/FVC ratio pretransplant, and the use of methotrexate as immune prophylaxis for GVHD (35). The syndrome is also commoner in recipients of HLA-nonidentical grafts. In a number of the reported cases, a precipitating event appears to have been an acute bacterial bronchitis.

4. Interstitial Pneumonitis

Interstitial pneumonitis occurring late posttransplant is almost entirely restricted to patients with chronic GVHD (8). Of 198 patients with extensive chronic GVHD, 28 developed late (beyond 100 days posttransplant) interstitial pneumonia (14%) (8). In most of these a microbial etiology was documented: in 19% cytomegalovirus; in 19% pneumocystis carinii; in 10% varicella-zoster virus; and in 29% miscellaneous organisms. Idiopathic interstitial pneumonia accounted for 23%.

It is possible that idiopathic interstitial pneumonia represents GVHD directly involving the lung. In support of this are reports of a lymphoid interstitial pneumonitis in patients with chronic GVHD, in whom no microbiological organism was documented and which responded to immune suppressive treatment (36).

5. Pulmonary Fibrosis

Widespread, although patchy pulmonary fibrosis has been reported as one of the primary manifestations of chronic GVHD, flaring after a gradual reduction of immune suppressive treatment (37,38). It is possible that this simply represented a later histologic evolution of the pathologic mechanism evident in lymphoid interstitial pneumonia. Of interest, however, is the fact that dense fibrosis, so characteristic of chronic GVHD in other tissues, can occur in the lung also.

In view of the different etiological mechanisms that can underlie interstitial pneumonitis in the patient with chronic GVHD, tissue diagnosis is essential for appropriate management.

G. Esophagus

While esophageal involvement by chronic GVHD appeared relatively common in the initial patients diagnosed in Seattle in the late 1970s, involvement of this organ is now rarely seen. Symptoms include dysphagia, painful swallowing, and severe retrosternal pain. Endoscopy shows a characteristic desquamation of the upper esophagus, although the distal esophagus can also be involved. A distinctive esophageal web formation can occur. Abnormalities of esophageal motility include aperistalsis and produce retrosternal pain due to acid reflux. Histologically the changes do not include the characteristic muscle or neuronal abnormalities seen in progressive systemic sclerosis (Chapter 32). Radiologic examination with barium is useful in identifying webs, narrowings, and strictures, but the typical desquamation is usually only detected by endoscopy (40). Manometric studies have shown that patients with chronic esophageal GVHD clear acid poorly and this may be a factor predisposing to the peptic esophagitis sometimes present. Treatment must be directed towards preventing the acid-peptic reflux as well as immunosuppression for the underlying GVHD.

H. Intestine

Unlike patients with acute GVHD, patients with chronic GVHD rarely have clinical manifestations of intestinal involvement. When this does occur, it is usually relatively responsive to therapy, again in contrast to gut involvement in acute GVHD. Occasionally, a severe clinical and histologic intestinal GVHD syndrome will develop, especially when prophylactic immune suppression is being tapered or stopped. Clinical manifestations are the same as in acute GVHD of the gut and include abdominal pain, diarrhea, and occasional anorexia, nausea, and vomiting. Cells of the immune system associated with the intestine are involved in chronic GVHD with reduced numbers of IgA-bearing plasma cells and hypocellularity of the Peyer's patches. In advanced cases of chronic extensive GVHD, patchy fibrosis of the lamina propria and striking fibrosis of the submucosa and serosa have been noted, extending from the stomach to the colon (41). Such cases are rarely, if ever, seen these days although fibrotic strictures of the small intestine can occur after 4-6 months of persistent gut GVHD syndrome (42). In two such patients the fibrosis was segmental rather than diffuse, and both patients required extensive small bowel resections because of obstructive symptoms.

Again, rarely observed, but reported in the early literature on human chronic GVHD is the occurrence of a bacterial overgrowth (stasis syndrome) in patients with diarrhea and malabsorption. The diagnosis is made on the quantitative culture of bacterial and fungi from jejunal fluid. This syndrome responds to therapy with oral antibiotics.

I. Muscuso-Skeletal System

1. Inflammatory Myositis

Occasional cases of polymyositis have been reported in patients with chronic GVHD (43-46). This has presented as severe proximal muscle weakness. Biopsy shows necrotic fibers, interstitial inflammation, and IgG deposits on immunofluorescent staining. It appears responsive to corticosteroid therapy.

2. Myasthenia Gravis

Likewise, there are a number of case reports now of myasthenia gravis developing after bone marrow transplantation in patients with chronic GVHD (47,48). This has often occurred after tapering or discontinuation of immunosuppressive therapy for previously evident chronic GVHD. Antibodies to the acetylcholine receptor are present and occasionally antibodies to striated muscles. This myasthenic syndrome usually responds satisfactorily to pyridostigmine (together with atrophine to minimize the latter's side effects) treatment in addition to immune suppressive treatment for the chronic GVHD. It appears that the acetylcholine receptor antibody remains elevated for a prolonged period, and therefore maintenance treatment with both immune suppression and pyridostigmine should be continued long term. Plasmapheresis may be temporarily required for respiratory failure. In several patients studied, serial peripheral blood and bone marrow studies of cytogenetic and red cell markers have shown evidence of donor cells only (47). None of the donors nor family members had evidence of neurologic or muscular disease pre- or posttransplant. Interestingly, 11 of 54 patients (without clinical myasthenia) whose serum was examined posttransplant were found to have low levels of antibodies against the acetylcholine receptor (49). Furthermore, in one patient the concentration of antibodies to the receptor was increased years before myasthenia became clinically manifest.

It should be remembered that a proximal myopathy can develop due to corticosteroid therapy itself. It should also be noted that cyclosporine is effective in the treatment of myasthenia gravis unassociated with chronic GVHD (50).

3. Tendonitis/Fasciitis

Rarely, the primary target organ in chronic GVHD will be the fascial sheaths of the muscle tendons, particularly of the arms and legs around the wrist and ankle joints and digits. Stiffness and restriction of movements are the prime symptoms and this involvement will usually respond to immunosuppressive therapy. The diffuse fasciitis may be associated with eosinophilia, thus mimicking primary eosinophilic fasciitis (51).

4. Arthritis

Arthralgias, particularly of the large proximal girdle joints, and a transient arthritis of large and small joints were reported in Shulman's study (2), but such involvement is rarely seen with current prophylactic and therapeutic immunosuppressive regimens.

J. Gynecologic Manifestations

The sicca syndrome can involve the vagina resulting in dryness, stricture formation, and stenosis (52). Surgical treatment of vaginal adhesions may be required.

It should be noted that dryness and atrophy of the vagina may frequently occur secondary to chemo-radiation induced ovarian failure. In the latter patients, replacement ovarian hormone therapy, both topically and orally, will produce resolution of these changes. (All women should be tested for the possibility of ovarian failure after marrow transplantation because of the long-term risk of osteoporosis developing if ovarian failure is present.)

K. Hemopoietic System

The bone marrow may show hypocellularity, plasmacytosis, megaloblastic change, or eosinophilia in patients with chronic GVHD (2). More recently, fibrosis involving the marrow that resulted in a leukoerythroblastic anemia and thrombocytopenia has been described (53) and indicates yet another organ in this disease in which fibrosis occurs and causes functional damage.

Eosinophilia is a well-known abnormality in patients with chronic GVHD, although its mechanism is not yet determined.

Thrombocytopenia is also well known (54) and represents a poor prognostic sign for survival in this patient population (55). Recently a treatment program of alternate day cyclosporine and prednisone has shown an improved salvage rate for these patients (Chapter 38) (56).

In regard to marrow reserve it should be noted that hemopoietic progenitor cells, particularly in the blood, are reduced in patients with chronic GVHD (57).

Table 4 Site and Type of Late Infections After Bone Marrow Transplantation

Site	Type	Number of episodes	Total number
Pulmonary			62
	Bacterial pneumonia	23	
	Interstitial pneumona	7	
	Fungal pneumonia	4	
	Bronchitis	25	
	Pleurisy	3	
Cutaneous			49
	Varicella-zoster	29	
	Herpes simplex	2	
	Wart	3	
	Cellulitis, boil	8	
	Paronychia	3	
	Fungal	4	
Ear, nose, and throat			84
	Bacterial pharyngitis, tonsillitis	11	
	Oral candida	20	
	Esophageal candida	1	
	Otitis media	16	
	Oral herpes simplex	6	
	Gingivitis	1	
	Tooth abscess	2	
	Sinusitis	27	
Systemic			17
	Bacterial sepsis	11	
	Infectious mononucleosis	1	
	Measles	1	
	Acute febrile illness	4	
Opthalmic			15
	Purulent conjunctivitis	12	
	Herpes simplex keratitis	3	
Genitourinary			13
	Cystitis	11	
	Vaginitis	2	
Central nervous system			3
	Meningitis	2	
	Herpes simplex encephalitis	1	
Miscellaneous			1
	Hyperalimentation line infection	1	
Total			244

Source: Ref. 6 with permission.

Table 5 Infecting Organisms in Late Infections After Bone Marrow Transplantation

Organism	Number of episodes	Total number
Bacterial		38
Gram-positive bacilli		
Pneumococcus	11	
Staph. aureus	10	
Group B streptococcus	8	
Gram-negative bacilli		
Pseudomonas	3	
Escherichia coli	2	
Klebsiella	1	
Miscellaneous		
Haemophilus influenzae	2	
Mycobacterium fortuitum	1	
Fungal		27
Candida	22	
Nocardia	2	
Aspergillus	2	
Tinea sp.	1	
Viral		49
Varicella-zoster[a]	29	
Herpes simplex[a]	15	
Cytomegalovirus	2	
Measles	1	
Respiratory syncytial virus	1	
Mycoplasma	1	
Total		114

[a]Not always isolated but presumed to be present on the basis of the clinical picture.
Source: Ref. 6 with permission.

L. Immune System

The lymph nodes, spleen, and thymus are major target organs for chronic GVHD, and the impact on the function of this system is reviewed fully in Chapter 36. Both cell-mediated and humoral immunity are severely affected, and the major clinical consequence is a marked susceptibility to infectious complications.

The dominant effect of chronic GVHD on the lymphoid system is severe and persistent lymphoid hypocellularity and atrophy (2,58,59). This may result in functional asplenia, as determined by radioisotope scanning of the spleen (60), which in turn helps explain the particular predisposition of patients with chronic GVHD to pneumococcal infections (5-7). Recovery of splenic function after a period of functional asplenia has been described (61).

Circulating autoantibodies are a well-known component of the chronic GVHD syndrome. In one report, the occurrence of antinuclear, antismooth muscle, and anti-

Table 6 Effect of Chronic GVHD and of Circulating Suppressor Cells on the Incidence of Late Infections After Marrow Transplantation

| | HLA-identical sibling transplant recipients without chronic GVHD | HLA-identical sibling transplant recipients with chronic GVHD | |
		Without nonspecific suppressor cells	With nonspecific suppressor cells
Patients studied	15	21	19
No late infections	7	2	0
1-2 late infections	10	6	9
3 or more late infections	8	13	10
Late VZ infection	6 (24%)	8 (38%)	9 (47%)
VZ at any time post transplant	11 (44%)	12 (57%)	15 (79%)
VZ at any time post transplant excluding patients <10 yr	10/19 (53%)	12/18 (67%)	14/17 (82%)
Fatal infection	0	1 (pseudomonas sepsis)	1 (measles pneumonia)

Abbreviations: GVHD = Graft-vs.-Host Disease; VZ = varicella-zoster.

Source: Ref. 6 with permission.

mitochondrial antibodies in patients with chronic GVHD was 80%, 82%, and 14%, respectively. Antiepidermal antibodies were present in 14%, but antinative DNA, antisoluble nuclear antigen, and anticentromere antibodies were not found (62). In a second study of 26 patients with GVHD, the incidence of antinuclear antibodies was 39% (63). In this study antibodies to double stranded DNA were present in 15%, to smooth muscle in 41%, and to nucleoli in 22%. The presence of multiple antibodies correlated with the severity of the GVHD. Although these antibodies are conventionally called "antibodies," they will in fact be alloantibodies if derived from donor-origin B cells (as is likely).

M. Infectious Complications

Chronic GVHD is the major determinant for the development of infectious complications occurring 6 months or later after allogeneic bone marrow transplantation (5,6,8). Chronic GVHD predisposes to bacterial infections and to interstitial pneumonia. Both bacterial infections and interstitial pneumonia are rare in patients without chronic GVHD. The site of infection, type of infection, and infecting organisms seen in this patient population are shown in Tables 4 and 5. The subgroup of patients with chronic GVHD in whom circulting nonspecific suppressor cells (64) were detected had the highest incidence of varicella-zoster infections of any patient cohort posttransplant (6). The effect of chronic GVHD and of circulating nonspecific suppressor cells in chronic GVHD patients on the risk of developing late infections and late varicella-zoster infections is shown in Table 6.

V. ORGANS WITH POSSIBLE CLINICAL INVOLVEMENT

A. Kidney

Recently two cases of minimal change nephrotic syndrome were reported in patients with chronic GVHD (65). The presenting features were edema and proteinuria, and renal pathology included an increase in the mesangial matrix, extensive coalescence of foot processes, and electron-dense deposits in the basement membrane with negative immuno-fluorescence staining. The renal manifestations responded to corticosteroid therapy. In another report, renal biopsy revealed a membranous glomerulonephritis in a patient developing nephrotic syndrome in association with chronic GVHD on withdrawal of cyclosporine treatment (66).

B. Central Nervous System

An infant transplanted for severe combined immune deficiency died at 133 days posttransplant. Autopsy examination of the brain showed focal lymphohistiocytic aggregates thought possibly to represent a previous unreported lesion of chronic GVHD (67).

Confirmation of the involvement of both kidney and the central nervous system by chronic GVHD must await further case reports.

VI. SUMMARY

Chronic Graft-vs.-Host Disease is a multisystem disorder that has had both positive and negative influences on quality of life and survival after allogeneic marrow transplantation. The positive influences stem from the associated graft-vs.-leukemia effect. The negative influences stem from the immune suppression and the connective tissue disorder effects. Much is known about its pathogenesis, but further investigation must be done to try to separate the graft-vs.-host from the graft-vs.-leukemia effects. The debilitated, end-stage, crippled, runted patient with chronic GVHD is now rarely seen due to earlier diagnosis and treatment consequent upon the introduction of routine monitoring for disease activity at 3 months posttransplant. Relatively effective treatment approaches have been devised both for standard-risk and high-risk chronic GVHD. Risk factors for development of chronic GVHD and for survival have been delineated. The challenge for the future lies in utilizing the graft-vs.-leukemic effect while minimizing the graft-vs.-host effect.

ACKNOWLEDGMENT

Supported in part by a grant from the Governement Employees Assistance to Medical Research Fund.

REFERENCES

1.   Atkinson K, Horowitz M, Gale RP, van Bekkum DW, Gluckman E, Good RA et al. Risk factors for chronic graft-vs.-host disease after HLA-identical sibling bone marrow transplantation. Blood 1990, in press.
2.   Shulman HM, Sullivan KM, Weiden PL, MacDonald G, Striker G, Sale G, Hackman R, Tsoi M, Storb R, Thomas E: Chronic graft-versus-host syndrome in man. A long term clinicopathological study of 20 Seattle patients. Am J Med 1980;69:204-217.
3.   Graze PR, Gale RP: Chronic graft-versus-host disease: a syndrome of disordered immunity. Am J Med 1979;66:611-620.

4. Sullivan KM, Shulman HM, Storb R, Weiden PL, Witherspoon RP, McDonald GB, Schubert MM, Atkinson K, Thomas E: Chronic graft-versus-host disease in fifty-two patients: adverse natural course and successful treatment with combination immunosuppression. Blood 1981;57:267-276.

5. Atkinson K, Storb R, Prentice RL, Weiden PL, Witherspoon RP, Sullivan K, Noel D, Thomas E: Analysis of late infections in 89 long term survivors of bone marrow transplantation. Blood 1979;53:720-731.

6. Atkinson K, Farewell V, Tsoi MS, Sullivan KM, Witherspoon RP, Thomas ED, Storb R: Analysis of late infections after human bone marrow transplantation. Role of non-specific suppressor cells in patients with chronic graft-versus-host disease and genotypic non identity between marrow donor and recipient. Blood 1982;60:714-720.

7. Winston DJ, Schiffman G, Wang DC, Feig S, Lin C, Marso E, Ho W,Young L, Gale R: Pneumococcal infections after human bone marrow transplantation. Ann Intern Med 1979;91:835-841.

8. Sullivan KM, Meyers JD, Flournoy N, Storb R, Thomas ED: Early and late interstitial pneumonia following human bone marrow transplantation. Int J Cell Cloning 1986;4:107-121.

9. Atkinson K, Horowitz M, Gale RP, Lee MB, Rimm AA, Bortin MM: Consensus among bone marrow transplanters for diagnosis, grading and treatment of chronic graft-versus-host disease. Bone Marrow Transplant 1989;4:247-254.

10. Sanders JE, Flournoy N, Thomas ED, Buckner CD, Lum LG, Clift RA, Appelbaum F, Sullivan K, Stewart P, Doney K, Storb R: Marrow transplant experience in children with acute lymphoblastic leukemia: an analysis of factors associated with survival, relapse and graft-versus-host disease. Med Pediat Oncol 1985;13:165.

11. Lazarus HM, Coccia PF, Hertzig RH, Graham-Pole J, Grose S, Strandjord S, Garden E, Cheung N, Spitzer T, Warm S: Incidence of acute graft-versus-host disease with and without methotrexate prophylaxis in allogeneic bone marrow transplant patients. Blood 1984;64:215.

12. Klingemann HG, Storb R, Fefer A, Deeg HJ, Appelbaum FR, Buckner CD, Cheever M, Greenberg P, Stewart P, Sullivan K, Witherspoon R, Thomas E: Bone marrow transplantation in patients 45 years and older. Blood 1986;67:770.

13. Shulman HM, Sale GE, Lerner KG, Barker A, Weiden P, Sullivan K, Gallucci B, Thomas E, Storb R: Chronic cutaneous graft-versus-host disease in man. Am J Path 1978;91:545-570.

14. Himes SR, Farmer ER, Burnes WH, Morrison W, Tutschka P, Walters L, Santos G: Bullous scleroderma-like changes in chronic graft-versus-host disease. Arch Dermatol 1985;121:1189-1192.

15. Garnis S, Billick RC, Srolovitz H: Eruptive vascular tumors associated with chronic graft-versus-host disease. J Am Acad Dermatol 1984;10:918-921.

16. Atkinson K, Biggs JC, Dodds AJ, Concannon A: Cyclosporin A associated hepatotoxicity after allogeneic bone marrow transplantation:differentiation from other causes of post transplant liver disease. Transplant Proc 1983;15:2761-2767.

17. Shulman HM, MacDonald GB: Liver disease after marrow transplantation. In *The Pathology of Bone Marrow Transplantation*, edited by Sale GE, Shulman HM. Masson, New York, 1984; pp. 104-135.

18. Snover DC, Weisdorf SA, Ramsay NK, McGlave P, Kersey JH: Hepatic graft-versus-host disease: a study of the predictive value of liver biopsy and diagnosis. Hepatology 1984;4:123-130.

19. Yau JC, Zander AR, Srigley JR, Vern R, Stroehlein J, Korinek J, Vellekoop L, Dicke K: Chronic graft-versus-host disease complicated by micronodular cirrhosis and esophageal varices. Transplant Proc 1986;41:129-130.

20. Schubert MM, Sullivan KM, Morton TH, Izutsu K, Peterson D, Fluornoy N, True-love E, Sale G, Buckner D, Storb R, Thomas E: Oral manifestations of chronic graft-versus-host disease. Arch Intern Med 1984;144:1591-1595.

21. Heimdahl A, Johnson G, Danielesson KH, Llonqvist B, Sundelin P, Ringden O: Oral condition of patients with leukemia and severe aplastic anaemia. Follow-up one year after bone marrow transplantation. Oral Surg Oral Med Oral Pathol 1985; 60:498-504.

22. Sale GE, Shulman HM, Schubert MM, Sullivan KM, Kopecky KJ, Hackman RC, Morton T, Storb R, Thomas E: Oral and opthalmic pathology of graft-versus-host disease in man: predictive value of the lip biopsy. Human Pathol 1981;12:1022-1030.

23. Izutsu KT, Sullivan KM, Schubert MM, Truelove E, Shulman H, Sale G, Morton T, Rice J, Witherspoon R, Storb R, Thomas E: Disordered salivary immunoglobulin secretion and sodium transport in human chronic graft-versus-host disease. Transplant Proc 1983;35:441-446.

24. Gratwohl AA, Moutsopoulos H, Chused TM, Akizuki M, Wolf R, Sweet J, Diesseroth A: Sjøgren-type syndrome after allogeneic bone marrow transplantation. Ann Intern Med 1977;87:703-706.

25. Jack MK, Hicks JD: Ocular complications in high dose chemoradiotherapy and marrow transplantation. Ann Opthalmol 1981;13:709-711.

26. Franklin R, Kenyon KR, Tutschka PJ, Saral R, Green WR, Santos GW: Ocular manifestations of graft-versus-host disease. Am Acad Opthalmol 1983;90:4-13.

27. Atkinson K, Bryant D, Biggs JC, Concannon A, Dodds AJ: Obstructive airways disease: a serious manifestation of chronic graft-versus-host disease after allogeneic bone marrow transplantation in man. Transplant Proc 1984;16:1018-1020.

28. Roca J, Granena A, Rodriguez-Roisin R, Alvarez P, Agusti-Vidal A, Rozman C: Fatal airway disease in an adult with chronic graft-versus-host disease. Thorax 1982;37:77-78.

29. Wyatt SE, Nunn P, Hows JM: Airways obstruction associated with graft-versus-host disease after bone marrow transplant. Thorax 1984;39:887-894.

30. Ralph DD, Springmeyer SC, Sullivan KM, Hackman RC, Storb R, Thomas ED: Rapidly progressive airflow obstruction in marrow transplant recipients. Possible association between obliterative bronchiolitis and chronic graft-versus-host disease. Am Rev Respir Dis 1984;129:641-644.

31. Kurzrock R, Zander A, Kanojia M, Vellekoop L, Spitzer G, Jagannath S, Schell S, Peters L, Dicke K: Obstructive lung disease after allogeneic bone marrow transplantation. Transplant Proc 1984;37:156-160.

32. Johnson FL, Stokes DC, Ruggerio D, Dalla-Pozza L, Callihan TR: Chronic obstructive airways disease after bone marrow transplantation. J Pediatr 1984;105:370-376.

33. Ostrow D, Buskard N, Hill RS, Vickars L, Churg A: Bronchiolitis obliterans complicating bone marrow transplantation. Chest 1985;87:828-830.

34. Rosenburg ME, Vercellotti GM, Snover DC, Herd D, McGlave P: Bronchiolitis obliterans after bone marrow transplantation. Am J Hematol 1985;18:325-328.

35. Clark JG, Schwartz DA, Flournoy N, Sullivan KM, Crawford SW, Thomas ED: Risk factors for airflow obstruction in recipients of bone marrow transplants. Ann Int Med 1987;107:648-656.

36. Perrault C, Cousineau S, D'Angelo G, Gyger M, Nepveu F, Boileau J, Bonny Y, Lacombe M, Lavellee R: Lymphoid interstitial pneumonia after allogeneic bone marrow transplantation. A possible manifestation of chronic graft-versus-host disease. Cancer Research 1985;55:1-9.

37. Atkinson K, Bryant D, Delprado W, Biggs JC: Widespread pulmonary fibrosis as a major clinical manifestation of chronic graft-versus-host disease. Bone Marrow Transplant 1989;4:129-132.

38. Raschko JW, Cottler-Fox M, Abbondanzo SL, Torrisi JR, Spitzer TR, Deeg HJ: Pulmonary fibrosis after bone marrow transplantation responsive to treatment with Prednisone and Cyclosporin. Bone Marrow Transplant 1990;4:201-205.

39. MacDonald GB, Sullivan KM, Schuffler MD, Shulman HM, Thomas ED: Esophageal abnormalities in chronic graft-versus-host disease in humans. Gastroenterology 1981; 80:914-921.

40. MacDonald GB, Sullivan MK, Plumley TF: Radiographic features of esophageal involvement in chronic graft-versus-host disease. Am J Roent 1984;142:501-506.

41. MacDonald GB, Sale GE: The human gastrointestinal tract after allogeneic marrow transplantation. In *The Pathology of Bone Marrow Transplantation*, edited by Sale GE, Shulman HM. Masson, New York, 1984; pp. 77-103.

42. Spencer GD, Shulman HM, Myerson D, Thomas ED: Diffuse intestinal ulceration after marrow transplantation: a clinical-pathological study of 13 patients. Hum Pathol 1990;in press.

43. Urbano-Marquez A, Estruch R, Grau JM: Inflammatory myopathy associated with chronic graft-versus-host disease. Neurology 1986;36:1091-1093.

44. Reyes MG, Noronha P, Thomas W, Heredia R: Myositis of chronic graft-versus-host disease. Neurology 1983;33:1222-1224.

45. Pier N, Dubowitz V: Chronic graft-versus-host disease presenting with polymyositis. Br Med J 1983;286:2024.

46. Anderson BA, Young PV, Kean WF, Ludwin SK, Galbraith PR, Anastassiades TP: Polymyositis in chronic graft-versus-host disease: a case report. Arch Neurol 1982; 39:188-190.

47. Smith CIE, Biberfeld RL, Christensson B, Gahrton G, Hammarstrom L, Lefvert A, Lonnquivst B, Matell G, Pirskanen R, Ringden O, Svanborg E: Myasthenia gravis after bone marrow transplantation: evidence for a donor origin. N Engl J Med 1983; 309:1565-1568.

48. Bolger GB, Sullivan KM, Spence AM, Appelbaum FR, Johnston R, Sanders JE, Deeg H, Witherspoon R, Doney K, Nims J, Thomas E, Storb R: Myasthenia gravis after allogeneic bone marrow transplantation: relationship to chronic graft-versus-host disease. Neurol 1986;36:1087-1091.

49. Smith CIE, Hammarstrom L, levert AK: Bone marrow grafting induces acetylcholine receptor antibody formation. Lancet 1985;1:978.

50. Elkharrat D, Goulon M, Gajdos P: Cyclosporine for myasthenia gravis. N Engl J Med 1987;317:770.

51. van den Bergh V, Tricot G, Fonteyn G, Dom R, Bulcke J: Diffuse fasciitis after bone marrow transplantation. Am J Med 1987;83:139-143.

52. Corson SL, Sullivan KM, Batzer F, August C, Storb R, Thomas ED: Gynecologic manifestations of chronic graft-versus-host disease. Obstet Gynecol 1982;60:488-492.

53. Atkinson K, Dodds A, Concannon A, Biggs JC: Late onset transfusion-dependent anaemia with thrombocytopenia secondary to marrow fibrosis and hypoplasia associated with chronic graft-versus-host disease. Bone Marrow Transplant 1987;2: 445-449.

54. First LR, Smith BP, Lipton J, Nathan DG, Rappeport JM: Isolated thrombocytopenia after allogeneic bone marrow transplantation: existence of transient and chronic thrombocytopenic syndromes. Blood 1985;64:368-374.

55. Sullivan KM, Witherspoon RP, Storb R, Weiden P, Fluornoy N, Dalberg S, Deeg HJ, Saunders J, Doney K, Appelbaum F, McGuffin R, MacDonald G, Meyers J, Schubert M, Shulman H, Sale G, Annasetti C, Loughran TP, Strom S, Nims, J, Thomas E: Prednisone and azothiaprine compared with prednisone and placebo for treatment of graft-versus-host disease: prognostic influence of prolonged thrombocytopenia after allogeneic marrow transplantation. Blood 1988;72:546-554.

56. Sullivan KM, Witherspoon RP, Storb R, Deeg HJ, Dahlberg S, Sanders JE, Appel-baum F, Doney K, Annasetti C, Weiden P, Loughran T, Hill R, Sheilds A, Yee G, Shulman N, Nims J, Strom S, Thomas E: Alternating day cyclosporine and predni-sone for treatment of high risk chronic graft-versus-host disease. Blood 1988;72: 555-561.

57. Atkinson K, Norrie S, Chan P, Zehnwirth B, Downs K, Biggs JC: Haemopoietic progenitor cell function after HLA-identical sibling bone marrow transplantation; influence of chronic graft-versus-host disease. Int J Cell Clon 1986;4:203-220.

58. van Bekkum DW: Graft-versus-host disease. In *Bone Marrow Transplantation. Biological Mechanisms and Clinical Practice*, edited by van Bekkum DW, Lowen-berg B. Marcel Dekker, Inc., New York, 1985; pp. 147-212.

59. Elkins WL: Cellular immunology and the pathogenesis of graft-versus-host reac-tions. Prog Allergy 1971;15:78-187.

60. Al-Eid MA, Tutschka PJ, Wagner HN, Santos GW, Tsan MF: Functional asplenia in patients with chronic graft-versus-host disease. J Nucl Med 1983;24:1123-1126.

61. Demetrakopoulos GE, Tsokos GC, Levine AS: Recovery of splenic function after GVHD-associated functional asplenia. Am J Hematol 1982;12:77-80.

62. Rouquette-Galley AM, Boyeldieu D, Gluckman E, Abuaf N, Combrisson A; Auto-immunity in 28 patients after allogeneic bone marrow transplantation: compari-son with Sjøgren syndrome and scleroderma. Br J Haematol 1987;66:45-47.

63. Lister J, Messner H, Keystone AE, Miller R, Fritzler MJ: Autoantibody analysis of patients with graft-versus-host disease. J Clin Lab Immunol 1987;24:19-23.

64. Tsoi MS, Storb R, Dobbs S, Kopecky K, Santos E, Weiden P, Thomas E: Non-specific suppressor cells in patients with chronic graft-versus-host disease after marrow grafting. J Immunol 1979;123:1970-1976.

65. Gomez-Garcia P, Herrara-Arroyo C, Torrez-Gomez A, Gomez-Caraska J, Aljama-Gar-cia P, Lopez-Rubio F, Martinez-Guiballe F, Ornez-Torez G, Rojas-Contreras R: Renal involvement in chronic graft-versus-host disease: a report of 2 cases. Bone Marrow Transplant 1988;3:357-362.

66. Hiess EC, Goldschmidt E, Santelli G, Sharpentier B, Machover D, Friess D: Mem-branous nephropathy in a bone marrow transplant recipient. Am J Kidney Dis 1988;11:188-191.

67. Rouah E, Gruber R, Shearer W, Armstrong D, Hawkins EP: Graft-versus-host disease in the central nervous system. A real entity? Am J Clin Pathol 1988;89: 543-546.

32

Pathology of Chronic Graft-vs.-Host Disease

Howard M. Shulman
Fred Hutchinson Cancer Research Center
University of Washington School of Medicine
Seattle, Washington

I. INTRODUCTION

In 1975, while a resident in pathology, I began to collect clinical and histologic data from 19 long-lived Seattle allogeneic marrow graft recipients in whom the GVHD process remained active. Our findings (1,2) and reports from other marrow transplant centers (3-13) clearly demonstrated that this late-occurring clinicopathological syndrome, which subsequently became known as chronic GVHD, was quite different from acute GVHD. In the 5 years since we published the monograph "Pathology of Bone Marrow Transplantation," which extensively illustrated and discussed chronic GVHD (14), additional pathologic abnormalities associated with chronic GVHD (C-GVHD) have been reported and a rapidly expanding body of knowledge has accumulated on the immunopathogenesis of C-GVHD. This chapter reviews some of those early highlights and presents newer findings in the pathology of chronic GVHD.

A number of generalizations serve as a useful guide to the pathology of chronic GVHD: (1) The biologic and histologic distinction of acute from chronic GVHD does not always coincide with the operational definition of chronic GVHD using 150 days after marrow transplant as the cut-off between acute and chronic GVHD. (2) Chronic GVHD has dynamic histologic features. In the early phase, the predominant findings are lymphoplasmacytic infiltration involving the epithelia and glands listed in Table 1. (3) The consequence of these early inflammatory changes are seen in the later phase where there is widespread fibrosis, stenosis, obliteration, or atrophy of the involved tissues. (4) Following a flare of chronic GVHD, the histologic changes, particulalry those in the epidermis and the liver, may be more closely akin to those of acute GVHD. Furthermore, in the absence of chronic inflammation, it may not be possible to distinguish active disease from residual late fibrotic damage. (5) Unlike acute GVHD, there is a rather extensive destruction of tubulo-alveolar glands and ducts and a corresponding clinical sicca syndrome. (6) Several infrequent soft tissue manifestations of chronic GVHD mimic the

Table 1   Organs Affected by Chronic GVHD

Epithelial and Mucosal Surfaces
    skin epidermis, dermal appendages, nails
    conjunctiva, ? cornea
    mouth, gingiva, and squamous mucous membranes
    esophagus
    vagina
    intestines and colon
        transiently during flare
        as an extension of preexisting severe acute GVHD
    ? bronchiolar respiratory epithelium
Glands and ducts
    small hepatic bile ducts
    sweat glands, breast ducts
    glands in esophageal mucosa
    glands in trachea and large airways
    periurethral glands
    salivary glands, major and minor
Soft Tissues
    muscle
    serosal surfaces
    synovium
    dermal collagen
    ? vessels
    ? glomeruli
Lymphoid Organs
    lymph nodes and peripheral associated lymphoid tissues
    thymus
    spleen

---

naturally occurring autoimmune collagen vascular disease, such as myositis, myasthenia gravis, and arthritis. Associated with these changes are the formation of autoantibodies. (7) Some changes of chronic GVHD appear to be largely the consequence of damage incurred during acute GVHD such as segmental intestinal ulceration, fibrosis, and stenosis. Persistent liver test abnormalities such as elevations of alkaline phosphatase and hyperbilirubinemia may also reflect damage to small bile ducts incurred mainly during acute rather than chronic GVHD. (8) The etiology of some late changes has not been resolved; GVHD, inflammation, or infection are all possibilities. Examples include the obliterative small airway lesions, idiopathic interstitial pneumonia, intramural esophageal fibrosis, and chronic active liver disease. (9) The overall Karnofsky score or number of organ systems involved by chronic GVHD has proven a more useful barometer of clinical outcome than grading the histologic lesions (15).

    In the following sections, the natural history of chronic GVHD in specific organ systems, pragmatic points relating to the diagnosis and management, and relevant information regarding pathogenesis within that organ system are presented.

    Table 1 contains a breakdown of the tissues targeted by GVHD, subdivided into their anatomic components. Several of these targets appear in more than one category. Similar histologic changes have been produced in several experimental allogeneic models of chronic GVHD (16-21). In general, the inflammatory changes, particularly those in the skin are less marked than in man.

II. SKIN INVOLVEMENT

A. Extensive Involvement

The skin and its appendages are the structures most commonly affected by chronic GVHD. Since early diagnosis and aggressive treatment have decreased the inflammatory component and have lessened the number of patients with severe end stage sclerodermatous alterations (15-22), the description of chronic cutaneous GVHD given here is in part historical. Patients with the extensive form of chronic GVHD (2,15), comprising approximately 80% of all chronic GVHD cases, have a generalized type of skin disorder which involves much of the skin surface including hair and nails (1). The early inflammatory phase has epidermal features resembling lichen planus and dermal changes resembling lupus profundus or generalized morphea (1). Grossly, the early skin lesions have several appearances: papulosquamous plaques, scarring alopecia, or dyspigmentation ranging from a diffuse, violaceous hue to reticulated hyperpigmentation and/or leukoderma (Fig. 1).

These different external appearances are in part related to increased blood flow, refraction of light through the thickened stratum cornea or parakeratotic layer, disturbances to the epidermal-melanin unit with irregular transfer of excessive melanin pigment to the keratinocytes, and melanin incontinence into the papillary dermis. Nail changes include periungual erythema thinning, thickening, grooving, opacification, and pterygium (1,23). Histologically, papulosquamous plaques represent epidermal thickening from hypertrophy and hyperplasia of keratinocytes, hyperkeratosis, and spotty parakeratosis. When lymphocytic inflammation along the dermal-epidermal junction is striking and accompanied by blunted, saw-tooth-like rete ridges, the term lichen planus-like GVHD is apt (7,9) (Fig. 2).

The appendageal inflammation around follicles, eccrine coils, and subcutis inflammation may be lymphocytic or lymphoplasmacytic and include scattered eosinophils. The inflammation may surround neurovascular bundles, but true leukocytoclastic vasculitis is rare. Damaged eccrine ducts develop squamous metaplasia and like the epidermis show individual cell necrosis. The marked blood flow, inflammation, and edema around the abundant eccrine coils in the hands and feet are responsible for violaceous palmar papules. Limited histologic study of the nails demonstrates damage to the matrix and germinal portion of the nail matrix which produces the nail plate (Raugi and Shulman, unpublished data).

The progression from the early to the late phase of generalized chronic GVHD is a continuum taking place from 3 months to 18 months. Major late changes are epidermal atrophy, destruction of dermal appendages, and fibrous remodeling of both the papillary and reticular dermis (Fig. 3). The dermal fibrosis begins first in the papillary or upper dermis and is often patchy following down along the tracts of the destroyed hair follicles. This distribution of dermal sclerosis differs from that of scleroderma where the process begins within the deep dermis or along the dermal subcutaneous junction (2).

Late fibrotic changes involving the reticular dermis include a coarsening and crowding of the collagen bundles which become straightened, elongated, and hypereosinophilic. Eventually both the reticular and the papillary dermis merge into a broad homogenous sclerotic zone. The dermal fibrosis results in straightening of the dermal subcutaneous

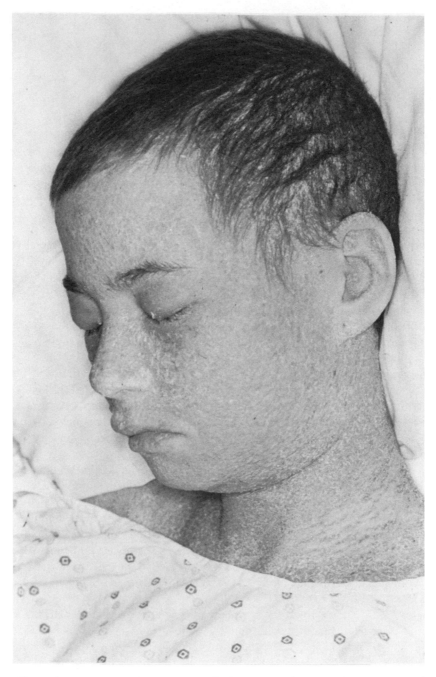

Figure 1   Early generalized chronic GVHD—generalized erythematous papulosquamous eruption.

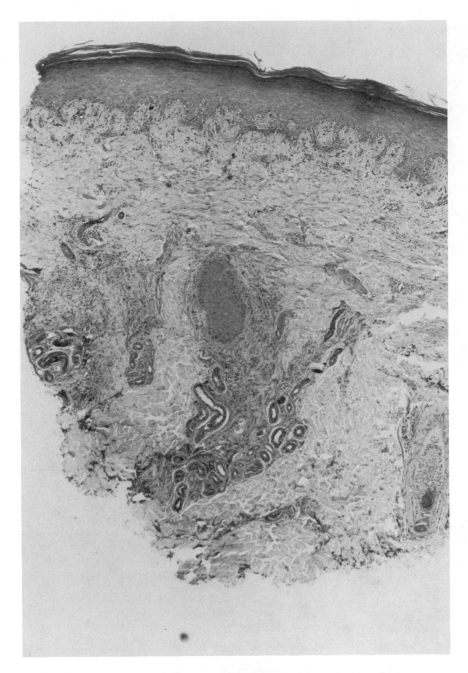

Figure 2 Early generalized chronic GVHD section through a papulosquamous eruption. Thickened epidermis with diffuse lichenoid inflammation has a lichen planus-like appearance. Dermis has a pronounced lymphoplasmacytoid inflammation about eccrine coils, ducts, and follicles.

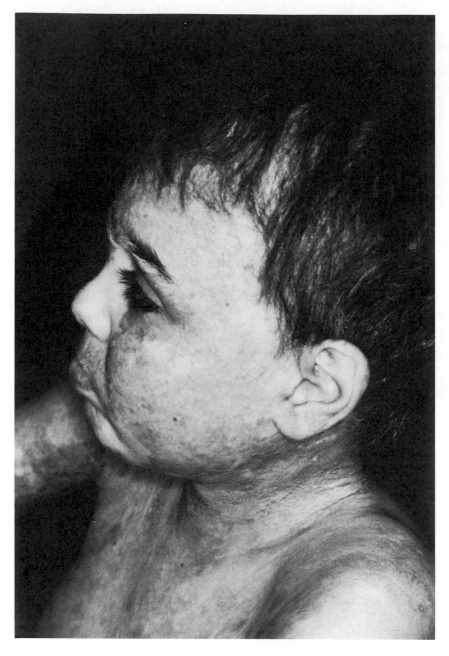

Figure 3 Late generalized chronic GVHD. Poikiloderma with dyspigmentation, scarring, alopecia, and tightness of skin.

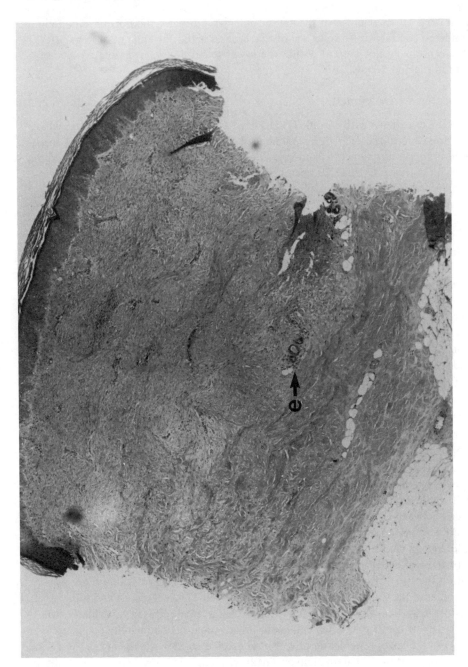

Figure 4 Late chronic GVHD. Widened upper dermis is fibroblastic, lower dermis is homogenized, and dermal-subcutaneous junction is straightened. Note remnant of eccrine unit (e).

junction (Fig. 4). As sclerosis of the dermal collagen proceeds, the fibrous remodeling may undergo contraction. The legacy of this process is the entrapment of large arteries which are normally not present within the lower rectal dermis and isolated erector pilorum in the mid dermis.

B. Localized Involvement

Ten to 20% of patients with chronic GVHD have a localized type of skin disease which has features of localized scleroderma and lichen sclerosis and atrophicus (1,6). Grossly, the lesions appear dyspigmented and atrophic (cigarette paper-thin epidermis) overlying irregular induration. These lesions can present in clusters which later coalesce as symmetrical hyperpigmented lesions, often in the corners of both eyes or as broad bands of induration on the trunk, and sometimes following the distribution of tight-fitting undergarments. This localized type of chronic GVHD usually is not associated with involvement of viscera other than liver. The course is generally indolent with spontaneous regression and some decrease of hyperpigmentation. The histologic abnormalities of these localized lesions can be overlooked because the early abnormality consists only of focal homogenization of dermal collagen bundles with little or no inflammatory change in the epidermis or its appendages. As the lesions run their course, the full thickness of the dermis becomes homogenized. Late localized lesions resemble late generalized chronic GVHD. Like true scleroderma (24), localized chronic GVHD may also show clinical regression with softening and lessening of pigmentation. There are no data to indicate whether certain HLA donor-recipient combinations are more frequently associated with either form of cutaneous chronic GVHD.

C. Diagnostic Caveats

Several pragmatic points relate to the diagnosis of cutaneous chronic GVHD. Chronic GVHD may not be temporally homogeneous; biopsy of more than one abnormal site may be indicated. Grading the degree of the cutaneous inflammation about the epidermis or the appendages has no prognostic value. The primary uses of skin biopsies are to help define the chronic GVHD as extensive or limited and to assess whether the C-GVHD process is active or inactive. In practice, this distinction may be difficult because an incomplete response to immunosuppressive therapy often results in more subtle changes. The presence of continuing vacuolar degeneration along the basal layer, even in the absence of intraepithelial lymphocyte infiltration and eosinophilic body formation, is an indication that the chronic GVHD is active. Assessment of C-GVHD skin biopsies is greatly aided if the skin biopsy is full thickness to include sweat glands and subcutis and is taken from an area which does not appear grossly normal. This is particularly true during a flare of the disease when cutaneous involvement may be patchy and centered primarily in the lower reticular dermis, around eccrine coils, or vessels in the subcutaneous fat. This type of deep dermal involvement with chronic GVHD has occasionally produced a rippled fibrotic appearance similar to eosinophilic fasciitis.

D. Immunopathology

The immunopathogenesis of chronic GVHD has been investigated by electron microscopy (25,26), immunofluorescence (27,28), immunophenotyping (29-32), and by a number of in vitro immunologic studies. Both humans (27,28) and rodents (18) with C-GVHD develop granular immune deposits of IgM and C3 along the dermal-epidermal junction. The appearance of these deposits coincides roughly with the onset of C-GVHD (28). These deposits are absent from the skin of syngeneic recipients and most allogeneic recipients without C-GVHD. The nature of the deposits whether alloimmune or an epiphenomenon has not been settled. Indirect immunofluorescence studies have demonstrated that the sera from patients with C-GVHD and other inflammatory skin diseases contain antibodies which react to epidermal antigens expressed along the basal keratinocytes (27). Patients with C-GVHD also contain circulating autoantibodies to cytoskeletal intermediate filaments (33). The highest titer of these antibodies were found in patients with early generalized lichen planus-like skin lesions. However, serum from patients with other autoimmune diseases such as polymyositis and primary biliary cirrhosis contains similar autoantibodies; therefore, they appear to be nonspecific markers of inflammation rather than evidence of the primary antibody response induced against the epidermis. In a rat model of C-GVHD, Beschorner et al. have concluded that the immune deposits are an epiphenomenon; the immune deposits occurred only in the chimeras which spontaneously develop C-GVHD, but not in those irradiated animals in which C-GVHD was adoptively transferred with sensitized spleen and marrow from animals with C-GVHD (18,34).

Chronic cutaneous GVHD appears to be a cell-mediated phenomena. Electronmicroscopic studies of the lymphocytic satellitosis lesions in chronic GVHD (the putative aggressor lymphocytes surrounding a keratinocyte target) show point contact between activated lymphocytes and keratinocytes and Langerhans cells, thought to indicate cytotoxic activity (25). Most immunophenotypic marker studies of human chronic GVHD indicate that the infiltrating skin mononuclear cells in chronic GVHD mark as CD8[+] (cytotoxic-suppressor) T lymphocytes (29-32), even in a study in which predominantly CD4[+] cells were infused with the donor marrow (35).

The effector cell-target interaction is likely a dynamic process involving the interaction of T-cell growth factors produced by the epidermis cells and regulatory cytokines secreted by the T cells (36-39). In vitro gamma interferon induces class II MHC antigens on keratinocytes (38), thereby stimulating T-cell blasts to proliferate (39). Gamma interferon treatment of keratinocytes also increases their susceptibility to undergo lysis by cytotoxic T lymphocytes (39). C-GVHD also causes a decrease in the number of Langerhans cells and leads to expression of HLA-DR on lesional keratinocytes (39). In vitro systems for studying keratinocyte proliferation and wound healing also demonstrate a dynamic process. Release of cytokines and growth factors can modulate the growth of keratinocytes and effect the appearance of the epidermis into either hyperproliferation and acanthosis or hypoproliferation and atrophy (37).

Studies indicate that the dermal fibrosis that obtains in chronic GVHD is a direct consequence of the chronic inflammatory process. First, fibrosis begins along the dermalepidermal interface in the papillary and adventitial (periappendageal) dermis associated with intense lichenoid inflammation (1,26). Second, in patients successfully treated with immunosuppressive therapy, the fibrosis and telangiectasia stop in the midportion of the reticular dermis (Fig. 5). Third, electron microscopic studies of early C-GVHD first show activated fibroblasts in the upper dermis (25). Claman has hypothesized that the dermal fibrosis of chronic GVHD may be facilitated by degranulation of vasoactive agents released from mast cells (40). The specific stimuli to degranulate have not been clarified. A murine model of C-GVHD generated across non-H-2-(minor)-histocompatibility barriers suggests that dermal fibroblasts may first be stimulated by donor T cells to proliferate (42). Later, these expanded fibroblasts synthesize collagen in response to release of the lymphokine IL-4 by T cells autoreactive to tissue HLA-DR expression.

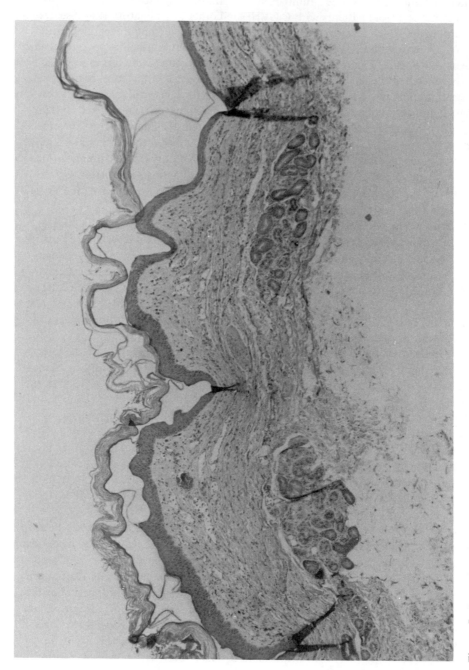

Figure 5 Late chronic GVHD arrested by immunosuppressive treatment. Epidermis is atrophic. The dermal fibrosis is confined to the upper portion, and the eccrine units are spared.

The murine model of C-GVHD by Parkman et al. does not readily explain the localized form of C-GVHD. However, skin biopsies from patients with naturally occurring localized scleroderma indicate that only certain subpopulations of fibroblasts may be responsible for the increased collagen synthesis (42). The process of cell selection or regulatory mechanisms which modulate fibroblast behavior to selectively produce collagen requires additional study.

III. GASTROINTESTINAL INVOLVEMENT

A. Esophagus

Gastrointestinal involvement in chronic GVHD is confined mainly to the squamous epithelium of the esophagus and underlying tubuloalveolar glands. Histologic changes involving the squamous mucosa is similar to that in the skin and mouth. As a consequence of inflammation, ulcerated esophageal surfaces may become opposed to each other and reepithelialized with weblike membranes forming strictures (14,43). Manometric studies in patients with esophageal desquamation indicate that they clear acid poorly and have nonspecific motor abnormalities. Occasional patients have developed perimuscular fibrosis analogous to that seen in scleroderma and in murine chronic GVHD (Fig. 6). Whether this mural fibrosis is secondary to contiguous mucosal or glandular inflammation as was suggested by a previous human study of esophageal C-GVHD (43) or is part of generalized visceral myopathy (18) is unsettled.

B. Small and Large Intestine

Mucosal disease of the stomach, intestines, and colon is unusual in chronic GVHD. When present it usually signifies persistence of damage incurred during acute GVHD. Occasionally during a flare of chronic GVHD there may be a transient diarrhea with focal crypt damage and individual cell necrosis, but generally this process is self-limited. Severe intestinal disease incurred during acute GVHD may result in localized segments of stenosis. In these areas, the epithelium is ulcerated, and the lamina propria and submucosa are fibrotic producing a stenotic obstruction (44).

Prior to the advent of early immunosuppressive therapy for chronic GVHD, several patients developed malabsorption, diarrhea, abdominal pain, and malnutrition (2,14). At autospsy, there was extensive fibrosis in the submucosal and subserosal regions of the intestines, along with hyalinization of submucosal vessels. Whether these changes represented residua of acute GVHD or were part of the generalized fibrosis seen in chronic GVHD was never clearly settled. Fortunately, this latter gut complication has become vanishingly rare to absent.

C. Liver

Roughly 90% of patients with chronic GVHD have abnormal liver function tests (LFT). Elevations of alkaline phosphatase are usually most striking, with lower elevations of bilirubin and hepatocellular enzymes. These LFT abnormalities are presumed to reflect chronic GVHD since they are rare in long-lived allogeneic survivors who have no other evidence of C-GVHD.

Chronic GVHD of the liver is a cholestatic hepatitis with segmental destructive bile duct lesions (14,45,46) (Fig. 7). Histologically, the distinction from acute GVHD is often

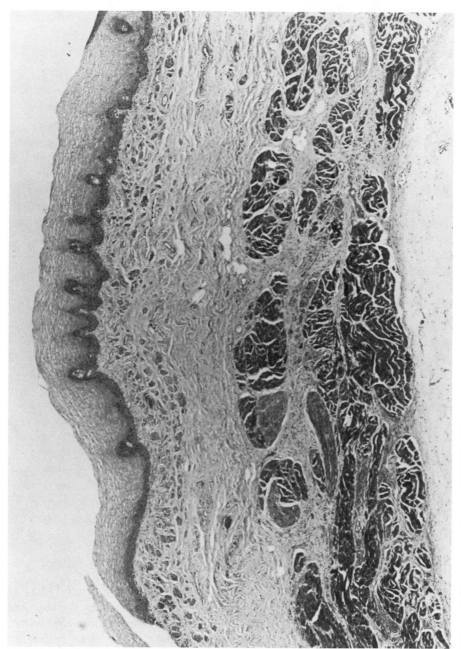

Figure 6 Esophageal chronic GVHD. There is extensive fibrosis in the submucosa and in between the muscularis circularis layers.

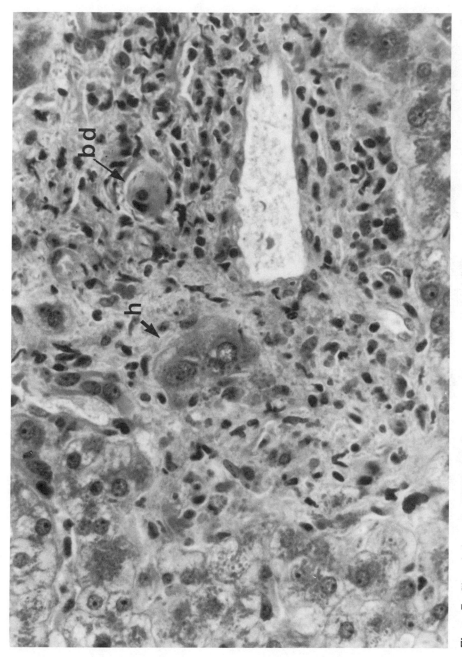

Figure 7 Chronic hepatic GVHD. Expanded portal space contains loosely scattered mononuclear cells and entrapped hepatocytes (h) and degenerative bile duct (bd). Bile duct has loss of nuclei and cellular outlines, hypereosinophilic cytoplasm, and intraepithelial lymphocytes.

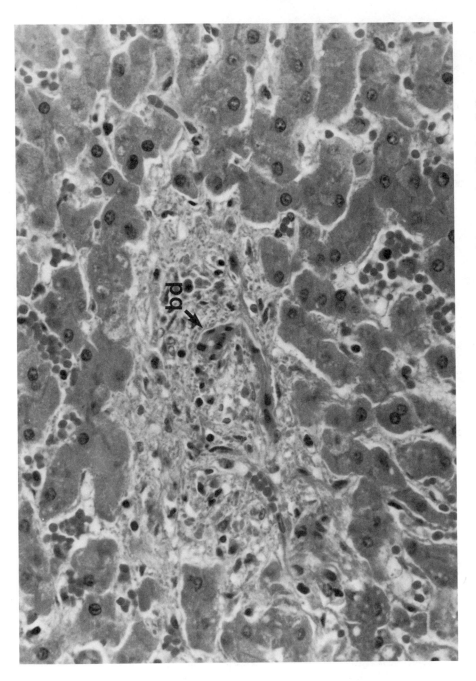

Figure 8   Chronic hepatic GVHD.   Enlarged portal space contains remnant of degenerative bile duct (bd).

blurred. Episodes of acute GVHD and flares of chronic GVHD have a similar appearance. The practical question facing clinicians and pathologists is whether persistent liver abnormalities or rising liver function tests in the presence of otherwise inactive chronic GVHD represent a flare of chronic hepatic GVHD or viral hepatitis. Differential diagnosis in such cases typically lies between non-A non-B viral hepatitis and chronic GVHD. Though cytomegalovirus infections are common, the hepatitis is usually anicteric and bile duct lesions such as those produced by GVHD are not encountered (47-49). Coded histologic studies comparing chronic GVHD to chronic hepatitides show that the histologic distinction is not always precise (45,46). Liver biopsies with periportal inflammation and proliferated bile ducts can be seen in either of the two conditions. Features such as segmental bile duct destruction, cytologically atypical bile ducts, and bile duct dropout favor a diagnosis of GVHD (Fig. 7). The common appearance of chronic hepatic GVHD under treatment is of relatively few inflammatory cells within hyalinized portal triads containing few or no bile ducts and striking hepatocellular canalicular cholestasis (Fig. 8).

Patients with hepatic chronic GVHD have a low propensity to develop cirrhosis. In the handful of such cases reported (14,50,51) non-A non-B viral hepatitis cannot be excluded. Expected rapid developments in the identification of the genomic code of non-A non-B viral hepatitis will presumably lead to development of diagnostic reagents which will detect the infectious agent in tissues. When that occurs reexamination of liver biopsies from patients with chronic GVHD should shed additional light on the distinction of chronic GVHD from non-A non-B viral hepatitis.

IV. SICCA SYNDROME

Chronic GVHD produces dryness and atrophy of mucous membranes with widespread destruction of secretory glands including those in the eyes, nose, upper alimentary airway, skin, and periurethral areas (3,4,9,14,52,53). Oral mucosal abnormalities associated with C-GVHD include noninfectious leukoplakia, reticulate vascularity, and mucosal atrophy with submucosal fibrosis (54-56). The glandular histology shows inflammatory destruction centered about the centrally draining ductal structure with secondary involution and destruction of the alveolar components of the glands (14) (Fig. 9). The similarity of this process in the minor salivary glands and the small bile ducts lead Epstein et al. to hypothesize that both chronic GVHD and primary biliary cirrhosis were part of a dry gland syndrome (57).

Oral labial biopsies are routinely obtained to confirm and classify the type of chronic GVHD and to monitor the efficacy of immunosuppressive therapy. The initial histologic schema as proposed by Sale et al. (52) included a two-tiered grading threshold schema. Grade I changes have mucosal and/or periductal lymphocytes. Grade II changes include intraepithelial lymphocytes plus some evidence of destruction of mucosal or ductal epithelium. The specificity of grade I changes is relatively (50%) low, while that of the grade II lesion is higher (75%) but still not pathognomonic. Accordingly, a diagnosis of extensive C-GVHD requires confirmatory evidence of C-GVHD in an additional site, e.g., skin, eye, liver.

In practice, the distinction of grade I from grade II changes is often difficult. Patients have often been on immunosuppressive therapy, and many of the cases involve borderline changes lying somewhere between grade I and grade II changes, with sparse inflammation and rare apoptotic bodies. Recently, Nakhlaeh et al. presented preliminary data demonstrating that patients with minimal mucosal changes and rare apoptotic cells

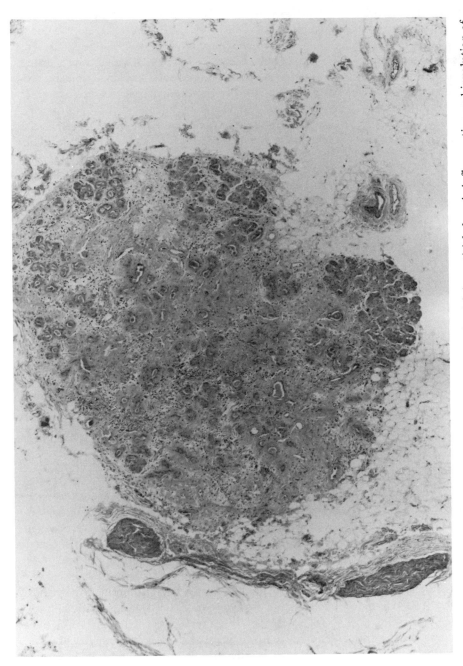

Figure 9 Lacrimal gland with chronic GVHD has duct ectasia with interstitial chronic inflammation and involution of glandular acini.

behaved in a fashion that was indistinguishable from patients with grade II biopsy changes (58). On the other hand, a negative mucosal epithelial biopsy did not exclude the possibility of grade II salivary gland changes. Therefore, a true negative lip biopsy requires both mucosa and minor salivary glands to be present.

V. RESPIRATORY INVOLVEMENT

Approximately 10% of patients with C-GVHD develop pulmonary complications exclusive of bacterial and viral infections. These complications include an obstructive small airway disease, idiopathic interstitial pneumonitis, and a progressive restrictive pulmonary fibrosis. The pathogenesis of these various pulmonary lesions, i.e., immunologic, infectious, or late chemoradiation toxicity has not been easy to separate. The evaluation has been hampered by the infrequency of these complications and from nonuniformity of diagnosis and treatment among different centers.

A. Obstructive Airways Disease

Five to 10% of patients with C-GVHD develop an indolent late-onset bronchodilator-resistant obstructive pulmonary disease associated with histologic lesions of bronchiolitis obliterans and constrictive bronchiolitis (59-61). These lesions are similar to those reported in association with collagen vascular diseases of rheumatoid arthritis (62) and Sjögren's syndrome (63). Up to 25% of all heart-lung allograft recipients develop similar pulmonary lesions (64).

The development of similar lesions in a rat lung transplant model (65) has tilted thinking toward immunologically mediated injury. In these studies, only the left lung was allografted and cyclosporine was omitted decreasing the likelihood of potentially confounding infections. In the experimentally allografted lung, the early changes of rejection consisted of a dense cuff of activated lymphocytes surrounding the bronchioles. Lymphocytic infiltration of the lamina propria and epithelium with individual cell necrosis of respiratory epithelial cells progressed to mucosal ulceration. This was followed by replacement of the submucosa and mucosa with granulation tissue.

In man, the small airway lesions tend to be temporarily homogeneous; thus, the histologic scenario of this lesion is based on piecing together lesions from different patients. This may, in fact, result in representing more than one type of disease process, as witnessed by the fact that one series included patients 49 to 602 days posttransplant (61). In patients with C-GVHD, the earliest pulmonary bronchiolar lesion may consist of lymphoid expansion of the bronchus-associated lymphoid tissue (BALT), a nonspecific finding that has been present at autopsy in a number of patients dying of C-GVHD (2). A more typical and characteristic bronchiolar lesion consists of a widened and edematous lamina propria, a partially to completely ulcerated epithelium, and a lumen containing desquamated debris and inflammatory cells (Fig. 10). In later stages as the airway disease progresses or undergoes repair, this exudate is incorporated into the fibroblastic lamina propria. The process may be eccentric, creating a fibroblastic tongue which extends into or obliterates the lumen (Fig. 10). If the fibrosis is concentric, a constrictive obliterative lesion results. Part or all of the surrounding bronchial smooth muscle may be destroyed leaving an irregular scar rich in blood vessels resembling a varix (Fig. 11). Elastic stains demonstrate the residual bronchial landmarks of these lesions. A less obvious finding is the marked reduction or absence of small bronchioles represented as scar

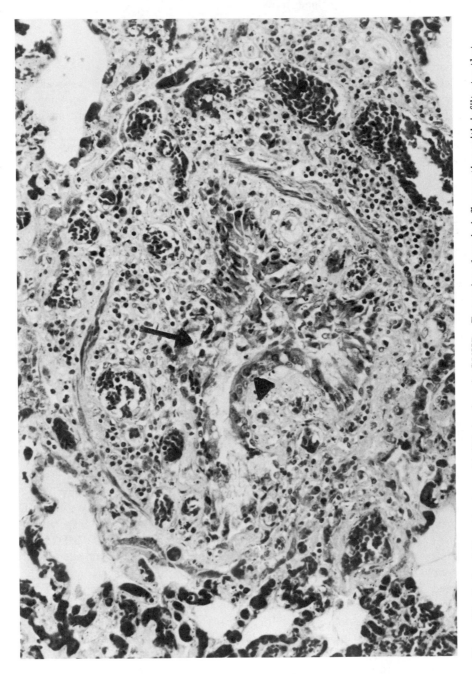

Figure 10 Early obliterative bronchiolitis in chronic GVHD. Extensive chronic inflammation with infiltrates that efface the mucosa (arrow). Eccentric fibroblastic submucosal tongue of granulation tissue is compressing the lumen (arrowhead).

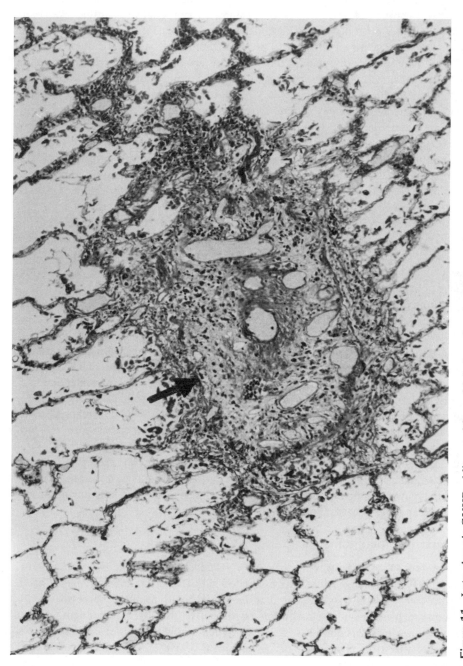

Figure 11 Late chronic GVHD obliterated bronchiole is replaced with constrictive fibrosis and dilated blood vessels. Remnant of bronchiolar smooth muscle surrounds the periphery (arrow).

tissue adjacent to pulmonary arterioles. Besides the small airway lesions, the large bronchioles often contain an acute inflammatory infiltrate, which likely represents a superinfection.

Repeated attempts by various bone marrow transplant centers to detect viral agents
associated with bronchiolitis obliterans, i.e., respiratory syncytial virus, influenza, parain-
fluenza, adenovirus, mycoplasma, and legionella, have been unsuccessful, though it should
be noted that some agents are difficult to isolate without molecular techniques.

Despite the absence of demonstrable infectious agents, there is much circumstantial
evidence that infections play an important role in this lesion. Respiratory infections occur from GVHD-induced immunodeficiency. Moreover, some chronic GVHD patients
have had improvement of airway symptoms following the elimination of chronic aspiration by esophageal dilatation. Infections can enhance immune reactions and the afferent
limb of GVHD by facultatively stimulating expression of class II MHC antigens (HLA-
DR) on epithelia, through release of gamma interferon (36,37,39,66). Experimentally,
a viral infection localized into the salivary glands of bone marrow transplanted rats resulted in more GVHD within these infected glands (67). Epithelial expression of class II
MHC antigens can be induced on bronchial epithelium (68,69), but whether the bronchial
respiratory epithelium is a primary target of GVHD is controversial. Beschorner et al.
have shown a positive statistical relationship between GVHD and lymphocytic infiltration
of respiratory epithelium of large airways termed lymphocytic bronchitis (70). However,
studies in a canine model of GVHD and human post mortem observation of accident victims have failed to confirm the specificity of these findings for GVHD (71).

Chronic GVHD produce immunodeficiency with an attendant increase in infections
by a variety of mechanisms (72). Previous studies have shown that patients with C-
GVHD have a decrease in salivary IgA (73) and a decrease in IgA-bearing plasma cells in
the gut (74). Recently, Hruban et al. have demonstrated that rejected lung allografts
have a corresponding decrease of the bronchus-associated lymphoid tissue (BALT), in
particular, IgA-bearing plasma cells (75). Given the parallels between lung rejection and
small airway disease associated with chronic GVHD, it seems reasonable to expect that
similar depletions of the BALT may arise with C-GVHD. Holland et al. found a positive
association between chronic GVHD, bronchiolitis obliterans and reduced serum IgG levels
(61). A local lack of respiratory IgG, especially of IgG_2 subclass, is associated with
chronic respiratory infections (76). Though IgG subclasses were not studied by Holland
et al., their findings are in keeping with the propensity for patients with chronic GVHD
to develop recurrent sinopulmonary infections, otitis media, and bacterial pneumonias to
common encapsulated bacterial organisms.

B. Interstitial Pneumonia

Approximately 4% of patients with chronic GVHD develop idiopathic interstitial pneumonias (IIP) (77). In some cases of IIP associated with C-GVHD the pulmonary infiltrates seen on chest X-ray have improved or disappeared with immunosuppressive therapy. In one such case from our institution, retrospective histologic studies demonstrated
a noninvasive cavitary aspergillosis suggesting a hypersensitivity reaction. Whether cases
of idiopathic interstitial pneumonia associated with C-GVHD have concomitant obstructive airway lesions is not clear.

A final confounding fact regarding IIP and C-GVHD is that some long-term allogeneic survivors transplanted for hematologic malignancy develop severe progressive restrictive pulmonary disease. This has occurred without any obvious C-GVHD and is pre-

sumably related to the late effects of pretransplant chemoirradiation conditioning (78). Histologically distinguishing this sort of end-stage pulmonary fibrosis from IIP associated with C-GVHD or unrecognized infection may not be possible.

VI. SOFT TISSUE INVOLVEMENT

Infrequently, patients with C-GVHD develop polymyositis, arthritis, or serositis (2,69, 80). The pathologic picture is of lymphoplasmacytic inflammation of the tissues. Myositis may be extensive and symptomatic or consist of patchy interstitial mononuclear cell infiltration without obvious symptoms. Involvement of other soft tissues including the kidneys and their vessels is controversial. Asymptomatic vascular and glomerular alterations have been reported, in association with chronic GVHD (2,3,81). However, these alterations, thickening and splitting of glomerular basement membranes, mesangial sclerosis, increased arterial interstitial smooth muscle matrix, and intimal proliferation have been found in patients who died of leukemic relapse after one or more years posttransplant (Shulman, unpublished data). In addition, small numbers of patients transplanted for hematologic malignancies without GVHD have developed renal insufficiency independent of cyclosporine, apparently as a manifestation of late chemoirradiation damage (82,83). In more recent times, the evaluation of the glomeruli and vessels has been further confounded by the long-term effects of cyclosporine on these structures (84).

VII. IMMUNE SYSTEM

Classically, the immune system is one of the primary targets of GVHD. Histologic study of the lymphoid organs in patients with C-GVHD has been confined to limited numbers of post mortem examination. The autopsy material reflects changes related to stress, patient age, previous TBI, immunosuppressive treatment, possibly the type of C-GVHD (extensive or localized), and the duration of survival. In general, most patients with C-GVHD have failed to develop secondary reactive germinal centers and have lymphopenia particularly noticeable in the paracortex of lymph nodes, malpighian corpuscles of the spleen, and the thymus (14) (Fig. 12).

Thymic damage instigated during acute GVHD is posited as one of the causes for immunodeficiency and immune dysregulation associated with C-GVHD (18,85,86). Experimentally, a chronic GVHD syndrome also develops in autologous or syngeneically engrafted rodents following cessation of cyclosporine treatment provided that thymic irradiation is given before the marrow transplant (87,88). Immunohistologic studies of the thymuses from rats with cyclosporine-induced syngeneic chronic GVHD indicates permanent damage to the thymic medulla (87). Evaluation of autopsy thymuses from human marrow transplant recipients by histology, histochemistry, and immunohistochemistry indicated that thymic injury was universally profound in the early posttransplant period, particularly in patients receiving total body irradiation (89). Patients with GVHD had additional individual thymic epithelial cell death. Long-term marrow allograft survivors displayed delayed reconstitution of normal thymic epithelium, although a few showed evidence of reconstitution of normal thymic architecture. Interestingly, the thymus gland of a teenager who died from an auto accident 4 years after regression of limited C-GVHD had a well-developed thymic gland. These studies suggest that thymic damage caused by GVHD can be reversible after the development of graft-host intolerance.

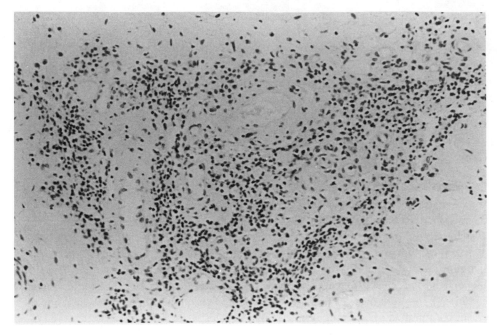

Figure 12 Fibrotic and atrophic thymus from a 12-year-old with extensive chronic GVHD one year posttransplant for aplasia. Patient had received neither immunosuppressive therapy nor total body irradiation pretransplant.

A consequence of GVHD-induced thymic injury may be the infrequent development of autoimmune phenomena such as myasthenia gravis, which has developed in several allografted patients with C-GVHD following cessation of corticosteroid therapy (90,91). Preliminary immunohistochemical studies on thymuses from patients with chronic GVHD demonstrate a relative increase of thymic myoid muscle cells (T. Kirchner, personal communication). Myoid cell express both the intra- and extracellular complete acetylcholine receptor domains and are presumably a key autoimmune target in the genesis of myasthenia gravis (92). In the presence of GVHD and thymic damage, thymic interdigitating dendritic cells may serve as antigen presenting accessory cells which present the complete acetylcholine receptor antigen on myoid cells to existing autoreactive thymic T cells, leading to the production of autoantibodies to the receptor and subsequently myasthenia gravis (85).

VIII. CONCLUSION

The histologic studies of chronic GVHD have provided a conceptional framework for clinical and laboratory investigations of the syndrome. Histopathology plays a pivotal role when used to monitor therapeutic efficacy of immunosuppressive therapy and distinguish active versus inactive chronic GVHD with residual damage. Immunohistologic studies of chronic GVHD have helped define the effector cells and targets of GVHD. Chronic GVHD is a valuable model for studying immunodeficiency and autoimmune states.

ACKNOWLEDGMENT

This research was supported by grants CA 18029, CA 15704, and HL 36444 awarded by the National Institutes of Health, DHHS.

NOTE ADDED IN PROOF

Nakhleh et al. have recently published new criteria for minimal histologic involvement with oral C-GVHD which improve the specificity of grade II changes and aid in the distinction from grade I (inconclusive changes). Biopsies graded as inconclusive had mild mucoasal inflammation with three or fewer apoptotic bodies, or salivary glands had less than 10% loss of acinar tissue or minimal to mild inflammation without ductal epithelial cell necrosis. When either mucosa and/or the salivary gland histology satisfied more stringent grade II criteria, 94-100% of patients had other organs involved by C-GVHD. The fate of their patients with histilogically inconclusive oral biopsies was less clear, as 33-50% still had changes associated with C-GVHD elsewhere. This study emphasizes a point previously made by Sale et al. (52), that improving a test's specificity involves a trade-off with lower sensitivity.

REFERENCES

1. Shulman HM, Sale GE, Lerner KG, Barker EA, Weide PL, Sullivan K, Gallucci B, Thomas ED, Storb R: Chronic cutaneous graft-versus-host disease in man. Am J Path 1978;91:545-570.
2. Shulman HM, Sullivan KM, Weiden PL, McDonald GB, Striker GE, Sale GE, Hackman RC, Tsoi M-S, Storb R, Thomas ED: Chronic graft-versus-host syndrome in man: a long term clinicopathologic study of 20 Seattle patients. Am J Med 1980; 69:204-217.
3. Graze PR, Gale RP: Chronic graft-versus-host disease: a syndrome of disordered immunity. Am J Med 1978;66:611.
4. Gratwohl AA, Moutsopoulos HM, Chused TM, Akizuki M, Wolf RO, Sweet JB, Deisseroth AB: Sjogren-type syndrome after allogeneic bone marrow transplantation. Ann Intern Med 1977;87:703-706.
5. Spielvogel RL, Ullman S, Goltz RW: Skin changes in graft-versus-host disease. South Med J 1976;69:1277-1281.
6. Van Vloten WA, Scheffer E, Dooren LJ: Localized scleroderma-like lesions after bone marrow transplantation in man: a chronic graft-versus-host reaction. Br J Dermatol 1977;96:337-341.
7. Saurat JH, Didier-Jean L, Gluckman E, Bussel A: Graft-versus-host reaction and lichen planus-like eruption in man. Br J Dermatol 1975;92:591-592.
8. Simes MA, Johansson E, Rapola J: Scleroderma-like graft-versus-host disease as late consequence of bone marrow grafting. Lancet 1977;2:831-832.
9. Lawley TJ, Peck GL, Moutsopoulos HM, Gratwohl AA, Diesseroth AB: Scleroderma, Sjogren-like syndrome, and chronic graft-versus-host disease. Ann Intern Med 1977;87:707-709.
10. Hood AF, Soter NA, Rappeport J, Gigli I: Graft-versus-host reaction: Cutaneous manifestations following bone marrow transplantation. Arch Dermatol 1977;113:1087-1091.
11. Kruger GRF, Berard GP, DeLellis RA, Graw RG Jr, Yankee RA, Leventhal BG, Rogentine GN, Herzig GP, Halterman RH, Henderson ES: Graft-versus-host disease: morphologic variation and differential diagnosis in 8 cases of HL-A matched bone marrow transplantation. Am J Pathol 1971;63:179-202.

12. Meuwissen HJ, Rodey G, McArthur J, Pabst H, Gatti R, Chilgren R, Hong R. Frommel D, Coifman R, Good RA: Bone marrow transplantation. Therapeutic usefulness and complications. Am J Med 1971;51:513-532.

13. Mathe G, Amiel JL, Schwarzenberg L. *Bone Marrow Transplantation and Leucocyte Transfusions*, edited by Kugelmass IN. Charles C. Thomas Publisher, Springfield, Illinois, 1971;p. 70.

14. Sale GE, Shulman HM: *The Pathology of Bone Marrow Transplantation*. Masson Inc., New York, 1984.

15. Sullivan KM, Shulman HM, Storb R, Weiden PL, Witherspoon RP, McDonald GB, Schubert MM, Atkinson K, Thomas ED: Chronic graft-versus-host disease in 52 patients: Adverse natural course and successful treatment with combination immunosuppression. Blood 1981;57:267-276.

16. Stastny P, Stembridge VA, Ziff M: Homologous disease in the adult rat, a model for autoimmune disease. I. General features and cutaneous lesions. J Exp Med 1963; 118:635-648.

17. Stastny P, Stembridge VA, Vischer T, Ziff M: Homologous disease in the adult rat, a model for autoimmune disease. II. Findings in the joints, heart, and other tissues. J Exp Med 1965;122:681-709.

18. Beschorner WE, Tutschka PJ, Santons GW: Chronic graft-versus-host disease in the rat radiation chimera. I. Clinical presentation, hematology, histology and immunopathology in long-term chimeras. Transplantation 1982;33:393-399.

19. Rappaport H, Khalil A, Halle-Pannenko O, Pritchard L, Dantchev D, Mathe G: Histopathologic sequence of events in adult mice undergoing lethal graft-versus-host reaction developed across H-2 and/or non-H-2 histocompatibility barriers. Am J Path 1979;96:121-142.

20. Hamilton BL, Parkman R: Acute and chronic graft-versus-host disease induced by minor histocompatibility antigens in mice. Transplantation 1983;36:150-155.

21. Atkinson K, Shulman HM, Deeg HJ, Weiden PL, Graham TC, Thomas ED, Storb R: Acute and chronic graft-versus-host disease in dogs given hemopoietic grafts from DLA-nonidentical littermates: two distinct syndromes. Am J Path 1982;108:196-205.

22. Sullivan KM, Witherspoon RP, Storb R, Deeg HJ, Dahlberg S, Sanders JE, Appelbaum FR, Doney KC, Weiden PL, Anasetti C, Loughran TP, Hill R, Shields A, Yee G, Shulman HM, Nims J, Strom S, Thomas ED: Alternating-day cyclosporine and prednisone for treatment of high-risk chronic graft-versus-host disease. Blood 1988; 72:555-561.

23. Esterly NB: (editorial) Nail dystrophy in dyskeratosis congenita and chronic graft-versus-host disease. Arch Dermatol 1986;122:506-507.

24. Black C, Dieppe P, Huskisson T, Hart FD: Regressive systemic sclerosis. Ann Rheumat Dis 1986;45:384-388.

25. Gallucci BB, Shulman HM, Sale GE, Lerner KG, Caldwell LE, Thomas ED: The ultrastructure of the human epidermis in chronic graft-versus-host disease. Am J Path 1979;95:643-662.

26. Janin-Mercier A, Saurat JH, Bourges M, Sohier J, Didier-jean L, Gluckman E: The lichen planus-like and sclerotic phases of the graft-versus-host disease in man: an ultrastructural study of six cases. Acta Derm Venerol (Stockh)1981;61:187-193.

27. Saurat JH, Didier-jean L, Beucher F, Gluckman E: Immunoflourescent tracing of cytoplasmic components involved in keratinocyte differentiation. Br J Dermatol 1978;98:155-163.

28. Tsoi M-S, Storb R, Jones E, Weiden PL, Shulman HM, Witherspoon R, Atkinson K, Thomas ED: Deposition of IgM and complement at the dermo-epidermal junction in acute and chronic graft-vs-host disease in man. J Immunol 1978;120:1485-1492.

29. Volc-Platzer B, Rappersberger K, Mosberger I, Hinterberger W, Emminger-Schmid-
    neier W, Radaskiewixz T, Wolff K: Sequential immunohistologic analysis of the skin
    following allogeneic bone marrow ransplantation. J Invest Dermatol 1988;91:162-
    168.
30. Fujii H, Ohashi M, Nagura H: Immunohistochemical analysis of oral lichen-planus-
    like eruption in graft-versus-host disease after allogeneic bone marrow transplanta-
    tion. Am J Clin Pathol 1988;89:177-186.
31. Muller C, Schuch K, Pawelec G, Wilms K, Wernet P: Immunohistology of graft-
    versus-host disease mediated skin lesions and its correlation to a large granular
    lymphocyte surface phenotype and function. Blut 1982;44:89-94.
32. Kaye VN, Neumann PM, Kersey J, Goltz RW, Baldridge BD, Michael AF, Platt JL:
    Identity of immune cells in graft-versus-host disease of the skin: analysis using
    monoclonal antibodies by indirect immunofluorescence. Am J Pathol 1984;116:
    436-440.
33. Tazzari PL, Gobbi M, Zauli D, Tassinari A, Crespi C, Miserocchi F, Dinota A, Bandini
    G, Ricci P, Tura S: Close association between antibodies to cytoskeletal intermedi-
    ate filaments and chronic graft-versus-host disease. Transplantation 1987;44:234-
    236.
34. Beschorner WE, Tutschka PJ, Santos GW: Chronic graft-versus-host disease in the
    rat radiation chimera. III. Immunology and immunopathology in rapidity induced
    models. Transplantation 1983;35:224-230.
35. Atkinson K, Cooley M, Farrelly H, O'Flaherty E, Ashby M, Biggs J: CD4+ T cells
    appear capable of initiating graft-versus-host disease across non-major histocom-
    patibility complex (MHC) barriers in man. Bone Marrow Transplantation 1987;2:
    79-84.
36. Bos JD, Kapsenberg ML: The skin immune system: Its cellular constituents and
    their interactions. Immunology Today 1986;7:235-240.
37. Morhenn VB: Keratinocyte proliferation in wound healing and skin diseases. Im-
    munology Today 1988;9:104-107.
38. Kupper TS, Lee F, Coleman D, Chodakewitz J, Flood P, Horowitz M: Keratinocyte
    derived T-cell growth factor (KTGF) is identical to granulocyte macrophage colony
    stimulating factor (GM-CSF). J Invest Dermatol 1988;91:185-188.
39. Niederwieser D, Aubock J. Troppmair J, Herold M, Schuler G, Boeck G, Lotz J,
    Fritsch P, Huber C: IFN-mediated induction of MHC antigen expression on human
    keratinocytes and its influence on in vitro alloimmune responses. J Immunol 1988;
    140:2556-2564.
40. Claman HN: Mast cell depletion in murine chronic graft-versus-host disease. J Invest
    Dermatol 1985;84;246-248.
41. Parkman R, Champagne J, DeClerck Y, Cooper M, Draper V, Walker S: Cellular
    interactions in graft-versus-host disease. Transplant Proc 1987;19:53-54.
42. Kahari VM, Sandberg M, Kalimo H, Vuorio T, Vuorio E: Identification of fibro-
    blasts responsible for increased collagen production in localized scleroderma by in
    situ hybridization. J Invest Dermatol 1988;90:664-670.
43. McDonald GB, Sullivan KM, Schuffler MD, Shulman HM, Thomas ED; Esophageal
    abnormalities in chronic graft-versus-host disease in humans. Gastroenterology 1981;
    80:914-921.
44. Spencer GD, Shulman HM, Myerson D, Thomas ED, McDonald GB: Diffuse intesti-
    nal ulcertation after marrow transplantation: a clinicopathologic study of 13 pati-
    ents. Hum Pathol 1986;17:621-633.
45. Shulman HM, Sharma P, Amos D, Fenster LF, McDonald GB: A coded histologic
    study of hepatic graft-versus-host disease after human bone marrow transplantation.
    Hepatology 1988;8:463-470.

46. Snover DC, Weisdorf SA, Ramsay NK, McGlave P, Kersey JH: Hepatic graft versus-host disease: A study of the predictive value of liver biopsy in diagnosis. Hepatology 1984;4:123-130.

47. Snover DC, Hutton S, Balfour HH, Bloomer JR: Cytomegalovirus infection of the liver in transplant recipients. J Clin Gastroenterol 1987;9:659-665.

48. Snover DC, Horwitz CA: Liver disease in cytomegalovirus mononucleosis: a light microscopal and immunoperoxidase study of six cases. Hepatology 1984;4:408-412.

49. Beschorner WE, Pino J, Boitnott JK, Tutschka PJ, Santos GW: Pathology of the liver with bone marrow transplantation. Effects of busulfan, carmustine, acute graft-versus-host disesse, and cytomegalovirus infection. Am J Pathol 1980;99:369-385.

50. Yau JC, Zander AR, Srigley JR, Verm RA, Stroehlein JR, Korinek JK, Vellekoop L, Dicke KA: Chronic graft-versus-host disease complicated by micronodular cirrhosis and esophageal varices. Transplantation 1986;41:129-130.

51. Knapp AB, Crawford JM, Rappeport JM, Gollan JL: Cirrhosis as a consequence of graft-versus-host disease. Gastroenterology 1987;92:513-519.

52. Sale GE, Shulman HM, Schubert MM, Sullivan KM, Kopecky KJ, Hackman RC, Morton TH, Storb R, Thomas ED: Oral and ophthalmic pathology of graft-versus-host disease in man: predictive value of the lip biopsy. Hum Pathol 1981;12:1022-1030.

53. Jack MK, Jack GM, Sale GE, Shulman HM, Sullivan HM: Ocular manifestations of graft-versus-host disease. Arch Ophthalmol 1983;101:1080-1084.

54. Schubert MM, Sullivan KM, Morton TH, Izutsu KT, Peterson DE, Flournoy N, Truelove EL, Sale GE, Buckner CD, Storb R, Thomas ED: Oral manifestations of chronic graft-versus-host disease. Arch Intern Med 1984;144:1591-1595.

55. Rodu B, Gockerman JP: Oral manifestations of the chronic graft-versus-host reaction. JAMA 1984;249:504-507.

56. Barrett AP, Bilous AM: Oral patterns of acute and chronic graft-versus-host disease. Arch Dermatol 1984;120:1461-1465.

57. Epstein O, Thomas HC, Scherlock S: Primary biliary cirrhosis is a dry gland syndrome with features of chronic graft-versus-host disease. Lancet 1980;1:1166-1168.

58. Nakhleh R, Miller W, Snover D: The significance of mucosal versus salivary gland changes in lip biopsies in the diagnosis of chronic graft-versus-host disease (C-GVHD). United States and Canadian Academy of Pathology, Annual Meeting, Washington, Abstract 389, 1988; p. 66A.

59. Ralph DD, Springmeyer SC, Sullivan KM, Hackman RC, Storb R, Thomas ED: Rapidly progressive air-flow obstruction in marrow transplant recipients. Am Rev Respir Dis 1984;129:641-644.

60. Urbanski SJ, Kossakowska AE, Curtis J, Chan CK, Hutcheon MA. Hyland RH, Messner H, Minden M, Sculier JP: Idiopathic small airways pathology in patients with graft-versus-host disease following allogeneic bone marrow transplantation. Am J Surg Pathol 1987;11:965-971.

61. Holland HK, Wingard JR, Beschorner WE, Saral R, Santos GW: Bronchiolitis obliterans in bone marrow transplantation and its relationship to chronic graft-versus-host disease and low serum IgG. Blood 1988;72:621-627.

62. Geddes DM, Corrin B, Brewerton DA, Davies RJ, Turner-Warwick M: Progressive airway obliteration in adults and its association with rhematoid disease. Quart J Med 1977;184:427-444.

63. Newball HA, Brahim SA: Chronic obstructive airway disease in patients with Sjogren's syndrome. Am Rev Respir Dis 1977;115:295-304.

64. Yousem S, Burke C, Billingham M: Pathologic pulmonary alterations in long-term human heart-lung transplantation. Hum Pathol 1985;16:911-923.

65. Tazelaar HD, Prop J, Niewenhuis P, Billingham ME, Wildevuur CR: Airway pathology in the transplanted rat lung. Transplantation 1988;45:864-869.
66. Unanue ER, Allen PM: Editorial: comment on the finding of Ia expression in non-lymphoid cells. Lab Invest 1986;55:123-125.
67. Rossie KM, Sheridan JF, Barthold SW, Tutschka PJ: Graft-versus-host disease and sialodacryadentis viral infection in bone marrow transplanted rats. Transplantation 1988;45:1012-1016.
68. Struhar D, Harbeck RJ, Horiuchi T, Edelson JD, Mason RJ: Class II antigens of the major histocompatibility complex are expressed in lung tissue of bleomycin treated rats and patients with idiopathic pulmonary fibrosis (IPF). Am Rev Respir Dis 1986;133:A144.
69. Romaniuk A, Prop J, Peterson A, Wildevuur CRH, Niewenhuis P: Expression of class II major histocompatibility complex antigens by bronchial epithelium in rat lung allografts. Transplantation 1987;44:209-214.
70. Beschorner WE, Saral R, Hutchins GM, Tutschka PJ, Santos GW: Lymphocytic bronchitis associated with graft-versus-host disease in recipients of bone marrow transplants. N Engl J Med 1978;299:1030-1036.
71. O'Brien KD, Hackman RC, Sale GE, Prentice R, Deeg J, Thomas ED, Storb R: Lymphocytic bronchitis unrelated to acute graft-versus-host disease in canine marrow graft recipients. Transplantation 1984;37:234-238.
72. Lum LG: The kinetics of immune reconstitution after human marrow transplantation. Blood 1987;69:369-380.
73. Izutsu KT, Sullivan KM, Schubert MM, Truelove EL, Shulman HM, Sale GE, Morton TH, Rice JC, Witherspoon RP, Storb R, Thomas ED: Disordered salivary immunoglobulin secretion and sodium transport in human chronic graft-versus-host disease. Transplantation 1983;35:441-446.
74. Beschorner WE, Yardley JH, Tutschka P, Santos G: Deficiency of intestinal immunity with graft-versus-host disease in humans. J Infect Dis 1981;144:38-46.
75. Hruban RH, Beschorner WE, Baumgartner WA, Achuff SC, Traill TA, Digennaro KA, Reitz BA, Hutchins GM: Depletion of bronchus-associated lymphoid tissue associated with lung allograft rejection. Am J Pathol 1988;132:6-11.
76. Reynolds HY: Immunoglobulin G and its function in the human repiratory tract. Mayo Clin Proc 1988;63:161-174.
77. Sullivan KM, Meyers JD, Fluornoy N, Storb R, Thomas ED: Early and later interstitial pneumonia following human bone marrow transplantation. Internat J Cell Cloning 1986;4:107-121.
78. Sullivan KM, Deeg HJ, Sanders JE, Shulman HM, Witherspoon RP, Doney KC, Appelbaum FR, Schubert MM, Stewart PS, Springmeyer S, McDonald GB, Storb R, Thomas ED: Late complications after marrow transplantation. Semin Hematol 1984;21:53-73.
79. Anderson BA, Young PV, Kean WF, Ludwin SK, Galbraith PR, Anastassiades TP: Polymyositis in chronic graft-versus-host disease. A case report. Arch Neurol 1982;39:188-190.
80. Reyes MG, Noronha P, Thomas W Jr, Heredia R: Myositis of chronic graft-versus-host disease. Neurology 1983;33:1222-1224.
81. Furst DE, Clements PJ, Graze P, Gale R, Roberts N: A syndrome resembling progressive systemic sclerosis after bone marrow transplantation. A model for scleroderma? Arthritis and Rheumatism 1979;22:904-911.
82. Guinan EC, Tarbell NJ, Niemeyer CM, Sallan SE, Weinstein HJ: Intravascular hemolysis and renal insufficiency after bone marrow transplantation. Blood 1988;72:451-455.

83. Bergstein J, Andreoli SP, Provisor AJ, Yum M: Radiation nephritis following total-body irradiation and cyclosphosphamide in preparation for bone marrow transplantation. Transplantation 1984;41:63-66.

84. Dische FE, Neuberger J, Keating J, Parson V, Calne RY, Williams R: Kidney pathology in liver allograft recipients after long-term treatment with cyclosporin A. Lab Invest 1988;58:395-402.

85. Shulman HM: Is graft-versus-host disease an alloimmune or autoimmune disorder? In *Clinical Aspects of Autoimmunity*, edited by Tan EM. Fones & Mann Projects Division, New York, 1988; pp. 18-30.

86. Seddik M, Seemayer TA, Lapp WS: T cell functional defect associated with thymic epithelial cell injury induced by a graft-versus-host reaction. Transplantation 1980; 29:61-66.

87. Beschorner WE, DiGennaro KA, Hess AD, Santos GW: Cyclosporine and the thymus: influence of irradiation and age on thymic immunopathology and recovery. Cell Immunol 1987;110:350-364.

88. Cheney RT, Sprent J: Capacity of cyclosporine to induce auto-graft-versus-host disease and impair intrathymic T cell differentiation. Transplant Proc 1985;17:528-530.

89. Muller-Hermelink HK, Sale GE, Borisch B, Storb R: Pathology of the thymus after allogeneic bone marrow transplantation in man. A histologic immunohistochemical study of 36 patients. Am J Pathol 1987;129:242-256.

90. Smith CIE, Aarli JA, Biberfield P, Bolme P, Christensson B, Gahrton G, Hammarstrom L, Lefvert A-K, Lonnqvist B, Matell G, Pirskanen R, Ringden O, Svanborg E: Myasthenia gravis after bone marrow transplantation. Evidence for a donor origin. N Engl J Med 1983;309:1565-1568.

91. Bolger GB, Sullivan KM, Spencer AM et al.: Myasthenia gravis after allogeneic bone marrow transplantation: relationship to chronic graft-versus-host disease. Neurology 1986;36:1087-1091.

92. Kirchner TH, Tzartos S, Hoppe F, Schalke B, Wekerle H, Muller-Hermelink HK: Pathogenesis of myasthenia gravis. Acetylcholine receptor-related antigenic determinants in tumor-free thymuses and thymic epithelial tumors. Am J Pathol 1988; 130:268-280.

93. Nakhleh RE, Miller W, Snover DC: Significance of mucosal vs salivary gland changes in lip biopsies in the diagnosis of chronic graft-vs-host disease. Arch Path Lab Med 1989;113:932-934.

33

Pathogenesis of Human Chronic Graft-vs.-Host Disease

Kerry Atkinson
St. Vincent's Hospital
Sydney, New South Wales, Australia

I. INTRODUCTION

The classical immunogenetic requirements for Graft-vs.-Host Disease (GVHD) were first laid down by Billingham in 1966 (1) and, although human chronic GVHD was first described 9 years later (2), it fits well within these requirements. The requirements are:

1. Genetically determined histocompatibility differences between the graft donor and the recipient.
2. The presence of immunocompetent cells in the graft which can recognize foreign histocompatibility antigens of the host and mount an immunologic reaction against cells bearing such antigens.
3. The inability of the host to react against, and reject, the donor graft.

Within this framework the pathogenetic mechanism of human chronic GVHD is composed of a number of different components, which together make up this complex multisystem clinical disorder. These components are summarized in Table 1 and will be dealt with individually.

II. INITIATION OF GVHD AFTER BONE MARROW TRANSPLANTATION

There is no doubt that the initiating event in the pathogenesis of GVHD after marrow transplantation is the activation of alloreactive mature donor T cells present in the graft by recipient cells expressing histocompatibility antigens that are not shared by the cells of the donor. The evidence for this came initially from experiments in rodent models of bone marrow transplantation in which the donor marrow was depleted of T cells by incubation with anti-T-cell antibody and complement prior to its infusion into the reci-

Table 1 Components in the Pathogenesis of Chronic GVHD

Initiation of antihost alloreactivity by activation of marrow donor T cells against histo-
    compatibility antigens not shared by the donor
Persisting antihost alloreactivity
Target organ damage by:
    Direct T-cell-mediated cytotoxicity
    Antibody and complement-mediated cytotoxicity
    Fibrosis secondary to leukokine production by T cells
    Inflammatory damage by cytotoxic cytokines (e.g., TNF)
Development of autoreactivity
Development of counterbalancing regulatory cells
Multifactorial immune deficiency

pient (3-6). Indeed the complete and permanent abrogation of GVHD by this mechanism in one such model indicated that T cells were both necessary and sufficient for the
initiation of GVHD (7). Subsequent refinements of these model systems demonstrated
that both CD4$^+$ T cells (class II MHC reactive) and CD8$^+$ T cells (class I reactive) were
each able to initiate GVHD, depending on the features of the histocompatibility barriers
between the donor and recipient murine strains involved (8-10). Further evidence for
the role of immune competent cells in the initiation of GVHD was obtained by the demonstration of a dose-response effect with increasing numbers of spleen cells in the hemopoietic graft producing increasing severity of GVHD (11).

    Similar observations have been made in human recipients of marrow transplants.
There is no doubt that T-cell depletion of the donor marrow can markedly decrease the
incidence and severity of subsequent acute and chronic GVHD (12-16). Additionally,
two centers have shown a direct relationship between the number of T cells infused after
the depletion procedure and the severity of subsequent acute GVHD (17,18). In one
study in which an anti-CD2 and an anti-CD8 monoclonal antibody were used (together
with rabbit complement) to produce T-cell depletion, the residual infused T cells were
of the CD4 phenotype, and since acute GVHD (albeit mild) occurred in these patients,
the inference was drawn that CD4$^+$ T cells are capable of inducing acute GVHD across
non-MHC barriers in man (19). The reciprocal experiment (depleting the marrow with an
anti-CD4 antibody) has not yet been reported. There is, thus, no doubt that donor T
cells play a major role in initiating acute and chronic GVHD in man. In view of this it
is not surprising that preceding acute GVHD has been shown to be the main determinant
for the subsequent development of chronic GVHD in man (20-22).

III. CONTINUING ANTIHOST ALLOREACTIVITY

Evidence for the continuing presence of circulating T cells sensitized to host (recipient)
alloantigens has been documented in patients with, but not in those without, chronic
GVHD (23). In genotypically HLA-identical sibling donor-recipient transplants, chimera
cells from patients with chronic GVHD were found to be reactive in mixed lymphocyte
culture (MLC) when stimulated by host peripheral blood lymphocytes that had been
cryopreserved pretransplant. Donor cells continued to show nonreactivity in MLC to
these same cryopreserved recipient cells. There was no difference between the MLC responses of patients with and without chronic GVHD to donor cells. These results repre-

sented the first evidence of involvement of cell-mediated immunity of the graft against the host in patients with chronic GVHD.

More recently, Goulmy has documented the presence of cytotoxic T cells specific for recipient minor histocompatibility antigens in patients with acute and chronic GVHD after HLA-identical sibling marrow transplantation (24). The highest initial levels of antihost cytotoxic T-cell activity were noted in patients with chronic GVHD. This activity developed either early posttransplant or at the time of discontinuation of prophylactic immunosuppression for GVHD.

The main questions, therefore, in the pathogenesis of chronic GVHD now center on the effector mechanisms, specifically on the ways in which target organ damage is related to the development of antihost alloreactivity.

IV. MECHANISMS OF TARGET ORGAN DAMAGE

There are a number of candidates for the pathologic mechanisms by which target organ damage is caused in chronic GVHD (Table 1).

A. T-Cell-Mediated Cytotoxicity

Several reports have described the presence in tissues of patients with chronic GVHD of a cellular infiltrate composed predominantly of $CD8^+$ cells (25-28). Furthermore, electron-microscopic examination of the skin in patients with chronic GVHD has shown lymphocytes in both broad zone and point contact with epidermal cells (29). Similar ultrastructural changes have been reported in a patient whose main manifestation of chronic GVHD was polymyositis: contacts were observed between lymphocytes and degenerated muscle fibers (30). Combining these two techniques, a recent study utilizing immune electron microscopy has described degeneration of keratinocytes to which $CD8^+$ cells were attached in five patients with chronic oral GVHD (31). The infiltrating cells were further shown to be $CD3^+$ and $CD8^+$, and in some cases expressed the interleukin 2 receptor ($CD25^+$).

B. Antibody and Complement-Mediated Cytotoxicity

The main site of histological damage in patients with skin GVHD is at the dermo-epidermal junction. In a study of 88 allogeneic marrow recipients, dermo-epidermal junctional deposits of IgM and the third component of complement were significantly associated with chronic GVHD (32). Eighty-six percent of patients with chronic GVHD showed heavy IgM deposits while light deposits were present in only 11% of healthy marrow donors, patients biopsied before transplantation, and patients without GVHD posttransplant. Additionally, Saurat (33) has demonstrated the presence of serum IgG specific for epidermal basal cells in two of four patients with chronic GVHD. It has been postulated that these dermal deposits are antibodies produced by donor cells in response to antigenic differences between donor and host.

C. Promotion of Fibrosis by Soluble T-Cell Products

Although no corresponding data have yet been produced in man, the revealing experiments of De Clerc and colleagues (34) demonstrating the production of leukokine from cells present in mice with chronic GVHD, which increased the amount of collagen secretion per fibroblast, are worthy of note. Additionally, a leukokine from T cells in mice with acute GVHD stimulated the proliferation of fibroblasts. Taken together, such growth factors are likely responsible for the fibrosis which is the hallmark of late stage organ damage in human chronic GVHD.

D. Other Possible Mechanisms

1. Increased Susceptibility of Epithelial Target Tissues

Expression of class II MHC gene products on epithelial cells in the skin and gut of rodents (35,36) undergoing GVHD, and in the skin (26,27) and liver (37) of patients with GVHD has been described. However, the bulk of these latter reports have included patients with acute rather than chronic GVHD. It is postulated that alloreactive T cells release gamma interferon in the local vicinity of the target epithelial cells, thus promoting their expression of HLA-DR antigens. This in turn may render these epithelial cells more susceptible to attack by class II reactive T cells of donor origin.

2. Large Granular Lymphocyte-Mediated Cytotoxicity

Although large granular lymphocytes have been postulated to play a role in the mechanism of skin damage in acute GVHD in rodents (38), such cells have not been prominent in histologic studies of patients with chronic GVHD.

3. Damage Mediated by Tumor Necrosis Factor

Although antibodies to tumor necrosis factor clearly decrease the severity of acute GVHD in rodents and improve their survival (39), corresponding data in humans with chronic GVHD have not yet been reported.

Additional components in the multifactorial pathogenesis of chronic GVHD include the development of autoreactivity, suppressor cell populations, and the characteristic severe immune deficiency.

V. AUTOREACTIVITY

While acute GVHD appears to be primarily an alloreactive disease and while alloreactivity is also clearly a component in human chronic GVHD, some features of autoreactivity have been described in human chronic GVHD and likely play a pathogenic role in the production of the disease. First, the systemic nature and protean manifestations of human chronic GVHD bear resemblance to a number of autoimmune connective tissue disorders including progressive systemic sclerosis, systemic lupus erythematosis, eosinophilic fasciitis, Sjögren's syndrome, and primary biliary cirrhosis. Second, circulating autoantibodies are a well-described feature of patients with clinical chronic GVHD (Chapter 31). Third, autoreactive T cells were clearly demonstrated to develop in chronic, but not acute, GVHD in the model system developed by Parkman and colleagues (40). This latter interesting finding provides an explanation for one of the central enigmas of the pathogenesis of GVHD, namely the widespread atrophy and hypocellularity of the lymphoid system. Without evidence for such an autoimmune antilymphocyte reaction, it is difficult to understand why the donor-antigen hemopoietic stem cells in the recipient's marrow cavity, which is usually normocellular, is unable to repopulate the recipient's lymphoid system. Again, corresponding data in man have not yet been reported.

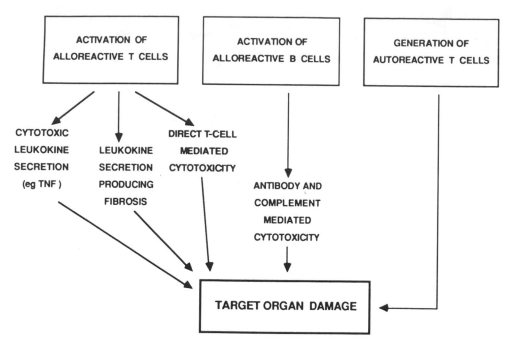

Figure 1 Mechanisms of target cell damage in chronic Graft-vs.-Host Disease.

VI. DEVELOPMENT OF REGULATION

Perhaps in an attempt to counterbalance the alloreactive and autoreactive cell populations described above, approximately 50% of patients with chronic GVHD develop detectable circulating T cells nonspecifically suppressive of mitogen and alloantigen induced proliferation (41). These cells are not detectable in long-term survivors without chronic GVHD, who, in contradistinction, develop circulating T cells specifically suppressive of antihost alloreactivity (42). It has been postulated that the graft-host tolerance exhibited by this latter patient population is mediated by these specific suppressor cells (42). It has been further postualted that patients with chronic GVHD are unable to produce such specific regulatory cells because of the histologic (43) and functional (44) damage to the thymus gland in patients with chronic GVHD. Further, these nonspecific suppressor cells may actually contribute to the multifactorial immune deficiency characteristic of patients with chronic GVHD, and indeed the highest incidence of varicella-zoster infections (79%) in patients given HLA-identical sibling marrow transplants is seen in that cohort of patients with chronic GVHD in whom circulating nonspecific suppressor cells are detectable (45).

The cascade of events involved, or postulated to be involved, in the pathogenesis of target cell damage in human chronic GVHD is illustrated in Figure 1.

VII. IMMUNE DEFICIENCY

Of equal importance to the target organ damage in patients with chronic GVHD is their marked susceptibility to infection. Chronic GVHD is the main determinant for infectious complications late posttransplant (45,56). The severe combined immune defi-

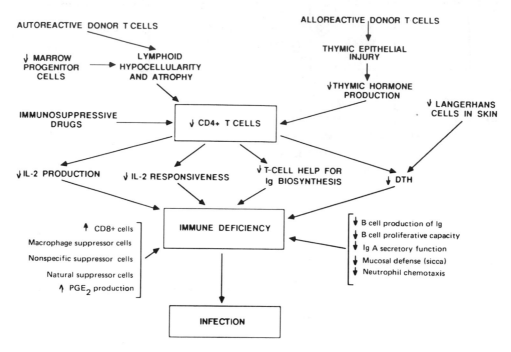

Figure 2 Components of the immune deficiency in chronic Graft-vs.-Host Disease.

ciency characteristic of chronic GVHD is well documented. The immune system itself (lymph nodes, spleen, and thymus) is a major target organ in chronic GVHD, presumably due to the bi-pronged attack by both autoreactive and alloreactive donor cells upon it. While the impact of chronic GVHD on both the immune and hemopoietic systems is fully dealt with elsewhere in this book (Chapter 36), the role of immune deficiency in the pathogenesis of the infections characteristic of the disease is central, and a graphical summary of the components of the immune deficiency in chronic GVHD is given in Figure 2.

ACKNOWLEDGMENT

Supported in part by a grant from the Government Employees Assistance to Medical Research Fund.

REFERENCES

1. Billingham RE: The biology of graft-versus-host reactions. In *The Harvey Lectures*, New York, Academic Press, 1966-67;62:21-78.
2. Saurat JH, Gluckman E, Bussel A, Didierjean L, Puissat A: The lichen planus-like eruption after bone marrow transplantation. Br J Dermatol 1975;93:675-681.
3. Rodt H, Thierfelder S, Eulitz M: Anti-lymphocytic antibodies and marrow transplantation. III. Effect of heterologous anti-brain antibodies on acute secondary disease in mice. Eur J Immunol 1974;4:15-19.

4. Muller-Ruchholtz W, Wottge HU, Muller-Hermelink HK: Bone marrow transplantation in rats across histocompatibility barriers by selective elimination of lymphoid cells in donor marrow. Transplant Proc 1976;8:537-541.

5. Korngold R, Sprent J: Lethal graft-versus-host disease after marrow transplantation across minor histocompatibility barriers in mice. Prevention by removing mature T cells from marrow. J Exp Med 1978;148:1687-1698.

6. Onoe K, Fernandez G, Good RA: Humoral and cell mediated immune responses in fully allogeneic marrow chimera mice. J Exp Med 1980;151:115-132.

7. Thierfelder S, Cobbold S, Kummer U, Waldman H, Schuh R: Anti-lymphocytic antibodies and marrow transplantation. VII. Two of nine monoclonal anti-Thy-1 antibodies used for pre-treatment of donor marrow suppressed graft-versus-host reactions without added complement. Exp Hematol 1985;13:948-955.

8. Korngold R, Sprent J: Features of T-cells causing H-2 restricted lethal graft-versus-host disease across minor histocompatibility barriers. J Exp Med 1982;155:872-883.

9. Hamilton BL: Experimental models of GVHD. J Cell Biochem 1986;(Suppl):211 (abstract).

10. Carmody L, Atkinson K, Cooley MA, Chapman G, Biggs JC, McKenzie I: Both class I and class II responsive T-cell subsets can separately initiate lethal graft-versus-host disease in incompatible murine radiation chimeras. Transplant Proc 1987;19:2876-2878.

11. Okunewick JP, Meredith RF, Brozovich B, Seeman PR, Magliere K: Exponential relationship between spleen cell concentration and fatal graft-versus-host response after transplantation of allogeneic spleen-marrow cell mixtures. Transplant Proc 1980;29:507-510.

12. Prentice HG, Blacklock HA, Janossy G, Gilmore JM, Price-Jones L, Tidman N, Trejdosiewiez L, Skeggs D, Ball S, Graphakos S, Patterson J, Ivory K, Hoffbrand A: Depletion of T-lymphocytes in donor marrow prevents significant graft-versus-host disease in matched allogeneic leukemia marrow transplant recipients. Lancet 1984;1:472-475.

13. Martin PJ, Hansen JA, Buckner CD, Sanders JE, Deeg HJ, Stewart P, Appelbaum F, Clift R, Fefer A, Witherspoon R, Kennedy M, Sullivan K, Storb R, Thomas E: Effects of in vitro depletion of T cells in HLA-identical allogeneic marrow grafts. Blood 1985;66:664-672.

14. Waldman NH, Polliak A, Hale G, Or R, Cividalli G, Weiss L, Weshler Z, Sammuel S, Manor D, Brautbar C, Rachmilewitz E, Slavin S: Elimination of graft-versus-host disease by in vitro depletion of alloreactive lymphocytes with a monoclonal rat anti-human lymphocyte antibody (Campath-I). Lancet 1984;2:483-485.

15. Filipovich AH, Vallera DA, Youle RL, Quinones R, Neville JRD, Kersey J: Ex-vivo treatment of donor marrow with anti-T cell immunotoxins for prevention of graft-versus-host disease. Lancet 1984;1:469-472.

16. Atkinson K, Biggs JC, Cooley MA, Farrelly H, O'Flaherty E, Raphael H, Ashby M, Conncannon A, Dodds A, Morgan G, McKenzie I: A comparative study of T-cell depleted and non-depleted marrow transplantation for haematological malignancy. Aust NZ J Med 1987;17:16-23.

17. Atkinson K, Farrelly H, Cooley MA, O'Flaherty E, Downs K, Biggs JC: Human marrow T cell dose correlates with severity of subsequent acute graft-versus-host disease. Bone Marrow Transplant 1987;2:51-57.

18. Kernan NA, Flomenberg N, Collings NH, O'Reilly R, Dupont B: Quantitation of T-lymphocytes in human marrow by a limiting dilution assay. Transplantation Proceedings 1985;40:317-322.

19. Atkinson K, Cooley MA, Farrelly H, O'Flaherty E, Ashby M, Biggs JC: CD4+T cells appear capable of initiating graft-versus-host disease across non-MHC barriers in man. Bone Marrow Transplant 1987;2:79-84.

20. Storb R, Prentice RL, Sullivan KM, Shulman HM, Deeg HJ, Doney KC, Buckner C, Clift R, Witherspoon R, Appelbaum F, Sanders J, Stewart P, Thomas E: Predictive factors in chronic graft-versus-host disease in patients with aplastic anaemia treated by marrow transplantation from HLA-identical siblings. Ann Intern Med 1983;98:461.

21. Ringdén O, Paulin T, Lonnqvst B, Nilsson B: An analysis of factors predisposing to chronic graft-versus-host disease. Exp Hematol 1985;13:1062-1067.

22. Atkinson K, Horowitz MM: Risk factors for chronic graft-versus-host disease. 1988; manuscript in preparation.

23. Tsoi MS, Storb R, Dobbs S, Medill L, Thomas ED: Cell mediated immunity to non-HLA antigens of the host by donor lymphocytes in patients with chronic graft-versus-host disease. J Immunol 1980;125:2258-2262.

24. Goulmy E, Blockland E, Pool J, Zwaan F, Vossen J, van Rood JJ: Minor transplantation antigens in man and their role in bone marrow transplantation. Proceedings. 12th International Congress of the Transplantation Society 1988;2:344 (abstract).

25. Atkinson K, Munro V, Vasak E, Biggs JC: Mononuclear cell subpopulations in the skin defined by monoclonal antibodies after HLA-identical sibling marrow transplantation. Br J Dermatol 1986;114:145-160.

26. Lampert IA, Janossy G, Suitters AJ: Immunological analysis of the skin in graft-versus-host disease. Clin Exp Immunol 1982;50:123-131.

27. Favrot M, Janossy G, Tidman N, Blacklock H, Lopez E, Bofill M, Lampert I, Morgenstern G, Powles R, Prentice H: T-cell regeneration after allogeneic bone marrow transplantation. Clin Exp Immunol 1983;54:59-72.

28. Muller C, Schuch K, Pawelec G, Wilms K, Wernet P: Immunohistology of graft-versus-host disease mediated skin lesions and its correlation to a large granular lymphocyte surface phenotype and function. Blut 1982;44:89-94.

29. Gallucci BB, Shulman HM, Sale GE, Lerner G, Caldwell LE, Thomas ED: The ultrastructure of the human epidermis in chronic graft-versus-host disease. Am J Pathol 1979;95:643-662.

30. Urbano-Marquez A, Estruch R, Grau JM, Granena A, Martin-Ortega E, Palou J, Rozman C: Inflammatory myopathy associated with chronic graft-versus-host disease. Neurol 1986;36:1091-1093.

31. Fuji IH, Ohashi M, Nagura H: Immuno-histochemical analysis of oral lichen planus-like eruption in graft-versus-host-disease after allogeneic bone marrow transplantation. Am J Clin Pathol 1988;89:177-186.

32. Tsoi MS, Storb R, Jones E, Weiden PL, Shulman H, Witherspoon RP, Atkinson K, Thomas E: Deposition of IgM and complement at the dermo-epidermal junction in acute and chronic graft-versus-host disease in man. J Immunol 1978;120:1485-1492.

33. Saurat JH, Gluckman E, Bonnetblanc J, Didierjean L, Bussel A, Puissant A: Charactères cliniques et biologiques des éruptions licheniennes après greffe de moëlle osseuse. Ann Dermatol Syphylig 1975;102:521.

34. DeClerc Y, Draper V, Parkman R: Clonal analysis of murine graft-versus-host disease. II Leukokines that stimulate fibroblast proliferation and collagen synthesis in graft-versus-host disease. J Immunol 1986;136:3549-3552.

35. Lampert IA, Suitters AG, Chisholm PM: Expression of Ia antigen on epidermal keratinocytes in graft-versus-host disease. Nature 1981;293:149-150.

36. Mason DW, Dallman M, Barclay AN: Graft-versus-host disease induces expression of Ia antigen in rat epidermal cells and gut epithelium. Nature 1981;293:150.

37. Niglio F, Pignatelli M, Mazzeo V, Baraldini M, Stefanini GF, Gaudigli G, Bandini G, Ricci P, Tura S, Gasbarrini G: Expression of major histocompatibility complex Class II antigens on bile duct epithelium in patients with hepatic graft-versus-host disease after bone marrow transplantation. J Hepatol 1987;5:182-189.

38. Guillen F, Ferrara J, Hancock W, Messadi D: Acute cutaneous graft-versus-host disease to minor histocompatibility antigens in a murine model. Lab Invest 1986; 55:35-42.
39. Piguet PF, Grau GE, Allet B, Vassalli P: Tumour necrosis factor/cachectin is an effector of skin and gut lesions of the acute phase of graft-versus-host disease. J Exp Med 1987;166:1280-1289.
40. Parkman R: Clonal analysis of murine graft-versus-host disease. I. Phenotypic and functional analysis of T lymphocyte clones. J Immunol 1986;136:3543-3548.
41. Tsoi MS, Storb R, Dobbs S, Kopecky K, Santos E, Weiden P, Thomas E: Non-specific suppressor cells in patients with chronic graft-versus-host disease after marrow grafting. J Immunol 1979;123:1970-1976.
42. Tsoi MS, Storb R, Dobbs S, Thomas ED: Specific suppressor cells in graft-versus-host tolerance of HLA-identical marrow transplantation. Nature 1981;292:355-357.
43. Shulman HM, Sullivan KM, Weiden PL, MacDonald G, Striker G, Sale G, Hackman R, Tsoi M, Storb R, Thomas E: Chronic graft-versus-host syndrome in man. A long term clinicopathological study of 20 Seattle patients. Am J Med 1980;69:204-217.
44. Atkinson K, Incefy GS, Sullivan K, Iwata T, Dardenne M, Ochs HD, Good R, Thomas E, Storb R: Low serum thymic hormone levels in patients with chronic graft-versus-host disease. Blood 1982;59:1073-1077.
45. Atkinson K, Farewell V, Tsoi MS, Sullivan KM, Witherspoon RP, Thomas ED, Storb R: Analysis of late infections after human bone marrow transplantation. Role of non-specific suppressor cells in patients with chronic graft-versus-host disease and genotypic non identity between marrow donor and recipient. Blood 1982;60:714-720.
46. Atkinson K, Storb R, Prentice RL, Weiden PL, Witherspoon RP, Sullivan KM, Noel D, Thomas E: Analysis of late infections in 89 long term survivors of bone marrow transplantation. Blood 1979;53:720-731.

34

Risk Factors for and Prevention of Human Chronic Graft-vs.-Host Disease

Kerry Atkinson
St. Vincent's Hospital
Sydney, New South Wales, Australia

I. RISK FACTORS FOR THE DEVELOPMENT OF CHRONIC GVHD

There are two published reports on factors predictive of the development of chronic Graft-vs.-Host Disease (GVHD) after allogeneic bone marrow transplantation (1,2). The first of these, from Seattle (1), was restricted to patients who were transplanted from an HLA-identical sibling donor for severe aplastic anemia. Binary logistic regression analysis identified three factors independently predisposing to the development of chronic GVHD in this population: (a) the presence of preceding moderate to severe acute GVHD and, in those patients without such prior acute GVHD, (b) increasing patient age, and (c) the use of viable donor buffy coat cells (in addition to the donor marrow given to prevent marrow graft rejection in patients with aplastic anemia).

These patients were prepared for transplant with cyclophosphamide 200 mg/kg, and of 110 evaluable patients (those living 6 months or longer posttransplant), 102 were given methotrexate as posttransplant immunosuppression, while 8 were given cyclosporine. When all 110 patients were analyzed together, acute GVHD of moderate to severe intensity was the major determinant for subsequent development of chronic GVHD, generating an estimated relative risk for development for chronic GVHD of 11.65. There were no other significant risk factors for those with prior acute GVHD of moderate or severe intensity. When, however, the analysis was restricted to patients who had either no acute GVHD or only mild acute GVHD, increasing patient age and the addition of buffy coat cell infusions were each significantly associated with the development of chronic GVHD. The effect of patient age was most strikingly seen in 68 patients with no evidence of acute GVHD: while none of 14 children aged 1 to 10 years without prior acute GVHD developed chronic GVHD, 11 of 24 adults did, including 5 of 6 aged 31 years or over.

Factors incorporated in the analysis, but found to show no significant association with the development of chronic GVHD, included the marrow cell dose, relative response in mixed lymphocyte culture, number of preceding erythrocyte and platelet transfusions, ABO group of donor and recipient, transplant year, duration and cause of aplastic anemia, infection status at admission, previous treatment with prednisone, HLA-A and HLA-B antigens of patients (and donors), and, surprisingly, sex match between donor and recipient and donor age.

Similar results were found in a study of 75 allogeneic transplant recipients reported from Stockholm (2). In bivariate analysis, significant factors associated with the development of chronic GVHD in this patient cohort were donor age over 17 years, recipient age over 17 years, preceding grade II-IV (moderate to severe) acute GVHD, the use of donor buffy coat cells, and a preceding cytomegalovirus infection. In multivariate analysis, however, only donor age above 17 years, preceding acute GVHD grade II-IV, and treatment with donor buffy coat cells were independently associated with the development of chronic GVHD. In fact, the number of patients given donor buffy coat in addition to donor marrow cells for severe aplastic anemia was only 5, and of the 4 long-term survivors, all developed chronic GVHD. Among HLA-identical donor recipient pairs (65 of the 75 total patients included in the study), patients with donors over 17 years of age had an actuarial incidence of chronic GVHD of 72% at 400 days posttransplant compared with a 27% incidence in recipients with donors under 17 years of age. Cytomegalovirus (CMV) infection was not a significant risk factor in multivariate analysis.

Factors not significant in this analysis included diagnosis, sex match between donor and recipient, the number of nucleated bone marrow cells infused, previous splenectomy and the type of chemical prophylaxis used to minimize the development of GVHD (methotrexate or cyclosporine).

The two preceding studies included a total of 75 and 24 patients developing chronic GVHD, respectively. A recent analysis from the International Bone Marrow Transplant Registry involved a study population of 2534 patients given HLA-identical sibling marrow transplants for either hematologic malignancy or severe aplastic anemia and reported to the Registry between 1982 and 1987 (3). Incorporated in this population was a cohort of 316 patients who developed chronic GVHD without preceding acute GVHD, i.e., their chronic GVHD was of the de novo onset type. This cohort of patients provided a unique opportunity to examine factors predisposing to the development of chronic GVHD independent of their association (if any) with acute GVHD. While prior acute GVHD was confirmed as being the overwhelming determinant for the development of subsequent chronic GVHD in those with moderate to severe acute GVHD, patient age and factors associated with the donor marrow assumed importance in patients with de novo chronic GVHD. In these patients, age greater than 20 years, donation from an alloimmune female to a male recipient and donation of T-replete (versus T-depleted) marrow were each independently significant in multivariate analysis. When all three of these factors were present, the probability of development of chronic GVHD at 3 years posttransplant was 55% (Table 1). Each of these 3 factors was also operative in patients with prior mild (grade I) acute GVHD, although the presence of all three factors in this patient group increased the probability of developing chronic GVHD to 75%.

In this analysis an alloimmune status of the donor was assumed for people who had received blood transfusions or for women who had had pregnancies prior to marrow harvest. The actuarial probability of developing de novo chronic GVHD at 3 years posttransplant ranged from 18% for 305 male recipients of nonalloimmune male marrow to 43%

Table 1 Risk Factors for the Development of Chronic GVHD

Risk factors	3-year probability of chronic GVHD (%)
None	12
A. Patient age > 20 years	18
B. T-cell-replete graft	20
C. Alloimmune female donor for male recipient	18
A and B	30
A, B, C	58

for 60 male recipients of alloimmune female marrow. The probability in 158 male recipients of nonalloimmune female marrow was 26%. In this cohort of patients without prior acute GVHD, the 3-year actuarial probability of developing chronic GVHD in those with donors less than 20 years of age was 18% compared to 34% in those with donors aged greater than 20 years. Also in this cohort the use of unmanipulated marrow together with posttransplant methotrexate with or without cyclosporine was associated with a 3-year probability of developing chronic GVHD of 29% compared to a probability of 22% in recipients of T-depleted marrow.

For patients who had evidence of prior acute GVHD the probability of developing subsequent chronic GVHD was 50% in those with grade II actue GVHD and 85% in those with grade III-IV acute GVHD (Table 2). In view of the previous suggestions of a correlation between CMV infection and the development of chronic GVHD (2,4), detailed analyses of the possible role of both clinical and subclinical (serologic) CMV infections pre- and posttransplant, as well as of the serological status of the donor, were carried out in this Registry analysis. There was no correlation between the presence of clinical CMV infection posttransplant and the subsequent development of chronic GVHD in the total patient population, either in those who developed no acute GVHD or in those who did develop acute GVHD. If posttransplant subclinical CMV infection was included in the analysis together with the presence of clinical CMV infection, a higher probability of developing chronic GVHD (48%) was found in patients with infection posttransplant com-

Table 2 Possibility of Development of Chronic GVHD According to Grade of Preceding Acute GVHD

Severity of preceding acute GVHD	3-year probability of chronic GVHD (%)
None	25
Mild	50
Moderate	58
Moderate-severe	77
Severe	85

pared those without (40%). However, such an association was no longer found when patients with and without prior acute GVHD were analyzed separately. Posttransplant CMV infection (clinical or subclinical) was highly correlated with the severity of acute GVHD in this study population, and once the latter variable was adjusted for, CMV infection was not associated with an increased risk of developing chronic GVHD. Specifically, CMV infection was not significantly associated with chronic GVHD in multivariate analysis. No effect on the development of chronic GVHD was associated with the CMV serologic status of the donor, nor with the presence of clinical or subclinical CMV infection in the recipient pretransplant.

Other variables not associated with the probability of developing chronic GVHD in this study included patient sex, patient race, the presence of pretransplant infection, use of laminar airflow rooms, the nucleated marrow cell dose, and the drug used to prevent GVHD in patients given T-replete marrow.

In summary, it appears clear that viable donor buffy coat cells increase the incidence of chronic GVHD in patients transplanted for severe aplastic anemia, while in those with hematologic malignancy, the severity of preceding acute GVHD is the overwhelming determinant in those who experience this complication. For those with no prior acute GVHD, increasing patient age and the combination of an alloimmune female donor for a male recipient are important predisposing factors. T-cell depletion of the donor marrow protects against the development of chronic GVHD.

Finally it should be noted that the use of booster marrow infusions for poor graft function has been associated with an almost universal incidence of chronic GVHD (5). In contrast, the risk of chronic GVHD after a second marrow transplant for recurrence of hematologic malignancy has been very similar to the risk after the first transplant (6).

II. RISK FACTORS FOR SURVIVAL

A number of factors have been identified as predisposing to mortality in patients with chronic GVHD (7). These include age greater than 20 years, prior grade II-IV acute GVHD, the progressive onset of chronic GVHD (i.e., acute merging into chronic GVHD), and failure to respond to 9 months of immune suppressive treatment for chronic GVHD. In addition, the presence of thrombocytopenia at the time of diagnosis of chronic GVHD is an indicator of poor prognosis (8). Mortality did not appear related to gender, acute GVHD prophylaxis, or time to start immune suppressive therapy for chronic GVHD.

III. PREVENTION OF CHRONIC GVHD

It is clear from the three studies of factors predisposing to the development of chronic GVHD that the best way to prevent chronic GVHD is to prevent or minimize acute GVHD. This is substantiated in the IBMTR study by the significantly lower incidence of chronic GVHD in recipients of T-cell-depleted grafts compared to those receiving nondepleted transplants. Additional reports to this effect have been recorded (9). Unfortunately, the increased incidence of graft rejection and increased recurrence rate of hematologic malignancy after T-cell-depleted transplantation currently negates any advantage to be gained by decreasing the incidence of acute and chronic GVHD.

Just as there has been no difference in the incidence of acute GVHD in prospective randomized trials comparing methotrexate and cyclosporine as single agents posttransplant, there has been no difference in the incidence of chronic GVHD in these studies

(10,11). However, the combination of methotrexate and cyclosporine appears superior in decreasing the incidence of acute GVHD compared to either cyclosporine alone (12) or methotrexate alone (13). Long-term follow-up reports are awaited to determine if this decrease in acute GVHD is accompanied by a decrease in chronic GVHD.

In the occasional situation in which more than one HLA-identical sibling is available as a marrow donor, male siblings should be chosen in preference to female, and younger males in preference to older males. When the only donor available is an allo-immune female and the recipient is male, strong consideration should be given to the use of a T-cell-depletion protocol, particularly if additional measures to minimize the chance of graft failure (such as the intravenous administration of monoclonal anti-T-cell antibodies or recombinant hemopoietic growth factors to the recipient pretransplant) are used.

Since chronic GVHD often occurs in temporal association with the cessation of pro-phylactic immunosuppressive treatment (such as methotrexate at day 102 posttransplant or prednisone at the end of a 9-month course of treatment for established chronic GVHD), it is likely, though not proven, that slow tapering of prophylactic chemical im-munosuppression will be beneficial compared to a more rapid or abrupt taper.

At the present time experimental procedures to minimize the development of chronic GVHD including the use of cultured thymic fragments (14), partially HLA-matched thymic epithelial cells (14), Thymosin fraction 5 (15), or Thymopentin (16) have not been effective in reducing the incidence of chronic GVHD, improving immuno-logic recovery, or altering long-term survival.

ACKNOWLEDGMENT

Supported in part by a grant from the Government Employees Assistance to Medical Research Fund.

REFERENCES

1. Storb R, Prentice RL, Sullivan KM, Shulman HM, Deeg HJ, Doney KC, Buckner CD, Clift R, Witherspoon R, Appelbaum F, Sanders J, Stewart P, Thomas E: Predictive factors in chronic graft-versus-host disease in patients with aplastic anemia treated by marrow transplantation from HLA-identical siblings. Ann Int Med 1983,98:461–466.
2. Ringden O, Paulin T, Lonnqvist B, Nilsson B: An analysis of factors predisposing to chronic graft-versus-host disease. Exp Hematol 1985;13:1062–1067.
3. Atkinson K, Horowitz M, Gale RP, van Bekkum DW, Gluckman E, Good RA, Jacobsen N, Kolb HJ, Parkman R, Rimm A, Ringden O, Rozman C, Sobicinski KA, Zwaan FE, Bortin MM: Risk factors for chronic graft-versus-host disease after HLA-identical sibling bone marrow transplantation. Manuscript submitted for publication.
4. Lonnqvist B, Ringden O, Wahren B, Gahrton G, Lundgren G: Cytomegalovirus infection associated with and preceding chronic graft-versus-host disease. Transplant Proc 1984;38:465–468.
5. Bolger GB, Sullivan KM, Storb R: Second marrow infusion for poor graft function following allogeneic marrow transplantation. Bone Marrow Transplant 1986;1:21-30.
6. Atkinson K, Biggs JC, Concannon A, Dodds A, Dale B, Norman J: Second mar-row transplants for recurrence of haematological malignancy. Bone Marrow Trans-plant 1986;1:159-166.

7. Sullivan KM, Witherspoon RP, Storb R, Weiden P, Fluornoy N, Dahlberg S, Deeg H, Sanders J, Doney K, Appelbaum F, McGuffin R, MacDonald G, Meyers J, Schubert M, Shulman H, Sale G, Annasetti C, Loughran TP, Strom S, Nims J, Thomas E: Prednisone and azathioprine compared with prednisone and placebo for treatment of chronic graft-versus-host disease: prognostic influence of prolonged thrombocytopenia after allogeneic marrow transplantation. Blood 1988;72:546-554.

8. Sullivan KM, Witherspoon RP, Storb R, Deeg HJ, Dahlberg S, Sanders JE, Appelbaum F, Doney K, Weiden P, Annasetti C, Loughran T, Hill R, Shields A, Shellman H, Nims J, Strom S, Thomas E: Alternating day cyclosporine and prednisone for treatment of high risk chronic graft-versus-host disease. Blood 1988;72:555-561.

9. Franceschini F, Butturini A, Gale RP: Clinical trials of T-cell depletion in bone marrow transplantation, in *Progress in Bone Marrow Transplantation*, edited by Gale RP, Champlin RE. Allan R Liss, New York, 1987; pp. 323-335.

10. Storb R, Deeg HJ, Fisher L, Appelbaum F, Buckner CD, Bensinger W, Clift R, Doney K, Irle C, McGuffin R, Martin P, Sanders J, Schoch G, Singer J, Stewart P, Sullivan K, Witherspoon R, Thomas E: Cyclosporine versus methotrexate for graft-versus-host disease prevention in patients given marrow grafts for leukemia. Long term follow-up of 3 controlled trials. Blood 1988;71:293-298.

11. Atkinson K, Biggs JC, Concannon AJ, Dodds A, Downs K, Ashby M: A prospective randomized trial of cyclosporine versus methotrexate after HLA-identical sibling marrow transplantation for patients with acute leukemia in first remission: analysis 2.5 years after last patient entry. Aust NZ J Med 1988;18:594-599.

12. Storb R, Deeg HJ, Whitehead J, Appelbaum F, Beatty P, Bensinger W, Buckner C, Clift R, Doney K, Farewell V: Marrow transplantation for leukemia. Methotrexate and cyclosporine compared with cyclosporine alone for prophylaxis of acute graft-versus-host disease after marrow transplantation for leukemia. N Engl J Med 1986;314:729-735.

13. Storb R, Deeg HJ, Farewell V, Doney K, Appelbaum F, Beatty P, Buckner R, Clift R, Hansen J, Hill R, Longton G, Lum L, Martin P, McGuffin R, Saunders J, Stewart P, Sullivan K, Witherspoon R, Thomas E: Marrow transplantation for severe aplastic anemia. Methotrexate alone compared to a combination of methotrexate and cyclosporine for prevention of acute graft-versus-host disease. Blood 1986;68:119-125.

14. Atkinson K, Storb R, Ochs HD, Goehle SG, Sullivan K, Witherspoon RP, Lum L, Tsoi M, Sanders K, Parr M, Thomas E: Thymus transplantation after allogeneic bone marrow grafting to prevent chronic graft-versus-host disease in humans. Transplant Proc 1982;33:168-173.

15. Witherspoon RP, Hersman J, Storb R, Ochs H, Goldstein A, McClure J, Weiden P, Thomas E: Thymosin fraction 5 does not accelerate reconstitution of immunologic reactivity after human marrow grafting. Br J Hematol 1983;55:595-608.

16. Witherspoon RP, Navari R, Storb R, Sullivan KM, Doney K, Beatty P, Lum L, Thomas E: Treatment of marrow graft recipients with thymopentin. Bone Marrow Transplant 1987;1:365-371.

35

Early Detection and Monitoring of Chronic Graft-vs.-Host Disease

Thomas P. Loughran, Jr., and Keith M. Sullivan
Fred Hutchinson Cancer Research Center
University of Washington School of Medicine
Seattle, Washington

I. INTRODUCTION

Chronic Graft-vs.-Host Disease (GVHD) is a major late complication of allogeneic marrow transplantation, occurring in 25-45% of patients surviving the transplantation procedure (1,2). Three forms of onset have been identified: (1) progressive chronic GVHD develops as a direct extension of acute GVHD, (2) quiescent chronic GVHD develops after resolution of acute GVHD, and (3) de novo chronic GVHD develops without preceding acute GVHD (3). The de novo form accounts for 20-30% of patients with chronic GVHD (3). The natural history of untreated extensive chronic GVHD is unfavorable, with less than 20% of patients surviving with Karnofsky performance scores ≥70% (2). However, early institution of immunosuppressive therapy has significantly increased disability-free survival (2,4,5). Therefore it is important that the onset of chronic GVHD be recognized early and treatment started before clinical deterioration. This chapter details the approach taken in Seattle for monitoring the onset of chronic GVHD and response to therapy.

II. DAY 100 SCREENING STUDIES. EARLY DIAGNOSIS

The clinical manifestations of chronic GVHD are protean and resemble the features of several autoimmune disorders (3). Organ involvement may include skin, oral mucosa, eyes, liver, esophagus, intestine, and lung (3,6). Before patients leave the transplant center to return to the care of their referring physicians, screening studies for chronic GVHD are performed at day 100 posttransplant (Table 1). Results of these studies are used to diagnose and stage the extent of chronic GVHD. Clinical chronic GVHD is defined as both histologic and clinical evidence of chronic GVHD, and may be either limited or extensive (3). In contrast to patients with untreated clinical extensive chronic

Table 1 Day 100 Screening Studies

Physical examination including skin and oral mucosa
Skin biopsy
Oral biopsy
Bone marrow aspiration
Schirmer's test
Liver function tests:
    alkaline phosphatase
    SGOT
    total bilirubin
Complete blood count with platelet count
Weight of patient

GVHD, patients with limited chronic GVHD have a favorable prognosis without therapy
(3). Subclinical chronic GVHD is defined as histologic evidence of chronic GVHD on both
skin and lip biopsies without symptoms or signs of clinical disease (4).

We completed recently an analysis of the value of these screening tests for predicting the subsequent development of clinically extensive chronic GVHD. One hundred
sixty-nine allogeneic marrow transplant recipients were evaluated prospectively with the
day 100 screening studies. Three groups of patients were defined: Group 1 patients (n =
78) were asymptomatic, had normal physical examinations at the time of screening, and
never developed evidence of chronic GVHD (minimum follow-up 8 years). Group 2 patients (n = 38) had symptoms and signs of chronic GVHD at the time of testing. Group
3 patients (n = 53) had normal physical examinations, similar to Group 1 patients, but
later developed clinical signs of extensive chronic GVHD. Positive screening studies
denoting chronic GVHD were seen not only in Group 2 patients, but also in Group 3
patients.

We studied this predictive value by univariate and multivariate analysis. In a Kaplan-Meier analysis several factors at day 100 posttransplant were significantly associated
with an increased probability of subsequently developing chronic GVHD in patients
who had normal physical examinations at the time of screening: (1) light microscopy
findings of chronic GVHD on skin (p = 0.0001) or oral (p = 0.0110) biopsies; (2) direct
immunofluorescent microscopy (7,8) findings on skin biopsy of abnormal complement
deposition in the dermal basement zone (p = 0.0153), or on oral biopsy of abnormal IgM
deposition in cytoid bodies (p = 0.0456) or decreased numbers of IgA plasma cells in the
immunocompetence area of labial tissue (p = 0.0006); (3) bilirubin values greater than
1.0 mg/dl (p = 0.0004); (4) older mean patient age (p = 0.0011); (5) previous II-IV acute
GVHD (p = 0.005); and (6) previous prednisone therapy after day 50 posttransplant
(p = 0.0014). Patients with normal physical examinations at day 100 posttransplant but
with skin biopsies showing chronic GVHD had an 85% probability of developing chronic
GVHD by 4 years posttransplant (95% confidence intervals, 67-100%). Conversely, the
probability of developing chronic GVHD within this time for patients with normal exam-
intions and negative skin biopsies was 36% (95% confidence intervals, 25-47%).

Earlier studies demonstrated the predictive value of oral biopsies for subsequent
development of chronic GVHD (9,10); however, these studies did not evelute results of
skin biopsies. We wished to determine which of the significant factors from the univari-

ate analysis acted as independent risk factors for developing chronic GVHD. In the first analysis, results of direct immunofluorescent microscopy were excluded, since these studies were performed in less than half of the Group 1 and Group 3 patients. Multivariate analysis showed that independent risk factors included: (1) light microsocopic findings of chronic GVHD on skin biopsy, relative risk 3.23 with 95% confidence intervals of 1.75 to 5.94 (p = 0.0002); and (2) previous history of grade II-IV acute GVHD, relative risk 3.12 with 95% confidence intervals 1.72 to 5.64 (p = 0.0002). The second model analyzed included results of direct immunofluorescent microscopy. Multivariate analysis showed that independent risk factors included: (1) light microscopic findings of chronic GVHD on skin biopsy, relative risk 5.96 with 95% confidence intervals of 1.95 to 18.19 (p = 0.0017); and direct immunofluorescent microscopic findings on oral biopsy of decreased numbers of IgA plasma cells in the immunocompetence area of labial tissue, relative risk 11.53 with 95% confidence intervals of 2.51 to 52.03 (p = 0.0017). A previous history of grade II-IV acute GVHD was not a significant independent risk factor for developing chronic GVHD when results of direct immunofluorescent microscopy were included in the analysis.

It is conceivable that patients identified as having subclinical chronic GVHD by day 100 screening studies might benefit from increasing rather than decreasing immunosuppressive therapy. A randomized trial which demonstrated the effectiveness of immunosuppressive therapy of chronic GVHD included patients who had only subclinical disease (4). Overall there was no benefit in early therapy for this group of patients since >70% of them developed clinical GVHD despite treatment. Moreover, relapse of malignancy was increased significantly in patients in whom chronic GVHD remained subclinical.

Nevertheless, day 100 screening studies remain valuable for patients transplated for malignant and nonmalignant diseases. Patients identified as having subclinical chronic GVHD need close monitoring as immunosuppressive therapy is tapered, so that effective treatment can be instituted early in the evolution of clinical chronic GVHD. Increasing immunosuppressive therapy at day 100 may be beneficial for patients identified as having subclinical chronic GVHD who were transplanted for nonmalignant diseases such as aplastic anemia or Thalassemia major or for patients with malignant diseases with low probability of relapse, such as acute myelogenous leukemia in first remission or chronic myelogenous leukemia in chronic phase. A randomized trial addressing this issue has been instituted in Seattle.

III. MONITORING: 2 MONTHS ON THERAPY

A randomized double-blind clinical trial demonstrated the effectiveness of immunosuppressive treatment of chronic GVHD (4). We were interested in determining whether results of skin biopsy obtained after 2 months of therapy could be correlated with eventual therapeutic response. One hundred twenty-six patients were entered onto the protocol; 81 had skin biopsies obtained at the 2-month interval. Of these 81 patients, 65 were evaluable for response (5 patients were excluded because of relapse, 5 because of nonrelapse death, and 6 because results of skin biopsies were indeterminate). A skin biopsy showing active chronic GVHD pathology was significantly associated with treatment failure after 9 months of therapy (p = 0.027) and also with overall treatment failure (p = 0.008). No association was demonstrated between pathologic skin biopsies and either flare of chronic GVHD or nonrelapse death (Table 2).

Table 2 Correlation of Results of Skin Biopsies Obtained After Two Months of Therapy to Clinical Outcome

	Results of skin biopsy		
Outcome	Normal	Chronic GVHD	Significance
1. Failure after 9 months of therapy	4/40	9/25	$p = 0.027$
2. Overall treatment failure	7/40	13/25	$p = 0.008$
3. Flare of chronic GVHD	10/40	6/25	n.s.
4. Nonrelapse death	8/45	6/29	n.s.

IV. MONITORING: 9 MONTHS ON THERAPY

After 9 months of therapy, patients are reevaluated in Seattle with the studies outlined in Table 1. Results of this evaluation are used to define response to treatment: (1) complete response—clinically inactive disease with both skin and oral biopsies showing no evidence of chronic GVHD pathology; (2) partial response—clinically inactive disease and no new organ involvement but with biopsies showing continued chronic GVHD activity; (3) failure—progressive disease after 2 months of treatment or stable disease with Karnofsky performance scores <50% at 9 months of treatment (4). Patients achieving a complete response have therapy discontinued. If clinical and histologic disease activity returns in these patients (i.e., a flare of chronic GVHD), then therapy is reinstituted for a another 9 months. If chronic GVHD symptoms remain clinically active and disabling after 18 months of therapy, then these patients are also considered as treatment failures. Patients failing to respond to therapy are considered for salvage therapy with immunosuppressive agents such as azathioprine or alternating day prednisone/cyclosporine (5).

V. MONITORING: SPECIAL SITUATIONS

A. Differential Diagnosis of Abnormal Liver Function Tests

Chronic liver disease is seen in approximately 90% of patients with chronic GVHD (3), with liver function tests showing a predominant cholestatic pattern. Other diseases involving the liver and developing after day 100 include chronic viral infections (non-A, non-B hepatitis, cytomegalovirus hepatitis, hepatitis B virus) and cyclosporine drug toxicity (11). In general, liver function tests start to improve within a month of starting immunosuppressive therapy but may remain abnormal for prolonged periods. Increasingly abnormal liver function tests after a month of therapy pose a difficult management problem, i.e., does this situation reflect inadequately treated chronic GVHD or a side effect of treatment (cyclosporine toxicity)? One empiric approach is to stop cyclosporine treatment for a week to see if there is any improvement in liver function tests. Alternatively, a liver biopsy can be performed, looking for specific signs of chronic GVHD such as reduction or absence of small bile ducts (12) or possibly cyclosporine toxicity (13,14) although its morphology remains poorly defined.

B. Detection of Obliterative Bronchiolitis

As long-term survival after marrow transplantation has increased, late complications such as the development of obstructive lung disease have become increasingly apparent (15-18).

Pathologic examination of lung tissue in these patients has shown bronchiolitis obliterans (15,16). Our recent multivariate analysis has shown that obstructive airway disease, as determined by forced expiratory volume at 1 second divided by forced vital capacity, was significantly associated with chronic GVHD (18). Since treatment of severe chronic obstructive lung disease resulting from obliterative bronchiolitis is not effective, early identificaton of such patients using pulmonary function tests may be important. Patients with early obstructive airway disease associated with chronic GVHD may benefit from increased immunosuppressive therapy, as has been shown in solid organ transplantation (19). In addition, prophylaxis with intravenous immunoglobulin may correct qualitative or quantitative deficiencies of serum IgG and IgG subclasses which contribute to the pathogenesis of obliterative bronchiolitis (20,21).

ACKNOWLEDGMENT

This work was supported by PHS grants number CA 18221, CA 18029, CA 09515, CA 15704 from the National Cancer Institute, and HL 36444 from the National Institute of Heart, Lung, and Blood, DHHS. Dr. Loughran is a Special Fellow of the Leukemia Society of America.

REFERENCES

1. Shulman HM, Sullivan KM, Weiden PL, McDonald GB, Striker GE, Sale GE, Hackman R, Tsoi M-S, Storb R, Thomas ED: Chronic graft-versus-host syndrome in man: A long-term clinicopathological study of 20 Seattle patients. Am J Med 1980;69:204-217.

2. Sullivan KM, Shulman HM, Storb R, Weiden PL, Witherspoon RP, McDonald GB, Schubert MM, Atkinson K, Thomas ED: Chronic graft-versus-host disease in 52 patients: Adverse natural course and successful treatment with combination immunosuppression. Blood 1981;57:267-276.

3. Sullivan KM: Acute and chronic graft-versus-host disease in man. Int J Cell Cloning 1986,4(Suppl 1):42-93.

4. Sullivan KM, Witherspoon RP, Storb R, Weiden P, Flournoy N, Dahlberg S, Deeg HJ, Sanders JE, Doney KC, Appelbaum FR, McGuffin R, McDonald GB, Meyers J, Schubert MM, Gauvreau J, Shulman HM, Sale GE, Anasetti C, Loughran TP, Strom S, Nims J, Thomas ED: Prednisone and azathioprine compared to prednisone and placebo for treatment of chronic graft-versus-host disease: Prognostic influence of prolonged thrombocytopenia after allogeneic marrow transplantation. Blood 1988; 72:546-554.

5. Sullivan KM, Witherspoon RP, Storb R, Deeg HJ, Dahlberg S, Sanders JE, Appelbaum FR, Doney KC, Weiden P, Anasetti C, Loughran TP, Hill R, Shields A, Yee G, Shulman H, Nims J, Strom S, Thomas ED: Alternating-day cyclosporine and prednisone for treatment of high-risk chronic graft-versus-host disease. Blood 1988;72: 555-561.

6. Schubert MM, Sullivan KM, Morton TH, Izutsu KT, Peterson DE, Flournoy N, Truelove EL, Sale GE, Buckner CD, Storb R, Thomas ED: Oral manifestations of chronic graft-host disease. Arch Intern Med 1984;144:1591-1595.

7. Saurat JH, Bonnetblanc JM, Gluckman E, Didierjean L, Bussel A, Puissant A: Skin antibodies in bone mrarrow transplanted patients. Clin Exp Dermatol 1976;1: 377-384.

8. Tsoi M-S, Storb R, Jones E, Weiden PL, Shulman H, Witherspoon R, Atkinson K, Thomas ED: Deposition of IgM and complement at the dermo-epidermal junction

in acute and chronic cutaneous graft-vs-host disease in man. J Immunol 1978;120: 1485-1492.

9. Sale GE, Shulman HM, Schubert MM, Sullivan KM, Kopecky KJ, Hackman RC, Morton TH, Storb R, Thomas ED: Oral and ophthalmic pathology of graft versus host disease in man: Predictive value of the lip biopsy. Hum Pathol 1981;12:1022-1030.

10. Janin-Mercier A, Devergie A, Arrago JP, Brocheriou C, Lemarchand-Venencie F, Rain JD, Gluckman E: Systemic evaluation of Sjögren-like syndrome after bone marrow transplantation in man. Transplantation 1987;43:677-679.

11. McDonald GB, Shulman HM, Sullivan KM, Spencer GD: Intestinal and hepatic complications of human bone marrow transplantation. Gastroenterology 1986;90:460-477, 770-784.

12. McDonald GB, Shulman HM, Wolford JL, Spencer GD: Liver disease after human marrow transplantation. Semin Liver Dis 1987;7:210-220.

13. Powles RL, Clink H, Sloane J, Barrett AJ, Kay HEM, McElwain TJ: Cyclosporin A for the treatment of graft-versus-host disease in man. Lancet 1978;ii:1327-1331.

14. Atkinson K, Biggs J, Dodds A Concannon A: Cyclosporine-associated hepatoxicity after allogeneic marrow transplantation in man. Differentiation from other causes of posttransplant liver disease. Transplant Proc 1983;15:2761-2767.

15. Ralph DD, Springmeyer SC, Sullivan KM, Hackman RC, Storb R, Thomas ED: Rapidly progressive air-flow obstruction in marrow transplant recipients: Possible association between obliterative bronchiolitis and chronic graft-versus-host disease. Am Rev Respir Dis 1984;129:641-644.

16. Kurzrock R, Zander A, Kanojia M, Vellekoop L, Spitzer G, Jagannath S, Schell S, Peters L, Dicke K: Obstructive lung disease after allogeneic bone marrow transplantation. Transplantation 1984;37:156-160.

17. Chan CK, Hyland RH, Hutcheon MA, Minden MD, Alexander MA, Kossakowski AE, Urbanski SJ, Fyles GM, Fraser IM, Curtis JE, Messner HA. Small-airways disease in recipients of allogeneic bone marrow transplants: An analysis of 11 cases and a review of the literature. Medicine 1987;66:327-340.

18. Clark JG, Schwartz DA, Flournoy N, Sullivan KM, Crawford SW, Thomas ED: Risk factors in airflow obstruction in recipients of bone marrow transplants. Ann Intern Med 1987;107:648-656.

19. Glanville AR, Baldwin JC, Burke CM, Theodore J, Robin ED: Obliterative bronchiolitis after heart-lung transplantation: Apparent arrest by augmented immunosuppression. Ann Intern Med 1987;107:300-304.

20. Sullivan KM. Immunoglobulin therapy in bone marrow transplantation. Am J Med 1987;83:34-45.

21. Holland HM, Wingard JR, Beschorner WE, Saral R, Santos GW. Bronchiolitis obliterans in bone marrow transplantation and its relationship to chronic graft-v-host disease and low serum IgG. Blood 1988;72:621-627.

36

Effects of Acute and Chronic Graft-vs.-Host Disease on Immune Recovery After Bone Marrow Transplantation

Lawrence G. Lum*
Medical College of Wisconsin
Milwaukee, Wisconsin

I. INTRODUCTION

Although bone marrow transplantation (BMT) is an accepted form of therapy for a number of malignant and nonmalignant disorders (1-4), the overall success of BMT is limited by graft failure, recurrent disease, nonmarrow organ toxicity, infections during the immunodeficiency following BMT, Graft-vs.-Host Disease (GVHD), and its related complications. Death due to infections caused by bacteria, viruses, fungi, and opportunistic organisms is one major reason for failure of BMT (5-10). Factors that impair the establishment of a competent immune system increase the probability of dying from an infectious complication. The misdirected reactions seen in acute and chronic GVHD are immunologically crippling. Together, the preparative chemoradiotherapy, the GVHD prophylaxis, GVHD itself and agents used to treat GVHD increase the susceptibility of recipients to infections and prolong the immunodeficiency seen after BMT. This chapter discusses how acute and chronic GVHD affect the kinetics of immune reconstitution after BMT. The effects of acute and chronic GVHD on cellular and humoral immune recovery in BMT recipients will be compared or contrasted with recipients who were not affected by GVHD.

II. GENERAL CONSIDERATIONS

A. The Effect of Time on Immune Reconstitution

The most important element in the development of donor-derived immunity is time after marrow grafting (11-17). Time is needed for stem cells to develop and repopulate the lymphopoietic and hematopoietic systems. However, a number of variables disrupt

---

* *Present affiliation*: Wayne State University, Detroit, Michigan

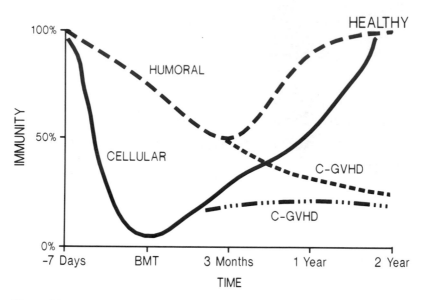

Figure 1 The kinetics of cellular and humoral immune reconstitution are shown for those who become long-term healthy marrow graft recipients and those who develop chronic GVHD (c-GVHD).

the orderly recapitulation of immune ontogeny. Regardless of the type of graft (autologous, syngeneic, or matched allogeneic), most recipients have a profound immunodeficiency during the first 3-6 months after BMT. Immune functions tend to recover sooner in autologous and syngeneic recipients than in allogeneic recipients (18-19). Generally speaking, underlying disease, conditioning regimen, prophylaxis and treatment of acute GVHD with immunosuppressive agents do not have major effects on immune reconstitution (20). Immune reconstitution is complete by 2 years postgrafting in most healthy recipients, whereas it is delayed in those with chronic GVHD. Figure 1 depicts the overall kinetics of immune reconstitution for humoral and cellular immunity for recipients with and without chronic GVHD.

Many studies have shown the presence of cytotoxic cells by phenotyping and functional assays early after BMT (21-27). First to appear after BMT are cytotoxic systems involving cells that exhibit natural killer (NK) activity, mitogen-induced cellular cytotoxicity, and antibody (Ab)-dependent cellular cytotoxicity. The immune state in the first 1 to 2 months postgrafting is analogous to primitive invertebrate immune systems wherein cytotoxicity is exhibited by mononuclear cells. Early cytotoxic and phagocytic functions mediated by granulocytes and monocytes are vital for survival. Transplant recipients are susceptible to overwhelming bacterial and fungal infections until granulocyte counts rise to approximately 500 cells/mm³ in spite of the liberal use of antimicrobial or antifungal agents. Recipients who fail to engraft or lose their grafts are likely to die of sepsis during prolonged periods of granulocytopenia.

The absolute numbers of T and B cells are normal around 3-4 months after BMT in most recipients who received HLA-identical related transplants (15-16,27-34). Suppressor activity is the predominant T-cell function seen in the first 3-6 months postgrafting regardless of the type of graft, the presence or absence of acute GVHD, the type of posttransplant immunosuppression, marrow manipulations, T-cell depletion, or preparative regimen. These findings are consistent with the high proportions of CD8$^+$ cells found early after grafting. One teleological explanation may be that the new immune system is attempting to develop tolerance. Increased suppressor activity mediated by the T cells of transplant recipients may be analogous to those in newborns.

B cells from the recipients fail to respond to neoantigens and cannot be activated to proliferate or differentiate into immunoglobulin (Ig)-secreting cells (35-44). On the other hand, preexisting donor immunity to recall antigens (Ags) can be transferred from donors to recipients and detected in the first several months after BMT (45-51). Mature T-cell functions such as helper activity (e.g., the secretion of lymphokines) for Ab synthesis do not develop until a year or more after BMT.

B. The Role of the Thymus

The role of thymic epithelium in the education of donor-derived T cells after BMT remains elusive. The higher incidence of chronic GVHD in older recipients suggest that the thymic microenvironment may be needed in educating T cells. In addition to recipient age, the preparative chemoradiotherapy may impair the ability of the thymus to function. A number of studies have tried to correct this problem by providing transplanted thymic epithelium, thymosin fraction V, pentapeptide thymopoietin, or varicella-zoster specific transfer factor to recipients, but they have not been successful in accelerating immune reconstitution or preventing GVHD (52-55).

C. Residual Host Immunity

Graft rejection in patients transplanted for aplastic anemia or patients who received T-cell-depleted bone marrows provide evidence for "host resistance." Host immunity persists in aplastic anemia patients since their conditioning regimens are less immunosuppressive than those transplanted for hematologic malignancies who receive additional immunosuppression in the form of radiotherapy. For example, aplastic anemia patients exposed to alloantigens due to transfusions prior to transplant have an increased rate of graft rejection. The immunobiology involved is exemplified by the fact that the rate of graft rejection in untransfused aplastic anemia patients is much lower than in their transfused counterparts (56-57).

Graft rejection in recipients who receive T-cell-depleted marrow shows that T-cell depletion can be problematic. Although vigorous depletion of T cells has decreased the incidence of acute GVHD, it has also increased the incidence of graft failure and recurrent leukemia (58-61). Graft failure may be due to radioresistant host cells that interfere with engraftment, proliferation, and differentiation of donor stem cells. The clinical results in recipients of T-cell-depleted marrow grafts show that T cells are needed to overcome resistance and to sustain engraftment. The reasons for sustained engraftment in recipients of T-cell-depleted marrow grafts in some institutions may be the result of increased pre- or posttransplant immunosuppression, high marrow cell dose, and higher numbers of T cells remaining in the marrow inoculum after T-cell depletion of the marrow inoculum (62). Residual radioresistant elements of host immunity may provide a protective role during the first several months postgrafting. Persistent host Abs to recall Ags may be transiently protective against childhood diseases. On the other hand, persistent host Abs to recall Ags may cause clinical problems such as hemolysis due to ABO blood group differences between the donor and recipient (17). When there are no differences between host and donor Ig spectrotypes or allotypes (51,63), the disappearance of host Abs and the emergence of donor Abs is difficult to evaluate.

D. Local Immunity

Along with the skin, the linings of the intestinal, respiratory, and urinary tracts provide important barriers that prevent the entry of pathogens. The preparative regimens damage each of these barriers. Not only is the integrity of the barriers altered, but resident lymphocytes are destroyed by the preparative regimens. The type of infections that occur during the first 3 months reflect impaired mucosal immunity and impaired secretion of fluids containing IgA, which may help protect against viral and bacterial infections. If impaired mucosal immunity is combined with impaired systemic immunity (11-14,16), the reason for the high incidence of life-threatening infections during the first few months after BMT is evident.

The skin and gut may be further damaged by infiltration with inflammatory cells that cause necrosis and denudation of these tissues during the process of acute GVHD. Seeding of the systemic circulation with pathogens from the gastrointestinal, respiratory, and urinary tracts accounts for most septic episodes. Until the skin and the mucosal linings are normal, the susceptibility to overwhelming sepsis is very high despite the use of prophylactic antibiotics, antiviral agents, laminar airflow rooms, and intravenous gammaglobulin.

Lip biopsies from recipients with chronic GVHD show histologic evidence of sialadenitis, stomatitis, or both with sialodochitis (64). Histologic involvement of the salivary glands in recipients with chronic GVHD is associated with low IgA levels, low salivary flow rates, and increased concentrations of sodium, albumin, and IgG (64).

E. The Role of Phagocytes

Marrow transplant recipients have no immunologic defense until their neutrophils begin to appear between 15 to 45 days postgrafting (65-67). Chemotaxis of neutrophils is impaired during the first 4 months after BMT (65). Chemotactic responses of neutrophils of recipients with severe acute GVHD, chronic GVHD, or infections were lower than those seen in the neutrophils of healthy recipients (65). Iodination capacity (the ability of neutrophils to phagocytose and activate oxygen dependent mechanisms of intracellular killing) was not different from controls during the early period (65). Obviously, without neutrophils, bacteria and fungal infections are life-threatening.

Monocytes of donor-origin can be found in peripheral blood as early as 41 days after BMT (68). Tissue fixed macrophages of donor-origin in the lung and liver can be detected by 80 days after BMT (69-70). Alveolar lavage macrophages had abnormal chemotaxis, phagocytosis, and cytotoxicity early postgrafting (71). Accessory functions such as IL-1 production (72), presentation of Ag (*Escherichia coli*) in proliferation assays (68), or supporting pokeweed mitogen (PWM) stimulated T-cell-dependent Ig production recover early after BMT (73). A few recipients with chronic GVHD had monocytes that suppressed Ig synthesis by normal T and B cells (73).

F. Cytotoxic Lymphocytes

Impaired NK activity or T-cell-mediated cytotoxicity directed at viruses may explain why roughly half of the recipients develop infections with the herpes group of viruses (6-8). Cytomegalovirus (CMV) infections account for 60% of the interstitial pneumonias that occur in the first 2 to 4 months postgrafting (8). Prophylaxis against CMV infections using i.v. gammaglobulin, CMV-immune globulin, acyclovir, and combinations thereof have met with limited success (74-80). Recently, a study showed that prophylactic acyclovir could significantly reduce infections with CMV (77). If used early after diagnosis, 9-(1,3-dihihydroxy-2-propoxymethyl) guanine (DHPG) for the treatment of documented systemic CMV infections has been reported to be useful (81-83). The long-term use of DHPG, however, is problematic due to its marrow suppressive activity.

NK activity against K562 or Chang cell targets, Ab-dependent cellular cytotoxicity, and mitogen-induced cellular cytotoxicity become normal in most recipients in the first 2 months after BMT (21-24,26). Many studies show increased absolute numbers of NK cell phenotypes (25-27,33,84-85). About 80% of the recipients have lymphocytes with normal cytotoxic functions by a year after BMT (21,23,26).

Development of Epstein-Barr virus (EBV)-induced lymphomas in recipients of T-cell-depleted grafts is likely due to impaired antiviral T-cell-mediated immunity (86-88). One group showed that the lack of HLA-restricted CMV-specific cytotoxic T-lymphocyte responses and NK-cell responses to CMV correlated with the development of fatal CMV infections (22).

III. ACUTE GVHD

A. The Clinical Problem of Acute GVHD

Misdirected alloreactive cytotoxic T cells or NK cells may be responsible for the development of acute GVHD when the transplanted immune system does not recognize host tissues as self, T lymphocytes attack the "foreign" antigens on recipient (host) tissues resulting in the graft-vs.-host reaction. This immunologic reaction may be due to non-HLA-antigenic differences between the donor and recipient or improper T-cell thymic education (89-94). Unfortunately, GVHD is a major clinical problem that limits the success of BMT due to the high mortality rate associated with it or its complications. About 50% of HLA-identical recipients who receive T-cell-containing grafts develop acute GVHD (3,4,89,90). Ten to 15% of all recipients die of acute GVHD or its related complications. Figure 2 depicts the multiple factors that play a role in determining successful short-term outcome in marrow graft recipients.

Acute GVHD can involve the skin, liver, and gut. Skin involvement can range from a mild erythrematous rash to blistering and bullae formation involving the full thickness of the skin. The histologic changes involve necrolysis leading to separation of the dermal-epidermal junction associated with infiltration of lymphocytes and the development of eosinophilic bodies (89-96). Impairment of liver functions can vary from mild elevations of bilirubin to markedly elevated levels of bilirubin, lactic dehydrogenase (LDH), alkaline phosphatase, and serum glutamic oxaloacetic transaminase (SGOT). Problems in the gastrointestinal tract include mild to severe nausea, vomiting, and diarrhea. Life-threatening diarrhea and gastrointestinal hemorrhage is seen in severe GVHD. Elevated levels of IgE have been reported to correlate with the presence of acute GVHD (97-99). However, prospective studies by others and ourselves did not reveal any direct correlations between the IgE levels and acute GVHD (100 and Henderson, unpublished). The role of IgE in the pathogenesis of acute GVHD remains controversial.

Some studies suggest that enterobacteria in the gut may augment the development of acute GVHD (101). It was postulated that enterobacteria share antigenic determinants with host epithelium and act as immune adjuvants to induce immune reactions directed at the gastrointestinal tract. Clinical observations support this hypothesis. First, recipients who have acute GVHD have more infections than those without acute GVHD (4,102). Second, recipients transplanted for aplastic anemia who were kept in laminar

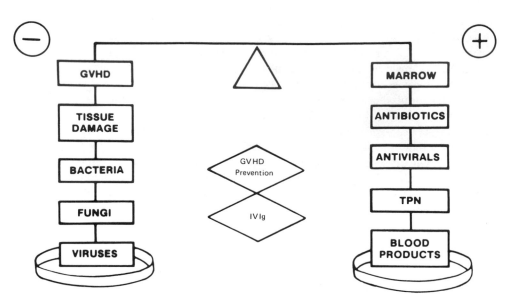

Figure 2 The balance between factors that could produce a negative outcome and factors that help produce a positive result in human bone marrow transplantation is critical for the first 2 to 3 months after BMT. Placed under the fulcrum are factors such as intravenous gammaglobulin (IVIg) and postgrafting immunosuppression (GVHD prevention) that could be beneficial or detrimental.

airflow rooms had less infections. Finally, the recipients had delayed onset of their acute GVHD (102).

B. Laboratory Findings in Acute GVHD

One study showed an association between decreased NK activity and severe viral infections; there was a correlation between high NK activity and the incidence of acute GVHD (23). The appearance of NK activity in the first months after BMT has been associated with acute GVHD (23). However, the conclusions of these studies are controversial. Some studies show no correlations between cytotoxic activity and the clinical findings of GVHD, infections, or recurrent leukemia (21). Studies are needed to determine if recipients of T-cell-depleted grafts are different from recipients who received T-cell-containing grafts in their recovery of cytotoxic cell functions. Explanations for the varied findings in cytotoxic assays include heterogeneous cytotoxic populations, differences in the recipients, differences in assay techniques, and the type of postgrafting immunosuppression.

Most healthy recipients have normal cell mediated lympholysis (CML) assays whereas those with acute or chronic GVHD have impaired CML assays (103). The defective lymphocyte responses in the CML assay may be due to reduced or absent IL-2 production by lymphocytes from recipients with chronic GVHD (103-104). The addition of exogenous IL-2 to cultures during the sensitization phase of the CML assays reconstituted cytotoxic activity in lymphocytes from recipients with chronic GVHD (103).

A series of studies suggest that T cells or Abs play a role in the graft-vs.-host reaction directed at host tissues bearing non-HLA Ags (92,93,105-110). Multiple attempts have been made to identify the cells or Abs that mediate acute GVHD. One study showed that T-cell clones isolated from skin biopsies from marrow recipients with acute GVHD could proliferate in response to host lymphocytes but were not cytotoxic to host lymphocytes (92). Others could not show that donor-derived lymphocytes would proliferate in response to cryopreserved host lymphocytes (105). Phenotyping and functional studies using skin biopsy-derived lymphocytes show heterogeneity in both the phenotypes and functions of the infiltrating cells (109). One promising approach is the development of predictive tests for acute GVHD (92,93,106-108,110). By culturing presensitized donor lymphocytes with recipient skin and evaluating the histologic changes seen after culture, it may be possible to use the findings to reliably predict acute GVHD before donor selection (93). Such a test will not only help select prospective donors but may also help customize the type of postgrafting immunosuppression.

IV. THE EFFECTS OF MANIPULATIONS TO PREVENT GVHD

The prevention or treatment of acute GVHD with immunosuppressive agents increases the susceptibility to infections by further suppressing the immune system. Methotrexate, cyclophosphamide, cyclosporin A (Cyclosporine), corticosteroids, anti-T-cell Abs, antithymocyte globulin, counterflow centrifugal elutriation, T-cell depletion, or combinations of the above have been used to prevent and treat GVHD (58-60,111-120). In a prospective trial, cyclosporine was superior to long-term methotrexate prophylaxis in regards to time to engraftment, amount of mucositis, platelet transfusion support, and length of hospital stay (20). However, there were no differences in immune recovery as measured by in vitro immune function tests (20). The combination of cyclosporine and short-term methotrexate (given 1, 3, 6, and 11 days postgrafting) was superior to cyclosporine alone in preventing acute GVHD and in improving survival (113). Figure 3 shows how T-cell depletion with or without additional postgrafting immunosuppression can lead to impaired immune reconstitution.

Although T-cell depletion of the marrow inoculum prevents acute GVHD in mice, adapting T-cell depletion of the marrow to man has been less than straightforward. Methods to remove T cells include treatment with antithymocyte globulin, anti-T cell monoclonal antibodies (MAb) and complement-mediated lysis, sheep erythrocyte rosetting, lectin agglutinin sedimentation, counterflow centrifugal elutriation, immunobeads linked with anti-T-cell MAbs, or magnetic beads linked to anti-T-cell MAb. Most reports show reductions in the overall incidence and severity of acute GVHD, but they also show an increase in the incidence of graft rejection, late graft loss, leukemic relapse, and secondary malignancies (58-61,86-88,119,121). On the other hand, some groups show reductions in acute GVHD associated with persistent engraftment (62,115,117). After counterflow centrifugal elutriation to deplete T cells from the marrow, one group showed sustained engraftment after adding 1×10^6 T cells/kg body weight of the recipient to the marrow inoculum (62). The general consensus is that vigorous T-cell depletion removes not only the T cells that mediate GVHD, but also T cells that may facilitate engraftment and mediate the graft-vs.-leukemia effect (122,123).

T cells or their precursors in the bone marrow inoculum may play a vital role in immune reconstitution. Based on the hypothesis that a T-cell subset mediates acute GVHD, several investigators depleted CD8[+] cells (Class I reactive) from the marrow graft

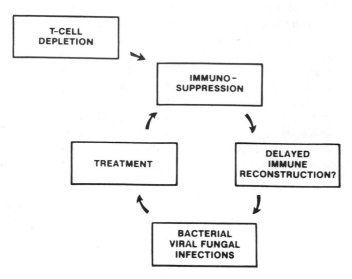

Figure 3 T-cell depletion to prevent GVHD may result in a cycle of immune suppression, the potential of delayed immune reconstitution, increased susceptibility to infections, and the use of antiviral or other agents that may lead to suppression of marrow function.

to prevent acute GVHD (124,125). Early results suggest that CD8$^+$ depletion may reduce the incidence and severity of acute GVHD; however, longer follow-up intervals are needed to assess the overall success of such manipulations. One study suggests that the incidence of fungal infections may be a greater problem after T-cell depletion (126), but the long-term effects of T-cell depletion on incidence of life-threatening infections and immune reconstitution remains to be determined.

V. THE EFFECTS OF ACUTE GVHD ON EARLY LYMPHOCYTE FUNCTIONS

A. Cellular Immunology

In recipients who received T-cell-containing grafts, T and B cells repopulate the marrow and the peripheral blood within the first 3 months after BMT. Absolute numbers and proportions of CD2$^+$ and CD3$^+$ cells are normal or near normal 3 to 4 months after BMT. The absolute number and proportions of the helper/inducer phenotype (CD4$^+$) in most BMT recipients is lower than normal and the absolute number and proportions of the suppressor/cytotoxic (CD8$^+$) cells is higher than normal resulting in low (<1.0) CD4/CD8 ratios (15, 26-35, 127-132). Studies on recipients who received T-cell-depleted marrow grafts show delayed recovery of functional T-cell precursor frequencies in the first 4 months after BMT (133). Preliminary results at the Medical College of Wisconsin (MCW) in T-cell-depleted grafts show the absolute numbers and proportions of CD2$^+$, CD3$^+$ and CD4$^+$ cells in the peripheral blood to be persistently low in the first year after BMT (Lum, unpublished observation).

Recipients of T-cell-containing grafts had inverted CD4/CD8 ratios regardless of the type of graft, age, infections, or presence or absence of acute GVHD. One early study using the TH2$^+$ subset specific antisera showed that patients with acute GVHD lacked TH2$^+$ cells and some recipients with chronic GVHD had TH2$^+$, Ia$^+$ T cells suggesting in vivo activation of T cells (134). Small numbers of immature T cells or thymocytes as defined by OKT10 have been found up to 12 months after BMT (29,30,129). Dual labeling studies in one investigation showed that CD8$^+$, CD11$^+$ (Leu 15) cells were increased in 11 of 12 short-term recipients and 6 of 11 recipients with chronic GVHD (131). Decreased CD4/CD8 ratios have been associated with viral infections, but remain an area of controversy between several groups (28-30,33). Some groups found a correlation between acute GVHD and low CD4/CD8 (31,32); however, other investigations show that most short-term autologous marrow graft recipients also have low CD4/CD8 ratios (135,136). Most investigators agree that recipients who develop chronic GVHD have persistently low CD4/CD8 ratios (15,30,35).

The expression of IL-2 receptors or DR antigens on peripheral blood T cells up to 3 months postgrafting is thought to be related to activation with alloantigens. The expression of IL-2 receptors defined by anti-CD25 (anti-Tac) MAb remains controversial (137,138). One report showed that >25% of the cells in peripheral blood expressed IL-2 receptors in recipients undergoing graft rejection or acute GVHD (139). In contrast, another group did not find CD25$^+$ cells postgrafting (30). Five of 12 short-term recipients of T-cell-containing grafts with and without acute GVHD expressed IL-2 receptors ranging from 1 to 12% (Lum, unpublished observation). The presence of OKT10 markers, DR antigens, IL-2 receptors, and inverted CD4/CD8 ratios may simply reflect early stages in T-cell ontogeny.

The upregulation of IL-2 receptors in BMT recipients may reflect in vivo activation of T cells that may precede GVHD or graft rejection. In an attempt to address this question, we measured free IL-2 receptors (in collaboration with Dr. David Nelson, Metabolism Branch, NCI) in serum samples from recipients who received T-cell-containing or T-cell-depleted grafts. Although some recipients had elevated circulating IL-2 receptor levels, there were no correlations between serum IL-2 receptor levels and the presence of acute GVHD or graft rejection. High circulating levels of IL-2 receptors may be a result of shedding of IL-2 receptors by proliferating myeloid cells.

Delayed type hypersensitivity as measured by skin tests to recall Ags is impaired during the first 3 months after BMT (140). Lymphocyte proliferative responses to alloantigens and mitogens are low but present during the first 3 to 6 months after BMT, and Ag-specific proliferative responses are impaired in recipients who received T-cell-containing grafts during the early period (11-14,16). During the early period, recipients cannot be sensitized to dinitrochlorobenzene (140). Studies on lymphocytes from recipients who received T-cell-depleted grafts showed impaired responses to mitogens, alloantigens, and specific Ag during the first 6 months or more after BMT (Lum, unpublished observations). These results may be due to T-cell depletion or the administration of immunosuppressive or marrow suppressive drugs or both. Impaired proliferative responses by T cells are consistent with the decreased numbers of T cells quantitated by limiting dilution assays that assess the frequency of proliferating T lymphocytes in the marrow inoculum (122,133,141).

In an attempt to determine whether posttransplant deficits in T-cell function documented by limiting dilution methods in allogeneic BMT recipients depend upon the genetic disparity at minor histocompatibility loci, Drs. R. Miller (Boston University) and H. Kaizer (Rush-Presbyterian-St. Lukes) are comparing responder frequencies in allorecipients to responses in recipients who were autografted with cryopreserved marrow. The early results suggest that autotransplant recipients show deficits at least as severe as those seen in allorecipients (Miller, personal communication).

A number of assay systems have been used to assess T-cell function in the regulation of polyclonal or specific Ab synthesis in short-term recipients of T-cell-containing marrow grafts after PWM, Protein A from *Staphylococcus aureus*, or EBV stimulation (36-39,142,143). After PWM stimulation, T cells from most short-term recipients could not provide helper activity to normal B cells and exhibited excess suppressor activity (36-39,131). Purified CD4$^+$ cells from these recipients failed to provide helper activity and their CD8$^+$ cells did not consistently exhibit suppressor activity in the PWM system (39).

Preliminary studies at MCW show that three-quarters of the short-term recipients who received T-cell-depleted marrow grafts had T cells that failed to help B cells produce Ig and exhibited excess suppressor activity in the presence of normal T and B cells. Our results suggest that T-cell depletion may retard T-cell maturation for functions such as the production of growth factors. One study showed that large granular lymphocytes from recipients of T-cell-depleted grafts spontaneously secreted IL-2, interferon gamma, and B-cell differentiation factor in the first 4-6 weeks after BMT (144).

On the other hand, the lack of suppressor/cytotoxic T cells responsible for regulating EBV driven clones may give rise to lymphomas in those who received T-cell-depleted marrow grafts (87,88). Studies using the EBV-driven Ig synthesis model system showed that T cells from recipients of T-cell-containing bone marrow did not suppress normal B cells while donor T cells normally suppress B-cell proliferation and differentiation (40). This lack of T-cell-mediated "immune surveillance" in the EBV system may be exacerbated in those who received T-cell-depleted grafts.

B. Humoral Immunity

Serum IgG and IgM levels return to normal or near normal levels in the first 4 months after BMT. Levels of IgA, on the other hand, take years to recover in recipients of HLA-identical T-cell-containing grafts (11-14,16). Recently, a study in autologous marrow graft recipients showed that IgM, IgG, and IgA levels recovered faster in recipients prepared using intensive thio-TEPA chemotherapy than in recipients prepared with cyclophosphamide and total body irradiation (145). The reason for elevated levels of IgE seen in some recipients remains controversial. One study suggests that elevated IgE levels are a part of the process of immune recovery and were associated but not directly correlated with acute GVHD (100). The effects of T-cell depletion, marrow-purging procedures, or mismatching at the MHC on recovery of IgG, IgM, and IgA levels are not known. Evaluation of this issue is confounded by the administration of CMV hyperimmune globulin or intravenous gamma globulin by many groups for CMV-infection prophylaxis during the first 3 months after BMT (74-78,145). Preliminary results from a recent prospective study suggests that the use of intravenous gamma globulin may actually decrease the incidence of acute GVHD (146). Total hemolytic complement, the third component of complement, and the fourth component of complement are normal by 3 months after BMT (16,19). The functions of the complement components and their interactions with other elements of the immune system are intact.

For years, many investigators thought there was no transfer of donor-derived immunity to recipients. Studies by us and others show that specific Ab titers can be detected in short-term marrow graft recipients with or without immunizing the donor or recipient pretransplant in the first 2 to 3 months after BMT.

Ab titers to tetanus toxoid (TT), diphtheria toxoid (DT), and measles virus (MV) were in the normal range in the first 100 days postgrafting in majority of recipients who received HLA-identical grafts (45,49). None of the recipients in the study group were boosted with recall Ags or received supplemental intravenous gammaglobulin. Two hundred and twenty-one of 235 short-term recipients had anti-TT titers; 176 of 232 (76%) had anti-DT titers; and 7 of 8 had anti-MV titers (45,49). Most of the Abs to recall Ags during the first 100 days postgrafting are likely produced by donor-derived B cells. A major component of the B-cell response may be from memory B cells that are activated by allogeneic effects, expand, and differentiate into plasma cells. Ag-specific help may not be required for these B cells to produce specific Ab. Other sources of Ab include passive Ab acquired via the transfusion of blood products and persistent host Abs. The contribution by persistent host Abs to titers 4 months after marrow grafting is essentially zero. The probability of finding host type isohemagglutinins in ABO-incompatible recipients is less than 20% 80 days after BMT and is essentially zero 120 days after BMT (17). On the other hand, Ig allotypes of donor origin can be documented as early as 113 days postgrafting (147). Since Ig allotypes of donor origin need to accumulate before they can be detected, synthesis of donor allotypes by B cells likely begins in the first 60 days postgrafting.

Ab responses to primary and secondary immunizations with neoantigens such as keyhole-limpet hemocyanin (KLH), pneumococcal polysaccharide Ags, and bacteriophage $\emptyset$X174 in allogeneic and syngeneic recipients is low or absent in the first 6 months postgrafting (16-17). Generally, recipients in the first 6 months to a year postgrafting are unresponsive to immunizations with neoantigens.

One group of studies shows that there is short-term transfer of Ag-specific immunity when the marrow donor is boosted prior to transplantation (46,51,63). One early study used specific anti-KLH and anti-yellow fever virus titers to confirm lymphoid engraftment in an identical twin recipient by immunizing the twin donor with KLH and yellow fever virus before BMT (148). Recently studies have used Ab spectrotyping to detect differences in isoelectric focusing patterns between donors and recipients to TT or DT to demonstrate the switch from the synthesis of host Abs to donor Abs (46,51,63). Both groups boosted the donors and recipients before transplant and the recipient after transplant with Ag to detect the specific Ab synthesis of donor origin.

Phenotyping data on the peripheral blood from recipients of T-cell-containing marrow grafts during the first 2-3 months after BMT show normal proportions and absolute numbers of B cells as determined by polyvalent antisera directed at surface Igs (13-14, 16). The expression of CD5$^+$ on human B cells in the first 30 days postgrafting suggests that B cells in early stages of maturation may circulate in BMT recipients (149).

Surface IgG, IgM, IgA, and IgD staining of B cells from marrow recipients who received T-cell-containing grafts showed that certain recipients did not have sIgG- or sIgA-bearing B cells (150). Others have shown that B cells from BMT recipients had higher numbers of primitive-IgM determinants per B cell than normal B cells (151). Recently, one study showed a dissociation between B-cell phenotypes and functions (152). Recipients who received T-cell-depleted grafts at Medical College of Wisconsin show increased proportions of sIgM- and sIgD-bearing B cells. Together, these data strongly suggest that B-cell development may be arrested at early maturational stages.

The phenotyping evidence for maturational arrest is supported by data from assays of B-cell function. In the early period, B cells from recipients fail to produce in vitro Ig (36,37,39,43,44,142,143,152,153). In T-dependent systems, B cells from short-term recipients who received T-cell-containing marrow grafts did not produce IgA, IgG, or IgM after PWM stimulation in the presence of normal helper T cells (39,153). B cells from short-term recipients did not produce anti-TT after TT-stimulation in the presence of donor helper T cells (47). In assays of B-cell activation, growth, and differentiation, B cells from short-term recipients who received T-cell-containing marrow grafts were inert (43,44,48). In another study, Ig synthesis by B cells was defective; however, B-cell proliferative responses were intact in recipients of T-cell-depleted HLA-matched grafts (154). In mismatched recipients, recovery of proliferative responses to mitogens was incomplete and delayed (154). With the exception of memory B cells that were triggered by "allogeneic effects" to produce Ig spontaneously, B cells from short-term recipients are unable to respond to normal T-cell signals.

VI. CHRONIC GVHD

A. The Clinical Problem of Chronic GVHD

The syndrome of chronic GVHD resembles autoimmune disorders such as systemic lupus erythrematosus, Sjögren's syndrome, lichen planus, eosinophilic fasciitis, and scleroderma. The clinical manifestations include skin lesions, buccal mucositis, keratoconjunctivitis, strictures of the esophagus and vagina, chronic liver disease, inflammation of the bowel, and failure to thrive. Circulating autoantibodies and deposition of Abs and complement in the skin support this analogy (155-164). Approximately 35-45% of recipients of HLA–identical marrow grafts develop chronic GVHD between 3 and 15 months after BMT (158,161,163,165). Recipient age is a major risk factor for the development of chronic GVHD.

The association of acute and chronic GVHD suggests that the pathogenesis of the two entities is related. Studies show that lymphocytes from long-term recipients are reacting against host Ags. Lymphocytes from long-term recipients exhibit unidirectional mixed lymphocyte culture (MLC) reactivity to host lymphocytes and specific cytotoxicity directed at host fibroblasts (164,166). Lymphocytes from recipients with chronic GVHD exhibited a higher proportion of MLC reactivity than those from healthy long-term recipients. Lymphocytes responsible for mediating the MLC anti-host reactivity were not detected in healthy recipients due to circulating specific suppressor T cells that suppressed responses of donor cells to trinitrophenol-modified host cells (168). The predominance of suppressor T cells in MLC systems (105,167-170) and the excessive suppressor T-cell activity in Ig production systems (35-39,41,42) may reflect the immature immune system's attempt to downregulate reactive T- and B-cell clones directed at non-HLA Ags. As mentioned earlier, lack of adequate thymic T-cell education may impair the clonal selection process and lead to the development of autoreactive clones resulting in chronic GVHD.

B. Cellular Immune Reconstitution

Healthy long-term recipients of T-cell-containing marrow grafts normalize the proportion and absolute numbers of CD4$^+$, CD3$^+$, and CD8$^+$ cells in their peripheral blood 6 months to a year after BMT. Recipients with chronic GVHD have persistently elevated proportions of CD8$^+$ cells and decreased proportions of CD4$^+$ cells in their peripheral blood (15,27-34,128). There is significant delay of T-cell subset recovery as defined by MAb OKT3, 4, 8, 10, and 11 in recipients of autologous marrow grafts after preparation with intensive thio-TEPA chemotherapy as compared to those who were prepared with cyclo-phosphamide and total body irradiation (145). Selective in vivo sequestration and con-sumption of CD4$^+$ cells by ongoing chronic GVHD reactions in the skin, liver, or gut may be responsible for the low numbers of circulating CD4$^+$ cells.

Delayed-type hypersensitivity to at least one of five recall skin test Ags can be de-tected by 4 years postgrafting in over 90% of all recipients who received T-cell-containing grafts (140). Similar patterns of skin test positivity to specific allergens in marrow donors was detected in long-term recipients who were skin test negative to the same allergens pretransplant (171). Proliferative responses to alloantigens, mitogens, and specific Ags are normal or near normal after 6 months after BMT in recipients who were unaffected with chronic GVHD (16). Proliferative responses of lymphocytes to mitogens in recipi-ents who received T-cell-depleted grafts at this institution are depressed for more than a year postgrafting. Longer follow-up and greater numbers of recipients who received T-cell-depleted marrow grafts will be needed to determine if there are differences between those with and without chronic GVHD.

Evaluation of T-cell functions in the PWM-stimulated Ig production system showed that T cells from long-term recipients failed to provide helper activity and exhibited ex-cessive suppressor activity (35-37,41,42). Function studies on purified T_{G+} and T_{G-} subsets revealed heterogeneous functions within each subset (172). Studies which used anti-CD4 and anti-CD8 MAbs and complement to negatively select CD8$^+$ and CD4$^+$ cells showed that the increased suppressor T-cell activity in the whole T-cell population was generally due to increased proportions of CD8$^+$ cells (35,173,174). The remarkable finding was that CD4$^+$ cells from recipients with chronic GVHD failed to provide helper activity, whereas CD4$^+$ cells from healthy recipients consistently provided helper activity (173,174).

T- and B-cell functions in long-term recipients were evaluated by using four differ-ent nonspecific activators of Ig synthesis to determine if there were differences between the functional profiles for the various subsets from one activator to another (173). The results show that the recovery pattern of CD4$^+$ helper activity from a particular recipient was different for each activator. The presence or absence of suppressor activity in CD8$^+$ cells was also a function of the activator used to stimulate Ig production. Recipients with chronic GVHD had delayed development of normal CD4$^+$ and CD8$^+$ T-cell functions in all systems. The heterogeneous functional responses seen in each T-cell subset suggest that there are a series of maturational stages within each phenotype. A recent study showed functional heterogeneity within the CD8$^+$ subset. The CD8$^+$, CD11$^-$ cells pro-vided helper activity and CD8$^+$, CD11$^+$ cells suppressed Ab production when cocultured with normal T and B cells stimulated with PWM (131). The ratio of CD11$^+$ to CD11$^-$ cells within the CD8$^+$ subset may determine whether unfractionated CD8$^+$ cells exhibit suppressor activity.

C. Humoral Immune Reconstitution

With the exception of IgA, serum Ig levels are in the normal range for healthy long-term recipients of T-cell-containing marrow grafts whereas those with chronic GVHD can have abnormal Ig levels for years after BMT. Healthy recipients of T-cell-containing marrow grafts can respond to primary and secondary immunizations with neoantigens such as KLH and bacteriophage ∅X174. In contrast, recipients with chronic GVHD re-main impaired in their primary and secondary Ab responses (17). Furthermore, the recipients with chronic GVHD fail to switch from IgM anti-$\emptyset$X174 synthesis to IgG synthesis.

Two-thirds of the healthy recipients who received T-cell-containing grafts had B cells that secreted Ig in the presence of normal T cells, and over 75% of those with chronic GVHD had B cells that failed to secrete Ig (35,41,42,173,174). One study showed that there are distinct functional groups of B cells in recipients, and these groups of B cells may represent different maturational stages of B cells (173). For instance, B cells from the same recipient may respond in one Ig synthesis system and not in another Ig synthesis system.

To further dissect B-cell functions, B cells from short-term and long-term recipients were studied using assays for B-cell activation, proliferation, and differentiation (175-177). B cells from some recipients could be activated with Staphylococcal Cowan I Bacteria, but would not proliferate or differentiate in the presence of T-cell factors (43,44, 152,178). In other recipients, B cells could proliferate to T-cell factors but could not secrete Ig. These defects were seen more frequently in recipients with chronic GVHD and not in B cells from normal controls. There was a high correlation between the failure of recipient B cells to produce Ig after costimulation with Staphylococcal Cowan I Bacteria and T-cell-replacing factors and low serum Ig levels (p = 0.0075) (43). Similar defects in B-cell proliferation and differentiation have been demonstrated in autologous BMT or recipients of peripheral blood stem cell transplants (44). A recent study showed that allogeneic matched recipients of T-cell-depleted grafts had B cells that could produce Ig by 5-6 months after BMT (154). Mismatched recipients, however, had prolonged deficits in recovery of their B-cell proliferative and differentiative functions. These results suggest that there are specific defects in the normal maturational pathways for B cells after BMT.

D. Transferred Immunity

The majority of long-term healthy recipients who received related HLA-identical T-cell-containing marrow grafts had anti-TT and anti-DT titers in the normal range without booster immunizations of the donor or recipients before or after marrow grafting (45, 59). None of the recipients received intravenous gammaglobulin supplementation. In long-term healthy recipients, 85 of 125 (68%) had anti-TT titers; 12 of 18 (67%) had anti-MV titers; and 62 of 104 (60%) had anti-DT titers. In recipients with chronic GVHD, 79 of 166 (48%) had anti-TT titers; 6 of 15 (40%) had anti-MV titers; and 40 of 136 (29%) had anti-DT titers (45,49).

Two-thirds of the healthy recipients of unrelated matched or related one Ag mismatched T-cell-containing grafts had anti-TT titers, and 37% of the same recipients had anti-DT titers (49). Chronic GVHD inhibits the development of transferred Ag-specific immunity from donors to recipients. Approximately 40% of the recipients of unrelated matched or related one Ag mismatched grafts had anti-TT titers in the normal range; 25% of the same recipients had anti-DT titers in the normal range. Several groups have reported transfer of viral-specific immunity from donors to recipients (179,180). One report documented transfer of anti-acetylcholine-receptor antibody from a donor to a recipient (181). Recipients of T-cell-depleted grafts have circulating Abs to recall Ags (49). Studies are needed to evaluate the transfer of specific immunity in HLA-disparate transplants with and without T-cell depletion in the absence of booster immunizations.

T and B lymphocytes from nonboosted long-term recipients produced in vitro anti-TT after TT-stimulation (47-49). In one study, helper activity for anti-TT synthesis could be detected, but recipient B cells did not secrete anti-TT (47). However, anti-TT synthesis was detected in cultures containing higher numbers of recipient T and B cells (50). These results show that T and B cells from recipients can collaborate in specific Ab synthesis even though their numbers may be low in peripheral blood. Others have shown that anti-TT synthesis can be induced in recipient B cells shortly after transplant if both donor and recipient are boosted (46,51,63). These results clearly show that memory cells can be transferred in the marrow inoculum. One group study showed that marrow B cells from marrow donors can be stimulated with PWM or TT to produce in vitro anti-TT with booster immunizations (182). Studies in our laboratory show that bone marrow mononuclear cells from nonboosted recipients 6 months or more after receiving T-cell-depleted marrow grafts produced in vitro anti-TT (unpublished). These results suggest that the bone marrow contains significant numbers of Ag-specific memory B cells.

VII. MODULATION OR ACCELERATION OF IMMUNE RECOVERY

Many attempts have been made to accelerate immune reconstitution. Thymic transplants were pursued since the development of chronic GVHD may be the result of low or absent thymic function in older (>30 years) recipients. The administration of thymosin fraction V and transplantation of thymic epithelium have not been successful (52,53). Clinical performance and laboratory measures of those who received transplanted thymic tissue were not different from controls who did not receive thymic transplants. It is likely that the amount of thymic tissue transplanted and type of concurrent immunosuppression was not enough for effective T-cell education. In order to boost varicella-zoster-specific immunity, varicella-specific transfer factor was given to prevent or attenuate varicella-zoster infections between 50 and 64 days after BMT without any modulating effects on reconstitution (54). Thymosin fraction 5 was also given after BMT to accelerate immune reconstitution without either beneficial or detrimental effects (53).

If donors were immunized with vaccines for CMV, the marrow inoculum would contain expanded populations of specific T and B cells. In this manner, transferred anti-CMV immunity could be boosted prior to transplant to protect the recipient after BMT. Alternatively, the marrow inoculum could be exposed to an Ag en route to the recipient. These approaches are supported by the data obtained using TT or hepatitis vaccine immunizations to boost donors and recipients before and after BMT in order to increase specific Ab production in recipients after BMT (46,51,63).

Recombinant interleukins will likely play a major role in accelerating the reconstruction of the immune system after BMT. However, a great deal of basic and clinical research is needed to understand the roles the interleukins play in the maturation and differentiation of hematopoietic and lymphopoietic cells before the recombinant molecules can be used successfully.

Future studies revolve around the issues of preventing infection, enhancing specific immunity, and accelerating immune reconstitution. An exciting new area will be the insertion of specific genes into the marrow cells or into specific lymphocyte subsets to reconstitute specific immune defects. This approach combined with the use of recombinant molecules to regulate or enhance the growth of certain cell populations may allow medical scientists to accelerate and modulate the process of immune reconstitution.

VIII.   RECOMMENDATIONS FOR REIMMUNIZATION

Some transplant groups have been reimmunizing their recipients. Current data suggest that many recipients are not protected from the "childhood diseases" if one simply equates protection with the presence of an Ab titer in the normal range. Transferred specific and herd immunity may explain why more recipients do not become infected with childhood diseases. Recipients who develop titers to recall Ags need not be reimmunized to the same Ags, whereas those who do not develop Abs titers need to be reimmunized. Healthy long-term recipients who do not have detectable Ab titers to recall Ags should be given a primary series (up to three immunizations) of tetanus toxoid, diphtheria toxoid, and inactivated polio (Salk) vaccine. We expect the immune system of those who are seronegative to respond to immunogens as if they were neoantigens. Recipients with chronic GVHD do not respond to immunizations and should be immunized after their chronic GVHD is resolved. The use of attenuated viral vaccines is not recommended.

IX.   SUMMARY

The development of the new donor-derived immune system after bone marrow transplantation (BMT) takes up to 2 years in healthy BMT recipients. Early after BMT, acute Graft-vs.-Host Disease (GVHD) and its treatment increase the susceptibility to overwhelming infections and retard the development of the immune system. The new system develops from a primitive state characterized by cytotoxic and suppressive functions and progresses to a mature state characterized by specialized lymphocyte functions such as lymphokine production, proliferation, and expression of growth factor receptors. These specialized functions develop in healthy long-term recipients, whereas the same functions are absent or impaired in those who develop chronic GVHD.

ACKNOWLEDGMENT

This work was supported in part by funds from the American Cancer Society (Grant #IM-536) and the Division of Hematology and Oncology, Departments of Medicine and Pediatrics, Medical College of Wisconsin and Wayne State University. I express my appreciation to Ms. Paula Zamiatowski and my wife, Carol Lum, for their assistance in the preparation of this manuscript.

REFERENCES

1.   Thomas ED, Storb R, Clift RA, Fefer A, Johnson FL, Neiman PE, Lerner KG, Glucksberg H, Buckner CD: Bone marrow transplantation. N Engl J Med 1975;292:832-843.
2.   Thomas ED, Storb R, Clift RA, Fefer A, Johnson FL, Neiman PE, Lerner KG, Glucksberg H, Buckner CD: Bone-marrow transplantation. N Engl J Med 1975;292:895-902.
3.   Lum LG, Storb R: Bone marrow transplantation. In *Principles of Organ Transplantation*, edited by Flye MW. WB Saunders, Philadelphia, 1988.
4.   Storb R, Thomas ED: Allogeneic bone-marrow transplantation. Immunol Rev 1983; 71:77-102.
5.   Winston DJ, Schiffman G, Wang DC, Feig SA, Lin C-H, Marso EL, Ho WG, Young

LS, Gale RP: Pneumococcal infections after human bone-marrow transplantation. Ann Intern Med 1979;91:835-841.

6. Atkinson K, Storb R, Prentice RL, Weiden PL, Witherspoon RP, Sullivan K, Noel D, Thomas ED: Analysis of late infections in 89 long-term survivors of bone marrow transplantation. Blood 1979.53:720-731.

7. Atkinson K, Meyers JD, Storb R, Prentice RL, Thomas ED: Varicella-zoster virus infection after marrow transplantation for aplastic anemia or leukemia. Transplantation 1980;29:47-50.

8. Neiman P, Wasserman RB, Wentworth BB, Kaug F, Lerner KG, Storb R, Buckner CD, Clift RA, Fefer A, Fass L, Glucksberg H, Thomas ED: Interstitial pneumonia and cytomegalovirus infection as complications of human marrow transplantation. Transplantation 1973;15:478-485.

9. Meyers JD: Infection in recipients of marrow transplants. In *Current Clinical Topics in Infectious Diseases*, edited by Remington JS, Swartz MN. New York, McGraw-Hill, 1985; pp. 261-292.

10. Bowden RA, Meyers JD: Infectious complications following marrow transplantation. Plasma Therapy & Transfusion Technology 1985;6:285-302.

11 Halterman RH, Graw RG Jr, Fuccillo DA, Leventhal BG: Immunocompetence following allogeneic bone marrow transplantation in man. Transplantation 1972; 14:689-697.

12. Fass L, Ochs HD, Thomas ED, Mickelson E, Storb R, Fefer A: Studies of immunological reactivity following syngeneic or allogeneic marrow grafts in man. Transplantation 1973;16:630-640.

13. Elfenbein GJ, Anderson PN, Humphrey RL, Mullens GM, Sensenbrenner LL, Wands JR, Santos GW: Immune system reconstitution following allogeneic bone-marrow transplantation in man: A multiparameter analysis. Transplant Proc 1976;8:641-646.

14. Gale RP, Opelz G, Mickey MR, Graze PR, Saxon A, for the UCLA Bone Marrow Transplant Team: Immunodeficiency following allogeneic bone-marrow transplantation. Transplant Proc 1978;10:223-227.

15. Witherspoon RP, Lum LG, Storb R: Immunologic reconstitution after human marrow grafting. Semin Hematol 1984;21:2-10.

16. Noel DR, Witherspoon RP, Storb R, Atkinson K, Doney K, Mickelson EM, Ochs HD, Warren RP, Weiden RL, Thomas ED: Does graft-versus-host disease influence the tempo of immunologic recovery after allogeneic human marrow transplantation? An observation on 56 long-term survivors. Blood 1978;51:1087-1105.

17. Witherspoon RP, Storb R, Ochs HD, Flournoy N, Kopecky KJ, Sullivan KM, Deeg HJ, Sosa R, Noel DR, Atkinson K, Thomas ED: Recovery of antibody production in human allogeneic marrow graft recipients: Influence of time posttransplantation, the presence or absence of chronic graft-versus-host disease, and antithymocyte globulin treatment. Blood 1981;58:360-368.

18. Shiobara S, Harada M, Mori T, Kodo H, Ishino C, Matsue K, Odaka K, Kondo K, Hattori K: Difference in posttransplant recovery of immune reactivity between allogeneic and autologous bone marrow transplantation. Transplant Proc 1982; 14:429-433.

19. Witherspoon RP, Kopecky K, Storb R, Flournoy N, Sullivan KM, Sosa R, Deeg HJ, Ochs HD, Cheever MA: Immunological recovery in 48 patients following syngeneic marrow transplantation for hematological malignancy. Transplantation 1982;33: 143-149.

20. Witherspoon RP, Deeg HJ, Lum LG, Ochs HD, Hansen JA, Thomas ED, Storb R: Immunologic recovery in human marrow graft recipients given cyclosporine or methotrexate for the prevention of graft-versus-host disease. Transplantation 1984; 37:456-461.

21. Livnat S, Seigneuret M, Storb R, Prentice R: Analysis of cytotoxic effector cell function in patients with leukemia or aplastic anemia before and after marrow transplantation. J Immunol 1980;124:481-490.

22. Quinnan GV Jr, Kirmani N, Esber E, Saral R, Manischewitz JF, Roger JL, Rook AH, Santos GW, Burns WH: HLA-restricted cytotoxic T lymphocyte and nonthymic cytotoxic lymphocyte responses to cytomegalovirus infection of bone marrow transplant recipients. J Immunol 1981;126:2036-2041.

23. Dokhelar M-C, Wiels J. Lipinski M, Tetaud C, Devergie A, Gluckman E, Tursz T: Natural killer cell activity in human bone marrow recipients. Early reappearance of peripheral natural killer activity in graft-versus-host disease. Transplantation 1981;31:61-65.

24. Lopez C, Kirkpatrick D, Sorell M, O'Reilly RJ, Ching C, and Bone Marrow Transplant Unit: Association between pre-transplant natural killer and graft-versus-host disease after stem-cell transplantation. Lancet 1979;2:1103-1107.

25. Charmot D, Ragueneau N, Olive D, Maraninchi D, Mawas C: Generation of CD8 cytolytic T cells early after autologous or allogeneic bone marrow transplantation. Bone Marrow Transplantation 1987;2:183-194.

26. Niederwieser D, Gastl G, Rumpold H, Marth C, Kraft D, Huber C: Rapid reappearance of large granular lymphocytes (LGL) with concomitant reconstitution of natural killer (NK) activity after human bone marrow transplantation (BMT). Br J Haematol 1987;65:301-305.

27. Linch DC, Knott LJ, Thomas RM, Harper P, Goldstone AH, Davis EG, Levinski RJ: T cell regeneration after allogeneic and autologous bone marrow transplantation. Br J Haematol 1983;53:451-458.

28. Atkinson K, Hansen JA, Storb R, Goehle S, Goldstein G, Thomas ED: T-cell subpopulations identified by monoclonal antibodies after human marrow transplantation. I. Helper-inducer and cytotoxic-suppressor subsets. Blood 1982;59:1292-1298.

29. Forman SJ, Nocker P, Gallagher M, Zaia J, Wright C, Bolen J, Mills B, Heckt T, Blume K: Pattern of T cell reconstitution following allogeneic bone marrow transplantation for acute hematological malignancy. Transplantation 1982;34:96-98.

30. Schroff RW, Gale RP, Fahey JL: Regeneration of T cell subpopulations after bone marrow transplantation: Cytomegalovirus infection and lymphoid subset imbalance. J Immunol 1982;129:1926-1930.

31. Friedrich W, O'Reilly RJ, Koziner B, Gebhard DR Jr, Good RA, Evans RL: T-lymphocyte reconstitution in recipients of bone marrow transplants with and without GVHD: Imbalances of T-cell subpopulations having unique regulatory and cognitive functions. Blood 1982;59:696-701.

32. Gratama JW, Maipal A, Oljans R, Zwaan FE, Verdonck LF, de Witte T, Vossen JMJJ, Bolhuis RLH, de Gast GC, Jansen J: T lymphocyte repopulation and differentiation after bone marrow transplantation. Early shifts in the ratio between T4+ and T8+ T lymphocytes correlate with the occurrence of acute graft-versus-host disease. Blood 1984;63:1461-1423.

33. Favrot M, Janossy G, Tidman N, Blacklock M, Lopez E, Bofill M, Lampert I, Morgenstein G, Powles R, Prentice HG, Hoffbrand AV: T cell regeneration after allogeneic bone marrow transplantation. Clin Exp Immunol 1983;54:59-72.

34. Van de Griend RJ, Astaldi A, Vossen JM, Dooren LJ, Schellekens PHA, Zwaan FE, Van De Ende A, Roos M, Roos D: T lymphocyte characteristics in bone marrow transplanted patients. I. Changes in biochemical properties that correlate with immunologic reconstitution. J Immunol 1981;126:636-640.

35. Lum LG, Orcutt-Thordarson N, Seigneuret MC, Storb R: The regulation of Ig synthesis after marrow transplantation: IV. T4 and T8 subset function in patients with chronic graft-versus-host disease. J Immunol 1982;129:113-119.

36. Pahwa SG, Pahwa RM, Friedrich W, O'Reilly RJ, Good RA: Abnormal humoral immune responses in peripheral blood lymphocyte cultures of bone marrow transplant recipients. Proc Natl Acad Sci USA 1982;79:2663-2667.

37. Korsmeyer SJ, Elfenbein GJ, Goldman CK, Marshall SL, Waldmann TA: B cell, helper T cell, and suppressor T cell abnormalities contribute to disordered immunoglobulin synthesis in patients following bone marrow transplantation. Transplantation 1982;33:184-186.

38. Dosch H-M, Gelfand EW: Failure of T and B cell cooperation during graft-versus-host disease. Transplantation 1981;31:48-50.

39. Witherspoon RP, Goehle S, Kretschmer M, Storb R: Regulation of immunoglobulin production after human marrow grafting: The role of helper and suppressor T cells in acute graft-versus-host disease. Transplantation 1986;41:328-335.

40. Okos AJ, Lum LG, Storb R: Epstein-Barr virus (EBV)-induced immunoglobulin (Ig) production and suppression by EBV immune T-cells in bone marrow transplant recipients. Blood (Suppl) 1983;62:227a (abstr).

41. Lum LG, Seigneuret MC, Storb R, Witherspoon RP, Thomas ED: In vitro regulation of immunoglobulin synthesis after marrow transplantation. I. T-cell and B-cell deficiencies in patients with and without chronic graft-versus-host disease. Blood 1981; 58:431-439.

42. Saxon A, McIntyre RE, Stevens RH, Gale RP: Lymphocyte dysfunction in chronic graft-versus-host disease. Blood 1981;58:746-751.

43. Matsue K, Lum LG, Witherspoon RP, Storb R: Proliferative and differentiative responses of B cells from human marrow graft recipients to T cell-derived factors. Blood 1987;69:308-315.

44. Kiesel S, Pezzutto A, Moldenhauer G, Haas R, Körbling M, Hunstein W, Dörken B: B-cell proliferative and differentiative responses after autologous peripheral blood stem cell or bone marrow transplantation. Blood 1988;72:672-678.

45. Lum LG, Munn NA, Schanfield MS, Storb R: The detection of specific antibody formation to recall antigens after human bone marrow transplantation. Blood 1986; 67:582-587.

46. Wimperis JZ, Brenner MK, Prentice HG, Reittie JE, Karayiannis P, Griffiths PD, Hoffbrand AV: Transfer of a functioning humoral immune system in transplantation of T-lymphocyte-depleted bone marrow. Lancet 1986;1:339-342.

47. Shiobara S, Lum LG, Witherspoon RP, Storb R: Antigen specific antibody responses of lymphocytes to tetanus toxoid after human marrow transplantation. Transplantation 1986;41:587-592.

48. Jin N-R, Lum LG: IgG anti-tetanus toxoid antibody production induced by Epstein-Barr virus from B cells of human marrow transplant recipients. Cell Immunol 1986; 101:266-273.

49. Lum LG, Noges JE, Beatty P, Martin PJ, Deeg HJ, Doney KC, Loughran T, Sullivan KM, Witherspoon RP, Thomas ED, Storb R: Transfer of specific immunity in marrow recipients given HLA-mismatched, T cell-depleted, or HLA-identical marrow grafts. Bone Marrow Transplant 1988;3:399-406.

50. Lum LG, Seigneuret MC, Storb R: The transfer of antigen-specific humoral immunity from marrow donors to marrow recipients. J Clin Immunol 1986;6:389-396.

51. Wimperis JZ, Brenner MK, Prentice HG, Thompson EJ, Hoffbrand AV: B cell development and regulation after T cell-depleted marrow transplantation. J Immunol 1987;138:2445-2450.

52. Atkinson K, Storb R, Ochs HD, Goehle S, Sullivan KM, Withespoon RP, Lum LG, Tsoi M-S, Sanders JE, Parr M, Stewart P, Thomas ED: Thymus transplantation after allogeneic bone marrow graft to prevent chronic graft-versus-host disease in humans. Transplantation 1982;33:168-173.

53. Witherspoon RP, Hersman J, Storb R, Ochs H, Goldstein AL, McClure J, Noel D, Weiden PL, Thomas ED: Thymosin fraction 5 does not accelerate reconstitution of immunologic reactivity after human marrow grafting. Br J Haematol 1983;55:595-608.

54. Bowden RA, Siegel MS, Steele RW, Day LM, Meyer JD: Immunologic and clinical responses to varicella-zoster-specific transfer factor following marrow transplantation. J Infect Dis 1985;152:1324-1327.

55. Witherspoon RP, Navari R, Storb R, Sullivan KM, Doney K, Beatty P, Lum LG, Thomas ED: Treatment of marrow graft recipients with Thymopentin. Bone Marrow Transplant 1987;1:365-371.

56. Storb R, Thomas ED, Buckner CD, Clift RA, Johnson FL, Fefer A, Glucksberg G, Giblett ER, Lerner KG, Neiman P: Allogeneic marrow grafting for treatment of aplastic anemia. Blood 1974;43:157-180.

57. Storb R, Thomas ED, Buckner CD, Clift RA, Deeg HJ, Fefer A, Goodell BW, Sale GE, Sanders JE, Singer J, Stewart R, Weiden PL: Marrow transplantation in thirty "untransfused" patients with severe aplastic anemia. Ann Intern Med 1980;92:30-36.

58. Martin PJ, Hansen JA, Buckner CD, Sanders JE, Deeg HJ, Stewart P, Appelbaum FR, Clift R, Fefer A, Witherspoon RP, Kennedy MS, Sullivan KM, Flournoy N, Storb R, Thomas ED: Effects of in vitro depletion of T cells in HLA-identical marrow grafts. Blood 1985;66:664-672.

59. Prentice HG, Blacklock HA, Janossy G, Bradstock KF, Skeggs D, Goldstein G, Hoffbrand AV: Use of anti-T-cell monoclonal antibody OKT3 to prevent acute graft-versus-host disease in allogeneic bone-marrow transplantation for acute leukaemia. Lancet 1982;1:700-703.

60. Filipovich AH, McGlave PB, Ramsay NK, Goldstein G, Warkentin PI, Kersey JH: Pretreatment of donor bone marrow with monoclonal antibody OKT3 for prevention of acute graft-versus-host disease in allogeneic histocompatible bone-marrow transplantation. Lancet 1982;1:1266-1270.

61. Goldman JM, Gale RP, Horowitz MM, Biggs JC, Champlin RE, Gluckman E, Hoffmann RG, Jacobsen SJ, Marmont AM, McGlave PB, Messner HA, Rimm AA, Rozman C, Speck B, Tura S, Weiner RS, Bortin MM: Bone marrow transplantation for chronic myelogenous leukemia in chronic phase: Increased risk for relapse associated with T-cell depletion. Ann Intern Med 1990;108:806-814.

62. Wagner JE, Donnenberg AD, Noga SJ, Cremo CA, Gao IK, Yin HJ, Vogelsang GB, Rowley S, Saral R, Santos GW: Lymphocyte depletion of donor bone marrow by counterflow centrifugal elutriation: Results of a phase I clinical trial. Blood 1988;72:1168-1176.

63. Saxon A, Mitsuyasu R, Steven R, Champlin RE, Kimata H, Gale RP: Designed transfer of specific immune responses with bone marrow transplantation. J Clin Invest 1986;78:959-967.

64. Izutsu KT, Sullivan KM, Schubert MM, Truelove EL, Shulman HM, Sale GE, Morton TH, Rice JC, Witherspoon RP, Storb R, Thomas ED: Disordered salivary immunoglobulin secretion and sodium transport in human chronic graft-versus-host disease. Transplantation 1983;35:441-446.

65. Sosa R, Weiden PL, Storb R, Syrotuck J, Thomas ED: Granulocyte function in human allogeneic marrow graft recipients. Exp Hematol 1980;8:1183-1189.

66. Territo MC, Gale RP, Cline MJ, and The UCLA Bone Marrow Transplantation Team: Neutrophil function in bone marrow transplant recipients. Br J Haematol 1977;35:245-250.

67. Clark RA, Johnson FL, Klebanoff SJ, Thomas ED: Defective neutrophil chemotaxis in bone marrow transplant patients. J Clin Invest 1976;58:22-31.

68. Tsoi M-S, Dobbs S, Brkić S, Ramberg E, Thomas ED, Storb R: Cellular interactions in marrow-grafted patients. II. Normal monocyte antigen-presenting and defective T-cell proliferative functions early after grafting and during chronic graft-versus-host disease. Transplantation 1984;37:556-561.

69. Thomas ED, Ramberg RE, Sale GE, Sparkes RS, Golde DW: Direct evidence for a bone marrow origin of the alveolar macrophage in man. Science 1976;192:1016-1018.

70. Gale RP, Sparkes RS, Golde DW: Bone marrow origin of hepatic macrophages (Kupffer cells) in humans. Science 1978;201:937-938.

71. Winston DJ, Territo MC, Ho WG, Miller MJ, Gale RP, Golde DW: Alveolar macrophage dysfunction in human bone marrow transplant recipients. Am J Med 1982;73:859-866.

72. Brkić S, Tsoi M-S, Mori T, Lachman L, Gillis S, Thomas ED, Storb R: Cellular interactions in marrow-grafted patients. III. Normal interleukin 1 and defective interleukin 2 production in short-term patients and in those with chronic graft-versus-host disease. Transplantation 1985;39:30-35.

73. Shiobara S, Witherspoon RP, Lum LG, Storb R: Immunoglobulin synthesis after HLA-identical marrow grafting: V. The role of peripheral blood monocytes in the regulation of in vitro immunoglobulin secretion stimulated by pokeweed mitogen. J Immunol 1984;132:2850-2856.

74. Winston DJ, Pollard RB, Ho WG, Gallagher JG, Rasmussen LE, Huang SN, Lin CH, Gossett TG, Merigan TL, Gale RP: Cytomegalovirus immune plasma in bone marrow transplant recipients. Ann Intern Med 1982;97:11-18.

75. Meyers JD, Leszczynski J, Zaia JA, Flournoy N, Newton B, Syndman DR, Wright GG, Levin MJ, Thomas ED: Prenvention of cytomegalovirus infection by cytomegalovirus immune globulin after marrow transplantation. Ann Intern Med 1983;98:442-446.

76. O'Reilly RJ, Reich L, Gold J, Kirkpatrick D, Dinsmore R, Kapoor N, Condie R: A randomized trial of intravenous hyperimmune globulin for the prevention of cytomegalovirus (CMV) infections following marrow transplantation: Preliminary results. Transplant Proc 1983;15:1405-1411.

77. Meyers JD, Reed RC, Shepp DH, Thornquist M, Dandliker PS, Vicary CA, Flournoy N, Kirk LE, Kersey JH, Thomas ED, Balfour HH Jr: Acyclovir for prevention of cytomegalovirus infection and disease after allogeneic marrow transplantation. N Engl J Med 1988;318:70-75.

78. Winston DJ, Ho WG, Lin CH, Bartoni K, Budinger MD, Gale RP, Champlin RE: Intravenous immunoglobulin for prevention of interstitial pneumonia after bone marrow transplantation. Ann Intern Med 1987;106:12-18.

79. Bowden RA, Sayers M, Flournoy N, Newton B, Banaji M, Thomas ED, Meyers JD: Cytomegalovirus immune globulin and seronegative blood products to prevent primary cytomegalovirus infection after marrow transplant. N Engl J Med 1986;314:1006-1010.

80. Kapoor N, Tutschka PJ, Copelan EA: Prevention of fatal CMV infection by administration intravenous gammaglobulin. Blood (Suppl) 1987;70:308a (abstr).

81. Ash RC, Turner P, Smith R, Chitambar C, Hansen R, Casper J, Haasler G: The use of 9(1,3-dihydroxy-2-propoxymethyl) guanine (ganciclovir, DHPG) and intravenous immunoglobulin (IVIG) in the treatment of serious cytomegalovirus (CMV) infections in thirty-one allogeneic bone marrow transplant (BMT) patients. Blood (Suppl) 1987;70:302a (abstr).

82. Reed EC, Dandliker PS, Meyers JD: Treatment of cytomegalovirus pneumonia with 9-[2-hydroxy-1-(hydroxymethyl) ethoxymethyl] guanine and high-dose corticosteroids. Ann Intern Med 1986;105:214-215.

83. Reed EC, Bowden RA, Dandliker PS, Meyers JD: Treatment of cytomegalovirus (CMV) pneumonia in bone marrow transplant (BMT) patients (PTS) with ganciclovir (GCV) and CMV immunoglobulin (CMV-IG). Blood 1987;70(Suppl):313a (abstr).

84. Parriera A, Smith J, Hows JM, Smithers SA, Apperley J, Rombos Y, Goldman JM, Gordon-Smith EC, Catovsky DJ: Immunological reconstitution after bone marrow transplant with Campath-1 treated bone marrow. Clin Exp Immunol 1987;67:142-150.

85. Leroy E, Calvo CF, Divine M, Gourdin M-F, Baujean F, Ben Aribia MH, Mishal Z, Vernant J-P, Farcet J-P, Senik A: Persistence of T8+/HNK-1+ suppressor lymphocytes in the blood of long-term surviving patients after allogeneic bone marrow transplantation. J Immunol 1986;137:2180-2189.

86. Shapiro RS, Pietryga D, Blazar BR, Greenberg J, McClain K, Kersey JH, Ramsay NKC, and Filipovich AH: B cell lymphoproliferative disorders following bone marrow transplantation. In *Progress in Bone Marrow Transplantation*. UCLA Symposium on Molecular and Cellular Biology, New Series, edited by Gale RP, Champlin R. New York, Alan R. Liss, Inc., 1987; Vol. 53, pp. 647-657.

87. Martin PJ, Shulman HM, Schubach WH, Hansen JA, Fefer A, Miller G, Thomas ED: Fatal Epstein-Barr virus-associated proliferation of donor B-cells after treatment of acute graft-versus-host disease with a murine anti-T cell antibody. Ann Intern Med 1984,101:310-315.

88. Bozdeck MS, Finlay JL, Trigg ME, Billing R, Hong R, Sugden W, Sondel W, Sondel PM: Monoclonal B-cell lymphoproliferative disorder following monoclonal antibody (CT2) T-cell depleted allogeneic bone marrow transplantation. Blood 1982;62 (Suppl):218a (abstr).

89. Deeg HJ, Storb R, Graft-versus-host disease: Pathophysiological and clinical aspects. In *Annual Review of Medicine*, edited by Creger WP. Palo Alto, CA, Annual Reviews 1984; Vol. 35, pp. 11-24.

90. Santos GW, Hess AD, Vogelsang GB: Graft-versus-host reactions and disease. Immunol Rev 1985;88:169-192.

91. Tsoi M-S: Immunological mechanisms of graft-versus-host disease in man. Transplantation 1982;33:459-464.

92. Reinsmoen NL, Kersey JH, Bach FH: Detection of HLA restricted anti-minor histocompatibility antigen(s) reactive cells from skin GVHD lesions. Hum Immunol 1984;11:249-257.

93. Vogelsang GB, Hess AD, Berkman AW, Tutschka PJ, Farmer ER, Convers PJ, Santos GW: An in vitro predictive test for graft versus host disease in patients with genotypic HLA-identical bone marrow transplants. N Engl J Med 1985;313:645-650.

94. van Bekkum DW, de Vries MJ: *Radiation Chimeras*, New York, Academic Press 1967; pp. 146-150.

95. Glucksberg H, Storb R, Fefer A, Buckner CD, Neiman PE, Clift RA, Lerner KG, Thomas ED: Clinical manifestations of graft-versus-host disease in human recipients of marrow from HLA-matched sibling donors. Transplantation 1974;18:295-304.

96. Grebe SC, Streilein JW: Graft-versus-host reactions: A review. Adv Immunol 1976; 22:119-221.

97. Walker SA, Rogers TR, Perry D, Hobbs JR, Riches PG: Increased serum IgE concentrations during infection and graft versus host disease after bone marrow transplantation. J Clin Pathol 1984;37:460-462.

98. Ringdén O, Persson U, Johansson SGO, Wilczek H, Gahrton G, Groth C-G, Lundgren B, Möller E: Markedly elevated serum IgE levels following allogeneic and syngeneic bone marrow transplantation. Blood 1983;61:1190-1195.

99. Saryan JA, Rappeport J, Leung DY, Parkman R, Geha RS: Regulation of human

immunoglobulin E synthesis in acute graft versus host disease. J Clin Invest 1983;71: 556-564.

100. Heyd J, Donnenberg AD, Burns WH, Saral R, Santos GW: Immunoglobulin E levels following allogeneic, autologous, and syngeneic bone marrow transplantation: An indirect association between hyperproduction and acute graft-v-host disease in allogeneic BMT. Blood 1988;72:442-446.

101. van Bekkum DW, Knaan S: Role of bacterial microflora in development of intestinal lesions from graft-versus-host reactions. J Natl Cancer Inst 1977;58:787-789.

102. Storb R, Prentice RL, Buckner CD, Clift RA, Appelbaum F, Deeg J, Doney K, Hansen JA, Mason M, Sanders JE, Singer J, Sullivan KM, Witherspoon RP, Thomas ED: Graft-versus-host disease and survival in patients with aplastic anemia treated by marrow grafts from HLA-identical siblings. Beneficial effect of a protective environment. N Engl J Med 1983;308:302-307.

103. Mori T, Tsoi M-S, Gillis S, Santos E, Thomas ED, Storb R: Cellular interactions is marrow-grafted patients. I. Impairment of cell-mediated lympholysis associated with graft-vs-host disease and the effect of interleukin 2. J Immunol 1983;130: 712-716.

104. Azogui O, Gluckman E, Fradelizi D: Inhibition of IL 2 production after human allogeneic bone marrow transplantation. J Immunol 1983;131:1205-1208.

105. Opelz G, Gale RP, and the UCLA Bone Marrow Transplant Team: Absence of specific mixed leukocyte culture reactivity during graft-versus-host disease and following bone marrow transplant rejection. Transplantation 1976;22:474-477.

106. Bagot M, Cordonnier C, Tilkin AF, Heslan M, Vernan TP, Dubertret L, Levey JP: A possible predictive test for graft-versus-host disease in bone marrow graft recipients: The mixed epidermal cell-lymphocyte reaction. Transplantation 1986; 41:316-319.

107. Berkman A, Farmer E, Tutschka P, Hess A, Santos G: Skin explant culture as a model for cutaneous graft-versus-host disease. Exp Hemat 1982;10:33-40.

108. Vogelsang GB, Hess AD, Silanskis M, Friedman K, Farmer E, Santos GW: Predictive models of graft versus host disease. In *Recent Advances and Future Directions in Bone Marrow Transplantation*, edited by Baum SJ, Santos GW, Takaku F. New York, Springer-Verlag 1988; pp. 141-144.

109. Kasten-Sportes C, Gluckman E, Azogui O: Heterogeneity of T lymphocytes infiltrating sites of acute and chronic graft versus host disease (GVHD) following human allogeneic bone marrow transplantation. Blood 1987;70(Suppl 1):308a (abstr).

110. Delmonte L, O'Reilly RJ, Kirkpatrick D, Kapoor N: In vitro model for detection of alloreactivity between HLA-matched donor-host pairs. Transplantation 1982; 34:100-103.

111. Rodt H, Kolb HJ, Netzel B, Haas RJ, Wilms K, Götze CB, Link H, and Thierfelder S: Effect of anti-T-cell globulin on GVHD in leukemic patients treated with BMT. Transplant Proc 1981;13:257-261.

112. Storb R, Deeg HJ, Thomas ED, Appelbaum FR, Buckner CD, Cheever MA, Clift RA, Doney KC, Flournoy N, Kennedy MS, Loughran TP, McGuffin RW, Sale GE, Sanders JE, Singer JW, Stewart PS, Sullivan KM, Witherspoon RP: Marrow transplantation for chronic myelocytic leukemia: A controlled trial of cyclosporine versus methotrexate for prophylaxis of graft-versus-host disease. Blood 1985;66: 698-702.

113. Storb R, Deeg HJ, Whitehead J, Appelbaum FR, Beatty P, Bensinger B, Buckner CD, Clift R, Doney K, Farewell V, Hansen J, Hill R. Lum L, Martin P, McGuffin R, Sanders J, Stewart P, Sullivan K, Witherspoon R, Yee G, Thomas ED: Marrow transplantation for leukemia: Methotrexate and cyclosporine compared with cy-

closporine alone for prophylaxis of acute graft versus host disease after marrow transplantation for leukemia. N Engl J Med 1986;314:729-735.

114. Reisner Y, Kapoor N, Kirkpatrick D, Pollack MS, Cunningham-Rundles S, Dupont B, Hodes MZ, Good RA, O'Reilly RJ: Transplantation for severe combined immunodeficiency with HLA-A, B, D, DR incompatible parental marrow cells fractionated by soy bean agglutinin and sheep red blood cells. Blood 1983;61:341-348.

115. de Witte T, Hoogenout J, de Pauw B, Holdrinet R, Janssen J, Wessels J, van Daal W, Hustinx T, Haanen C: Depletion of donor lymphocytes by counterflow centrifugation successfully prevents acute graft-versus-host disease in matched allogeneic marrow transplantation. Blood 1986;67:1302-1308.

116. Waldmann H, Polliak A, Hale G, Or R, Cividalli G, Weiss L, Weshler Z, Samuel S, Manor D, Brautbar C, Rachmilewitz EA, Slavin SJ: Elimination of graft-versus-host disease by in-vitro depletion of alloreactive lymphocytes with a monoclonal rat anti-human lymphocyte antibody (Campath-1). Lancet 1984;2:483-486.

117. Hervé P, Cahn JY, Flesch M, Plouvier E, Racadot E, Noir A, Couteret Y, Goldstein G, Bernard A. Lenys R, Bresson JL, Leconte des Floris R, Peters A: Successful graft-versus-host disease prevention without graft failure in HLA-identical allogeneic bone marrow transplantations with marrow depleted of T cells by monoclonal antibodies and complement. Blood 1987;69:388-393.

118. Storb R, Deeg HJ, Farewell V, Doney K, Appelbaum F, Beatty P, Bensinger W, Buckner CD, Clift R, Hansen J, Hill R, Longton G, Lum L, Martin P, McGuffin R, Sanders J, Singer J, Stewart P, Sullivan K, Witherspoon R, Thomas ED: Marrow transplantation for severe aplastic anemia: Methotrexate alone compared to a combination of methotrexate and cyclosproine for prevention of acute graft-versus-host disease. Blood 1986;68:119-125.

119. Apperley JF, Jones L, Hale G, Waldmann H, Hows J, Rombos Y, Tsatalas C, Marcus RE, Goolden AWG, Gordon-Smith EC, Catovsky D, Galton DAG, Goldman JM: Bone marrow transplantation for patients with chronic myeloid leukaemia: T-cell depletion with Campath-1 reduces the incidence of graft-versus-host disease but may increase the risk of leukaemic relapse. Bone Marrow Transplant 1986;1: 153-166.

120. Martin PJ, Hansen JA, Buckner CD, Sanders JE, Deeg HJ, Stewart P, Appelbaum FR, Clift R, Fefer A, Witherspoon RP, Kennedy MS, Sullivan KM, Flournoy N, Storb R, Thomas ED: Effects of in vitro depletion of T cells in HLA-identical allogeneic marrow grafts. Blood 1985;66:664-672.

121. Zutter MM, Martin PJ, Sale GE, Shulman HM, Fisher L, Thomas ED, Durnam DM: Epstein-Barr virus lymphoproliferation after bone marrow transplantation. Blood 1988;72:520-529.

122. Truitt RL, Ash RC: Manipulation of T-cell content in transplanted human bone marrow: Effect on GVH and GVL reactions. In *Progress in Clinical and Biological Research, Cellular Immunotherapy of Cancer*, vol. 244, edited by Truitt RL, Gale RP, Bortin MM. New York, Alan R. Liss, Inc. 1987; pp. 409-421.

123. Weiden PL, Sullivan KM, Flournoy N, Storb R, Thomas ED, and the Seattle Bone Marrow Transplant Team: Antileukemic effect of chronic graft-versus-host disease: Contribution to improved survival after allogeneic marrow transplantation. N Engl J Med 1981;304:1529-1533.

124. Atkinson K, Cooley M, Farrelly H, O'Flaherty E, Concannon A, Dodds A, Biggs J: T4+ cells can initiate human graft-versus-host disease: A pilot study of T cell depletion. Exp Hemat Soc 1986;325 (abstr).

125. Champlin R, Ho W, Lee K, Giorgi J, Gajewski J, Gale RP, Feig SJ: Selective depletion of CD8 cytotoxic/suppressor cells for prevention of graft-versus-host

disease (GVHD) following bone marrow transplantation (BMT). Blood 1987;70 (Suppl 1):318a (abstr).

126. Pirsch JD, Maki DG: Infectious complications in adults with bone marrow transplantation and T-cell depletion of donor marrow. Ann Intern Med 1986;104:619-631.

127. Pelliniemi T-T, Alanko S, Salmi TT, Toivanen A: Reappearance of activated T suppressor (CD8+, HLA-DR+) preceded a relapse of acute lymphoblastic leukemia after bone marrow transplantation. Blood 1987;70(Suppl 1):312a (abstr).

128. Smith BR, Rappeport JM, Burakoff SJ, Ault KA: Clinical correlates of unusual circulating lymphocytes appearing post marrow transplantation. In *Progress in Bone Marrow Transplantation*, edited by Gale RP, Champlin R. New York, Alan R. Liss, Inc., 1987; pp. 659-663.

129. de Bruin HG, Astaldi A, Leupers T, van de Griend RJ, Dooren LJ, Schellekens PTA, Tanke HJ, Roos M, Vossen JM: T lymphocyte characteristics in bone marrow-transplanted patients. II. Analysis with monoclonal antibodies. J Immunol 1981; 127:244-251.

130. Charmot D, Ragueneau M, Olive D, Maraninchi D, Mawas C: Generation of CD8 cytolytic T cells early after autologous or allogeneic bone marrow transplantation. Bone Marrow Transplant 1987;2:183-194.

131. Klingemann H-G, Lum LG, Storb R: Phenotypical and functional studies on a subtype of suppressor cells (CD9+/CD11+) in patients after bone marrow transplantation. Transplantation 1987;44:381-386.

132. Fox R, McMillan R, Spruce W, Tani P, Mason D, and the Scripps Clinic Bone Marrow Transplantation Team: Analysis of T lymphocytes after bone marrow transplantation using monoclonal antibodies. Blood 1982;60:578-582.

133. Daley JP, Rozans MK, Smith BR, Burakoff SJ, Rappeport JM, Miller RA: Retarded recovery of functional T cell frequencies in T cell-depleted bone marrow transplant recipients. Blood 1987;70:960-964.

134. Reinherz EL, Parkman R, Rappeport J, Rosen FS, Schlossman SF: Aberrations of suppressor T cells in human graft-versus-host disease. N Engl J Med 1979;300: 1061-1068.

135. Verdonck LF, de Gast GC: Is cytomegalovirus infection a major cause of T cell alterations after (autologous) bone-marrow transplantation? Lancet 1984;1:932-935.

136. Buckner CD, Stewart PS, Bensinger W, Clift R, Appelbaum F, Martin P, Sanders J, Fefer A, Lum L, Storb R, Hill R, Thomas ED: Critical issues in autologous marrow transplantation for hematologic malignancies. In *Recent Advances in Bone Marrow Transplantation*, edited by Gale RP. New York, Alan R. Liss, Inc. 1983; pp. 599-613.

137. Uchiyama T, Broder S, Waldmann T: A monoclonal antibody (anti-TAC) reactive with activated and functionally mature human T cells. I. Production of anti-TAC monoclonal antibody and distribution of TAC(+) cells. J Immunol 1981; 126:1393-1398.

138. Uchiyama T, Nelson DL, Fleisher TA, Waldmann TA: A monoclonal antibody (anti-TAC) reactive with activated and functionally mature human T cells. II. Expression of TAC antigen on activated cytotoxic killer T cells, suppressor cells, and on one of two types of helper T cells. J Immunol 1981;126:1398-1403.

139. Anderson MJ, Rappeport JM, Ault KA, Burakoff SJ, Smith BR: Clinical correlates of unusual circulating lymphocytes appearing post marrow transplantation (BMT). Blood 1985;66(Suppl):251a (abstr).

140. Witherspoon RP, Matthew D, Storb R, Atkinson K, Cheever M, Deeg HJ, Doney J, Kalbfleisch J, Noel D, Prentice R, Sullivan KM, Thomas ED: Recovery of in vivo

cellular immunity after human marrow grafting. Transplantation 1984;37:145-150.

141. Rozans MK, Smith BR, Emerson S, Crimmins M, Laurent G, Teichert T, Burakoff SJ, Miller RA: Functional assessment of T cell depletion from bone marrow prior to therapeutic transplantation using limiting dilution culture methods. Transplantation 1986;42:380-387.

142. Ringdén O, Witherspoon R, Storb R, Ekelund E, Thomas ED: B cell function in human marrow transplant recipients assessed by direct and indirect hemolysis-in-gel assays. J Immunol 1979;123:2729-2734.

143. Ringdén O, Witherspoon RP, Storb R, Ekelund E, Thomas ED: Increased in vitro B-cell IgG secretion during acute graft-versus-host disease and infection. Observations in 50 human marrow transplant recipients. Blood 1980;55:179-186.

144. Brenner MK, Reittie JE, Grob J-P, Wimperis JZ, Stephens S, Patterson J, Hoffbrand AV, Prentice HG: The contribution of large granular lymphocytes to B cell activation and differentiation after T-cell-depleted allogeneic bone marrow transplantation. Transplantation 1986;42:257-261.

145. Miller G, Burkeholder S, Stone MJ, Fay JW: Immune recovery after intensive Thio-TEPA chemotherapy compared to cyclophosphamide-total body radiotherapy and autologous marrow transplantation for neoplastic disease. Blood 1987;70 (Suppl 1):312a (abstr).

146. Sullivan KM, Kopecky K, Jocom J, Buckner CD, Counts G, Meyers JD, Petersen FB, Bowden R, Witherspoon RP, Storb R, Thomas ED: Antimicrobial and immunomodulatory effects of intravenous immunoglobulin in bone marrow transplantation. Blood 1988;72(Suppl 1):392a (abstr).

147. Witherspoon RP, Schanfield MS, Storb R, Thomas ED, Giblett ER; Immunoglobulin production of donor origin after marrow transplantation for acute leukemia or aplastic anemia. Transplantation 1978;26:407-408.

148. Starling KA, Falletta JM, Fernbach DJ: Immunologic chimerism as evidence of bone marrow graft acceptance in an identical twin with acute lymphocytic leukemia. Exp Hematol 1975;3:244-248.

149. Antin JH, Ault KA, Rappeport JM, Smith BR: B lymphocyte reconstitution after bone marrow transplantation. Leu 1 antigen defines a distinct population of B lymphocytes. J Clin Invest 1987;80:325-331.

150. Lum LG: A review: The kinetics of immune reconstitution after human marrow transplantation. Blood 1987;69:369-380.

151. Elfenbein GJ, Bellis MM, Ravlin HM, Santos GW: Phenotypically immature Bu cells in the peripheral blood after bone marrow grafting in man. Exp Hematol 1982;10:551-559.

152. Kagan JM, Champlin RE, Saxon A: B-cell dysfunction following human marrow transplantation: Functional-phenotypic dissociation in the early posttransplant period. Blood 1989;74:777.

153. Witherspoon RP, Lum LG, Storb R, Thomas ED: In vitro regulation of immunoglobulin synthesis after human marrow transplantation. II. Deficient T and non-T lymphocyte function with 3-4 months of allogeneic, syngeneic, or autologous marrow grafting for hematologic malignancy. Blood 1982;59:844-850.

154. Keever CA, Small TN, Flomenberg N, Heller G, Pekle K, Black P, Pecora A, Gillio A, Kernan NA, O'Reilly RJ: Immune reconstitution following bone marrow transplantation: Comparison of recipients of T cell-depleted marrow with recipients of conventional marrow grafts. Blood 1989;73:1340-1350.

155. Graze PR, Gale RP: Chronic graft versus host disease: A syndrome of disordered immunity. Am J Med 1979;66:611-620.

156. Saurat JH, Didier-Jean L, Gluckman E, Bussel A: Graft-versus-host reaction and lichen planus-like eruption in man. Br J Dermatol 1975;92:591-592.

157. Tsoi M-S, Storb R, Jones E, Weiden PL, Shulman H, Witherspoon RP, Atkinson K, Thomas ED: Deposition of IgM and complement at the dermoepidermal junction in acute and chronic graft-versus-host disease in man. J Immunol 1978;120:1485-1492.

158. Sullivan KM, Shulman HM, Storb R, Weiden PL, Shulman H, Witherspoon RP, Atkinson K, Thomas ED: Chronic graft-versus-host disease in 52 patients: Adverse natural course and successful treatment with combination immunosuppression. Blood 1981;57:267-276.

159. Shulman HM, Sullivan KM, Weiden PL, McDonald GB, Striker GE, Sale GE, Hackman R, Tsoi MS, Storb R, Thomas ED: Chronic graft-versus-host syndrome in man. A long-term clinicopathological study of 20 Seattle patients. Am J Med 1980;69:204-217.

160. Lawley TJ, Peck GL, Moutsopoulous HM, Gratwohl AA, Deisseroth AB: Scleroderma, Sjögren-like syndrome, and chronic graft-versus-host disease. Ann Intern Med 1977;87:707-709.

161. Sullivan KM, Storb R, Witherspoon R, Shulman H, Deeg HJ, Schubert M, Doney K, Appelbaum R, Tsoi MS, Sale G, Sanders J, McDonald G, Thomas ED: Biology and treatment of chronic graft-versus-host disease. In *Recent Advances in Bone Marrow Transplantation*, edited by Gale RP. Alan R Liss, Inc., New York, 1983; pp. 331-342.

162. Schulman HM, Sale GE, Lerner KG, Barker EA, Weiden PL, Sullivan K, Gallucci B, Thomas ED, Storb R: Chronic cutaneous graft-versus-host disease in man. Am J Pathol 1978;91:545-570.

163. Sullivan KM: Acute and chronic graft-versus-host disease in man. Int J Cell Cloning 1986;4(Suppl 1):42-93.

164. Tsoi M-S, Storb R, Dobbs S, Medill L, Thomas ED: Cell-mediated immunity to non-HLA antigens of the host by donor lymphocytes in patients with chronic graft-vs-host disease. J Immunol 1980;125:2258-2262.

165. Storb R, Prentice RL, Sullivan KM, Schulman HM, Deeg HJ, Doney KC, Buckner CD, Clift RA, Witherspoon RP, Appelbaum FA, Sanders JE, Stewart PS, Thomas ED: Predictive factors in chronic graft-versus-host disease in patients with aplastic anemia treated by marrow transplantation from HLA-identical siblings. Ann Intern Med 1983;98:461-466.

166. Tsoi M-S, Storb R, Weiden P, Santos E, Kopecky KJ, Thomas ED: Sequential studies of cell inhibition of host fibroblasts in 51 patients given HLA-identical marrow grafts. J Immunol 1982;128:239-242.

167. Tsoi M-S, Storb R, Dobbs S, Kopecky KJ, Santos E, Weiden PL, Thomas ED: Nonspecific suppressor cells in patients with chronic graft-vs-host disease after marrow grafting. J Immunol 1979;123:1970-1976.

168. Tsoi M-S, Storb R, Dobbs S, Thomas ED: Specific suppressor cells in graft-host tolerance of HLA-identical marrow transplantation. Nature 1981;292:355-357.

169. Atkinson K, Farewell V, Storb R, Tsoi MS, Sullivan KM, Witherspoon RP, Fefer A, Clift R, Goodell B, Thomas ED: Analysis of late infections after human bone marrow transplantation: Role of genotypic nonidentity between marrow donor and recipient and of nonspecific suppressor cells in patients with chronic graft-versus-host disease. Blood 1982;60:714-720.

170. Harada M, Ueda M, Nakao S, Kondo K, Odaka K, Shiobara S, Matsue K, Mori T, Matsuda T, and the Kanazawa University Bone Marrow Transplant Team: Nonspecific suppressor T cells cause decreased mixed lymphocyte culture reactivity in bone marrow transplant patients. J Immunol 1986;137:428-432.

171. Agosti JM, Sprenger JD, Lum LG, Witherspoon RP, Fisher LD, Storb R, Henderson WR: Transfer of allergen-specific IgE-mediated hypersensitivity with bone marrow transplantation. N Engl J Med 1988;319:1623-1628.

172. Lum LG, Seigneuret MC, Orcutt-Thordarson N, Ostenson RC, Storb R: Immuno-globulin production after marrow transplantation. III. The functional heterogeneity of Fc-IgG receptor positive and negative T cell subpopulations. Clin Exp Immunol 1982;48:675-684.

173. Lum LG, Seigneuret MC, Orcutt-Thordarson N, Noges JE, Storb R: The regulation of immunoglobulin synthesis after HLA-identical bone marrow transplantation: VI. Differential rates of maturation of distinct functional groups within lymphoid subpopulations in patients after human marrow grafting. Blood 1985;65:1422-1433.

174. Lum LG, Seigneuret MC, Orcutt-Thordarson N, Froelich TL, Storb R: Functional diversity in OKT4 and OKT8 subsets from long-term survivors after HLA-identical marrow grafting. Diagn Immunol 1983;1:179-187.

175. Muraguchi A, Fauci AS: Proliferative responses of normal human B lymphocytes: Development of an assay system for B cell growth factor (BCGF). J Immunol 1982;129:1104-1108.

176. Jelinek DF, Lipsky PE: The roles of T cells in activation, cell cycle progression, and differentiation of human B cells. J Immunol 1985;134:1690-1701.

177. Howard M, Paul WE: Regulation of B cell growth and differentiation by soluble factors. Ann Rev Immunol 1983;1:307-333.

178. Matsue K, Lum LG, Storb R: Effect of recombinant interleukin 2 (rIL2) on B cell responses in marrow transplant recipients. Int Soc Exp Hemat 1987;15:473 (abstr).

179. Wahren B, Gahrton G, Linde A, Ljungman P, Lonnqvist B, Ringdén O, Sundqvist V-A: Transfer and persistence of viral antibody-producing cells in bone marrow transplantation. J Infect Dis 1984;150:358-365.

180. Ljungman P, Lonnqvist B, Gahrton G, Ringdén O, Wahren B: Cytomegalovirus-specific lymphocyte proliferation and in vitro cytomegalovirus IgG synthesis for diagnosis of cytomegalovirus infections after bone marrow transplantation. Blood 1986;68:108-112.

181. Smith CIE, Aarli JA, Biberfeld P, Bolme P, Christensson B, Gahrton G, Hammarstrom L, Lefvert AK, Lonnqvist B, Matell G, Priskanen R, Ringdén O, Svanborg E: Myasthenia gravis after bone-marrow transplantation. N Engl J Med 1983;309:1565-1568.

182. Kodo H, Gale RP, Saxon A: Antibody synthesis by bone marrow cells in vitro following primary and booster tetanus toxoid immunizations in humans. J Clin Invest 1984;73:1377-1384.

37

Effects of Chronic Graft-vs.-Host Disease on Growth and Development

Jean E. Sanders
Fred Hutchinson Cancer Research Center
University of Washington School of Medicine
Seattle, Washington

I. INTRODUCTION

Since the first marrow transplants were performed in the early 1970s, the success of this procedure has steadily improved (1). The use of this therapeutic technique for a large number of children and young adults with malignant and nonmalignant hematologic disorders has resulted in an ever increasing number of long-term survivors. When an HLA-identical sibling donor is available for the young patient with aplastic anemia, marrow transplantation is the treatment of choice (2-11). For some patients with hematologic malignancies, marrow transplantation results in an improved disease-free survival compared to conventional treatment (12-32), and it represents the only possible cure for children with severe immune deficiency disorders, thalassemia major, or some metabolic diseases (33-39). As autologous marrow transplantation is used more frequently (40), and the pool of suitable marrow donors is expanded to include related and unrelated individuals who are partially or fully HLA matched with the recipient (41-44), the ability to use this procedure for an even larger number of patients will further increase its application.

The agents used in marrow transplant preparative regimens are designed to suppress the patient's immune system and eradicate the underlying disorder. These agents commonly include high dose cyclophosphamide (CY) given alone or in combination with other chemotherapy agents, such as busulfan (BU), or in combination with total body irradiation (TBI) or total lymphoid irradiation (TLI). These treatment modalities are likely to have an impact on endocrine function. In children the secretions of the endocrine glands act as catalysts to the normal growth potential of the body (45). Some are growth-promoting, such as pituitary growth-stimulating hormone and androgens. Others, such as thyroid hormone, androgens, and estrogens, promote maturation. The adrenal glucocorticoids are antagonistic to growth. Since normal growth and development require a balance of these hormones, it may be anticipated that abnormal hormone function will affect subsequent growth and development of children and young adults.

As described in other chapters of this book, chronic Graft-vs.-Host Disease (GVHD) is a systemic disorder which affects multiple organ systems. It has features of a number of autoimmune diseases and requires prolonged treatment with immunosuppressive agents, often with glucocorticoids, to control its manifestations. The young child requires normal function of all organs and normal metabolism in order for optimal growth to occur. When there is significant major organ dysfunction, such as liver, kidney, or pulmonary insufficiencies, normal growth is precluded due to impairment of tissue metabolism in all parts of the body. In the growing child, when this constellation of disorders is added to the endocrine dysfunction which may occur following the preparative regimen, abnormal or subnormal growth and development may be expected.

This chapter will review the late effects of the transplant preparative regimens and the effects of chronic GVHD and its treatment on the subsequent growth and development of children after marrow transplantation.

II. PREPARATIVE REGIMENS

The chemotherapy given prior to marrow transplantation must be immunosuppressive enough to permit engraftment. When CY only is given, doses of 200 mg/kg are needed to achieve adequate immunosuppression and engraftment (2-10). This regimen is often given to patients with aplastic anemia as 50 mg/kg/day for 4 consecutive days. Patients with other nonmalignant hematologic disorders, such as thalassemia major or Wiscott-Aldrich disease, require more aggressive marrow ablation to eliminate the abnormal clone and provide adequate immunosuppression. This has most recently been achieved with the use of BU, 14-16 mg/kg total dose given in divided doses over 4 days and followed by CY, 200 mg/kg (33-35). Children with metabolic disorders have required BU, 20 mg/kg total dose and 240 mg/kg of CY (38,39). Current survival figures show that 60-80% of children transplanted for nonmalignant hematologic diseases become long-term disease-free survivors.

Marrow transplant preparative regimens for the majority of patients with malignant hematologic disorders and solid tumors have included high dose CY or high dose cytosine arabinoside or etoposide with TBI (12-33). The doses of chemotherapy and TBI used in these regimens must be high enough to suppress the patient's immune system and also destroy the patient's underlying malignant disorder without producing unacceptable non-marrow organ toxicity. TBI has been given in various ways with dose rates ranging from 5-26 rads/min. The most common ways of administering TBI are either in single exposure doses of 750-1000 rads, or fractionated exposures over 3 to 7 consecutive days for total doses of 1200-1600 rads. Some preparative regimens for patients with nonmalignant hematologic disorders include only 200-300 rads of TBI, others 750 rads of TLI (4,5,11). For patients with hematologic malignancies, current survival figures vary between 15% and 70%, depending on the stage of the malignancy at the time of transplantation.

In addition to the irradiation given during the marrow transplant preparative regimen, many children have previously received cranial, cranio-spinal, or testicular irradiation. Although the chemotherapy these children have received prior to transplantation has not been demonstrated to adversely effect growth, cranial irradiation and cranio-spinal irradiation have been associated with growth hormone (GH) deficiency and decreased spinal growth (46-48). Testicular irradiation has produced testicular function abnormalities (49).

Table 1 Thyroid Function After Marrow Transplantation

Preparative regimen	TSH (% abnormal)	T4 (% abnormal)	Years follow-up (median)	Reference
CY	1/50 (2%)	1/50 (2%)	9	56
BU, CY	0/100 (0%)	0/100 (0%)	3	57
CY, 750 rads TLI	13/37 (35%)	3/37 (85)	4	11
CY, 1000 rads TBI	19/67 (28%)	9/67 (13%)	8	56,58
CY, 1000 rads TBI	10/23 (56%)	2/23 (9%)	3	59
CY, 1000 rads TBI	14/28 (50%)	0/28 (0%)	2	60
CY, 1200–1575 rads TBI	13/113 (12%)	3/113 (3%)	4	56,58
1320 rads TBI, CY	4/19 (21%)	0/19 (0%)	3	61

Abbreviations: TSH = Thyroid stimulating-hormone; T4 = thyroxine; CY - cyclophosphamide; BU = busulfan. TLI = total lymphoid irradiation; TBI = total body irradiation.

III. THYROID FUNCTION

Little is known about the effects of chemotherapy on thyroid function, but irradiation to the thyroid gland has been associated with development of compensated (covert) hypothyroidism, overt hypothyroidism, thyroiditis, and thyroid neoplasms (50-55). After irradiation the onset of thyroid dysfunction usually begins as asymptomatic compensated hypothyroidism within the first year in 31-53% of children and progresses to overt hypothyroidism in 6-25% over the next 5-10 years. Untreated compensated hypothyroidism may be a factor in the development of neoplastic thyroid disease after irradiation (55). Hypothyroidism also contributes to diminished linear growth.

Thyroid function including levels of thyroid stimulating hormone (TSH) and thyroxine (T4) has been determined in long-term surviving patients after transplantation (Table 1). Among the 50 patients with aplastic anemia who were prepared with CY, only one patient developed abnormal thyroid function (56). This idiopathic thyroiditis occurred in a 14-year-old boy 10 years after marrow transplant. This patient was one of 20 who previously had chronic GVHD. The 1% incidence of idiopathic thyroiditis in normal school age children is similar to that observed after CY. It is not possible to determine whether the development of this patient's thyroiditis is related to his previous chronic GVHD. Similar thyroid function studies have been performed in 100 patients after BU and CY preparative regimens and transplantation for thalassemia major. All patients had normal TSH and T4 levels before and after transplantation (57).

Among 37 children and young adults surviving after high dose CY and 750 rads single exposure TLI, 13 (35%) have developed compensated hypothyroidism with elevated TSH and normal T4 levels (Table 1) (11). Primary hypothyroidism occurred in 3 of the 37 (8%). Following marrow transplant preparative regimens containing TBI, thyroid dysfunction has been reported to occur in 12-56% of children (56,58-61). The highest incidence has been observed among patients receiving 1000 rads single exposure TBI, with 28-56% of children reported to have elevated TSH. Patients who received fractionated exposure TBI have lower incidences of abnormal thyroid function: 12-21% of patients develop elevated TSH, but only 3% have overt hypothyroidism with elevated TSH and low T4 levels. No series has found the development of these thyroid function abnormalities to be related to the presence of chronic GVHD.

IV. ADRENOCORTICAL FUNCTION

Long-term effects of chemotherapy or irradiation (or both) to the adrenal glands have not been reported for children receiving conventional treatments. Subnormal stimulated cortisol levels have been observed after central nervous system prophylaxis (62). The ACTH and cortisol responses after insulin stimulation have been normal in 50 children transplanted following TBI containing regimens (60,61). Plasma 11-desoxycortisol (Compound S) levels have been measured after metyrapone stimulation in 140 children who received marrow transplantation following CY only or high-dose chemotherapy and TBI (56,58). Although this single test did not permit discrimination between primary and secondary adrenal insufficiency, subnormal 11-desoxycortisol levels were found in 4% of patients receiving CY only and in 8-16% of patients receiving single or fractionated exposure TBI, respectively. These differences were not statistically significant. Similarly, there was no correlation with patient age, sex, previous cranial irradiation, or chronic GVHD.

V. GROWTH HORMONE AND GROWTH VELOCITY

Central nervous system irradiation has been associated with growth hormone (GH) deficiency, deficiency of growth hormone releasing factor, or both (46,47). The incidence of this appears to be related to the child's age and the total irradiation dose given (62-65). A dose of more than 3000 rads to the pituitary has been estimated to be the threshold for impairment of GH production. Among children receiving similar doses of cranial irradiation, results of GH production studies differ (66). This may be due to the use of various GH stimuli, the presence of growth hormone releasing factor deficiency, or variations in time intervals between irradiation and GH determinations. Both normal and subnormal growth rates have been observed. Among these patients, inconsistent responses to treatment with exogenous GH have been noted (63,67,68). In general, children surviving long term after leukemia treatment that did not include cranial irradiation have growth rates that are normal or near normal (69,70). Irradiation of growing bones produces epiphyseal, metaphyseal and diaphyseal injury which affects bone growth (71). The degree of impairment is related to patient age, site irradiated, total dose, and dose schedule received (72). The severity of the effect appears to increase with increasing irradiation dose, lengthening postirradiation interval and younger age at time of treatment. Doses of 1500-4400 rads to the entire spine result in suppression of spinal growth.

Following marrow transplant preparative regimens that utilized CY only or BU with CY, normal growth rates have been observed, but GH levels have rarely been determined (56,57). When tested, these children always had normal GH levels. Some children with chronic GVHD did have a lower growth velocity rate during the time of chronic GVHD therapy. This, however, reverted to normal, and catch-up growth occurred once the chronic GVHD was controlled and therapy was stopped.

GH levels have been determined following insulin, arginine, or L-dopa in at least 132 children who had received transplant preparative regimens containing TBI (56,58,60,61, 73,74). Overall 73 of the 132 (55%) had subnormal GH production. GH deficiency was present in 80-90% of those who had received previous cranial irradiation, but was found in less than half of those who had not received cranial irradiation prior to TBI. Growth velocity was less than normal for age in all patients. During the first 2 years after TBI, patients without chronic GVHD grew significantly better than those with chronic GVHD (58). Patients with chronic GVHD who also had previous cranial irradiation had the poorest growth rates. These patients did not demonstrate catch-up growth after treatment was stopped and chronic GVHD was no longer active. This observation may be explained by the growth-suppressive effects of glucocorticoids (75). Failure to achieve catch-up growth after completion of treatment, however, suggests that other factors, such as GH deficiency and irradiation effects on long bones, contribute to the decreased growth rates. Chronic GVHD abnormalities of liver, and kidney abnormalities secondary to cyclosporine therapy for chronic GVHD, may decrease the production of somatomedin C, a growth hormone dependent serum factor synthesized in these organs. No data are yet available regarding somatomedin C levels in patients with chronic GVHD either during or following treatment. Therapy with GH has been given to more than 25 patients. Patients have improved growth velocity with treatment, but the improvement in growth rates has been less than usually observed in nonirradiated GH-deficient children.

VI. PUBERTAL DEVELOPMENT

A. Chemotherapy

Significant effects on gonadal hormone production and germ cell viability have been observed after treatment for malignancy (76-80). Variables which are important include patient sex, type of therapy (irradiation or chemotherapy), dosage and duration of treatment, age, and sexual maturity. Most chemotherapy treated childhood leukemia survivors have normal pubertal progression and reproductive function. Elevated serum follicle stimulating hormone (FSH) levels and abnormal testicular histology have been observed in boys given CY prior to or during puberty (81). The germinal epithelium of the prepubertal testes is susceptible to cytotoxic-induced damage resulting in aplasia, higher serum FSH levels and abnormal testicular histology. Doses >350 mg/kg of CY have resulted in azoospermia; doses >14 g have resulted in permanent sterility; doses of 200 mg/kg or less result in minimal alteration of spermatogenesis. Primary ovarian failure has been reported following administration of more than 500 mg/kg CY to prepubertal girls (76,79,82).

Thirty-five children (20 girls and 15 boys) who were prepubertal when given 200 mg/kg of CY and transplantation for aplastic anemia are now more than 12 years of age and evaluable for onset of puberty (Table 2) (56,58). Normal development of secondary sexual characteristics occurred in 33 of these 35 (94%). Among the 20 girls, menarche occurred between 11 and 16 (median 13) years of age in 19; one girl had primary ovarian failure. The 19 who developed normally had normal gonadotropin levels. The one who did not had elevated FSH and luteinizing hormone (LH) levels as well as low estradiol levels and received estrogen/progesterone supplementation. Two of the 19 girls have married and had one normal child each. Semen analysis in 7 of the 15 boys demon-

Table 2 Pubertal Development After Transplantation

Preparative regimen	Patients with no chronic GVHD		Patients with chronic GVHD
Cyclophosphamide[a]			
Prepubertal at transplant	35		9
current age ≥ 13 years	28		7
development:			
normal	27		6
delayed	1	p = N.S.	1
Total Body Irradiation[b]			
prepubertal at transplant	95		47
current age ≥ 13 years	46		26
development:			
normal	26		5
delayed	20	p = 0.004	21

[a]From Ref. 56.
[b]From Refs. 56 and 58.

strated normal sperm counts in 5 and azoospermia in 2. Gonadotropin levels were normal in all boys. One of these young men has fathered a child. Nine girls and 4 boys have been evaluated for pubertal development following the transplant preparative regimen containing BU and CY (57). All of these patients had elevated gonadotropin levels, suggesting that it is BU alone, or when it is combined with CY that results in greater gonadal damage than CY alone. Chronic GVHD did not influence pubertal development in either the CY patients or the BU/CY patients.

B. Irradiation

Irradiation of the prepubertal gonad has been studied in boys (83). If irradiation is given while the boys are still prepubertal, little change in gonadotropin levels is observed. After the child attains puberty, however, irradiation results in both germinal epithelial and Leydig cell damage with elevated FSH and LH levels and decreased testosterone levels. Prepubertal boys who have been given 2400 rads testicular irradiation have delayed development of secondary sexual characteristics and elevated gonadotropin levels with low testosterone values (49,84). The effect of irradiation on the prepubertal ovary has not been carefully studied. In the postpubertal young female, studies have suggested that the dose of irradiation necessary to produce permanent sterility is related to patient age (77).

Following TBI, 41 girls who were prepubertal at the time of transplant and were followed until they were more than 12 years of age were evaluable for pubertal development (56,58,60,61). Delayed development was observed in 27 (66%). All of these girls had primary ovarian failure with elevated FSH and LH levels and low estradiol levels. They have needed therapy with estrogen and progesterone for secondary sex characteristic development. The girls who did develop normally all achieved menarche between the ages of 11 and 15 years and all had normal gonadotropin and estradiol levels. Similarly, 31 of 52 (60%) evaluable boys had delayed or absent development of puberty (56,58,60,61). Gonadotropin levels and testosterone levels were normal in those boys whose development was normal, but in all boys where development was delayed, gonadotropin levels were either elevated or prepubertal, and testosterone levels were low for age. Boys who had received additional testicular irradiation all had primary testicular failure with markedly elevated LH and FSH and very low testosterone levels. Thus, the incidence of gonadal failure was similar for both sexes; the majority will have delay in onset and progression of development of puberty. No difference was observed with respect to gonadal failure and the type of TBI administered. A summary of the only series comparing development of children with and without chronic GVHD is shown in Table 2 (56,58). Delayed development was significantly more frequent among patients who had chronic GVHD (21 of 26) compared to patients who did not have chronic GVHD (20 of 46) (p = 0.004).

VII. GONADAL FUNCTION POST-PUBERTY

A. Chemotherapy

Treatment with alkylating agents in adult women may impair reproductive function (85). Ovarian atrophy has been noted following treatment with BU (86). Results of ovarian biopsies in women who received CY demonstrate a loss of ova, suggesting that CY acts directly on the oocyte (87). The potential reversibility of this loss is related to the age of the patient and the total dose of CY received. The number of oocytes normally decreases steadily with age. Since the alkylating agents act by first order kinetics, equivalent drug doses in older patients whose ova are more depleted than those of younger patients may explain why the likelihood of infertility is increased in older women. A total dose of 5.2 gm CY given to a 40-year old woman will result in ovarian failure, whereas a total dose of 20 gm given to women less than 30 years of age is needed to produce ovarian failure (76). An evaluation of 49 women transplanted following CY demonstrated that all developed amenorrhea after transplant (88-92). All 33 patients who were between the ages of 13 and 26 years at transplant had ovarian function recovery 3 to 42 months after 200 mg/kg CY and transplantation. Of the 16 who were between 26 and 38 years of age, 5 recovered ovarian function, 4 had transient recovery of ovarian function, and 7 developed primary ovarian failure. The women who recovered ovarian function had normal FSH, LH, and estradiol levels. Nine of thse women have had 12 pregnancies, which resulted in 8 live births. Statistical analysis demonstrated that increasing patient age was the only factor significantly associated with development of ovarian failure (89). Chronic GVHD, which may affect vaginal mucosa, was not a factor associated with ovarian recovery or fertility after CY.

The predominant gonadal lesion after alkylating agent therapy in the adult male is localized to the germinal epithelium (76). Germinal aplasia, absent spermatogonia and spermatozoa have been noted in biopsy specimens from male patients treated with CY (93,94). This lesion usually produces an elevated FSH level and azoospermia with LH and testosterone levels remaining normal. Age is not a factor in development of this testicular compromise, but total dose of CY received is. Patients who receive more than 18 gm CY total dose develop azoospermia, but those who receive less than 250 mg/kg of CY given in low doses of CY for short periods of time develop oligospermia which is often reversible (95). However, recovery of spermatogenesis may occur after a period of a year or more after discontinuation of CY. Evaluation of testicular function in 53 men surviving more than one year after CY shows that nearly all have normal LH and testosterone levels, and 32 of the 53 have normal FSH levels (88,96). Semen analyses have been performed on only a few of these men, but 17 of 26 evaluated had normal sperm counts and motility. Ten of these men have fathered 11 children.

B. Irradiation

Impairment of ovarian function following irradiation to the ovary is related to the age of the woman at time of irradiation, or more precisely, the number of oocytes remaining at the time of irradiation (97). In women less than 40 years of age, doses of 800 rads result in 70% of the women becoming permanently sterilized. Fractionated irradiation doses of up to 2000 rads result in more than 50% of women 20-30 years of age developing ovarian failure. Following marrow transplant regimens containing 750 rads TLI administered in a single exposure or TBI administered in single exposures of 1000 rads or fractionated exposures of 1200-1575 rads, 139 women developed primary ovarian failure with elevated FSH and LH levels and low estradiol levels. Five women, all less than 26 years old at time of irradiation, had recovering ovarian function 3-4 years after 1200 rads fractionated TBI (88,89). Their LH, FSH, and estradiol levels all returned to normal. One of two women less than 26 years old at time of CY and TLI administration also had ovarian function recovery (96). Statistical analysis demonstrated that patient age and receiving 1200 rads fractionated TBI were factors associated with recovery (89). Chronic GVHD did not influence ovarian function recovery. More than half of the women with primary ovarian failure had symptoms of menopause with vasomotor instability, insomnia, osteoporosis, vaginitis, and vaginal atrophy. In addition, women with chronic GVHD developed vaginal strictures and webs secondary to vaginal involvement by chronic GVHD. Treatment with cyclic estrogen and progesterone controlled the menopause symptoms. Vaginal dilatation and control of chronic GVHD were needed in addition to systemic hormone therapy for the women with chronic GVHD. In rare cases, the webs across the vaginal opening were complete and needed to be surgically removed.

In the adult male, the magnitude and duration of irradiation effects on spermatogenesis depend upon the total dose received (77). Doses as low as 200 rads produce germinal epithelial damage resulting in decreased sperm counts and elevated FSH levels (98-100). Leydig cell damage usually does not occur until higher doses of irradiation and even then the testosterone levels remain normal. After doses of 200-300 rads, FSH levels and sperm counts have returned to normal after approximately 3 years, but after doses of 400-600 rads, 5 or more years are needed before testicular function returns to normal. When irradiation is administered in fractionated exposures, the effect may be more profound than when it is administered as a single exposure (101). The total irradiation dose above which recovery never occurs has not been firmly established, but few patients have been documented to have recovery above doses of 800 rads. Following TBI and marrow transplantation, 114 men have been evaluated at intervals of 1-14 years. They all demonstrated normal testosterone levels, 80% had normal LH levels, and 21% had normal FSH levels (88,96). Semen analysis showed no sperm in 62 of 64 men who submitted samples. Two men did have sperm counts of more than 15 million/ml, but not until more than 6 years after TBI. One of these men has fathered 3 normal children. Chronic GVHD did not influence testicular function.

VIII. SUMMARY

These evaluations of growth and development demonstrate that the development of endocrine function abnormalities which may influence growth and development rarely occur after preparative regimens with CY only. The impact of chronic GVHD for these children and young adults is not great with respect to growth since once the chronic GVHD is controlled and treatment stopped, normal catch-up growth takes place. Chronic GVHD does not impact upon the ability of these children to mature or to have gonadal function recovery after transplant. However, after regimens containing TBI, multiple endocrine functional abnormalities may occur. Abnormalities which are not influenced by chronic GVHD are thyroid function and adrenal function. Longitudinal growth velocity and development of puberty are influenced not only by TBI, but also by the presence of chronic GVHD and perhaps also by its treatment. Chronic GVHD treatment regimens which utilize immunosuppressive therapy other than glucocorticoids are needed to differentiate between the negative influence of therapy and underlying chronic GVHD on growth and development. All of these children must be followed carefully in order to detect the endocrine abnormalities and to initiate appropriate hormone supplementation which may allow for improved growth and development.

ACKNOWLEDGMENT

This investigation was supported by PHS grant Numbers HL36444 awarded by the National Heart, Lung and Blood Institute, CA 18029, CA 26828, CA 18221, CA 09515, and CA 15704 awarded by the National Cancer Institute, DHHS.

REFERENCES

1. Bortin MM, Rimm AA: Increasing utilization of bone marrow transplantation. Transplantation 1986;42(Suppl 3):229-234.
2. Camitta BM, Thomas ED, Nathan DG, Gale RP, Kopecky KJ, Rappeport JM, Santos G, Gordon-Smith EC, Storb R: A prospective study of androgens and bone marrow transplantation for treatment of severe aplastic anemia. Blood 1979;53:504-514.
3. Storb R, Thomas ED, Weiden PL, Buckner CD, Clift RA, Fefer A, Fernando LP, Giblett ER, Goodell BW, Johnson FL, Lerner KG, Neiman PE, Sanders JE: Aplastic anemia treated by allogeneic bone marrow transplantation: A report on 49 new cases from Seattle. Blood 1976;48:817-841.
4. UCLA Bone Marrow Transplant Team: Bone-marrow transplantation in severe aplastic anemia, Lancet 1976;ii:921-923.
5. Bortin MM, Gale RP, Rimm AA for the Advisory Committee of the International Bone Marrow Transplant Registry: Allogeneic bone marrow transplantation for 144 patients with severe aplastic anemia. JAMA 1981;245:1132-1139.
6. Storb R, Thomas ED, Buckner CD, Clift RA, Deeg HJ, Fefer A, Goodell BW, Sale GE, Sanders JE, Singer J, Stewart P, Weiden PL: Marrow transplantation in thirty "untransfused" patients with severe aplastic anemia. Ann Intern Med 1980;92:30-36.
7. Storb R, Doney KC, Thomas ED, Appelbaum F, Buckner CD, Clift RA, Deeg HJ, Goodell BW, Hackman R, Hansen JA, Sanders J, Sullivan K, Weiden PL, Witherspoon RP: Marrow transplantation with or without donor buffy coat cells for 65 transfused aplastic anemia patients. Blood 1982;59:236-246.
8. Elfenbein GJ, Mellits ED, Santos GW for the Johns Hopkins Bone Marrow Transplant Program: Engraftment and survival after allogeneic bone marrow transplantation for severe aplastic anemia. Transplant Proc 1983;15;1412-1416.
9. Storb R, Deeg HJ, Farewell V, Doney K, Appelbaum F, Beatty P, Bensinger W, Buckner CD, Clift R, Hansen J, Hill R, Longton G, Lum L, Martin P, McGuffin R, Sanders J, Singer J, Stewart P, Sullivan K, Witherspoon R, Thomas ED: Marrow transplantation for severe aplastic anemia: Methotrexate alone compared to a combination of methotrexate and cyclosporine for prevention of acute graft-versus-host disease. Blood 1986;68:119-125.
10. Sanders JE, Whitehead J, Storb R, Buckner CD, Clift RA, Mickelson E, Appelbaum FR, Bensinger WI, Stewart PS, Doney K, Sullivan K, Deeg HJ, Witherspoon RP, Thomas ED: Bone marrow transplantation experience for children with aplastic anemia. Pediatrics 1986;77:179-186.
11. McGlave PB, Haake R, Miller W, Kim T, Kersey J, Ramsay NKC: Therapy of severe aplastic anemia in young adults and children with allogeneic bone marrow transplantation. Blood 1987;70:1325-1330.
12. Thomas ED, Buckner CD, Banaji M, Clift RA, Fefer A, Flournoy N, Goodell BW, Hickman RO, Lerner KG, Neiman PE, Sale GE, Sanders JE, Singer J, Stevens M, Storb R, Weiden PL: One hundred patients with acute leukemia treated by chemotherapy, total body irradiation, and allogeneic marrow transplantation. Blood 1977;49:511-533.
13. Thomas ED, Sanders JE, Flournoy N, Johnson FL, Buckner CD, Clift RA, Fefer A, Goodell BW, Storb R, Weiden PL: Marrow transplantation for patients with acute lymphoblastic leukemia in remission. Blood 1979;54:468-476.
14. Johnson FL, Thomas ED, Clark BS, Chard RL, Hartmann JR, Storb R: A comparison of marrow transplantation with chemotherapy for children with acute lymphoblastic leukemia in second or subsequent remission. N Engl J Med 1981;305:846-851.

15. Woods WG, Nesbit ME, Ramsay NKC, Krivit W, Kim TH, Goldman A, McGlave PB, Kersey JH: Intensive therapy followed by bone marrow transplantation for patients with acute lymphoblastic leukemia in second or subsequent remission: Determination of prognostic factors (A report from the University of Minnesota Bone Marrow Transplant Team). Blood 1983;61:1182-1189.
16. Dinsmore R, Kirkpatrick D, Flomenberg N, Sulati S, Kapoor N, Shank B, Reid A, Groshen S, O'Reilly RJ: Allogeneic bone marrow transplantation for patients with acute lymphoblastic leukemia. Blood 1983,62:381-388.
17. Zwaan FE, Hermans J, Barrett AJ, Speck B: Bone marrow transplantation for acute lymphoblastic leukemia: A survey of the European group for bone marrow transplantation (E.G.B.M.T.). Br J Hematol 1984;58:33-42.
18. Sanders JE, Flournoy N, Thomas ED, Buckner CD, Lum LG, Clift RA, Appelbaum FR, Sullivan KM, Stewart P, Deeg HJ, Doney K, Storb R: Marrow transplant experience in children with acute lymphoblastic leukemia: An analysis of factors associated with survival, relapse and graft-versus-host disease. Med Pediatr Oncol 1985; 13:165-172.
19. Sanders JE, Thomas ED, Buckner CD, Doney K: Marrow transplantation for children with acute lymphoblastic leukemia in second remission (Concise Report). Blood 1987;70:324-326.
20. Brochstein JA, Kernan NA, Groshen S, Cirrincione C, Shank B, Emanuel D, Laver J, O'Reilly RJ: Allogeneic bone marrow transplantation after hyperfractionated total-body irradiation and cyclophosphamide in children with acute leukemia. N Engl J Med 1987,317:1618-1624.
21. Thomas ED, Buckner CD, Clift RA, Fefer A, Johnson FL, Neiman PE, Sale GE, Sanders JE, Singer JW, Shulman H, Storb R, Weiden PL: Marrow transplantation for acute nonlymphoblastic leukemia in first remission. N Engl J Med 1979;301:597-599.
22. Powles RL, Morgenstern G, Clink HM, Hedley D, Bandini G, Lumley H, Watson JG, Lawson D, Spence D, Barrett A, Jameson B, Lawler S, Kay HEM, McElwain TJ: The place of bone-marrow transplantation in acute myelogenous leukaemia. Lancet 1980,i:1047-1050.
23. Kersey JH, Ramsay NKC, Kim T, McGlave P, Krivit W, Levitt S, Filipovich A, Woods W, O'Leary M, Coccia P, Nesbit ME: Allogeneic bone marrow transplantation in acute nonlymphoblastic leukemia: A pilot study. Blood 1982;60:400-403.
24. Santos GW, Tutschka PJ, Brookmeyer R, Saral R, Beschorner WE, Bias WB, Braine HG, Burns WH, Elfenbein GJ, Kaizer H, Mellits D, Sensenbrenner LL, Stuart RK, Yeager AM: Marrow transplantation for acute nonlymphocytic leukemia after treatment with busulfan and cyclophosphamide. N Engl J Med 1983;309:1347-1353.
25. Dinsmore R, Kirkpatrick D, Blomenberg N, Gulati S, Kapoor N, Brockstein J, Shank B, Reid A, Groshen S, O'Reilly RJ: Allogeneic bone marrow transplantation for patients with acute non-lymphoblastic leukemia. Blood 1984;63:649-656.
26. Appelbaum FR, Dahlberg S, Thomas ED, Buckner CD, Cheever MA, Clift RA, Crowley J, Deeg HJ, Fefer A, Greenberg PD, Kadin M, Smith W, Stewart P, Sullivan K, Storb R, Weiden P: Bone marrow transplantation or chemotherapy after remission induction for adults with acute nonlymphoblastic leukemia–A prospective comparison. Ann Intern Med 1984;101:581-588.
27. Sanders JE, Thomas ED, Buckner CD, Flournoy N, Stewart PS, Clift RA, Lum L, Bensinger WI, Storb R, Appelbaum FR, Sullivan KM: Marrow transplantation for children in first remission of acute nonlymphoblastic leukemia: An update. Blood 1985,66:460-462.

28. Clift RA, Buckner CD, Thomas ED, Kopecky KJ, Appelbaum FR, Tallman M, Storb R, Sanders J, Sullivan K, Banaji M, Beatty PS, Bensinger W, Cheever M, Deeg J, Doney K, Fefer A, Greenberg P, Hansen JA, Hackman R, Hill R, Martin P, Meyers J, McGuffin R, Neiman P, Sale G, Shulman H, Singer J, Stewart P, Weiden P, Witherspoon R: The treatment of acute non-lymphoblastic leukemia by allogeneic marrow transplantation. Bone Marrow Transplantation 1987;2:243-258.

29. Thomas ED, Clift RA, Fefer A, Appelbaum FR, Beatty P, Bensinger WI, Buckner CD, Cheever MA, Deeg HJ, Doney K, Flournoy N, Greenberg P, Hansen JA, Martin P, McGuffin R, Ramberg R, Sanders JE, Singer J, Stewart P, Storb R, Sullivan K, Weiden PL, Witherspoon R: Marrow transplantation for the treatment of chronic myelogenous leukemia. Ann Intern Med 1986;104:155-163.

30. Sanders JE, Buckner CD, Thomas ED, Fleischer R, Sullivan KM, Appelbaum FR, Storb R: Allogeneic marrow transplantation for children with juvenile chronic myelogenous leukemia (Concise Report). Blood 1988;71:1144-1146.

31. Appelbaum FR, Storb R, Ramberg RE, Shulman HM, Buckner CD, Clift RA, Deeg HJ, Fefer A, Sanders J, Self S, Singer J, Stewart P, Sullivan K, Witherspoon R, Thomas ED: Treatment of preleukemic syndromes with marrow transplantation. Blood 1987;69:92-96.

32. Appelbaum FR, Sullivan KM, Buckner CD, Clift RA, Deeg HJ, Fefer A, Hill R, Mortimer J, Neiman PE, Sanders JE, Singer J, Stewart P, Storb R, Thomas ED: Treatment of malignant lymphoma in 100 patients with chemotherapy, total body irradiation and marrow transplantation. J Clin Oncol 1987;5:1340-1347.

33. Thomas ED, Buckner CD, Sanders JE, Papayannopoulou T, Borgna-Pignatti C, De Stefano P, Sullivan KM, Clift RA, Storb R: Marrow transplantation for thalassemia. Lancet 1982;ii:227-229.

34. Lucarelli G, Galimberti M, Izzi T, Delfini C, Manna M, Agostinelli F, Baronciani D, Giorgi C, Angelucci E, Giardini C, Politi P, Manenti F: Marrow transplantation for thalassemia following busulphan and cyclophosphamide. Lancet 1985;i;1355-1357.

35. Lucarelli G, Galimberti M, Polchi P, Angelucci E, Baronciani D, Giardini C, Manenti F, Politi P, Durazzi SMT, Albertini F, Muretto P: Bone marrow transplantation for thalassemia. The experience of Pesaro. In *Advances and Controversies in Thalassemia Therapy: Bone Marrow Transplantation and Other Approaches*, edited by Buckner CD, Gale RP, Lucarelli G. New York: Alan R. Liss, Inc. 1989; p. 163-171.

36. Groth CG, Ringdén O: Transplantation in relation to the treatment of inherited disease. Transplantation 1984;38:319-327.

37. O'Reilly RJ, Brochstein J, Dinsmore R, Kirkpatrick D: Marrow transplantation for congenital disorders. Semin Hematol 1984;21(suppl 3):188-221.

38. Shaw PJ, Hugh-Jones K, Hobbs JR, Downie CJC, Barnes R: Busulphan and cyclophosphamide cause little early toxicity during displacement bone marrow transplantation in fifty children. Bone Marrow Transplantation 1986;1:193-200.

39. Hobbs JR: Displacement bone marrow transplantation and immunoprophylaxis for genetic diseases. Adv Intern Med 1988;33:81-118.

40. Kersey JH, Weisdorf D, Nesbit ME, LeBien TW, Woods WG, McGlave PB, Kim T, Vallera DA, Goldman AI, Bostrom B, Hurd D, Ramsay N: Comparison of autologous and allogeneic BMT for treatment of high-risk refractory ALL. N Engl J Med 1987;317:461-466.

41. Clift RA, Beatty PG, Thomas ED, Buckner CD, Weiden P, McGuffin R for the Seattle Marrow Transplant Team: Marrow transplantation from mismatched donors for the treatment of malignancy. Transplant Proc 1985;17:445-446.

42. Beatty PG, Clift RA, Mickelson EM, Nisperos B, Flournoy N, Martin PJ, Sanders JE, Stewart P, Buckner CD, Storb R, Thomas ED, Hansen JA: Marrow transplantation from related donors other than HLA-identical siblings. N Engl J Med 1985; 313:765-771.

43. Beatty PG, Di Bartolomeo P, Storb R, Clift RA, Buckner CD, Sullivan KM, Doney K, Appelbaum FR, Anasetti C, Witherspoon R, Sanders J, Stewart P, Martin PJ, Ciancarelli M, Hansen JA, Thomas ED: Treatment of aplastic anemia with marrow grafts from related donors other than HLA geneotypically matched siblings. Clinical Transplantation 1987;1:117-124.

44. Buckner CD, Sanders JE, Anasetti C, Beatty P, Hansen JA, Storb R, Clift RA, Thomas ED: Donors other than HLA—identical siblings. In *Advances and Controversies in Thalassemia Therapy: Bone Marrow Transplantation and Other Approaches*, edited by Buckner CD, Gale RP, Lucarelli G. New York: Allan R. Liss, Inc., 1989, p. 383-390.

45. Lowrey GJ: *Growth and Development of Children*, 8 ed. Year Book Medical Publishers, Chicago, 1986.

46. Shalet SM: Irradiation-induced growth failure. Clin Endocrinol Metab 1986;15: 591-606.

47. Hakami N, Mohammad A, Meyer JW: Growth and growth hormone of children with acute lymphoblastic leukemia following central nervous system prophylaxis with and without cranial irradiation. Am J Pediatr Hematol Oncol 1980;2:311-316.

48. Meadows AT, Silber J: Delayed consequences of therapy for childhood cancer. Cancer Journal for Clinicians 1985;35:271.

49. Shalet SM, Horner A, Ahmed SR, Morris-Jones PH: Leydig cell damage after testicular irradiation for lymphoblastic leukemia. Med Pediatr Oncol 1985;13:65-68.

50. Green DM, Brecher MD, Yakar D, Blumenson LE, Lindsay AN, Voohes ML, MacGillivray M, Freeman AI: Thyroid function in pediatric patients after neck irradiation for Hodgkin disease. Med Pediatr Oncol 1980;8:127.

51. Razack MS, Sako K, Shimaoka K, Getaz EP, Rao U, Parthasanathy KL: Radiation-associated thyroid carcinoma. J Surg Oncol 1980;14:287-291.

52. Schneider AB, Bekerman C, Favus M, Trohman LA, Gonzalez C, Rao UY, Sievertsen G, Pinsky S: Continuing occurrence of thyroid nodules after head and neck irradiation. Relation to plasma thyroglobulin concentration. Ann Intern Med 1981;94: 176-181.

53. Prentice RL, Kato H, Yoshimoto K, Mason M: Radiation exposure and thyroid cancer incidence among Hiroshima and Nagasaki residents. NCI 1982;62:207-212, Monograph.

54. Fleming ID, Black TL, Thompson EI, Pratt C, Rao B, Hustu O: Thyroid dysfunction and neoplasia in children receiving neck irradiation for cancer. Cancer 1985;55: 1190-1194.

55. Maxon HR: Radiation-induced thyroid disease, in *Medical Clinics of North America*, Vol. 69, No. 5, 1985, pp. 1049-1061.

56. Sanders, JE, Buckner CD, Sullivan K, Doney K, Appelbaum F, Witherspoon R, Anasetti C, Storb R, Thomas ED: Growth and development after bone marrow transplantation. In *Advances and Controversies in Thalassemia Therapy: Bone Marrow Transplantation and Other Approaches*, edited by Buckner CD, Gale RP, Lucarelli G. New York, Alan R. Liss, Inc., 1989; p. 273-280.

57. Manenti F, Galimberti M, Lucarelli G, Polchi P, DeSantis V, Tanas R, Vullo C, Ruggiero L: Growth and endocrine function after bone marrow transplantation for thalassemia major. In *Advances and Controversies in Thalassemia Therapy: Bone Marrow Transplantation and Other Approaches*, edited by Buckner CD, Gale RP, Lucarelli G. New York: Alan R. Liss, Inc., 1989; p. 273-280.

58. Sanders JE, Pritchard S, Mahoney P, Amos D, Buckner CD, Witherspoon RP, Deeg HJ, Doney KC, Sullivan KM, Appelbaum FR, Storb R, Thomas ED: Growth and development following marrow transplantation for leukemia. Blood 1986;68:1129-1135.

59. Sklar CA, Kim TH, Ramsay NKC: Thyroid dysfunction among long-term survivors of bone marrow transplant. Am J Med 1982;73:688-694.

60. Bolme P, Borgström, Carlstrom K: Endocrine changes in children after allogeneic bone marrow transplantation, in 27th Annual Meeting European Society for Pediatric Endocrinology, Abstract 57; 1988.

61. Redman JR, Bajorunas DR, Shank B, O'Reilly RJ: Endocrine dysfunction following successful bone marrow transplantation. Blood 1985;66(Suppl 1):261a.

62. Oliff A, Bode U, Bercu BB, DiChiro G, Graves V, Poplack DG: Hypothalmic-pituitary dysfunction following CNS prophylaxis in acute lymphocytic leukemia: Correlation with CT scan abnormalities. Med Pediatr Oncol 1979;7:141-145.

63. Romshe CA, Zipf WB, Miser A, Miser J, Sotos JF, Newton WA: Evaluations of growth hormone release and human growth hormone treatment in children with cranial irradiation-associated short stature. J Pediatr 1984;104:177-182.

64. Shalet SM, Beardwell CG, Pearson D, Morris-Jones PH: The effect of varying dose doses of cerebral irradiation on growth hormone production in childhood. Clin Endocrinol 1976;5:287-290.

65. Shalet SM, Price DA, Beardwell CG, Morris-Jones PH, Pearson D: Normal growth despite abnormalities of growth hormone secretion in children treated for acute leukemia. J Pediatr 1979;94:719-722.

66. Romshe CA, Zipf WB, Miser A, Miser J, Sotos JF, Newton WA: Evaluation of growth hormone release and human growth hormone treatment in children with cranial irradiation-associated short stature. J Pediatr 1984;104:177-181.

67. Winters RS, Green OC: Irradiation-induced growth hormone deficiency: Blunted growth response and accelerated skeletal maturation to growth hormone therapy. J Pediatr 1985,106:609-612.

68. Bercu BB, Shulman D, Root AW, Spiliotis BE: Growth hormone (GH) provocative testing frequently does not reflect endogenous GH secretion. J Clin Endocrinol Metab 1986;63:709-716.

69. Berry DH, Elders MJ, Crist W, Land V, Lui V, Sexauer AC, Dickinson L: Growth in children with acute lymphocytic leukemia: A Pediatric Oncology Group study. Med Pediatr Oncol 1983;11:39-45.

70. Robison LL, Nesbit ME Jr, Sather HN, Meadows AT, Ortega JA, Hammond GD: Height of children successfully treated for acute lymphoblastic leukemia: A report from the late effects study committee of Children's Cancer Study Group. Med Pediatr 1985,13:14-21.

71. Parker RG, Berry HC: Late effects of therapeutic irradiation on the skeleton and bone marrow. Cancer 1976;37:1162-1171.

72. Probert JC, Parker BR: The effects of radiation therapy on bone growth. Radiology 1975;114:155-160.

73. Ranke MB, Blum WF, Dopfer R, Niethammer K: Growth-related hormonal changes after allogeneic bone marrow transplantation in children and adolescents. In 27th Annual Meeting European Society for Paediatric Endocrinology, Abstract 59; 1988.

74. Borgström B, Bolme P: Growth and growth hormone in children after bone marrow transplantation. Horm Res 1988;30:98-100.

75. Rosenfeld RL, Furlanetto R, Boch D: Relationship of somatomedin-C concentrations to pubertal changes. J Pediatr 1983;103:723-726.

76. Shalet SM: Effects of cancer chemotherapy on gonadal function of patients. Cancer Treat Rev 1980;7:131-152.

77. Ash P: The influence of radiation on fertility in man. Br J Radiol 1980;53:271-278.

78. Kay H, Mattison D: How radiation and chemotherapy affect gonadal function. Contemp Obstet Gynecol 1985;109:106-115.

79. Siris ES, Leventhal BG, Vaitukaitis TL: Effects of childhood leukemia and chemotherapy on puberty and reproductive function in girls. N Engl J Med 1976;294: 1143-1146.

80. Maguire L: Fertility and cancer therapy. Postgrad Med 1979;65(Suppl 5):293-295, 298-299.

81. Lentz RD, Bergstein J, Steffes MW, Brown DR, Prem K, Michael AF, Vernier RL: Postpubertal evaluation of gonadal function following cyclophosphamide therapy before and during puberty. J Pediatr 1977;91:385-394.

82. Nicosia SV, Matus-Ridley M, Meadows AT: Gonadal effects of cancer therapy in girls. Cancer 1985,55:2364-2372.

83. Shalet SM, Beardwell CG, Jacobs HS, Pearson D: Testicular function following irradiation of the human prepubertal testes. Clin Endocrinol 1978;9:483-490.

84. Blatt J, Sherins RJ, Niebrugge D, Bleyer WA, Poplack DG: Leydig cell function following treatment for testicular relapse of acute lymphoblastic leukemia. J Clin Oncol 1985;3:1227-1231.

85. Uldall PR, Kerr DNS, Tacchi D: Amenorrhea and sterility. Lancet 1972;i:693-694.

86. Belohorsky B, Siracky J, Sandor L, Klauber E: Comments on the development of amenorrhea caused by Myleran in cases of chronic myelosis. Neoplasia 1960;4:397-402.

87. Warne GL, Fairley KF, Hobbs JB, Martin FIR: Cyclophosphamide-induced ovarian failure. N Engl J Med 1973;289:1159-1162.

88. Sanders JE, Buckner CD, Leonard JM, Sullivan KM, Witherspoon RP, Deeg HJ, Storb R, Thomas ED: Late effects on gonadal function of cyclophosphamide, total-body irradiation, and marrow transplantation. Transplantation 1983;36:252-255.

89. Sanders JE, Buckner CD, Amos D, Levy W, Appelbaum FR, Doney K, Storb R, Sullivan KM, Witherspoon RP, Thomas ED: Ovarian function following marrow transplantation for aplastic anemia or leukemia. J Clin Oncol 1988;6:813-818.

90. Hinterberger-Fischer M, Hinterberger W, Kos M, Kahls P, Schwarzinger I, Geissler K, Hajek-Rosenmayr A, Hocker P, Lechner K: Three successful pregnancies and deliveries after bone marrow transplantation for severe aplastic anemia (SAA). In European Cooperative Group for Bone Marrow Transplantation XIII, Annual Meeting of the EBMT and III Annual Meeting of EBMT Nurses Group, 1987;58:59 (Abstract).

91. Jacobs P, Dubovsky DW: Bone marrow transplantation followed by normal pregnancy. Am J Hematol 1981;11:209-211.

92. Schmidt H, Ehninger G, Dopfer R, Waller HD: Pregnancy after allogeneic bone marrow transplantation because of severe aplastic anemia, in European Cooperative Group for Bone Marrow Transplantation XIII, Annual Meeting of the EBMT and III Annual Meeting EBMT Nurses Group, 1987;50:55 (abstract).

93. Etteldorf JN, West CD, Pitcock JA, Williams DL: Gonadal function, testicular histology and meiosis following cyclophosphamide therapy in patients with nephrotic syndrome. J Pediatr 1976;88:206-212.

94. Fairley KF, Barrie JU, Johnson W: Sterility and testicular atrophy related to cyclophosphamide therapy. Lancet 1972;i:568-569.

95. Buchanan JD, Fairley KF, Barrie JU: Return of spermatogenesis after stopping cyclophosphamide therapy. Lancet 1975;ii:156-157.

96. Sklar CA, Kim TH, Ramsay NKC: Testicular function following bone marrow transplantation performed during or after puberty. Cancer 1984;53:1498-1501.

97. Lushbaugh CC, Casarett GW: The effects of gonadal irradiation in clinical radiation therapy: a review. Cancer 1976;37:1111-1120.

98. Mandl AM: The radiosensitivity of germ cells. Biol Rev 1964;39:288-297.

99. Rowley MJ, Leach DR, Warner GA, Heller CG: Effect of graded doses of ionizing radiation on the human testes. Radiat Red 1974;59:665-678.

100. Sandeman TF: The effects of x irradiation on male human fertility. Br J Radiol 1966;39:901-907.

101. Shapiro E, Kensella TJ, Makuch RW, Fraass BA, Gladstein E, Rosenberg SA, Sherin RJ: Effects of fractionated irradiation on endocrine aspects of testicular function. J Clin Oncol 1985;3;1232-1239.

38

Treatment of Extensive Human Chronic Graft-vs.-Host Disease

Kerry Atkinson
St. Vincent's Hospital
Sydney, New South Wales, Australia

I. INTRODUCTION

Without treatment only 20% of patients with extensive chronic Graft-vs.-Host Disease (GVHD) will become long-term survivors with a reasonable quality of life (Karnofsky score equal to or greater than 70%). However, with greater physician awareness of the disease, monitoring to detect the disease early and the early institution of effective immunosuppressive therapy has radically changed the outlook for these patients. The end-stage patient with severe wasting, sclerodermatous skin changes resulting in joint contractures, and frequent and often fatal infections, is now rarely, if ever, seen. The current hallmark of therapy for standard risk patients is prednisone, and for high-risk patients is prednisone and cyclosporine on an alternate-day basis. Of equal importance in achieving a satisfactory therapeutic outcome is the prophylactic use of cotrimoxazole, shown to decrease both the incidence of late bacterial infections and late interstitial pneumonitis in patients with established chronic GVHD. Of apparent value in patients refractory to prednisone or cyclosporine is the use of thalidomide and ultraviolet A phototherapy used in conjunction with psoralen as a photosensitizer. Shown to be of little or no value in therapy have been a number of other treatments including electron beam therapy, hydroxyquinolone, antithymocyte globulin, thymosin, transfer factor, plasma exchange, and marrow donor lymphocyte infusions.

II. NEED FOR TREATMENT

The initial Seattle classification of human chronic GVHD (1) differentiated limited from extensive GVHD (Chapter 31). Such differentiation has proved useful clinically and has been shown to be well accepted (2). The cohort of patients with limited chronic GVHD often do not need any immunosuppressive therapy. An example would be a patient with an asymptomatic, though often marked, elevation of serum alkaline phosphatase concentration due to chronic hepatic GVHD. Another example would be the patient with mild cutaneous dyspigmentation. These nonindications for therapy are relative rather than absolute, however; for example, a woman with facial hyperpigmentation may find it causes her considerable cosmetic distress, and she and her physician will need to decide whether this constitutes a sufficient indication for the institution of an immunosuppressive regime that can have considerable toxicity. Whether or not such patients with limited chronic GVHD receive immunosuppressive therapy, it would seem advisable to continue prophylactic cotrimoxazole treatment in them for as long as signs of active disease are present. Some centers employ a dose of one double strength tablet twice daily every day (3). In our center we have had no serious infectious complications on a regime that utilizes this dose on a twice weekly basis.

In contrast, extensive chronic GVHD should be treated. This is clearly demonstrated by the outcome of such patients who are not treated: of 13 patients with extensive chronic GVHD who received no treatment, 5 died of chronic GVHD: 2 with identified infections (staphylococcal septicemia and cytomegalovirus pneumonia) and 3 during sudden febrile illnesses (cultures or autopsy not obtained) (4). By one year posttransplant, 6 of 9 survivors were disabled by contractures. None subsequently showed evidence of spontaneous improvement of skin disease or contractures and basically became crippled.

III. TREATMENT OF STANDARD RISK EXTENSIVE CHRONIC GVHD

The cornerstone of therapy for this patient group is oral prednisone given for a duration of 9 months. This is based on the only randomized placebo-controlled clinical trial in chronic GVHD patients reported to date (3). In this study a double-blind comparison of prednisone plus placebo was compared to prednisone plus azathioprine as early treatment for extensive chronic GVHD. The dose of azothiaprine was 1.5 mg/kg/day, and the dose of prednisone was started at 1 mg/kg/day in divided doses for 2 weeks prior to tapering to an alternate-day scheme of prednisone 1 mg/kg every other day by week 9 of the 36-week protocol. All patients received cotrimoxazole one double strength tablet twice daily. The 63 patients randomized to each treatment group were well matched for prognostic factors; 11% of patients in each group had only subclinical chronic GVHD at all stages. The following criteria were used to judge treatment response:

No response: Progressive disease after 2 months of treatment or stable disease with persisting Karnofsky scores <50% after 9 months of treatment.
Partial response: Clinically inactive chronic GVHD, but biopsies show continuing GVHD activity with no new organ involvement after 9 months of therapy.
Complete response: Clinically inactive disease and biopsies showing no GVHD activity after 9 months of therapy.

Overall, treatment with prednisone alone resulted in fewer infections and better survival than prednisone plus azathioprine, although response of the GVHD was similar in both groups. A complete response of the chronic GVHD was seen in 33% of those given prednisone and placebo, compared to 37% in those given prednisone and azathioprine. A partial response was seen in 29% and 27%, respectively. No response was seen in 24% and 8%, respectively, while 14% of patients in the prednisone and placebo group died or relapsed before 9 months of therapy was completed, compared to 29% in the prednisone and azathioprine group. Twenty-three of 63 patients in the prednisone and placebo group died (minimun follow-up 3.8 years after transplant), while 33 of 63 patients in the prednisone and azothiaprine group died. The increased mortality in the latter group was due to an increased rate of fatal infectious complications (Table 1). Recurrence of hematological malignancy occurred in 14/63 in the prednisone and placebo group, and 10/63 in the prednisone and azathioprine group (not significant). The incidence of non-relapse mortality was significantly increased in azathioprine recipients. Actuarial survival was 61% in those receiving prednisone + placeob and 47% in those receiving prednisone and azathioprine (Fig. 1). In the prednisone and placebo group, 34 of 40 survivors had a Karnofsky performance score between 90 and 100% compared to 26 of 30 patients in the prednisone and azathioprine arm. A flare of the chronic GVHD after treatment was stopped was seen in 9 of the 21 complete responders given prednisone and placebo, and in 6 of the 23 complete responders given prednisone and azathioprine. Primary sites for flare included the skin in 10 patients, liver in 4, mouth in 1, eye in 1, and muscle in 1. All those with a flare of their chronic GVHD had therapy reinstituted for another 9 months. At the time of the report, 81% of the survivors were continuing off treatment free of chronic GVHD.

Hepatic abnormalities and significant marrow suppression were not more common in the azathioprine arm.

Interestingly, patients whose chronic GVHD remained subclinical through the treatment course had a significantly increased probability of relapse (55%) compared to patients whose chronic GVHD was manifested clinically throughout its course (28%). This increased recurrence rate of leukemia nullified any survival advantage that might have been gained by treating subclinical disease, and treatment should be reserved only for those with clinical evidence of chronic GVHD.

Thus, while this study showed that patients with chronic GVHD in the standard risk category had fewer infections and better survival if treated with prednisone compared to prednisone and azathioprine, there was still much room for improvement.

Table 1 Causes of Death in Patients Given Prednisone or Prednisone and Azathioprine as Treatment for Chronic GVHD

Cause of death	Prednisone + placebo (n = 63)	Prednisone + azathioprine (n = 63)
Infection	6	19
Recurrent malignancy	14	10
Graft-vs.-Host Disease	1	1
Respiratory failure	1	1
Heart failure	0	1
Hemorrhage	0	1
Suicide	1	0

Source: Ref. 3.

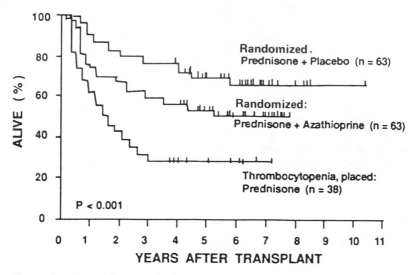

Figure 1 Actuarial survival of patients with chronic graft-versus-host disease random-ized to receive prednisone and placebo or prednisone and azathioprine, or placed on prednisone due to the presence of thrombocytopenia. Tick marks indicate patients alive. (Reproduced by permission from Ref. 3.)

IV. TREATMENT OF HIGH RISK CHRONIC GVHD

Several factors have been identified to delineate a cohort of patients with high risk chronic GVHD. These include the presence of thrombocytopenia ($<100,000/\mu l$), failure to respond to 9 months of immunosuppressive therapy as treatment for chronic GVHD, and patients whose chronic GVHD develops as part of a clinical continuum from acute GVHD (i.e., no quiescent interval)—the so called "progressive" type of chronic GVHD (5). The reason for the poor prognosis in patients with thrombocytopenia remains un-clear. Treatment with prednisone alone in thrombocytopenic chronic GVHD patients is unsatisfactory, with only 26% of such patients alive 5 years posttransplant (3). More en-couraging results have recently been reported by Sullivan et al. using a combination of prednisone was 1 mg/kg on alternate days and cyclosporine 6 mg/kg 12 hourly on alter-tients with high-risk extensive chronic GVHD were included in the study. The dose of prednisone was 1 mg/kg on alternate days and cyclosporine 6 mg/kg/12 hourly on alter-nate days. Again, cotrimoxazole one double strength tablet twice daily was given each day. Forty of the patients were given primary treatment for thrombocytopenic chronic GVHD, the median platelet count (range) being 35 (7-87) X $10^3/\mu l$. Twenty-one pa-tients received this protocol after failing initial therapy with prednisone with or without azathioprine. The 4-year actuarial survival posttransplant was 51% in those treated for primary thrombocytopenic chronic GVHD, and 67% in those treated after failing initial therapy. At the end of the 9-month treatment regime, 17 of the 61 patients had had a complete response, 20 a partial response, while 8 had no response, and 16 had died or relapsed. Nineteen of the 40 patients in the primary treatment group died as did 6 of the 21 in the salvage treatment group. The most common cause of death was interstitial pneumonia, with other deaths being due to recurrence of hematological malignancy (5 patients), progressive chronic GVHD without infection (5 patients), other infections

(4 patients), organ failure (3 patients), and hemorrhage (2 patients). Patients with thrombocytopenic chronic GVHD, who had persisting thrombocytopenia at the completion of 9 months of treatment, had particularly poor long-term survival: all four patients with 9-month platelet counts less than 100,000/μl subsequently died, compared to four subsequent deaths in 25 patients with 9-month values greater than 100,000/μl. As in the previous Seattle study (3), failure to respond to 9 months of treatment and the progressive type of onset of chronic GVHD were associated with increased mortality in this study.

At the time of the report, 21 of the 40 patients receiving this protocol as primary therapy were surviving as were 15 of 21 in the salvage therapy arm. Sixteen of the 21 patients in the first arm and 9 of the 15 patients in the salvage arm had Karnofsky performance scores of 90-100%, while 2 and 3, respectively, had Karnofsky scores of less than 70%. The median duration of the protocol therapy was 14 and 20 months, respectively, in the two groups, with 9 patients in each group still on therapy at the time of the report. Eighteen and 7 patients, respectively, in the two groups had stopped therapy, but only 12 and 6, respectively, were still off therapy at the time of the report. The median duration of therapy was 23 and 11 months, respectively. Survival of patients in the two groups is shown in Figure 2.

Toxicity of therapy in the 61 patients was as follows: hypertension (>140/100) 13; nephrotoxicity (creatinine > 2.0) 9; severe nausea 7, in 2 of whom cyclosporine had to be discontinued; aseptic necrosis 5; seizures or other neurological complications 4; diabetes mellitus 3. Additionally, infections were common with 35 (57%) of the 62 patients developing one or more of the following infections: 16 episodes of varicella-zoster; 8 episodes of interstitial pneumonia (3 cytomegalovirus, 3 pneumocystis carinii, and 2 idiopathic); 12 episodes of bacteremia (1 pneumococcal, 6 staphylococcal, and 5 gram-negative organism); 9 episodes of bacterial pneumonia; 10 episodes of sinusitis and 3 of otitis media, 3 episodes of septic arthritis, 3 of cellulitis, 3 fungal infections, and 1 cytomegalovirus retinitis. In summary, the combination of prednisone and cyclosporine

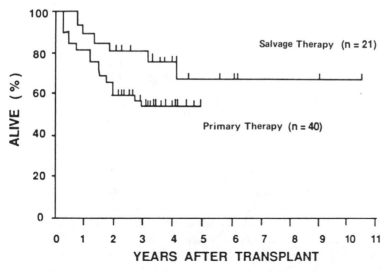

Figure 2 Actuarial survival of patients with high risk chronic graft-versus-host disease treated with prednisone and cyclosporine. (Reproduced by permission from Ref. 5.)

appears to have improved the prognosis for patients with high-risk chronic GVHD compared to that conferred by prednisone alone. Again, however, it is clear that there is ample room for further improvement.

V. OTHER COMBINATION IMMUNOSUPPRESSIVE REGIMES

A combination of prednisone and cyclophosphamide appeared as effective as prednisone and azathioprine in an early pilot study from Seattle (4). The dose of cyclophosphamide was 1.5 mg/kg/day. However, hemorrhagic cystitis was seen in 3 of 7 patients receiving 99-462 days of cyclophosphamide. The combination of prednisone and procarbazine (1.5 mg/kg/day) appeared less effective than prednisone and cyclophosphamide or prednisone and azathioprine: three of 6 patients showed no response to therapy (4).

VI. INEFFECTIVE THERAPIES FOR EXTENSIVE CHRONIC GVHD

No benefit was seen in 6 patients given antithymocyte globulin of either rabbit or goat origin at a dose of 7 mg IgG/kg on alternate days for six doses (4). Likewise the use of donor lymphocyte infusions, thymosin injections, transfer factor, hydroxychloroquine, and dermal electron beam radiation showed no benefit when each modality were evaluated (each in 2 of 10 total patients) (3,6).

VII. TREATMENT OF REFRACTORY CHRONIC GVHD

A small but definite minority of patients with extensive chronic GVHD do not respond to either prednisone alone or prednisone in combination with cyclosporine. Several modalities of treatment have been reported anecdotally from different centers suggesting some efficacy in this difficult situation. These modalities include thalidomide, the use of ultraviolet A phototherapy together with psoralen (PUVA), and penicillamine.

VIII. THALIDOMIDE

Although best known for its use as a sedative and antinausea agent in pregnant women with the consequent production of severe congenital malformations in babies born to these women, thalidomide has considerable immunosuppressive capacity. Its use in GVHD has been pioneered by the marrow transplant team at Johns Hopkins University, Baltimore (7,8) (see Chapter 15). Preliminary experiments showed thalidomide to be effective in treating GVHD produced in rat recipients of MHC-mismatched hemopoietic grafts (7). Subsequently, a trial of thalidomide was initiated in patients with prednisone/ azathioprine resistant chronic GVHD, or in those with high-risk chronic GVHD defined as those having poor Karnofsky performance status, thrombocytopenia, leukopenia, hyperbilirubinemia, or low IgG values (8). Thalidomide was administered as a 100 mg tablet every 6 hours with tapering of other GVHD medications after the first 6 weeks of therapy. Encouragingly, the first two patients on therapy for 3 months or longer had a significant and continued response to thalidomide, including the resolution of sclerodermatous cutaneous chronic GVHD. The subsequent three patients, who at the time of the report had received thalidomide for less than 3 months, also appeared to be responding, including a patient with sicca syndrome and one with myasthenia gravis. Serum levels of thalidomide measured by high performance liquid chromatography indicated a sustained level of drug 6-12 hours after the initial dose. Currently, upward escalation of the thalidomide dose is being tried with daily doses reaching 1200-1600 mg.

Anecdotally, we have seen a similar response with partial resolution of long-standing sclerodermatous cutaneous and subcutaneous fibrotic changes in two patients with chronic GVHD, not responding to prednisone and cyclosporine. Again the improvements were seen within 3 months of starting thalidomide.

Clearly, when this medication is utilized in female recipients, warning must be given on the dangers of conception. Most, though not all, of such recipients will have chemotherapy or chemo-radiation induced ovarian failure and should be already receiving ovarian hormone replacement therapy as prophylaxis for osteoporosis or for post-menopausal symptoms.

Some drowsiness is seen initially with thalidomide. The reported occurrence of peripheral neuropathy due to thalidomide has not yet been described in this small marrow transplant population.

IX. PSORALEN AND ULTRAVIOLET A PHOTOTHERAPY (PUVA)

The use of PUVA for the treatment of chronic GVHD resistant to conventional immuno-suppression was also pioneered by the Baltimore group (9,10). Again using the rat model of marrow transplantation, it was found that those animals given ultraviolet B irradiation to one side of the back before marrow allografting developed histologically less severe GVHD on the irradiated side (9). Subsequently a single patient given ultraviolet A irradiation for chronic cutaneous GVHD, together with the photosensitizer 8-methoxy-psoralen, showed improvement. We have treated a number of patients with chronic GVHD involving the mouth or the skin (11) and find it useful in over half those patients in whom it is tried. In the reported study (11), all three patients had shown skin or mouth GVHD refractory to prednisone and cyclosporine, and the third had also proven refractory to antithymocyte globulin and cyclophosphamide. All three patients responded to PUVA therapy. The response was longer lasting in two patients who had 24 and 28 treatments, respectively, for chronic oral GVHD. One patient given PUVA for cutaneous GVHD only received 10 treatments because of intervening infection. PUVA therapy decreased the degree of lichenoid striae, healed the large long-standing tongue ulcer present in one of the patients, and reversed the severe dry mouth present in the third patient. In patients with skin involvement, erythema has resolved.

Before PUVA, therapy patients should undergo opthalmological examination (for cataracts) and have a full blood count, biochemical screen, and antinuclear antibody test. Oral 8-methoxypsoralen 0.6 mg/kg is given 2 hours before exposure to the UVA radiation. During irradiation the patient lies supine under a bank of light tubes with their eyes protected. For total body skin exposure, the front is exposed first and then the back. For irradiation of the oral cavity, either the patient's head can be tilted to the side with the mouth wide open and the cheeks partially everted with a finger or, if available, a UVA pencil light can be inserted into the oral cavity. Treatment is normally given 4 days each week (Monday, Tuesday, Thursday, and Friday) unless evidence of erythema occurs, when it should be delayed. In our practice the dose for mouth irradiation is 0.75 J each day. The dose for skin irradiation is started at 0.75 J and is increased to 1.25 J to the trunk with additional exposures of 0.75 J to the palms and soles. Protection from sunlight for 24 hours after taking oral psoralen should be provided by UVA-protecting sunglasses.

Biopsies taken of the mouth or skin at the end of PUVA treatment still showed histological evidence of mild to moderate GVHD in each of our three patients with hydropic degeneration of the basal layer, eosinophilic bodies and a lymphocytic infiltrate in the epithelium and corium. Immunoperoxidase staining of these sections showed a complete absence of both Langerhans cells (as described in patients with chronic GVHD previously (12)) and, interestingly, of CD4[+] and CD8[+] cells.

Ultraviolet as opposed to gamma irradiation is known to diminish the immunogenic potential of cells that stimulate an immune response in vitro (13). It is currently unknown, however, whether the PUVA therapy in these patients works by inactivating residual recipient immunogenic mononuclear cells or donor origin GVHD effector cells (T or otherwise), or both.

PUVA therapy appears to be a useful therapeutic adjunct in patients with moderate or severe cutaneous or oral GVHD. It also allows subsequent dose reduction of conventional immune suppressive agents. Since an increased incidence of neoplasia has been reported with its use in other skin conditions (for example, psoriasis), it should only be used in the GVHD population as a last resort.

X. PENICILLAMINE

A single case report has appeared describing the successful treatment of chronic cutaneous GVHD with penicillamine (14). The patient was a 20-year-old with severe aplastic anemia given an HLA-identical sibling marrow transplant. Prophylaxis for GVHD was with methotrexate, but shortly after its discontinuation at day 100, the patient developed chronic GVHD involving the skin. Despite corticosteroid therapy, the skin manifestations progressed to dyspigmentation, ulceration, and joint contractures. Azathioprine was added without success. Penicillamine was then initiated at a dose of 125 mg b.d. and continued for 2 years. Within 2 months the skin began to improve with complete healing of skin ulceration and softening of the fibrosis. The fixed flexion joint deformities completely resolved.

Penicillamine was used in this case because of a beneficial report from its use in the treatment of progressive systemic sclerosis (15). Unfortuntely no other reports on its use in chronic GVHD have appeared at the present time.

XI. PREVENTION OF INFECTION

Of equal importance to the use of effective immunosuppression in managing patients with chronic GVHD is the prophylactic administration of cotrimoxazole to minimize the risk of infection to which these patients are so susceptible (see Chapter 28). Cotrimoxazole is effective in decreasing both the number of bacterial infections, particularly with encapsulated organisms (such as pneumococcus and haemophilus influenzae), and the incidence of interstitial pneumonia.

The standard dose used in Seattle is one double strength tablet twice daily every day. However, it appears from the experience of several centers (City of Hope, Duarte and St. Vincent's Hospital, Sydney) that a twice weekly regimen is equally effective. Our own practice is to administer the tablets on Monday and Thursday of each week. This less frequent regime has the advantage of cheapness, less likelihood of marrow suppression, and lesser risk of nephrotoxicity if utilized in conjunction with cyclosporine. Gastrointestinal intolerance on this twice weekly regime is virtually never encountered.

Patients with chronic GVHD should remain on prophylactic contrimoxazole for as long as they are receiving immunosuppressive therapy (and probably for 2 months after the cessation of such therapy) or while there is any evidence of activity of the chronic GVHD.

Occasional hypersensitivity to cotrimoxazole (in particular the sulphamethoxazole component) occurs. For such patients either an attempt at desensitization to cotrimoxazole can be made using increasing doses of cotrimoxazole syrup or an alternative antibiotic may be employed. Most commonly this is an oral cephalosporin or oral penicillin. Additionally, a monthly infusion or inhalation dose of pentamidine should be employed for pneumocystis carinii prophylaxis.

The importance of prophylactic cotrimoxazole is emphasized by the not infrequent observation of flares of infectious complications when the cotrimazole is discontinued (16).

XII. VACCINATION

The humoral immune response to specific immunizing antigens such as bacteriophage ϕX174, KLH, and pneumococcal polysaccharide remains grossly impaired in patients with chronic GVHD as compared to long-term survivors without GVHD (17). For this reason it seems pointless at the present time to recommend vaccination for patients with chronic GVHD. Furthermore, vaccination with any live virus is contraindicated in view of the possibility that the attenuated virus strains used in such vaccines may disseminate and cause clinical disease. In fact it is curious that measles and polio (as well as tetanus, diptheria, and pertussis) are remarkably infrequent after marrow transplantation. Tetanus vaccination or boosting is recommended if an individual is specifically at risk for this infection. Likewise the inactivated Salk polio vaccine (but not the attenuated Sabin vaccine) would be useful for those at risk during outbreaks of polio.

ACKNOWLEDGMENT

Supported in part by a grant from the Government Employees Assistance to Medical Research Fund.

REFERENCES

1. Shulman HM, Sullivan KM, Weiden PL, MacDonald G, Striker G, Sale G, Hackman R, Tsoi M, Storb R, Thomas E: Chronic graft-versus-host syndrome in man. A long term clinicopathological study of 20 Seattle patients. Am J Med 1980;69: 204-217.
2. Atkinson K, Horotitz M, Gale RP, Lee MB, Rimm AA, Bortin MM. Consensus among bone marrow transplanters for diagnosis, grading, and treatment of chronic graft-versus-host disease. Bone Marrow Transplant 1989;4:247-254.
3. Sullivan KM, Witherspoon RP, Storb R, Weiden P, Flournoy N, Dahlberg S, Deeg HJ, Sanders J, Doney K, Appelbaum F, McGuffin R, MacDonald G, Meyers J, Schubert M, Shulman H, Sale G, Anasetti C, Loughran TP, Strom S, Nims J, Thomas E: Prednisone and azothioprine compared with prednisone and placebo for treatment of chronic graft-versus-host disease: prognostic influence of prolong thrombocytopenia after allogeneic marrow transplantation. Blood 1988;72: 546-554.

4. Sullivan KM, Shulman HM, Storb R, Weiden PL, Witherspoon RP, McDonald GB, Schubert MM, Atkinson K, Thomas E: Chronic graft-versus-host disease in fifty-two patients: adverse natural course and successful treatment with combination immunosuppression. Blood 1981;57:267-276.

5. Sullivan KM, Witherspoon RP, Storb R, Deeg HJ, Dahlberg S, Sanders JE, Appelbaum F, Doney K, Weiden P, Anasetti C, Loughran T, Hill R, Shields A, Shellman H, Nims J, Strom S, Thomas E: Alternating day cyclosporine and prednisone for treatment of high risk chronic graft-versus-host disease. Blood 1988;72:555-561.

6. Shulman HB, Sale GE, Lerner KG, Barker EA, Weiden PL, Sullivan K, Gallucci B, Thomas ED, Storb R: Chronic cutaneous graft-versus-host disease in man. Am J Pathol 1978;92:545-570.

7. Vogelsang GB, Hess AD, Gordon G, Santos GW, Saral R, Santos G: Treatment and prevention of acute graft-versus-host disease with thalidomide in a rat model. Transplan Proc 1986;41:644-647.

8. Vogelsang GB, Hess AD, Ling C, Brundrett RB, Colvin OM, Wingard JR: Thalidomide therapy of chronic graft-versus-host disease. Blood 1987;70:315a (abstr).

9. Glazier A, Morrison WL, Buchanan C, Hess AD, Tutschka PJ: Suppression of epidermal graft-versus-host disease with ultraviolet radiation. Transplan Proc 1984;37: 211-213.

10. Hymes SR, Morrison WL, Farmer ER, Walters LL, Tutschka PJ, Santos GW: Methoxsalen and ultraviolet A radiation in treatment of chronic cutaneous graft-versus-host reaction. J Am Acad Dermatol 1985;12:30-37.

11. Atkinson K, Weller P, Ryman W, Biggs JC: PUVA therapy for drug-resistant graft-versus-host disease. Bone Marrow Transplant 1986;1:227-236.

12. Atkinson K, Munro V, Vasak E, Biggs JC: Mononuclear cell subpopulations in the skin defined by monoclonal antibodies after HLA-identical sibling marrow transplantation. Br J Dermatol 1986;114:145-160.

13. Lafferty KJ, Andrus L, Prowse SJ: Role of lymphokine and antigen in the control of specific T cell responses. Immunol Rev 1980;51:279-314.

14. Summerfield GP, Bellingham AJ, Bunch C, Woodrow JC: Successful treatment of chronic cutaneous graft-versus-host disease with penicillamine. Clin Lab Haemat 1983;5:313-318.

15. Herbert CM, Linderberg KA, Jayson MIV, Bailey AJ: Biosynthesis and maturation of skin collagen and scleroderma and the effect of D-penicillamine. Lancet 1974;1: 187-192.

16. Atkinson K, Farewell V, Tsoi MS, Sullivan KM, Witherspoon RP, Thomas ED, Strob R: Analysis of late infections after human bone marrow transplantation. Role of non-specific suppressor cells in patients with chronic graft-versus-host disease and genotypic non identity between marrow donor and recipient. Blood 1982;60:714-720.

17. Witherpsoon RP, Storb R, Ochs HD, Fluornoy N, Kopecky KJ, Sullivan KM, Deeg HJ, Sosa R, Noel D, Atkinson K, Thomas E: Recovery of antibody production in human allogeneic marrow graft recipients: influence of time post-transplantation, the presence or absence of chronic graft-versus-host disease and antithymocyte globulin treatment. Blood 1981;58:360-368.

39

Graft-vs.-Leukemia Effects in Clinical Bone Marrow Transplantation

Paul L. Weiden*
The Virginia Mason Clinic
Seattle, Washington

Mary M. Horowitz
Medical College of Wisconsin
Milwaukee, Wisconsin

I. INTRODUCTION

The possibility that a marrow graft might be associated with an antitumor effect was one of the early indications for initiating clinical use of bone marrow transplantation in the treatment of hemopoietic malignancies. Adoptive immunotherapy is the term used to encompass this immune-mediated antitumor effect of allogeneic marrow transplantation (1,2). Evidence for such an antitumor effect of adoptively transferred cells has come from various animal tumor models reviewed in Chapter 10. These studies establish in a variety of transplantable tumor models that cells in the donor bone marrow can recognize and destroy host malignant cells bearing tumor-associated or histocompatibility antigens or both. Evidence for the existence of a graft-vs.-tumor effect in human marrow graft recipients has been difficult to obtain, in part because of the difficulty of manipulating and controlling GVHD and in part because of the large number of other variables that influence the results of clinical bone marrow transplantation.

It is, nevertheless, clear that long-term disease-free survival can be obtained following transplantation in man using either syngeneic (identical twin), allogeneic (generally histocompatible siblings), or autologous (self) donor bone marrow. These apparent cures may simply reflect the antileukemic activity of intensive chemoradiotherapy prior to infusion of the marrow graft. Alternatively, by analogy with experimental animal studies, the graft itself may contribute an antitumor effect. The target antigens for such an antitumor effect could be either leukemia or other tumor-associated antigens or minor histocompatibility antigens present on malignant cells. An antitumor effect against leukemia antigens could be exerted by either a syngeneic or allogeneic graft, while an antileukemic effect against minor histocompatibility antigens could be exerted only by allogeneic bone marrow, as part of either clinically evident or subclinical GVHD.

Present affiliation: Fred Hutchinson Cancer Research Center, Seattle, Washington

In the present chapter, we shall first review the limited case reports which indicate in individual patients an association between clinical GVHD and apparent regression of malignancy. We will next review single institution reports exploring the relationship between leukemia relapse and donor source in recipients of allogeneic, syngeneic, and autologous transplants, and the relationship between leukemia relapse and clinically evident GVHD. We will then review attempts to decrease or augment GVHD and the resulting effect on leukemia recurrence. Finally, we will turn to an analysis of data submitted to the International Bone Marrow Transplant Registry (IBMTR) by over 150 bone marrow transplant teams between January 1978 and June 1987. A recent analysis of this extensive database provides additional evidence for a graft-vs.-leukemia effect in clinical bone marrow transplantation.

II. CASE REPORTS

In 1978, Odom and colleagues described two patients who underwent marrow transplantation for acute lymphoblastic leukemia (3). The course of each patient was characterized by: (1) early relapse of leukemia following engraftment of donor marrow, (2) subsequent achievement of remission at the time of diagnosis of clinically significant GVHD in the absence of specific antileukemic therapy, and (3) later leukemic relapse which occurred primarily in extramedullary sites with little or no involvement of bone marrow, lymph nodes, liver, and spleen. Cytogenetic studies in both cases documented that the posttransplant leukemic relapses involved host cells, while the marrow cells and peripheral blood lymphocytes were of donor origin. Cell-mediated cytotoxicity performed by mixing the peripheral blood lymphocytes of one of the recipients with autologous lymphoblasts was markedly positive. Thus both patients experienced prolonged bone marrow remissions in the face of active extramedullary leukemia, a clinical and pathological syndrome which Odom and colleagues concluded represented graft-vs.-leukemia reactions.

In their first patient, however, the marrow contained 72% lymphoblasts on day 27 posttransplantation and was morphologically normal on day 35, but the patient received rabbit antithymocyte globulin from day 24 to day 35. In the second patient, marrow aspiration on day 33 after transplantation contained 90% leukemic cells and on day 48 was free of leukemic cells. During this interval the patient had a rash, but only on day 42 did GVHD progress to involve the liver and become clinically significant. Thus, in each of the cases reported by Odom and colleagues, there was an extraordinarily rapid change in the marrow, i.e., from 50-90% leukemia cells to complete remission in 8-13 days, and in each case extramedullary leukemia progressed in spite of apparent marrow remission.

Recently, Petersen and colleagues described a patient with Burkitt's lymphoma who had failed to obtain a remission with conventional chemotherapy but achieved a complete remission following conditioning with cytosine arabinoside and total body radiation and infusion of HLA–identical sibling marrow (4). Complete remission was demonstrated by normal marrow morphology and cytogenetics. On day 33 posttransplant, however, the patient relapsed with 25% circulating Burkitt's cells and 10 of 20 marrow cells displaying a clonal cytogenetic abnormality in host cells that had been present pretransplant. No further chemotherapy was given, but cyclosporine (which had been administered as GVHD prophylaxis) was discontinued on day 34. Concurrent with the development of GVHD the patient's circulating Burkitt's lymphoma cells disappeared, and a complete remission was documented by normal marrow morphology and cytogenetics on day 92 posttransplantation. Because of progressive GVHD, cyclosporine and prednisone were instituted with subsequent improvement of GVHD. Twenty days later recurrent disease was detected, and the patient succumbed to progressive tumor.

These isolated case reports and other anecdotal cases of which the authors are aware are intriguing but inconclusive. There are also numerous and unreported occasions following allogeneic marrow transplantation where immunosuppressive medication has been discontinued in the hope that a clinically significant graft versus tumor effect might be observed, alas without clinical benefit.

III. SINGLE INSTITUTION DATA

A. Syngeneic Marrow Grafts

In 1979, the Seattle group examined the relationship between relapse of leukemia and GVHD in 46 recipients of identical twin (syngeneic) marrow, 117 recipients of HLA-identical sibling (allogeneic) marrow with no or minimal GVHD, and 79 recipients of allogeneic marrow with moderate-to-severe acute or chronic GVHD (5). The relative relapse rate was 2.5 times less in allogeneic marrow recipients with GVHD than in allogeneic recipients without it (p < 0.01) or than in syngeneic marrow graft recipients. This apparent antileukemic effect was more marked in patients with lymphoblastic than non-lymphoblastic leukemia and in those who received transplants during relapse rather than during remission and was most evident during the first 130 days after transplantation. A Cox proportional hazards regression model was used to estimate the effect of various factors simultaneously on the rate of relapse of leukemia. If only the influence of type of marrow graft (i.e., syngeneic or allogeneic) was considered, the relapse rate among recipients of allogeneic marrow was 0.68 times that among recipients of syngeneic marrow (95% confidence interval 0.44 to 1.06, p < 0.10). Taken alone, this analysis suggests that allogeneic marrow transplantation per se provides an antileukemic effect.

If the presence of moderate-to-severe GVHD was considered in addition, however, there was no significant difference between the relapse rate of syngeneic and allogeneic marrow recipients, whereas the relapse rate of patients with significant GVHD was only 0.43 times that of patients with no or only mild GVHD. This analysis suggests that the major difference between allogeneic and syngeneic marrow recipients was attributable to the presence of allogeneic marrow recipients with moderate or severe GVHD. Stated another way, this early analysis was consistent with the likelihood that there is a graft-vs-leukemia effect as part of GVHD and that this antitumor effect was not observed in allogeneic recipients without significant GVHD or in syngeneic graft recipients. Clearly, this does not address the question of whether or not all marrow transplants, including those from syngeneic donors or allogeneic donors not associated with significant GVHD, have a possible antitumor effect directed against leukemia antigens (as distinct from minor histocompatibility antigens).

More recently, the Seattle group has updated its syngeneic marrow transplantation experience by comparing the probability of relapse in 53 syngeneic versus 785 allogeneic marrow recipients (6). The syngeneic and allogeneic marrow recipient groups did not differ significantly in the relative representation of ALL versus ANL, age, or in the interval between diagnosis and marrow transplantation. All patients were in second or subsequent remission or relapse at the time of transplant, although the relative numbers of syngeneic and allogeneic graft recipients in remission versus relapse was not stated. Leu-kemia relapse was observed in 75% of the syngeneic but only 62% of the allogeneic marrow recipients (p < 0.0001). Further analysis of the leukemia relapse rates after syngeneic versus allogeneic marrow transplantation suggest that the antileukemic effect associated with allogeneic marrow transplantion is observed in patients with ANL as well as in patients with ALL, though this effect is not seen by the Seattle group in pa-tients with ANL transplanted in first remission. In a similar fashion, patients with chronic myelogenous leukemia transplanted in the chronic phase do not appear to exhibit any difference in relapse rates after allogeneic versus syngeneic marrow transplantation.

Gale and Champlin in 1984 pooled allogeneic and syngeneic transplant experience from several groups in a manner that allowed one to identify individually the experience of the transplant groups from UCLA, Johns Hopkins, Memorial Sloan Kettering Cancer Center, and the Royal Marsden Hospital (7). The combined report compares relapse rates in 31 syngeneic transplants with those in 339 allogeneic (HLA-identical sibling) trans-plants managed with similar chemotherapy. All patients had ANL in first remission. The actuarial relapse rate in the syngeneic transplants was 59 ± 20% (95% confidence interval) compared with 18 ± 4% in the allogeneic transplants. The experience of each institution considered individually is consistent with the combined results.

A graft-vs.-leukemia effect of allogeneic transplantation is not the only possible explanation for the higher relapse rate observed in syngeneic marrow recipients. For example, syngeneic marrow recipients do not receive posttransplant immunosuppression to suppress GVHD. Although the doses and agents utilized have only modest anitleuke-mic activity, one cannot exclude a significant antileukemic effect against a small num-ber of residual leukemia cells sublethally damaged by high doses of drugs and irradiation administered before transplantation. A second possibility is that recurrent leukemia in syngeneic transplant recipients represents not recurrence of host leukemia, but rather de novo induction of leukemia in donor cells, since there obviously is no way to distinguish donor from host cells in the syngeneic transplant setting. This possibility cannot be en-tirely excluded but nevertheless seems unlikely, particularly since all syngeneic donors, thus far, remain normal without evidence of leukemia. The final and most likely possi-bility is that the difference observed between syngeneic and allogeneic marrow grafts represents an antileukemic effect associated with transplantation of allogeneic marrow, either as part of GVHD or as a distinct graft-vs.-leukemia effect.

B. Autologous Marrow Grafts

Comparison of relapse rates in recipients of autologous versus allogeneic marrow trans-plants is made difficult by the possibility that leukemia relapse in recipients of autolo-gous marrow could be the result of viable leukemia cells reinfused with the marrow graft. Nevertheless, the study of Kersey et al. provides additional circumstantial evidence for the existence of a graft-vs.-leukemia effect in recipients of allogeneic marrow transplants with GVHD by comparing results in allogeneic transplant recipients to those observed in recipients of autologous marrow (8). Ninety-one patients with high-risk ALL in first or subsequent remission were treated with high-dose chemoradiotherapy. Forty-six patients received allogeneic (HLA-identical sibling), and 45 patients without a matched donor received their own marrow taken during remission and purged of leukemic cells with use of monoclonal antibodies. Posttransplant relapse of leukemia was the most frequent cause of treatment failure. Relapses occurred in an estimated 37% of patients with allo-geneic grafts in whom GVHD developed, 75% of patients with allogeneic grafts in whom

GVHD did not develop, and 79% of patients who received autologous grafts. Although allogenic graft recipients tended to have a lower remission number than autograft recipients (65% versus 42% in first or second remission), the differences in relapse rates between the groups persisted after adjustment for remission number. The interval before relapse was significantly shorter in the autologous marrow group than in the allogeneic marrow groups. The fraction of "cured" patients was estimated to be 20% in the autologous marrow group and 27% in the allogeneic marrow groups, a difference which was not statistically significant. The authors indicated that the earlier and more frequent relapses in recipients of autologous marrow were probably "partly due" to the absence of a graft-vs.-leukemia effect, since patients in whom GVHD developed had a lower probability of relapse. The observation that recipients of autologous marrow had a similar relapse rate to those recipients of allogeneic marrow who did not develop GVHD suggests that the marrow relapses in the patients with autologous grafts occurred primarily because of resistant disease in the marrow, rather than reinfusion of viable leukemia cells with the marrow.

C. Allogeneic Marrow Grafts

As discussed above, in 1979 the Seattle group initially reported that the relative leukemic relapse rate was 2.5 times less in allogeneic marrow recipients with GVHD than in recipients without it (5). Survival of all patients was comparable, however, since the lesser probability of recurrent leukemia in patients with GVHD was offset by a greater probability of other causes of death. In fact, there was no significant difference in survival among the three patient groups, i.e., syngeneic graft recipients, allogeneic recipients with no or mild GVHD, or allogeneic graft recipients with moderate-to-severe GVHD.

In a subsequent report, the Seattle group reported an apparent decrease in both incidence of moderate-to-severe acute GVHD and its associated acute mortality (9). This trend, in conjunction with the absence of any change over time in the apparent antileukemic effect associated with GVHD, resulted in improvement in survival for some allogeneic marrow transplant recipients with acute GVHD. This was true for patients with ALL transplanted in leukemic remission or relapse and patients with ANL transplanted in leukemic relapse. For patients transplanted in 1976 and before, survival plateaued at approximately 15% regardless of GVHD status. For patients transplanted in 1977 and 1978, however, survival was better for all patients and clearly for patients with grades II to IV acute GVHD (55%) than for those without GVHD (30%). These observations were the first to suggest that the existence of a graft-vs.-leukemia effect might not only decrease the likelihood of leukemia recurrence, but also might result in improved survival.

Two distinct GVHD syndromes were subsequently recognized in recipients of allogeneic marrow transplants as discussed elsewhere in this volume. In 1981, the Seattle group reported that chronic as well as acute GVHD was associated with a lower relapse rate and improved survival in acute leukemia patients transplanted with allogeneic marrow among those who survived the first 150 days in remission. One hundred and sixty-three patients with ANL or ALL in remisson or relapse who received marrow transplants from HLA–identical sibling donors between 1970 and 1979 were selected from the entire group of Seattle marrow transplant recipients because they were alive with their disease in remission 150 days after transplantation. Kaplan-Meier product limit estimates of the probability of recurrent leukemia or survival were determined in four patient groups: acute GVHD (grade II-IV) only, extensive chronic GVHD only, both acute and chronic GVHD, and neither acute or chronic GVHD. The probability of being in remission plateaued after 4 years for all patient groups and was highest in patients who had both acute and chronic GVHD (88%), intermediate in those with either acute (57%) or chronic (66%) GVHD, and lowest in those without any GVHD (38%). Chronic GVHD increased the probability of being in remission, both in patients with and without acute GVHD. The rate of leukemic relapse in patients in whom chronic GVHD developed was 0.31-0.36 times the rate of relapse in patients in whom chronic GVHD did not develop (p < 0.005) and was not affected by any of 20 potential prognostic variables including disease status at the time of transplant. Survival was superior in patients with chronic GVHD only (80%), intermediate and approximately equivalent in patients with acute GVHD with or without subsequent chronic GVHD (56% and 50%, respectively) and was poorest in patients with neither acute nor chronic GVHD (29%). Overall, the probability of survival in patients with chronic GVHD was 2.1 times greater than in patients without chronic GVHD (p = 0.01). However, it should be noted that the improved survival associated with GVHD applies only to patients who survive in remission for 150 days posttransplant. Since most GVHD-related deaths occur prior to this time, the overall impact of GVHD upon posttransplant survival cannot be assessed from this analysis.

In 1987, the Seattle group further updated their observed relationship of acute and chronic GVHD to relapse of acute leukemia following allogeneic marrow transplantation (11). Four hundred and fifty-four patients with acute leukemia who received allogeneic marrow transplants in Seattle between 1970 and 1986 survived in remission 150 days after receiving HLA-identical marrow. Of these, 252 patients had ANL in remission or relapse, and 202 had ALL in remission or relapse. Again, Kaplan-Meier product limit estimates of the probability of recurrent leukemia or survival were determined. Recurrence of leukemia following transplantation was observed in 28% of patients developing moderate to severe (grade II-IV) acute GVHD and 48% of patients with no or mild (grade 0-I) acute GVHD (p < 0.003). Relapse was observed in 34% of patients developing clinical extensive chronic GVHD and 45% of patients free of chronic GVHD (p = 0.0001). The incidence of recurrent leukemia was 28% in patients developing both acute and chronic GVHD and 52% in patients free of both acute and chronic GVHD (p = 0.0001). Among patients with ANL or ALL transplanted in relapse, the probability of recurrent leukemia was 74% without acute or chronic GVHD, 45% with acute and chronic GVHD, 35% with only acute GVHD, and 34% with only chronic GVHD (p = 0.0001). Five-year actuarial survival in these four GVHD groups were 25%, 34%, 59%, and 62%, respectively (p < 0.009). Among patients with ANL transplanted in first remission, however, GVHD had an adverse affect on survival and no influence on relapse. With 114 of these patients now surviving 5-15 years after marrow grafting, these remissions appear to be durable. Thus, these updated observations confirmed the earlier observations that both acute and chronic GVHD were associated with an apparent graft-vs.-leukemia effect and improved long-term survival in patients with ANL or ALL transplanted in relapse among patients who survive in remission 150 days posttransplant. No antileukemic effect of GVHD, however, could be demonstrated in patients transplanted while in remission.

The Seattle group has also reviewed the results of patients transplanted for chronic myelogenous leukemia (CML) to determine whether an apparent graft-vs.-leukemia effect could be identified (12). Among 123 patients with CML in chronic phase, GVHD had an adverse affect on survival and no influence on relapse. Among 45 patients with CML transplanted in accelerated phase or blast crisis, the probability of relapse was 65% without acute or chronic GVHD and 36% with acute and/or chronic GVHD (p < 0.01). Five-year actuarial survivals were 24% and 50%, respectively (p = 0.5). Thus, both acute and chronic GVHD were associated with a graft-vs-leukemia effect and apparent improved long-term survival in patients with CML in accelerated phase or blast crisis, but no antileukemic effect was observed in patients transplanted during chronic phase.

The Seattle group's experience also permits some consideration of the severity of chronic GVHD required to result in a statistically identifiable clinical graft-vs.-leukemia effect. A randomized double-blind comparison of prednisone and placebo versus prednisone and azathioprine as early treatment of extensive chronic GVHD was undertaken between January 1980 and December 1983 (13). One hundred and sixty-four evaluable patients were entered on this trial. Clinical chronic GVHD was diagnosed when both histologic and clinical evidence of chronic GVHD were present. Subclinical chronic GVHD was defined as histologic evidence of chronic GVHD on both skin and oral biopsies without signs or symptoms of clinical disease. Overall, 38% of patients entered into this trial started treatment when chronic GVHD was still subclinical. Seventy percent of these patients with subclinical disease at diagnosis, however, developed clinical chronic GVHD during treatment. Thus, in only 12% of the 164 evaluable patients did chronic GVHD remain subclinical throughout therapy. Patients who had subclinical chronic GVHD throughout treatment, however, had a 55% probability of relapse as compared with 28% and 25% rates of relapse, respectively, in patients with clinical or subclinical going to clinical chronic GVHD ($p = 0.0003$). These results suggest that chronic GVHD, like acute GVHD, must be clinically evident and significant in order to exert a clinically detectable graft-vs.-leukemia effect. The observation that the clinical severity of GVHD is directly related to the ability to detect a graft-vs.-leukemia effect suggests that, in man, the apparent graft-vs.-leukemia effect may be difficult to separate from GVHD.

Other single institutions have also reviewed their experience in order to investigate the possibility of a graft-vs.-leukemia effect. The results of 58 consecutive patients with acute leukemia who underwent marrow transplantation at UCLA between February 1974 and March 1978 from HLA-matched allogeneic donors were reported by McIntyre and Gale (14). The actuarial relapse rate was 62% in patients with no or grade I GVHD compared to 20% in patients with grade III to IV GVHD ($p = 0.05$). In this early study involving relatively few patients, the lower risk of leukemia relapse in patients with moderate-to-severe GVHD did not result in any improvement in survival, results similar to the early Seattle experience during the same time period.

At the University of Minnesota, 40 remission patients with high-risk ALL were treated with cyclophosphamide and fractionated total body irradiation, followed by marrow infusion from HLA-identical donors (15). After a median follow-up of more than 3 1/2 years, 13 patients were alive (11 relapse-free) between 2 and 4 1/2 years following transplantation. Not age, sex, remission number, extramedullary leukemia, nor white blood cell count at diagnosis were statistically significant as a predictor of relapse-free survival. Patients who developed acute GVHD, however, were found to have a significant reduction in risk of relapse and a trend toward improved disease-free survival. Specifically, 71% of patients with grades I-IV GVHD were relapse-free compared to 52% of patients with no GVHD ($p < 0.04$). Forty percent of patients with grades I-IV GVHD survived relapse-free 4 years posttransplant compared to 19% of patients without GVHD ($p = 0.11$). It should be recognized that the numbers of patients in this analysis are relatively small, i.e., 17 patients with acute GVHD and 23 without. Nevertheless, in both univariate and multivariate analysis the sole significant predictor of relapse-free outcome was the presence of acute GVHD. The authors concluded that this observation most likely reflects a graft-vs.-leukemia effect of GVHD, though the antileukemia efficacy of GVHD treatment could contribute to the observed results.

Chronic GVHD has also been associated with a significant graft-vs.-leukemia effect in results reported from Genova (16). Seventy-eight patients with acute or chronic leukemia in remission or relapse were conditioned with high-dose chemoradiotherapy and received HLA–identical sibling marrow. Among 57 patients who survived 100 or more days and thus were at risk for chronic GVHD, the probability of being in remission was 87% for patients with chronic GVHD and 37% for those without chronic GVHD (p = 0.00004). In addition, there was a survival advantage for patients with chronic GVHD compared to patients without chronic GVHD (73% versus 36%, respectively, p = 0.0009). It must be recognized, however, that these results represent a heterogeneous group of patients with different diagnoses and different rates of leukemic relapse.

Somewhat contrary results have been reported by Brochstein et al. at Memorial Sloan-Kettering Cancer Center (17). Ninety-seven children with either ALL or ANL received hyperfractionated total body radiation and high-dose cyclophosphamide, followed by marrow transplantation from HLA-identical sibling donors. The only pretransplant factor that significantly affected outcome was disease status at the time of transplantation, i.e., patients in early remission had better disease-free survival than patients in later remissions or relapse. The overall incidence of acute GVHD was 57% and that of chronic GVHD was 34%. The posttransplantation relapse rate, however, was not affected by the presence of *acute* GVHD in any disease category (p = 0.14 by log rank test after stratification according to risk group; actual data not given). However, there did appear to be an association between the presence of *chronic* GVHD and reduced incidence of relapse, when both high-risk and low-risk patient groups were examined jointly (p < 0.04). The data as presented do not permit analysis of the influence of GVHD on overall survival, although since GVHD had only a marginal influence on leukemia recurrence and was associated with higher nonleukemic mortality, the influence was likely to be negative. Thus, in this series no association between acute GVHD and a reduced risk of posttransplantation relapse was found, though there was an association between the presence of chronic GVHD and a lower relapse rate.

D. Manipulation of GVHD and Its Influence Upon Recurrence of Leukemia

The observation that acute and chronic GVHD are associated with a lesser likelihood of leukemic relapse and possibly greater likelihood of overall survival in some patient groups stimulated investigators to attempt to alter the transplantation regimen so that patients at high risk for leukemia relapse could benefit from the apparent anitleukemic effect of GVHD. For example, the likelihood of relapse after transplantation from HLA-identical siblings approaches 80% in the absence of acute or chronic GVHD for patients with leukemia transplanted during relapse or blast crisis (11). The Seattle group, therefore, attempted to amplify a graft-vs.-host leukemia effect by deletion of GVHD prophylaxis after allogeneic marrow transplantation in patients less than 30 years of age with advanced leukemia (18,19). Sixteen such patients who received marrow grafts from HLA-identical siblings without posttransplant immunosuppression were compared to 44 age and disease-matched controls who received methotrexate to prevent GVHD. All 60 patients were prepared with cyclophosphamide and total body irradiation. Grades II-IV acute GVHD developed in all 15 engrafted patients not given immunosuppression compared to 10 of 44 engrafted recipients who received methotrexate (p < 0.0001). The onset of GVHD was more rapid in the patients not given methotrexate (median onset day 8 compared to day 18 in the methotrexate group; p = 0.005). Despite the severity of GVHD in patients not given immunosuppression, there was no statistically significant difference in the probability of recurrent leukemia (41% versus 38%). The probability of death from causes other than recurrent malignancy was 58% without immunosuppression and 34% in the methotrexate group (p = 0.1). Actuarial 3-year relapse-free survival was 25% in patients who did not receive immunosuppression and 41% in the patients who received methotrexate (p = 0.3). In this small group of patients the presence of early, severe acute GVHD was increased by the deletion of immunosuppression, but no apparent influence on recurrent leukemia was seen.

These results, however, are contrary to those reported in preliminary form by Elfenbein et al. (20). These investigators treated 58 recipients of HLA-identical allogeneic marrow with posttransplant immunosuppression, including methotrexate, and compared these results with 27 patients who received no GVHD prophylaxis. Acute GVHD (grades II-IV) was observed in 32% of methotrexate-treated patients and 70% of patients who did not receive prophylaxis (p < 0.005). Chronic GVHD was observed in 29% of methotrexate treated patients and in 30% of patients given no prophylaxis. Relapse occurred in 18% of methotrexate treated recipients and in none of the no-prophylaxis patients (p < 0.05). The actuarial probability of survival at 2 years was 30% for methotrexate-treated patients and 51% for no-prophylaxis patients. Thus, in the experience of Elfenbein et al., methotrexate regimens given posttransplantation decreased the likelihood of acute GVHD, but patients who did not receive prophylaxis suffered fewer relapses and appeared to be somewhat more likely to survive. Therefore, there may be a role for attenuation of immunosuppression by reducing drug dose or schedule in patients with advanced leukemia in an attempts to promote a graft-vs-leukemia effect. Such an experimental approach should be confined, however, to patients with advanced leukemia at high risk for relapse and should be approached with caution since treatment of acute GVHD is difficult, and the fatality associated with severe acute GVHD and associated infections is high.

Early on, it was noted that treatment of acute GVHD was largely unsatisfactory, while treatment of chronic GVHD was associated with more encouraging results with apparent decreases in disability and mortality (21). It was reasoned, therefore, that attempts to increase the incidence of chronic GVHD in allogeneic marrow recipients who are at high risk for leukemic relapse would be more appealing than attempts to increase the incidence of acute GVHD. The observation that infusions of nonirradiated donor peripheral blood buffy coat cells in addition to bone marrow cells in patients transplanted for the treatment of aplastic anemia were associated with an increased incidence of chronic GVHD (22) suggested one potential approach. Thus, between December 1980 and July 1984, 109 patients with advanced hematologic malignancies were entered into a Seattle study designed to determine if the antileukemic effect of GVHD could be amplified, thereby improving long-term survival (23). The study was designed to test whether a graft-vs.-leukemia effect could be safely augmented by promoting GVHD, either by shortening the duration of posttransplantation immunosuppression or by infusing viable donor buffy coat cells. Patients were randomized to receive intermittent methotrexate for 102 days posttransplant (44 patients, group 1), an abbreviated 11-day course of methotrexate (40 patients, group 2), or methotrexate for 102 days plus viable buffy coat cells (25 patients, group 3). All 109 patients were prepared with cyclophosphamide and total body irradiation, and given marrow from HLA-identical siblings. The probability of grades II-IV acute GVHD was increased in both recipients of abbreviated methotrexate and donor buffy coat cells: the incidence was 25% in group 1, 59% in group 2, and 82% in group 3 (p = 0.0001). The incidence of chronic GVHD, however, did not differ significantly: 33%, 51%, and 44%, respectively (p = 0.3). The probability of recurrent malignancy at 5 years did not differ among the groups (38%, 45%, and 33%, respectively). The probability of nonrelapse mortality at 5 years was 33% in group 1, 45% in group 2, and 64% in group 3, due primarily to infections complicating GVHD. Thirty-nine of the 109 patients survived with a median follow-up of 5.1 years. Actuarial disease-free survival at 5 years was 41% in group 1, 30% in group 2, and 24% in group 3 (p = 0.3). This study demonstrated that abbreviating methotrexate prophylaxis or adding donor buffy coat cells increased the incidence of acute GVHD and nonrelapse mortality but failed to influence the likelihood of recurrent leukemia. Unexpectedly there was no apparent increase in the incidence of chronic GVHD in patients in groups 2 and 3 despite a significant increase in acute GVHD. Failure to increase the incidence of chronic GVHD in these patients could explain why recurrent leukemia was not decreased, since it would appear that chronic GVHD is most likely to be associated with a clinically beneficial graft-vs.-leukemia effect, i.e., a lesser likelihood of leukemic relapse combined with an increased likelihood of survival.

E. Marrow Depletion of T Cells

Since acute GVHD is thought to be largely mediated by donor T lymphocytes that react against disparate recipient histocompatibility antigens, one attractive approach to prevent GVHD is to eliminate T lymphocytes from the donor marrow before transplantation. This technique is effective in preventing acute GVHD across both major and minor histocompatibility barriers in mice (24,25) and has also been used effectively in randomly bred dogs (26). Because several uncontrolled studies had suggested that transplantation of T-cell-depleted donor marrow might reduce the risk of acute GVHD in man, the UCLA group undertook a randomized, prospective, double-blind trial to assess the effects of ex-vivo depletion of T lymphocytes from donor bone marrow using a monoclonal anti-T-cell antibody and complement (27). Forty patients were studied; all were patients with acute leukemia in remission or with CML in chronic or accelerated phase who underwent marrow transplantation from HLA-identical siblings between May 1983 and September 1984. Patients were conditioned with high-dose cyclophosphamide or cytosine arabinoside, followed by total body irradiation. Patients receiving T-cell-depleted bone marrow had a lower incidence of acute GVHD than control patients (3 of 20 versus 13 of 20; p = 0.004), and mortality due to acute GVHD was reduced. Five patients in the T-cell-depletion group developed graft failure, while all control patients had sustained engraftment (p < 0.005). Clinically apparent relapse of leukemia occurred in 7 patients from the T-cell-depletion group and in only 2 control patients (p not significant). Cytogenetic evidence of residual leukemia was also detected in the 5 patients with graft failure without overt relapse. If the patients with graft failure and only cytogenetic evidence of leukemic relapse are considered as having relapses, then the actuarial relapse rate is significantly higher in the T-cell-depleted group than in controls (60%, i.e., 12 of 20, compared to 10%, i.e., 2 of 20, p = 0.007). These data must be regarded as preliminary because of the relatively small number of patients within each diagnostic and remission group category but nevertheless suggest that depletion of T lymphocytes from the donor bone marrow abrogated a graft-vs.-leukemia effect in parallel to reducing the incidence of acute GVHD.

Apperley and colleagues have reported similar results (28). Between December 1983 and November 1985, they treated 39 patients with CML by chemoradiotherapy and transplantation from HLA-identical sibling donors using marrow that had been depleted of T cells in vitro using the rat monoclonal antibody Campath-I. Twenty-eight patients were in chronic phase (good risk group) and 11 patients were in more advanced phases of the disease (accelerated phase or blast crisis, poor-risk group). Acute GVHD occurred in 11% of good-risk and in 55% of poor-risk patients. In the good-risk patients, hematologic evidence of relapse was seen in four, and cytogenetic evidence of persisting or relapsed leukemia (i.e., Philadelphia chromosome positive marrow metaphases more than 6 months after transplant) was seen in three additional patients. In comparison with a historical control group of good-risk patients transplanted with untreated marrow between February 1981 and December 1983, the incidence of acute GVHD has reduced significantly (p < 0.001), but the risk of leukemia relapse, including patients with only cytogenetic evidence of relapse, was increased (p < 0.005).

Although T-cell depletion used in this manner appears to be associated with an increased risk of leukemia relapse, the mechanism by which T-cell depletion predisposed to relapse remains unclear. Clearly, this could simply be the result of the influence of T-cell depletion upon the occurrence and severity of GVHD. However, as an alternative possibility a role of T lymphocytes in the absence of GVHD, i.e., a graft-vs.-leukemia effect independent of GVHD, has been postulated by Butturini and Gale (29). These authors, based on their review of the literature, indicated that the actuarial relapse rate of leukemia following bone marrow transplantation for CML is 50% following T-cell depletion, 25% in syngeneic marrow recipients, 15% in HLA-identical marrow recipients without GVHD, and 5% in allogeneic marrow recipients with GVHD. They suggested that the antileukemic effect associated with bone marrow transplantation and distinct from GVHD should be referred to as graft-vs.-leukemia effect. They suggested that the increased risk of leukemia relapse in recipients of T-cell-depleted marrow is probably related in part to a loss of the antileukemic effect of GVHD. However, they contend this cannot be the full explanation since the relapse rate in T-cell-depleted transplants is substantially higher than that observed in recipients of syngeneic transplants (given unmanipulated marrow), indicators that T-cell depletion must increase relapse via a different mechanism. For example, activated T cells might release factors which either inhibit the growth or are cytotoxic to CML stem cells. Alternatively, T cells might compete with CML stem cells following radiation and bone marrow transplantation, or leukemia stem cells might be less dependent on T-cell growth factors than normal cells, thereby favoring the growth of CML stem cells and increasing the likelihood of leukemia relapse.

Another study was presented by Pollard and colleagues from the Royal Marsden Hospital in England (30). In a preliminary report, they noted that only 5 of 11 patients with ANL in first remission who received T-cell-depleted allogeneic HLA—identical sibling marrow following chemoradiotherapy remained in remission (actuarial probability = 40%) compared to 16 of 70 patients treated during a comparable interval who received untreated donor marrow and 6 months of cyclosporine (actuarial probability of remission = 70%, p < 0.025). The incidence of GVHD that required treatment in the cyclosporine-treated patients was 69% compared to only 18% in the Campath-I group. The authors felt that their data supported the hypothesis that GVHD may be associated with an antileukemic effect in ANL.

Gale and Reisner have considered the interrelationship among graft rejection, GVHD, and a graft-vs.-leukemia effect (31). They postulate that the most important determinant of graft rejection and GVHD is the extent of genetic disparity between donor and recipient. Thus, individuals most likely to reject their graft are also those most likely to get GVHD. Graft rejection and GVHD are both clearly recognized and accepted clinical syndromes. The third immunologic aspect of marrow transplantation, i.e., graft-vs.-leukemia effect, remains more controversial. Nevertheless, the chance of a graft-vs.-leukemia effect is also likely to be correlated with the degree of antigenic disparity between normal cells of the donor and leukemic cells of the recipient. If recipient leukemic cells display all the histocompatibility antigens present on their normal counterparts, one would predict a direct correlation between GVHD and graft-vs.-leukemia. If leukemia-specific antigens exist, however, GVHD may be distinguishable and may not correlate precisely with a graft-vs.-leukemia effect.

IV. ANALYSIS OF GRAFT-vs.-LEUKEMIA EFFECT FROM THE INTERNATIONAL BONE MARROW TRANSPLANT REGISTRY

The International Bone Marrow Transplant Registry (IBMTR) includes data from patients transplanted in over 150 centers worldwide. This represents approximtely 75% of currently active bone marrow transplant teams and more than 50% of all patients transplanted since the early 1970s. Since the Seattle transplant group does not currently submit data to the IBMTR, the results described above for the Seattle group are not included in the results of the IBMTR, while results of most other transplant groups are included. This affords the opportunity to examine evidence for graft-vs.-leukemia effects in two large, independent databases.

Data for the [2254] patients with early leukemia (ALL and ANL in first remission and CML in chronic phase) reported to the IBMTR between January 1978 and June 1988 were examined for evidence of graft-vs.-leukemia effects (32). The population included 1783 recipients of non-T-cell-depleted HLA-identical sibling allografts, 401 recipients of T-cell-depleted HLA-identical sibling allografts, and 70 recipients of syngeneic (identical twin) grafts. A variety of pretransplant conditioning regimens was used for these patients with more than 90% receiving total body radiation and cyclophosphamide. Conditioning regimens were similar for non-T-cell depleted, T-cell depleted, and syngeneic graft recipients.

The analysis was designed to detect graft-related antileukemia activity in association with GVHD and in the absence of clinically detectable GVHD. Patients were categorized into six groups: (1) recipients of non-T-cell-depleted allografts who were not diagnosed as having acute or chronic GVHD; (2) recipients of non-T-cell-depleted allografts with grades I-IV acute but not chronic GVHD; (3) recipients of non-T-cell-depleted allografts with chronic but not acute GVHD; (4) recipients of non-T-cell-depleted allografts with both acute and chronic GVHD; (5) recipients of transplants from genetically identical twins; and (6) recipients of T-cell-depleted allografts with or without acute or chronic GVHD. The actuarial probability of relapse at 3 years ranged from $7 \pm 3\%$ (95% confidence interval) for recipients of non-T-cell-depleted allografts who developed both acute and chronic GVHD to $46 \pm 15\%$ for recipients of syngeneic marrow. The differing antileukemia effects of the transplants could not be explained on the basis of pretransplant cytotoxic therapy.

The problem of assessing the effect of GVHD upon outcome is complex. Patients must survive sufficiently long to be at risk for acute GVHD and longer to be at risk for chronic GVHD. Consequently, the group of patients without GVHD includes those who relapse or die before GVHD can develop as well as those who survive without developing this complication. The group of patients with only acute GVHD includes patients with severe acute GVHD who do not survive sufficiently long to be at risk for chronic GVHD as well as those who survive but do not develop chronic GVHD. In this study, changes in GVHD status with time after transplant were accommodated by assigning patients into the three GVHD comparison groups desribed above in a time-dependent fashion (33). All patients were considered to be in the "no GVHD" group at day 0. Patients were assigned to the "acute GVHD only" group at the time of onset of acute GVHD and their subsequent survival and relapse experience compared to patients who survived a similar length of time without developing GVHD. Patients who later developed chronic GVHD were reassigned from the "acute GVHD only" group into the "both acute and chronic GVHD" group at the time chronic GVHD was diagnosed. Patients who developed de novo chronic GVHD were assigned to the "no GVHD" group until chronic GVHD developed and were then assigned to the "chronic GVHD only" group. By using a time-dependent model, rather than selecting patients who survive the early transplant period, the overall impact of GVHD on outcome can be estimated. Relative risks of relapse were then calculated using a multivariate proportional hazards regression model which also adjusted for patient age, presenting leukocyte count and posttransplant immunosuppressive therapy to prevent GVHD, i.e., methotrexate, cyclosporine, corticosteroids, or combination thereof.

A decreased risk of relapse was observed in patients who developed GVHD. Recipients of non-T-cell-depleted allografts who developed only acute GVHD had a risk of relapse 0.68 times as high as patients who received non-T-cell-depleted allografts and did not develop GVHD ($p = 0.03$); those with de novo chronic GVHD had a risk of 0.43 ($p = 0.01$); and those with both acute and chronic GVHD had a risk of 0.33 ($p = 0.0001$). This is consistent with the studies described above showing an antileukemia effect of GVHD. Similarities and differences were observed in regards to the effect of GVHD upon relapse for different leukemias. Acute GVHD alone was associated with a significantly decreased risk of relapse in ALL (relative risk 0.36, $p = 0.004$) but not in ANL or CML (relative risks 0.78 and 1.15 respectively, $p = NS$). In ALL, ANL, and CML, the lowest risk of relapse was observed in patients with both acute and chronic GVHD. It may be that the duration of active GVHD (generally longest in patients with both acute and chronic GVHD) is important in determining the magnitude of its antileukemia effect. Alternatively, since patients with more severe acute GVHD are more likely to develop chronic GVHD, it may be that patients with both acute and chronic GVHD have more severe GVHD overall. A relationship between severity of GVHD and relapse was observed in this study. When patients with only acute GVHD, only chronic GVHD, and both acute and chronic GVHD were analyzed separately, relapse risk decreased with increasing severity of GVHD. Despite its antileukemia effect, GVHD did not improve leukemia-free survival except in the group of patients who had mild acute and chronic GVHD. These patients had a risk of treatment failure 0.53 times as high as patients without GVHD ($p = 0.02$). Overall, however, patients with acute GVHD only (relative risk 1.84, $p = 0.0001$) and both acute and chronic GVHD (relative risk 1.79, $p = 0.0001$) had risks of treatment failure that was not significantly different from patients without GVHD (relative risk 1.19, $p = 0.45$).

To determine whether allogeneic grafts had a graft-vs.-leukemia effect in the absence of GVHD, recipients of grafts from identical twins were compared to recipients of non-T-cell-depleted allografts without GVHD. Syngeneic graft recipients had a risk of relapse 2.09 times as high as allograft recipients without GVHD (p = 0.005). This was accounted for primarily by a higher risk of relapse among patients with ANL who received syngeneic grafts (relative risk 2.58, p = 0.008). Patients with ALL and CML who received syngeneic grafts had risks of relapse that were not significantly different from the risk in recipients of allografts who did not develop GVHD. The mechanism of graft-vs.-leukemia reactions in the absence of GVHD in patients with ANL is unknown and cannot be determined by this type of analysis. It may be that leukemia-associated antigens, unable to be recognized by host immune cells or genetically identical immune cells from a syngeneic donor, can be recognized by immunocompetent cells from an allogeneic donor. Alternatively, the difference may be due to nonspecific cytotoxic effects of subclinical GVHD, directed at minor histocompatibility antigens, in allograft recipients. As in the study by Fefer et al. described above, it is not possible to exclude an increased susceptibility to leukemia in genetically identical donor cells. However, as in that study, leukemia did not develop in any of the 70 twin donors. Why this effect is seen only in ANL is uncertain.

Indirect evidence for an important role of the bone marrow graft in eradicating leukemia can be obtained by investigating changes in relapse rates after manipulation of the graft. The effect of T-cell depletion on relapse risk, independent of its effect on GVHD, was examined in this study by comparing relapse rates in recipients of T-cell-depleted allografts with relapse rates in recipients of non-T-cell-depleted allografts who did not develop GVHD. An increased risk (relative risk 1.76, p = 0.002) was observed in recipients of T-cell-depleted marrow. This increase was largely attributable to a strikingly high relapse risk in CML patients who received T-cell-depleted marrow (relative risk 5.14, p = 0.0001). Although the risk was increased in ALL and ANL, the difference was not statistically significant for these diseases. This contrasts with the graft-vs.-leukemia effect of allogeneic, non-T-cell-depleted grafts without GVHD as compared to syngeneic grafts which was most striking in ANL, suggesting different mechanisms. This effect is presumably mediated by T cells themselves but may possibly be due to some other cell or factor affected by T-cell depletion. T cells in non-T-cell-depleted grafts could contribute directly to the graft-vs.-leukemia effect or indirectly by facilitating engraftment or producing lymphokines that activate other effector cell mechanisms.

Although relapse rates after T-cell-depleted transplants were compared to relapse rates in patients who received non-T-cell-depleted transplants and did not develop GVHD, it is possible that patients without clinically detectable GVHD have a range of subclinical GVHD which differs between T-cell-depleted and non-T-cell-depleted grafts. This might account for the difference in relapse risk. To address this question, recipients of T-cell-depleted grafts with clinical GVHD were compared to recipients of non-T-cell-depleted marrow with GVHD using a regression model which adjusted for the severity of GVHD. Even among patients with clinical evidence of GVHD, T-cell-depleted grafts were associated with a significantly higher risk of relapse (relative risk 2.29, p = 0.0001) than non-T-cell-depleted grafts. In fact, the risk of relapse for patients who received T-cell-depleted grafts and developed GVHD was similar to the risk for patients who received non-T-cell-depleted grafts and did not develop GVHD. It appears that GVHD can compensate partially for the absence of some antileukemia effect removed by T-cell depletion.

The data from IBMTR, therefore, support an antileukemia effect of bone marrow transplantation in early leukemia that may have three separate components: (1) antileukemia activity associated with clinically evident GVHD; (2) antileukemia activity mediated by allogeneic (but not syngeneic) donor cells that can operate in the absence of GVHD; and (3) antileukemia activity independent of GVHD mediated presumably by both allogeneic and syngeneic donor cells that is weakened or abrogated by T-cell depletion.

V. CONCLUSIONS

Several studies over the past decade have documented a clinically relevant graft-vs.-leukemia effect. This effect is associated with both the acute and chronic forms of GVHD and is particularly noticeable in patients at high risk for relapse. It appears to be more difficult in man than in murine models to separate GVHD from a graft-vs.-leukemia effect. Any successful attempt aimed at the prevention of GVHD is likely to increase the incidence of leukemic relapse. Results fom T-cell-depletion studies and from syngeneic transplantation suggest that there is a T-cell-mediated graft-vs.-leukemia effect not associted with clinically apparent GVHD. Further studies are necessary to determine whether a transplant-mediated effect can be engineered which is directed at leukemia cells but does not induce GVHD with its associated morbidity and mortality.

ACKNOWLEDGMENTS

Support for this investigation was provided by grant CA 40053 from the National Cancer Institute, DHHS, contracts N01-AI-625330 from the National Institute of Allergy and Infectious Diseases, DHHS, B16-084-US from the Commission of European Communities and grants from the William Randolph Hearst Foundation, Ambrose Monell Foundation, Elsa U. Pardee Foundation, RGK Foundation, Sandoz Research Institute, Joan and Jack Stein, the Swiss Cancer League and Xoma Corporation.

REFERENCES

1. Mathe G, Amiel JL, Schwarzenberg L, Cattan A, Schneider M: Adoptive immunotherapy of acute leukemia: Experimental and clinical results. Cancer Res 1965; 25:1525-1531.
2. Fefer A, Einstein AB, Cheever MA: Adoptive chemoimmunotherapy in cancer in animals: A review of results, principles and problems. Ann NY Acad Sci 1976; 277:492-504.
3. Odom LF, August CS, Githen JH, Humbert JR, Morse H, Peakman D, Sharma B, Rusnale SL, Johnson FB: Remission of relapsed leukaemia during graft-versus-host reaction. Lancet 1978:ii;537-541.
4. Petersen FB, Appelbaum FR, Bigelow CL, Buckner CD, Clift RA, Sanders JE, Storb R, Sullivan KM, Weiden PL, Fefer A, Thomas ED: High-dose cytosine arabinoside, total body irradiation and marrow transplantation for advanced malignant lymphoma. In Bone Marrow Transplantation, 1989; in press.

5. Weiden PL, Flournoy N, Thomas ED, Prentice R, Fever A, Buckern CD, Storb R: Antileukemic effect of graft-versus-host disease in human recipients of allogeneic marrow grafts. N Engl J Med 1979;300:1068-1073.

6. Fefer A, Sullivan KM, Weiden P, Buckner CD, Schoch G, Storb R, Thomas ED: Graft versus leukemia effect in man: The relapse rate of acute leukemia is lower after allogeneic than after syngeneic marrow transplantation. In *Cellular Immunotherapy of Cancer*, edited by Truitt RL, Gale RP and Bortin MM. New York: A. R. Liss, 1987; pp. 401-408.

7. Gale RP, Champlin RE: How does bone-marrow transplantation cure leukaemia? Lancet 1984;ii:28-29.

8. Kersey JH, Weisdorf D, Nesbit MW, LeBien TW, Woods WG, McGlave PB, Kim T, Vellera DA, Goldman AI, Bostrom B, Hurd D, Ramsay NKC: Comparison of autologous and allogeneic bone marrow transplantation for treatment of high-risk refractory acute lymphoblastic leukemia. N Engl J Med 1987;317:461.

9. Weiden PL, Flournoy N, Sanders JE, Sullivan KM, Thomas ED: Antileukemic effect of graft-versus-host disease contributes to improved survival after allogeneic marrow transplantation. Transplant Proc 1981;13:248-251.

10. Weiden PL, Sullivan KM, Flournoy N, Storb R, Thomas ED: Seattle Marrow Transplant Team. Antileukemic effect of chronic graft-versus-host disease. Contribution to improved survival after allogeneic marrow transplantation. N Engl J Med 1981; 304:1529-1533.

11. Sullivan KM, Fefer A, Witherspoon R, Storb R, Buckner CD, Weiden P, Schoch G, Thomas ED: Graft-versus-leukemia in man: Relationship of acute and chronic graft-versus-host disease to relapse of acute leukemia following allogenic bone marrow transplantation. In *Cellular Immunotherapy of Cancer*, edited by Truitt RL, Gale RP, Bortin MM. New York: A. R. Liss, 1987; pp. 391-399.

12. Sullivan KM, Weiden PL, Storb R, Witherspoon RP, Fefer A, Fisher L, Buckner CD, Anasetti C, Appelbaum FR, Badger C, Beatty P, Bensinger W, Berenson R, Bigelow C, Cheever MA, Clift R, Deeg HJ, Doney K, Greenberg P, Hansen JA, Hill R, Loughran T, Martin P, Neiman P, Petersen FB, Sanders J, Singer J, Stewart P, Thomas ED: Influence of acute and chronic graft-versus-host disease on relapse and survival after bone marrow transplantation from HLA-identical siblings as treatment of acute and chronic leukemia. Blood 1989;73;1720-1728.

13. Sullivan KM, Witherspoon RP, Storb R, Weiden P, Flournoy N, Dahlberg S, Deeg HJ, Sanders JE, Doney KC, Appelbaum FR, McGuffin R, McDonald GB, Meyers J, Schubert MM, Gauvreau J, Shulman HM, Sale GE, Anasetti C, Loughran TP, Strom S, Nims J, Thomas ED: Prednisone and azathoprine compared with prednisone and placebo for treatment of chronic graft-versus-host disease: Prognostic influence of prolonged thrombocytopenia after allogeneic marrow transplantation. Blood 1988; 72:546-554.

14. McIntyre R, Gale RP: Relationship between graft-versus-leukemia and graft-versus-host in man—UCLA experience. In *Graft-Versus-Leukemia in Man and Animal Models*, edited by Okunewick J, Meredith R. Boca Raton, FL: CRC Press 1981; pp. 1-9.

15. Weisdorf DJ, Nesbit ME, Ramsay NKC, Woods WG, Goldman AI, Kim TH, Hurd DD, McGlave PB, Kersey JH: Allogeneic bone marrow transplantation for acute lymphoblastic leukemia in remission: Prolonged survival associated with acute graft-versus-host disease. J Clin Oncol 1987;5:1348-1355.

16. Bacigalupo A, VanLint MT, Frassmi F, Marmont A: Graft-versus-leukaemia effect following allogeneic bone marrow transplantation. Brit J Hemat 1985;61:749-750.

17. Brochstein JA, Kernan NA, Groshen S, Cirrincione C, Shank B, Emanuel D, Laver J, O'Reilly RJ: Allogeneic bone marrow transplantation after hyperfractionated total-

body irradiation and cyclophosphamide in children with acute leukemia. N Engl J Med 1987;317:1618-1624.

18. Sullivan KM, Deeg HJ, Sanders J, Losterman A, Amls D, Shulman H, Sale G, Martin P, Witherspoon R, Appelbaum FR, Doney K, Stewart P, Meyers J, McDonald GB, Weiden P, Fefer A, Buckner CD, Storb R, Thomas ED: Hyperactue graft-v-host disease in patients not given immunosuppression after allogeneic marrow transplantation. Blood 1986;67:1172-1175.

19. Sullivan KM, Storb R, Witherspoon RP, Weiden PL, Anasetti C, Appelbaum FR, Beatty P, Buckner CD, Deeg HJ, Doney K, Fisher L, Loughran TP, Martin P, Meyers J, McDonald GB, Sanders J, Shulman H, Stewart P, Thomas ED: Deletion of immunosuppressive prophylaxis after marrow transplantation increased hyperacute graft-versus-host disease but does not influence chronic graft-versus-host disease or relapse in patients with advanced leukemia. Clin Transplantation 1989;3:5-11.

20. Elfenbein G, Graham-Pole J, Weiner R, Goedert T, Gross S: Consequences of no prophylaxis for acute graft-versus-host disease after HLA-identical bone marrow transplantation (abstract). Blood 1987;70(Suppl 1):305a.

21. Sullivan KM, Shulman HM, Storb R, Weiden PL, Witherspoon RP, McDonald GB, Schubert MM, Atkinson K, Thomas ED: Chronic graft-versus-host disease in 52 patients: Adverse natural course and successful treatment with combination immunosuppression. Blood 1981;57:267-276.

22. Storb R, Doney KC, Thomas ED, Appelbaum F, Buckner CD, Clift RA, Deeg HJ, Goodell BW, Hackman R, Hansen JA, Sanders J, Sullivan K, Weiden PL, Witherspoon RP. Marrow transplantation with or without donor buffy coat cells for 65 transfused aplastic anemia patients. Blood 1982;59:236-246.

23. Sullivan KM, Storb R, Buckner CD, Fefer AF, Fisher L, Weiden PL, Witherspoon RP, Appelbaum FR, Banaji M, Hansen J, Martin P, Sanders JE, Singer J, Thomas ED: Graft-versus-host disease as adoptive immunotherapy in patients with advanced hematologic neoplasms. N Engl J Med 1989;320;828-834.

24. Vallera DA, Soderling CCB, Calrson GJ, Kersey JH: Bone marrow transplantation across major histocompatibility barriers in mice: effect of elimination of T cells from donor grafts by treatment with monoclonal Thy-1.2 plus complement or antibody alone. Transplantation 1981;31:218-222.

25. Korngold R, Sprent J: Lethal graft-versus-host disease after bone marrow transplantation across minor histocompatibility barriers in mice: prevention by removing mature T cells from marrow. J Exp Med 1978;148:1687-1698.

26. Kolb HJ, Reider I, Rodt H, Netzel B, Grosse-Wilde H, Scholz S, Schaffer E, Kolb H, Thierfelder S: Antilymphocytic antibodies and marrow transplantation: VI. Graft-versus-host tolerance in DLA-incompatible dogs following in vitro treatment of bone marrow with absorbed antithymocyte globulin. Transplantation 1979;27:242-245.

27. Mitsuyasu RT, Champlin RE, Gale RP, Ho WG, Lenarsky C, Winston D, Selch M, Elashoff R, Giorgi JV, Wells J, Terasaki P, Billing R, Feig S: Treatment of donor bone marrow with monoclonal anti-T-cell antibody and complement for the prevention of graft-versus-host disease: A prospective, randomized, double-blind trial. Ann Intern Med 1986;105:20-26.

28. Apperley JF, Jones L, Hale G, Waldmann H, Hows J, Rombos Y, Tsatalas C, Marcus RE, Goolden AWG, Gordon-Smith EC, Catovsky D, Galton DAG, Goldman JM: Bone marrow transplantation for patients with chronic myeloid leukaemia: T-cell depletion with Campath-1 reduces the incidence of graft-versus-host disease but may increase the risk of leukaemic relapse. Bone Marrow Transplantation 1986;1:53-66.

29. Butturini A, Gale RP: The role of T-cells in preventing relapse in chronic myelogenous leukemia. Bone Marrow Transplantation 1987;2:351-354.

30. Pollard CM, Powles RL, Millar JL, Shepherd V, Milan S, Lakhani A, Zuiable A, Trele-
    aven J, Helenglass G: Leukaemic relapse following Campath-1 treated bone marrow
    transplantation for leukaemia. Lancet 1986;ii:1343-1344.
31. Gale RP, Reisner Y: Graft rejection and graft-versus-host disease: Mirror images.
    Lancet 1986;i:1468-1470.
32. Horowitz MM, Gale RP, Sondel PM, Goldman JM, Kersey J, Kolb H-J, Rimm AA,
    Ringden O, Rozman C, Speck B, Truitt RL, Zwaan FL, Bortin MM: Graft-versus-
    leukemia reactions following bone marrow transplantation in humans. Blood 1990,
    in press.
33. Prentice RL, Kalbfleish JP, Peterson AV, Flournoy N, Farewell VT, Breslow NE:
    The analysis of failure times in the presence of competing risks. Biometrics 1978;
    34:541-553.

Index